D1609246

Cardiovascular Magnetic Resonance Imaging

CONTEMPORARY CARDIOLOGY

CHRISTOPHER P. CANNON, MD
SERIES EDITOR

ANNEMARIE M. ARMANI, MD
EXECUTIVE EDITOR

CARDIOVASCULAR MAGNETIC RESONANCE IMAGING

Edited by

RAYMOND Y. KWONG, MD, MPH

*Instructor of Medicine, Harvard Medical School,
Director, Cardiac Magnetic Resonance Imaging,
Cardiovascular Division,
Department of Medicine,
Brigham and Women's Hospital,
Boston, Massachusetts*

Foreword by

PETER LIBBY, MD

*Mallinckrodt Professor of Medicine,
Chief, Cardiovascular Medicine,
Harvard Medical School,
Brigham and Women's Hospital,
Boston, Massachusetts*

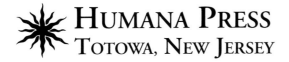

HUMANA PRESS
TOTOWA, NEW JERSEY

The content and opinions expressed in this book are the sole work of the authors and editors, who have warranted due diligence in the creation and issuance of their work. The publisher, editors, and authors are not responsible for errors or omissions or for any consequences arising from the information or opinions presented in this book and make no warranty, express or implied, with respect to its contents.

Due diligence has been taken by the publishers, editors, and authors of this book to assure the accuracy of the information published and to describe generally accepted practices. The contributors herein have carefully checked to ensure that the drug selections and dosages set forth in this text are accurate and in accord with the standards accepted at the time of publication. Notwithstanding, as new research, changes in government regulations, and knowledge from clinical experience relating to drug therapy and drug reactions constantly occurs, the reader is advised to check the product information provided by the manufacturer of each drug for any change in dosages or for additional warnings and contraindications. This is of utmost importance when the recommended drug herein is a new or infrequently used drug. It is the responsibility of the treating physician to determine dosages and treatment strategies for individual patients. Further it is the responsibility of the health care provider to ascertain the Food and Drug Administration status of each drug or device used in their clinical practice. The publisher, editors, and authors are not responsible for errors or omissions or for any consequences from the application of the information presented in this book and make no warranty, express or implied, with respect to the contents in this publication.

Production Editor: Amy Thau
Cover design by Karen Schulz
Cover Illustration: See preface

For additional copies, pricing for bulk purchases, and/or information about other Humana titles, contact Humana at the above address or at any of the following numbers: Tel.: 973-256-1699; Fax: 973-256-8341; or visit our Website: www.humanapress.com

This publication is printed on acid-free paper. ∞
ANSI Z39.48-1984 (American National Standards Institute) Permanence of Paper for Printed Library Materials.

Printed in the United States of America.   10   9   8   7   6   5   4   3   2   1
eISBN 978-1-59745-306-6

Library of Congress Cataloging-in-Publication Data

Available upon request

To my family, for their unconditional love and support

and

*To my teachers, patients, and students, from whom
I have learned so much.*

Foreword

Cardiovascular magnetic resonance imaging is maturing as a clinical tool in contemporary cardiovascular medicine. This imaging modality has become an important part of hospital-based practice. Yet, magnetic resonance imaging promises to offer even more to the cardiovascular practitioner in the future as instrumentation evolves and the manifold potential of magnetic resonance technology as applied to the cardiovascular system advances.

Magnetic resonance imaging already excels as a modality for definition of cardiovascular anatomy. Magnetic resonance imaging in particular offers information difficult to obtain from other sources regarding complex congenital cardiovascular anomalies and rigorous and quantitative aspects of regional ventricular function. Vascular angiography by magnetic resonance imaging has in many cases replaced traditional contrast angiography as the diagnostic modality of choice for non-coronary atherosclerosis and other vascular diseases. While the assessment of luminal stenosis by coronary magnetic resonance angiography remains challenged by resolution, and cardiac and respiratory motion, this technique can reliably assess the anatomic course of coronary anomaly. A new 3-dimensional volumetric technique combined with parallel imaging may advance this challenging application in the future.

Beyond anatomy, magnetic resonance imaging can offer metabolic information through spectroscopy and add molecular and cellular information. Indeed, the use of paramagnetic nanoparticles already discloses phagocytic capacity of cells in vivo. It is likely that many more magnetic resonance probes of cellular and molecular function will evolve in the coming years to advance magnetic resonance imaging beyond anatomy and perfusion studies to glean important biochemical and molecular information about the heart and vessels.

In addition to providing a rapidly evolving tool for cardiovascular diagnosis, magnetic resonance imaging may become increasingly important in guiding cardiovascular interventions. Already used in electrophysiologic laboratories, the use of MR technology in hybrid diagnostic/therapeutic applications will doubtless find a place in cardiovascular practice going forward.

The state-of-the-art compilation of expert contributions in this volume edited by Dr. Raymond Y. Kwong describes normal and pathologic anatomy of the cardiovascular system as assessed by magnetic resonance imaging. Functional techniques such as myocardial perfusion imaging, assessment of flow velocity, and other functional assessments receive important emphasis in this collection. The exciting area of atherosclerosis plaque imaging and targeted magnetic resonance imaging likewise receive emphasis in this volume. Taken together, *Cardiovascular Magnetic Resonance Imaging* covers all of the important aspects of magnetic resonance imaging of the cardiovascular system and lays a firm foundation for following its future evolution.

The proliferation of specialized imaging modalities for the cardiovascular system such as magnetic resonance imaging, radionuclide techniques, ultrasonographic examinations, and emerging optical modalities have led to a fragmentation of skills among various specialists. A multi-disciplinary work such as *Cardiovascular Magnetic Resonance Imaging* represents a goal for future integration. Dr. Kwong has assembled authors with expertise in cardiology, radiology, physics, and engineering, as well as physiology and bio-chemistry to explicate the various aspects of this complex field. As we move forward in cardiovascular imaging, we must not lose sight of our goal to answer the patient-based questions in the most effective and expeditious manner. We must not lose sight of the cardiovascular imaging examination as a consultation. We must strive to deploy our technology in the most cost-effective manner. Cross-training of cardiovascular imagers in multiple modalities will foster the ethos of performing the best examina-tion to answer the questions rather than using the tool at hand. The future flourishing and realization of the full potential of cardiovascular imaging technologies will require rethinking of traditional departmental and disciplinary boundaries. The vision for the future for non-invasive cardiovascular imaging in general, and magnetic resonance in particular, will benefit immeasurably from an interdisciplinary and seamlessly integrated approach.

As amply demonstrated in *Cardiovascular Magnetic Resonance Imaging*, this modality will provide an important bulwark of such an integrated program in cardiovascular imaging. The information assembled here will help the practitioner use this important modality in the most informed manner to answer the clinical questions at hand.

Peter Libby, MD
Mallinckrodt Professor of Medicine,
Chief, Cardiovascular Medicine,
Harvard Medical School,
Brigham and Women's Hospital,
Boston, Massachusetts

Preface

Since the successful invention of the first magnetic resonance imaging (MRI) system by Damadian et al. for cancer diagnosis three decades ago, the medical use of MRI has developed rapidly applicable to a wide range of diseases. Since the first attempt to image the heart with MRI in the early 1980s, extensive hardware and software advances overcame the initial obstacles of gating a rapidly beating heart and long acquisition times. Over the past years, cardiovascular MRI has become a crucial tool in many routine clinical cardiac diagnoses, with the advantage of providing not only structural but also a multitude of functional or physiologic data that are adjunctive or even superior to conventional imaging tools.

Cardiovascular Magnetic Resonance Imaging comprises the efforts of a team of international authors from different disciplines who contributed a broad range of expertise to the current field of cardiovascular MRI. Throughout the production of this book, the emphasis has been on comprehensive, scientifically accurate, and clear explanations of the many components of this rapidly advancing field. We aim to maintain a balance between technical basis, cardiac physiology, clinical validation, and available prognostic implications to enhance the educational value of this reference textbook. Radiologists, cardiologists, internists, and residents and fellows with interests in cardiovascular MRI may benefit from the range of materials discussed in this book. The accompanying CD/DVD aims to provide an improved interactive learning experience by including many clinical case presentations.

While plenty remains to be explored in unleashing the full potential of magnetic resonance technology in imaging the heart, the field of cardiovascular MRI has experienced steady growth, with balanced emphases in both technical improvement and clinical application. This first edition of *Cardiovascular Magnetic Resonance Imaging* is intended to serve as a practical introductory resource in helping our readers overcome the startup challenges in this field.

To better illustrate the versatility of cardiac MRI, we designed the front cover of this book to include multiple cardiac MRI techniques. Going in a counter-clockwise fashion: cine steady-state free precession imaging in a patient with severe mitral regurgitation; delayed enhancement imaging of myocardial infarction with the heart contained in a restraint device in a large animal; quantitative analysis of regional left ventricular function by displacement encoding stimulating echo technique (DENSE); and a 3D high-resolution visualization of the ascending aortic blood flow in a normal subject (courtesy of Drs. Michael Jerosen-Herold, Frederick Chen, Anthony Aletras, and Michael Markl, respectively).

I wish to express my appreciation to the editors at Humana Press for the opportunity to undertake this project and for their outstanding help and support in bringing *Cardiovascular Magnetic Resonance Imaging* to fruition. I am especially grateful to my mentors and colleagues around the world in the field of magnetic resonance imaging who have contributed these important chapters. I hope you enjoy reading this book.

Raymond Y. Kwong, MD, MPH

Contents

Contributors

HASSAN ABDEL-ATY, MD • *Senior Fellow, Stephenson CMR Centre at the Libin Cardiovascular Institute of Alberta, University of Calgary, Calgary, Alberta, Canada*

ANTHONY H. ALETRAS, PhD • *Laboratory of Cardiac Energetics, National Heart, Lung and Blood Institute, National Institutes of Health, US Department of Health and Human Services, Bethesda, Maryland*

MOUAZ AL-MALLAH, MD • *Fellow in Cardiovascular Imaging, Brigham and Women's Hospital, Boston, Massachusetts*

ANDREW E. ARAI, MD • *Senior Investigator, National Heart, Lung and Blood Institute, National Institutes of Health, US Department of Health and Human Services, Bethesda, Maryland*

VIGNENDRA ARIYARAJAH, MD • *Fellow in Cardiovascular Magnetic Resonance Imaging, Cardiovascular Division, Department of Medicine, Brigham and Women's Hospital, Boston, Massachusetts*

LEON AXEL, MD, PhD • *Professor of Radiology, Medicine, and Physiology and Neuroscience, NYU Medical Center, New York, New York*

DAVID A. BLUEMKE, MD, PhD • *Associate Professor, Radiology and Medicine, Johns Hopkins University School of Medicine, Clinical Director, MRI, Baltimore, Maryland*

RENÉ M. BOTNAR, PhD • *Professor of Biomedical Imaging, Technical University Munich, Munich, Germany*

PAUL A. BOTTOMLEY, PhD • *Russell H. Morgan Professor of Radiology, The Johns Hopkins University School of Medicine, The Johns Hopkins Hospital, Baltimore, Maryland*

LAWRENCE M. BOXT, MD, FACC • *Professor of Clinical Radiology, Albert Einstein College of Medicine of Yeshiva University, Chief, Division of Cardiac MRI and CT, Division of Cardiology and Department of Radiology, North Shore University Hospital, Manhasset, New York*

SHELTON CARUTHERS, PhD • *Clinical Scientist, Philips Medical Systems, St. Louis, Missouri*

TIMOTHY F. CHRISTIAN, MD • *Professor of Medicine and Radiology, Director of Cardiac Magnetic Resonance Imaging, University of Vermont, Burlington, Vermont*

ADAM L. DORFMAN, MD • *Instructor, Department of Pediatrics, Harvard Medical School, Department of Cardiology, Children's Hospital Boston, Boston, Massachusetts*

KEVIN J. DUFFY, MD • *Fellow in Cardiovascular Medicine, University of Pennsylvania School of Medicine, Philadelphia, Pennsylvania*

FREDERICK H. EPSTEIN, PhD • *Associate Professor of Radiology and Biomedical Engineering, University of Virginia, Charlottesville, Virginia*

HALE ERSOY, MD • *Instructor of Radiology, Harvard Medical School, Cardiovascular Magnetic Resonance Imaging and Computed Tomography, Boston, Massachusetts*

VICTOR A. FERRARI, MD • *Associate Professor of Medicine and Radiology, University of Pennsylvania School of Medicine, Associate Director, Noninvasive Imaging Laboratory, Hospital of the University of Pennsylvania, Philadelphia, Pennsylvania*

MATTHIAS G. FRIEDRICH, MD • *Associate Professor of Medicine, University of Calgary, Director, Stephenson CMR Centre at the Libin Cardiovascular Institute of Alberta, Calgary, Alberta, Canada*

TAL GEVA, MD • *Associate Professor of Pediatrics, Harvard Medical School, Chief, Division of Cardiac Imaging, Department of Cardiology, Children's Hospital Boston, Boston, Massachusetts*

HENRY R. HALPERIN, MD, MA • *Professor, Division of Cardiology, Department of Medicine, Johns Hopkins University School of Medicine, Baltimore, Maryland*

CHRISTOPHER J. HARDY, PhD • *Physicist, GE Global Research, Niskayuna, New York*

THOMAS H. HAUSER, MD, MMSc, MPH • *Instructor in Medicine, Harvard Medical School, Director, Nuclear Cardiology, Beth Israel Deaconess Medical Center, Boston, Massachusetts*

GLENN A. HIRSCH, MD • *Instructor of Medicine, Cardiology Division, The Johns Hopkins University School of Medicine, The Johns Hopkins Hospital, Baltimore, Maryland*

LI-YUEH HSU, DSc • *Staff Scientist, National Heart, Lung and Blood Institute, Bethesda, Maryland*

DAVID C. ISBELL, MD • *Fellow in Cardiovascular Disease, University of Virginia Health System, Charlottesville, Virginia*

MICHAEL JEROSCH-HEROLD, PhD • *Associate Professor of Medicine, Cardiac Physicist, Advanced Imaging Research Center, Oregon Health Sciences University, Portland, Oregon*

MAUNG M. KHIN, MD • *Fellow in Cardiovascular Magnetic Resonance Imaging, Brigham and Women's Hospital, Department of Medicine, Cardiovascular Division, Boston, Massachusetts*

W. YONG KIM, MD, PhD • *Associate Professor of Cardiovascular Magnetic Resonance, Magnetic Resonance Center, Institute of Clinical Medicine and Department of Cardiology, Aarhus University Hospital, Skejby Sygehus, Aarhus, Denmark*

SAMUEL ALBERG KOCK, MScBE, PhD STUDENT • *Magnetic Resonance Research Center, Institute of Clinical Medicine, Aarhus University Hospital, Skejby Sygehus, Aarhus, Denmark*

CHRISTOPHER M. KRAMER, MD • *Professor of Medicine and Radiology, University of Virginia Health System, Associate Chief, Cardiovascular Division and Director, Cardiac Magnetic Resonance, Charlottesville, Virginia*

RAYMOND Y. KWONG, MD, MPH • *Instructor of Medicine, Harvard Medical School, Co-director, Cardiac Magnetic Resonance Imaging and Computed Tomography, Cardiovascular Division, Department of Medicine, Brigham and Women's Hospital, Boston, Massachusetts*

HILDO J. LAMB, MD, MSc, PhD • *Senior President, Radiology, Leiden University Medical Center, Leiden, The Netherlands*

GREGORY LANZA, MD, PhD • *Associate Professor of Medicine and Biomedical Engineering, Washington University, St. Louis, Missouri*

ROBERT J. LEDERMAN, MD • *Investigator, Cardiovascular Branch, Division of Intramural Research, National Heart, Lung, and Blood Institute, National Institutes of Health, Bethesda, Maryland*

RUTH LIM, MD • *Fellow, Body and Cardiovascular Radiology, New York University Medical Center, New York, New York*

MARTIN J. LIPTON, MD • *Professor of Radiology, Harvard Medical School, Director of Education, Staff Radiologist, Department of Radiology, Brigham and Women's Hospital, Boston, Massachusetts*

BRUNO MADORE, PhD • *Assistant Professor of Radiology, Harvard Medical School, Brigham and Women's Hospital, Boston, Massachusetts*

WARREN J. MANNING, MD • *Professor of Medicine and Radiology, Harvard Medical School, Section Chief, Non-Invasive Cardiac Imaging, Beth Israel Deaconess Medical Center, Boston, Massachusetts*

MICHAEL MARKL, PhD • *Senior Scientist, Department of Diagnostic Radiology, Medical Physics, Director Cardiovascular MRI, Freiburg, Germany*

EIKE NAGEL, MD • *German Heart Institute Berlin, Director, Cardiovascular Magnetic Resonance Imaging, Berlin, Germany*

SAMAN NAZARIAN, MD • *Instructor and Fellow, Division of Cardiology, Department of Medicine, Johns Hopkins University School of Medicine, Baltimore, Maryland*

ANNE MORAWSKI NEUBAUER, MS • *Graduate Student, Biomedical Engineering, Washington University, St. Louis, Missouri*

BERNARD P. PAELINCK, MD, PhD • *Cardiologist, Department of Cardiology, University Hospital Antwerp, Edegem, Belgium*

DANA C. PETERS, PhD • *Instructor in Medicine, Harvard Medical School, Beth Israel Deaconess Medical Center, Boston, Massachusetts*

ANDREW J. POWELL, MD • *Assistant Professor, Department of Pediatrics, Harvard Medical School, Director, Cardiovascular Magnetic Resonance Imaging, Department of Cardiology, Children's Hospital Boston, Boston, Massachusetts*

MARTIN PRINCE, MD, PhD • *Professor of Radiology, Weill Medical College of Cornell University, Columbia College of Physicians and Surgeons, Chief of MRI, New York Hospital, New York, New York*

FRANK RYBICKI, MD • *Assistant Professor of Radiology, Harvard Medical School, Director, Cardiovascular Computed Tomography, Department of Radiology, Brigham and Women's Hospital, Boston, Massachusetts*

HAJIME SAKUMA, MD • *Associate Professor, Department of Radiology, Mie University Hospital, Tsu City, Mie Prefecture, Japan*

JEANETTE SCHULZ-MENGER, MD • *Assistant Professor, Charite, University Medicine Berlin, Director of Cardiac Magnetic Resonance, Franz Volhard Clinic, Berlin, Germany*

SERVET TATLI, MD • *Staff Radiologist, Department of Radiology, Brigham and Women's Hospital, Boston, Massachusetts*

RACHEL M. WALD, MD • *Instructor, Department of Pediatrics, Harvard Medical School, Department of Cardiology, Children's Hospital Boston, Boston, Massachusetts*

RALF WASSMUTH, MD • *Physician Scientist, Charite, University Medicine Berlin, Senior Investigator of Cardiac Magnetic Resonance, Franz Volhard Clinic, Berlin, Germany*

ROBERT G. WEISS, MD • *Professor of Medicine and Radiology, The Johns Hopkins University School of Medicine, The Johns Hopkins Hospital, Baltimore, Maryland*

HAN WEN, PhD • *Senior Investigator, National Heart, Lung and Blood Institute, Bethesda, Maryland*

SAMUEL A. WICKLINE, MD • *Professor of Medicine, Biomedical Engineering, Physics, and Cellular Biology, Washington University, St. Louis, Missouri*

PATRICK WINTER, PhD • *Assistant Professor of Medicine and Affiliate in Biomedical Engineering, Washington University, St. Louis, Missouri*

Companion CD/DVD

This CD-ROM contains a video and image viewing application with over 60 individual video clips corresponding to the chapters in this book. The application is compatible with most Mac and PC computers.

PC Users:

The application "HP_CMRI.exe" should launch automatically on most Windows computers when the disc is inserted into your computer. If the application does not start after a few moments, simply double-click the application "HP_CMRI.exe" located on the root of this CD-ROM.

Mac Users:

OSX: Double-click the application "HP_CMRI OSX" after inserting the CD-ROM. The Mac OSX operating system does not support an auto-start feature.

The following hardware and software are the minimum required to use this CD-ROM:
- **For Microsoft Windows:** An Intel Pentium II with 64 MB of available RAM running Windows 98, or an Intel Pentium III with 128 MB of available RAM running Windows 2000 or Windows XP. A monitor set to **1024 x 768** or higher resolution.
- **For Macintosh OS X:** A Power Macintosh G3 with 128 MB of available RAM running Mac OS X 10.1.5, 10.2.6 or higher. A monitor set to **1024 x 768** or higher resolution.

1 Basic MRI Physics

Anthony H. Aletras

INTRODUCTION

Magnetic resonance imaging (MRI) basic physics can be described at many different levels, ranging from purely descriptive all the way to quantum mechanics. Here, MRI physics is dealt with mostly in a descriptive manner, and simple mathematics are introduced only if necessary. The simple vector-based model for representing the magnetization is presented because it can deal with most aspects of MRI without the additional complexity of quantum mechanics. In this chapter, nuclear magnetic resonance (NMR) signal generation and its properties are discussed first. Subsequently, image formation in terms of localizing the NMR signal in three dimensions is presented.

SPINNING

Clinical MRI is based on imaging mostly water (and to a lesser extent the fat), which is abundant in physiological tissues. The water molecule contains two hydrogen atoms, which eventually will generate the MRI signal. The hydrogen atom (Fig. 1) consists in turn of a negatively charged electron and a nucleus, which contains a single positively charged proton. The MRI signal is generated from this nucleus, hence the use of the word *nuclear* in NMR.

In its simplest representation, one can consider the nucleus/proton as a tiny magnet (with a north and a south pole like any magnet) that spins along its axis (Fig. 2). These tiny tissue

From: *Contemporary Cardiology: Cardiovascular Magnetic Resonance Imaging*
Edited by: Raymond Y. Kwong © Humana Press Inc., Totowa, NJ

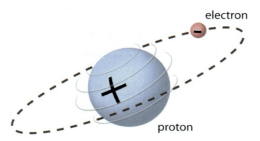

Fig. 1. The hydrogen atom consists of an electron and the nucleus, which contains one proton.

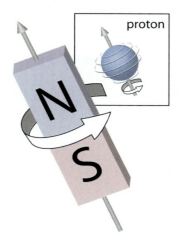

Fig. 2. The proton behaves like a spinning magnet with a north and a south pole; hence, we refer to it as a spin.

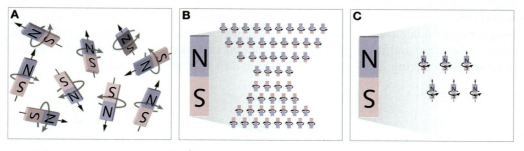

Fig. 3. (A) Spins are randomly oriented in the absence of an external magnetic field. **(B)** In the presence of an external magnetic field Bo, the spins align parallel or anti-parallel to it. **(C)** The difference between the parallel minus the anti-parallel spins represents the spins that will create detectable magnetic resonance signal.

magnets, which are called *spins*, are normally oriented randomly (Fig. 3A), but when brought close to a strong magnet (i.e., within a strong external magnetic field) they align along (parallel) or in the opposite direction (antiparallel) of it (Fig. 3B). The parallel orientation is slightly favored over the antiparallel, resulting in a small excess of spins along the parallel direction (approximately 1 in 1 million). These excess spins are the only ones that will eventually yield a signal (Fig. 3C) that can be later turned into images. This makes MRI a relatively insensitive method, and it is fortunate that there is an abundance of water in the

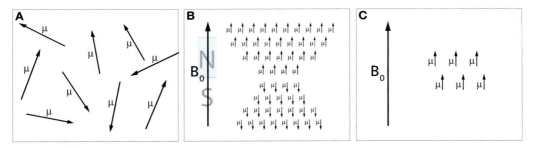

Fig. 4. (A) Spins, represented by μ vectors, are randomly oriented in the absence of an external magnetic field. **(B)** The external magnetic field is represented by a long vector, B_0. The spins (represented by the short vectors μ) align parallel or anti-parallel to B_0. **(C)** The difference between the parallel minus the anti-parallel vectors/spins will create detectable magnetic resonance signal.

body to compensate for this cancellation between spins. One can increase this small excess number of spins that produce signal by increasing the strength of the external magnet.

To avoid displaying small magnets in the figures that follow, each magnet is represented by a vector. The north pole of each magnet will correspond to the arrowhead and the south pole to the arrow tail. The length of each vector will correspond to the strength of each magnet. Therefore, Fig. 3 can now be redrawn as Fig. 4. Note that to distinguish these magnets, the letter μ is assigned to each spin and B_0 is used to describe the external magnetic field. A typical clinical scanner has a magnetic field strength of $B_0 =$ 1.5 *T*. For comparison, the earth's magnetic field is 0.00005 T. The magnet's B_0 field is created in such a way that it has the same strength over the volume of the body that we wish to image; in other words, it is a *homogeneous magnetic field*.

This description has ignored the actual spinning of the tiny tissue magnets/spins for the sake of simplicity but at the expense of accuracy. A better way to describe these spins is actually to take into account the spinning, which results in an arrangement of spins on the surface of a parallel and an antiparallel cone relative to the magnetic field B_0 (Fig. 5A) with properties as described. To help with the representation of the three-dimensional (3D) cones onto the two dimensions of the page, we put the cones into a 3D coordinate system and align the main static field along the z-axis of that system. This also results in the alignment of the two cones also along the z-axis. This Cartesian 3D coordinate system is called the *laboratory frame of reference*.

Note that the spins in Fig. 5 are not stationary but rather are *precessing* about the main magnetic field B_0; in other words, they run along the surface of the two cones like spinning tops. Because the parallel cone has a few more spins on it, one can redraw only those excess spins that have the potential to generate MRI signal (Fig. 5B). The speed with which the spins precess about the external magnetic field increases as the strength of B_0 increases. This is described by the following relationship, the *Larmor equation*:

$$\nu_0 = \gamma B_0 \tag{1}$$

The Larmor equation states that the type of nucleus involved, as described by its *gyromagnetic ratio* γ, is important for determining the speed of precession. For the hydrogen nucleus, it is 42.58 MHz/T, which results in a precessional speed (i.e., *frequency*) of approximately $\nu_0 = 64$ MHz (or 64 million rotations on the cone surface per second) for a typical clinical MRI scanner (1.5 T). The importance of this spinning/precession will become evident. It is most important to remember that spins want to precess about an external static magnetic field and that the frequency of precession is given by the Larmor equation.

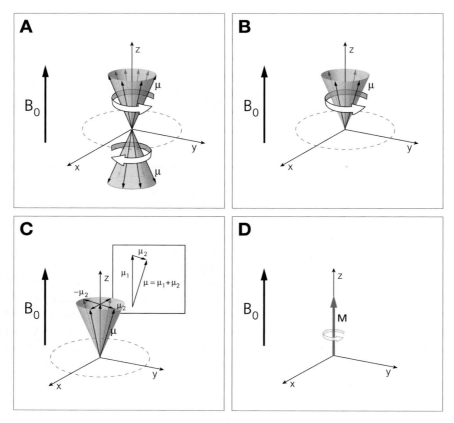

Fig. 5. (A) The spins actually precess on the surface of a parallel and an anti-parallel cone. **(B)** The excess spins precess on the surface of the parallel cone. **(C)** Each spin μ has components along the z-axis and on the base of the cone. The components lying on the base of the cone add up to zero. **(D)** The components along the z-axis add constructively to form the main magnetization vector M.

The excess spin cone seen in Fig. 5B can be further simplified if we notice that the vector components lying on the base of that cone cancel out (Fig. 5C). This happens because the spins randomly and uniformly occupy the surface of the cone since there is no particular reason for them to concentrate at one particular point of the cone surface. As a result, each of the vector components at the base of the cone has its counterpart pointing in the opposite direction; the net sum of all adds to zero. Because all components at the base cancel out, only the components along the z-axis remain. These constructively add together to form the net magnetization vector M (Fig. 5D).

From this point on, we will be dealing with the net magnetization vector M rather than the individual spins. As we use the net magnetization vector M to describe the MRI physics, do not forget that there is an inherent tendency for M to precess about magnetic fields in the same way that individual spins precess about magnetic fields. It is only when M is fully aligned with the z-axis (i.e., along with the main magnetic field B_0) that this precession is not visible to us.

What we have done so far is to place our patient inside the MRI scanner, which provides the static main magnetic field B_0, and to align the net magnetization vector M of the patient's tissue water along that field. We still have not collected information or signals from the patient.

THE MAGNETIC RESONANCE SIGNAL

The creation of the magnetic resonance (MR) signal is based on bringing the net magnetization vector M down onto the transverse xy-plane, away from the z-axis. This is done by applying a secondary magnetic field B_1. This magnetic field B_1 is applied for a brief period of time, on the order of a few thousandths of a second (about 1–5 ms), and this is why it is considered a pulse. B_1 is part of a pulse of radio frequency (RF), which is similar to what commercial radio stations emit to deliver news and music.

The magnetic field B_1 has one other characteristic that makes it different from B_0: it is not static but rather it rotates with a frequency v_1 perpendicular to the main magnetic field B_0. Therefore, B_1 is rotating onto the xy-plane of the laboratory frame of reference as seen in Fig. 6A. The rotation of B_1 needs to be at the same frequency (i.e., rotational speed) that the spins precess. In other words, B_1 needs to be *on-resonance* with the spins, which precess at the Larmor frequency:

$$v_1 = v_0 \tag{2}$$

The net magnetization M has to precess about the newly introduced rotating magnetic field B_1 while at the same time continuing to precess about the static magnetic field B_0. The path that the net magnetization M will follow while the resonance condition (Eq. 2) is satisfied can be seen in Fig. 6B.

This beehive trajectory is not easily seen as the result of two independent precessions of M about the two magnetic fields. To better visualize this motion, the rotating frame of reference is introduced. This new frame of reference views things as if one is seated onto the B_1 vector and is rotating with it (Fig. 6C). Of course, as a result, in the rotating frame of reference B_1 seems not to be moving at all, and it is aligned with the x-axis. Note that nothing really changes; it is only our perspective of things that changes. It is the equivalent of jumping onto a merry-go-round and not seeing the rotation of the horses anymore compared to standing off of the merry-go-round. Also, any precession of M about B_0, which happens at the same rotational speed because it is on-resonance, is also invisible to us while in the rotating frame of reference; because v_o is zero, it is as if B_0 is not there anymore (*see* Eq. 1). This is why when drawing the rotating frame of reference we do not include B_0 in it. From now on, whenever B_0 is not present know that we are inside the rotating frame of reference; any other notation is irrelevant.

In the rotating frame of reference (Fig. 6C), the precession about B_1 is the only motion visible to us. Because the net magnetization M must precess about B_1 and because M is perpendicular to B_1, the first part of this precession is a rotation on the zy-plane. If B_1 is removed while M crosses the transverse plane, that is, while M is on the y-axis, then we can detect the signal it creates (Fig. 6D). The B_1 has caused M to rotate from the z-axis to the y-axis; that is, a 90° rotation has occurred, and therefore B_1 is called a 90° RF pulse.

Signal detection is easier to see in the laboratory frame of reference (Fig. 6E) in which M precesses; do not forget that M behaves as a rotating magnet, and because of its rotation it can induce a voltage onto a loop of wire according to Faraday's law. This voltage is the MR signal, and we can record it at will. Note that because of the rotation of M at the Larmor frequency the signal we record at the loop of wire (i.e., our antenna) has a sinusoidal waveform as seen in Fig. 7A. This signal is called the *free-induction decay* (FID); for now, we ignore the fact that it is decaying with time, that is, that its size (also known as *amplitude*) diminishes with time.

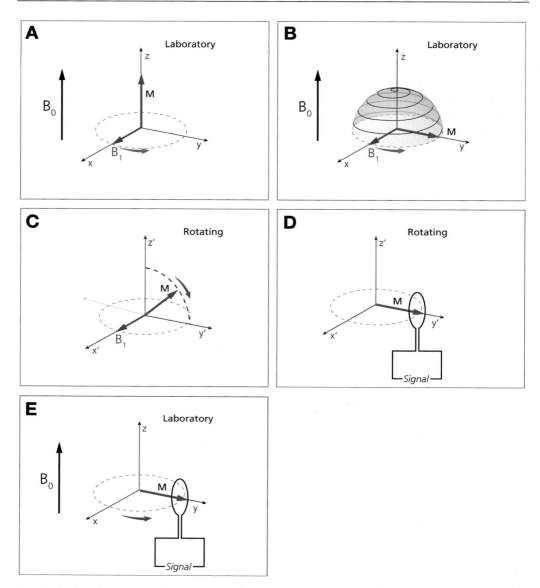

Fig. 6. (A) The RF pulse is represented in the Laboratory Frame of Reference as a vector B_1 spinning onto the xy-plane with a frequency v_1. **(B)** While B_1 is applied, the net magnetization vector precesses both about B_1 and B_0 in a beehive manner towards the xy-plane. **(C)** In the Rotating Frame of Reference (which rotates at a frequency of v_1) the RF pulse vector B_1 appears to be stationary. Also, B_0 is invisible in the Rotating Frame of Reference. Therefore, the net magnetization vector M appears to precess/rotate only about B_1. When M reaches the y'-axis, B_1 is removed so as to accomplish a total of 90° rotation of M. **(D)** In the Rotating Frame of Reference the net magnetization produces a signal onto a wire antenna. **(E)** In the Laboratory Frame of Reference the net magnetization produces an oscillating signal onto the wire antenna due to the rotation of M (Faraday's law).

Note that Fig. 7A shows the signal in the laboratory frame of reference (Fig. 6E) (i.e., at our antenna). If one observed the signal in the rotating frame of reference (Fig. 6D), then the waveform would be as seen in Fig. 7B, which is the equivalent of listening to the music of a radio station from our radio's speaker rather than trying to listen to it by

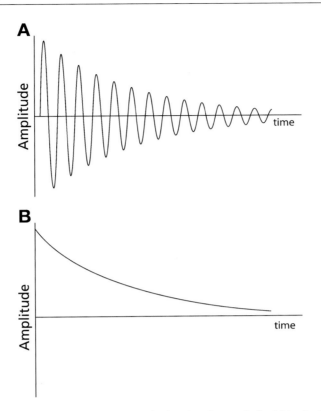

Fig. 7. (A) The oscillating free induction decay is the signal recorded within the laboratory frame of reference (Fig. 6E). **(B)** The non-oscillating free induction decay is the signal recorded within the rotating frame of reference (Fig. 6D).

foolishly placing an antenna in our ear. Again, it is all a matter only of how we perceive things. However, to be able to listen to the music (i.e., observe in the rotating frame of reference) we do need the radio receiver. Part of the MRI scanner is such a radio receiver. The signal, rather than being directed to a speaker, is saved in digital form to the computer's memory.

This sequence of events to create an FID is called the *one-pulse experiment,* and it is depicted in a *pulse sequence diagram* (Fig. 8). This is the most rudimentary experiment and consists of just switching on the 90° RF pulse for a short period of time, then switching it off, followed by turning on the receiver to acquire the MR signal, then turning it off.

RELAXATION TIMES: T_1, T_2, AND T_2^*

The MR signal in Fig. 7 is decaying with time until we can no longer observe any signal. This is happening as a result of two processes. First, the spins themselves are small magnets, and they interact with each other. This creates microscopic changes in the overall magnetic field that the spins experience; as a result, according to the Larmor equation, spins that constitute the net magnetization vector M (Fig. 9A) will precess with slightly different rotational speeds (Fig. 9B). Some spins will move faster, some slower, resulting in the slow decomposition of the net magnetization vector because the spins no longer precess in a coherent synchronized manner.

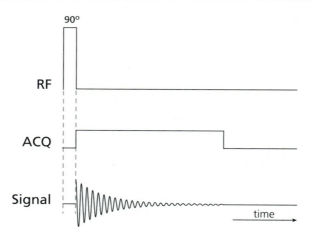

Fig. 8. The one pulse experiment pulse sequence diagram.

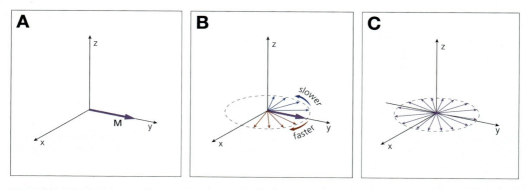

Fig. 9. (A) Following a 90° RF pulse along the *x*-axis, the magnetization vector M lies onto the *y*-axis. **(B)** The spins that comprise M will precess at faster and slower speeds due to spin-spin inter-actions. Dephasing will set in. **(C)** After some time, complete dephasing will occur so that the net sum of all spins is zero.

In other words, as time goes by, the spins will acquire a different rotational angle (or *phase*) relative to each other because of their slightly different rotational speeds (or fre-quencies). This is called *dephasing*, and it is the result of increasing randomness (or increasing entropy). These *spin-spin* interactions cause the eventual obliteration of the MR signal (Fig. 9C); in fact, the spins return to the randomness they had before the RF was pulsed (Fig. 5C). This type of relaxation mechanism, which depends only on spin-spin interactions, is referred to as T_2 *relaxation*.

However, the signal in Fig. 7 also decays as a result of an imperfectly homogeneous static magnetic field B_0. The effect is similar to that seen in Fig. 9 in that the macro-scopic B_0 inhomogeneity causes the individual spins to precess at different frequencies; as a result, M is destroyed because of dephasing. Note that no matter how good a static magnetic field we can create, the introduction of the human body into the field causes local inhomogeneity. Usually the MRI scanners have hardware that can be used for try-ing to correct these local inhomogeneities to some extent by what is called *shimming* of the field. The relaxation mechanism, which depends on spin-spin interactions and the additional B_0 field inhomogeneities, is referred to as T_2^* (T_2-star) *relaxation*. It is important to note that both T_2 and T_2^* only occur while the net magnetization vector M is on the *xy*-transverse plane (Fig. 9). While M is along the *z*-axis, these two relaxation processes do not happen.

The signal loss over time that is seen in the FID is dependent on T_2^* relaxation, and it follows an exponential decay:

$$M_{XY}(t) = M_{XY(t=0)}e^{-t/T_2^*} \tag{3}$$

Equation 3 states that the magnetization observed at time zero ($M_{XY(t=0)}$) on the transverse plane will decay exponentially according to the elapsed time t and a time constant T_2^*. For example, the myocardium has a T_2^* of approximately 20 ms. After time 3 T_2^*, 95% of the signal will be lost; after 5 T_2^*, 99.3% of it will be lost. This shows that the acquisition window (Fig. 8) for the one-pulse experiment should be adjusted accordingly in length because after 60 ms essentially no signal is acquired.

When the field inhomogeneities are not considered, the relaxation occurs more slowly, at a rate that is determined by a T_2 time constant (rather than T_2^*). This is also an exponential decay but a slower one according to T_2, which is about 50 ms in the myocardium.

$$M_{XY}(t) = M_{XY(t=0)}e^{-t/T_2} \tag{4}$$

In this case, the signal could potentially be acquired over a longer period of time (150 ms). Unfortunately, the magnetization in the one-pulse experiment is experiencing T_2^* relaxation, not T_2. We can use a different experiment, the *spin echo*, to acquire an MR signal that decays with T_2 and exploit the longer acquisition windows. Spin echoes are described in the next section.

So far, we have seen how the signal decays when the magnetization is on the transverse plane. We have not seen yet how the net magnetization vector recovers along the *z*-axis to its original state. This occurs via energy exchange between the spins and their surrounding environment (i.e., the lattice), hence the term *spin-lattice relaxation*. In other words, the spins release their excess energy to the lattice. This is a process that occurs along the *z*-axis only, and it is independent of the spin-spin relaxation, which occurs on the transverse plane. One can think of the net magnetization M growing along the *z*-axis as time goes by (Fig. 10). Remember that following a 90° RF pulse the entire M was on the *xy*-plane, and no magnetization remained along *z*; this is why M grows along the *z*-axis from zero to its maximum starting value. Spin-lattice relaxation occurs at a relatively slow rate according to the time constant T_1:

$$M_Z(t) = M_{Z(t=\infty)}[1 - e^{-t/T_1}] \tag{5}$$

Equation 5 states that the magnetization along the *z*-axis increases exponentially with time until it reaches its maximum after a long time. For the myocardium, T_1 is about 900 ms. After 3 T_1, the magnetization reaches 95% of its maximum value; after 5 T_1, it reaches 99.3% of its maximum. This means that we have to wait approximately 3 seconds or longer if we want to start the one pulse experiment again. Given that our signal is lost within only 60 ms because of T_2^*, this is indeed a long time to wait before the experiment can be repeated.

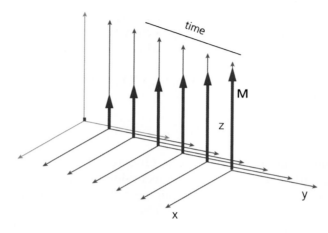

Fig. 10. T_1 relaxation: over time, the magnetization recovers along the z-axis from zero to its maximum value.

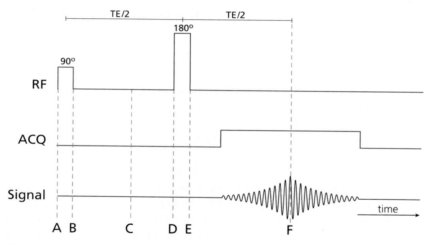

Fig. 11. The spin echo pulse sequence diagram. Note that the time-points A–F correspond to Figures 12A–12F.

SPIN ECHOES

We saw that the one-pulse experiment results in acquiring an FID, which reflects T_2^* decay. True T_2 decay can only be observed by creating and acquiring a spin echo rather than an FID. Figure 11 presents the pulse sequence diagram that describes this process. Observe that the signal is not acquired right after the 90° RF pulse (time-point B) but rather a waiting period (TE/2) is introduced, followed by an 180° RF pulse, which is in turn followed by the acquisition at the right time.

Let us see how the net magnetization responds to this type of a pulse sequence (Fig. 12). Note that the time-points A–F in Fig. 11 correspond to the letters A–F used in Fig. 12. Initially, M is aligned along the z-axis (Fig. 12A), and it responds to the 90° B_1 pulse, which is along the x-axis, by moving onto the y-axis of the transverse plane (Fig. 12B). On the transverse plane, M experiences signal loss caused by spin-spin

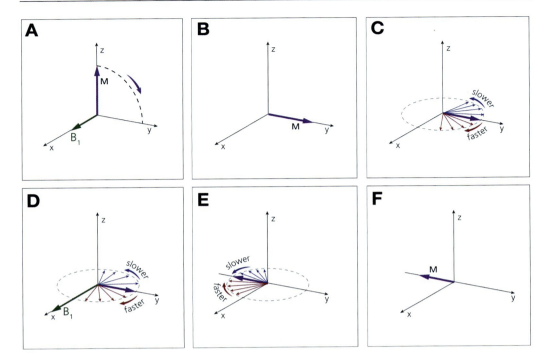

Fig. 12. (A) A 90° pulse along the *x*-axis forces the magnetization vector to move onto the *zy*-plane towards the *y*-axis. **(B)** Once the RF pulse is over all the spins are coherently adding up to form the net magnetization vector along the *y*-axis. **(C)** As time elapses, the spins dephase due to B_0 field inhomogeneities (spin-spin interactions are ignored for this example). The faster spins acquire positive phase while the slower spins lag behind and acquire negative phase. **(D)** A 180° pulse along the *x*-axis is applied. **(E)** The spins rotate onto the other side of the *xy*-plane. (Figure 13 shows why this happens) The spins continue to move with their respective speeds. **(F)** At time equal to TE all the spins rephase along −*y*.

interactions and additional loss caused by dephasing as a result of static magnetic field (B_0) inhomogeneities. Because spin-spin-related signal loss will always occur (according to T_2), we choose not to depict it here, but rather we focus our attention only on the extra dephasing caused by static field inhomogeneities (Fig. 12C); that is, we are concentrating on the "star" that turns T_2 into T_2^*. Some spins that comprise M will move faster (red; running clockwise) and some slower (blue; running counterclockwise); dephasing occurs during the TE/2 waiting period (Fig. 12C). Then, a 180° B_1 pulse along the *x*-axis is introduced (Fig. 12D), causing the dephasing spins to be rotated onto the other side of the *xy*-plane, as seen in Fig. 12E.

Let us discuss why such a rotation occurs by means of Fig. 13, and we will return to Figs. 11 and 12 in the next paragraph. First, take the red/faster spin closer to the *y*-axis (Fig. 12D) and copy it in Fig. 13A so that we can see how it responds to the 180° pulse. This spin can be decomposed into its *x*- and *y*-axis components as seen in Fig. 13B. The *x*-axis component is aligned with the 180° RF pulse (Fig. 13C) and does not move. However, the *y*-axis component (Fig. 13C) will have to rotate/precess about B_1 by 180° because it is perpendicular to it and ends up along −*y* (Fig. 13D). If we now recombine the *x* and *y* components (Fig. 13E), we can see the ending position of the

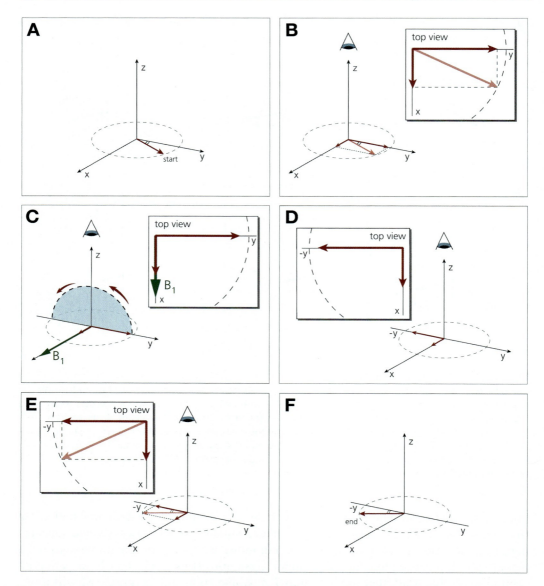

Fig. 13. (**A**) One of the fast moving spins is copied here from Figure 12C. (**B**) This spin vector has two components: one along the *x*-axis and one along the *y*-axis. (**C**) The 180° pulse along the *x*-axis forces the *y* component to rotate towards −*y*. The *x*-component does not move at all. (**D**) At the end of the RF pulse the two components are along *x* and −*y*. (**E**) These two components add together. (**F**) The ending position of the vector after the RF pulse is over.

spin (Fig. 13F) as a result of the 180° pulse. Similarly, we can apply the same rules to determine where the rest of the spins will end up.

Returning to Figs. 11 and 12, following the removal of the 180° pulse, the spins continue to rotate faster (red) or slower (blue) (Fig. 12E). If we wait for the same amount of time that it took them to dephase initially (i.e., TE/2), then they will rephase along −*y*, and the field inhomogeneity-related dephasing will no longer be visible (Fig. 12F). The time for rephasing the signal is the echo time (TE), and it is measured from the 90° RF pulse. This is the formation of a spin echo at time TE. The 180° pulse causes the apparent sign change (from positive to negative) to any phase accumulated prior to its application, so that the net phase adds to zero. Note that dephasing will take place after TE, and the signal will decay past TE (Fig. 11, signal axis). Only the top of the spin echo reflects true T_2 decay over the time TE. So, to measure the T_2 of tissues, multiple experiments are usually run at different echo times, and the amounts of decay of the acquired spin echoes are plotted against time before fitting the data with an exponential curve.

GRADIENTS AND GRADIENT ECHOES

Gradient echoes are also a secondary type of signal, similar in that respect to spin echoes. However, gradient echoes are not created by 180° RF pulses but rather with the application of gradient magnetic fields. A *gradient magnetic field* refers to a magnetic field that adds to or subtracts from the main static magnetic field B_0 a small amount of field strength. The amount added or subtracted depends on the particular location in space of the tissue of interest, and it is proportional to the distance from the center or the magnet (i.e., the *isocenter*). There are three different gradient magnetic fields one can apply at will: G_X, G_Y, and G_Z. These can be seen in the rotating frame of reference in Fig. 14A–C, respectively.

Let us take G_Y as an example (Fig. 14B) to try to understand how gradients work. In the absence of any gradient field, the spins would experience the same static magnetic field no matter where they are located in 3D space. In this case of the rotating frame of reference, the magnetic field strength would be zero because we choose to ignore B_0 (unlike the laboratory frame of reference, for which B_0 is visible). By applying a gradient magnetic field (Fig. 14B) along the y-direction (i.e., G_Y), what we do is modify the magnetic field such that at $y = 0$ the field is still zero; at $y = 1$ the field is slightly positive; at $y = 2$ the field is twice as positive as it was at $y = 1$; at $y = 3$ the field is three times as positive as it was at $y = 1$; and so on. Similarly, at $y = -1$ the field is slightly negative (i.e., spins would rotate in the opposite direction as at $y = 1$ but with the same rotational speed); at $y = -2$ the field is twice as strong as it was at $y = -1$; at $y = -3$ the field is three times as strong as it was at $y = -1$; and so on.

One can see now that, according to the Larmor equation, there is a particular rotational speed (also known as the *precessional frequency*) associated with each particular point on the y-axis. Given a spin's frequency of precession, one can figure out where on the y-axis that particular spin is located. Conversely, given a location on the y-axis one can predict what the precessional speed will be for a spin at that location. The gradient strength is measured in Tesla/meter, which shows basically how rapidly the field changes when moving from $y = 0$ to $y = 1$. Typical gradient strengths on state-of-the-art MR scanners are 0.040 T/m. One can see that this is relatively small compared to the static magnetic field of 1.5 T. However, such strength is sufficient to create a spread of frequencies; that is, spins at different locations on the y-axis will be precessing at different speeds. It is important to realize that the change in the field, when G_Y is applied, occurs as we move up and down the y-axis, but that we always are adding or subtracting to the main field B_0 along its direction, which is along the z-axis. A similar description to can be visualized for G_X or G_Z.

Do not forget that a gradient magnetic field is a known inhomogeneity we chose to impose on the tissues we are imaging. Indeed, with gradients, we force the B_0 field to

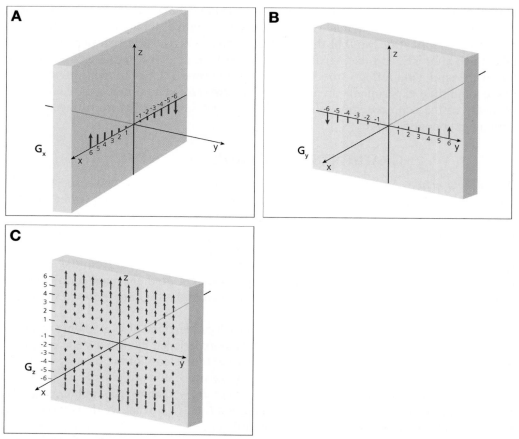

Fig. 14. (A) A G_X gradient magnetic field modifies the *z*-oriented static field depending on *x*-position. **(B)** A G_Y gradient magnetic field modifies the *z*-oriented static field depending on *y*-position. **(C)** A G_Z gradient magnetic field modifies the *z*-oriented static field depending on *z*-position.

change across space; that is, we create a deliberate (and known) B_0 inhomogeneity. This may not make much sense right now because we know that this will cause further signal decay to T_2^*, but we will show how we can use gradients both for creating gradient echoes and for imaging.

For the more mathematically inclined, the Larmor equation (Eq. 1) in the laboratory frame of reference in the presence of gradient fields becomes

$$\nu_0 = \gamma(B_0 + G_X x + G_Y y + G_Z z) \tag{6}$$

One can see how the gradients G_X, G_Y, and G_Z add to the main magnetic field B_0 depending on their strength and the distance of the tissue from the isocenter, that is, according to the tissue's *xyz*-location in space.

Gradient echoes can be created by gradient pulses with the sequence seen in Fig. 15 (the time-points A–F in Fig. 15 correspond to the labels A–F of Fig. 16). Note the addition of three more time axes that reflect the strength of the gradient fields along the *x*-, *y*-, and *z*-directions. The tissue is excited by a 90° B_1 pulse (Fig. 16A), which brings the net magnetization vector M from the *z*-axis down to the *y*-axis (Fig. 16B). Note that the

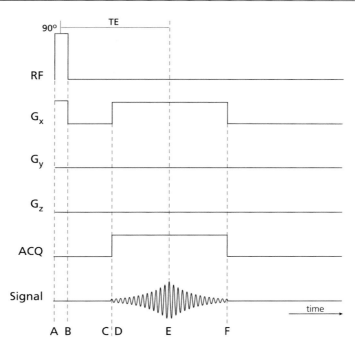

Fig. 15. The gradient echo pulse sequence diagram. Note that the time-points A-F correspond to Figures 16A–16F.

net magnetization of each location along the *x*-axis has been individually drawn in Fig. 16 so that we can monitor separately what happens at each location. A significant B_0 inhomogeneity is then introduced by turning on a brief negative G_X gradient pulse (Fig. 15, time-point B). This causes additional dephasing of the signal to that expected by T_2^* alone. In fact, for a typical MR scanner, gradient dephasing is about 1000 times larger than the dephasing attributed to T_2^*. As a result, by the time the negative gradient pulse is over (Fig. 15, time-point C), the signal is obliterated (Fig. 16C) as a result of spins moving faster (red) and slower (blue) in response to the negative gradient pulse.

Do not forget that we have control over the polarity and the strength of the gradients. So, we next turn on the G_X gradient with the same strength but with positive polarity (Fig. 15, time-point D). This causes dephasing in the opposite direction, in other words, *rephasing*. Spins that were fast now become slow and vice versa (Fig. 16D) because it is the gradient polarity that determines their speeds. If we wait until the positive gradient is applied for the same amount of time and at the same absolute strength as the negative gradient, then full rephasing will occur, and the top of a gradient echo will be seen (Fig. 16E and Fig. 15, time-point E). The time interval from the 90° RF pulse to the top of the gradient echo is called the *echo time*, TE. Of course, if the positive G_X gradient pulse continues to play out (Fig. 15, time interval E–F), then the spins will continue dephasing, and signal destruction will occur (Fig. 16F). An entire gradient echo then will have been formed.

It is important to note that, even though we managed to refocus at the top of the echo any dephasing done by the negative and positive G_X gradient pulses, we have not been able to rephase any dephasing caused by T_2^*. This is because we do not have any means for changing the polarity of the T_2^*-related B_0 inhomogeneities in a gradient echo

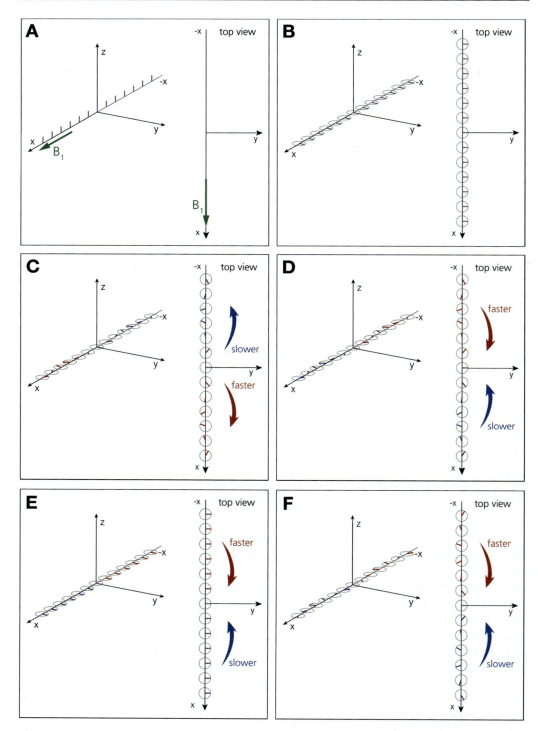

Fig. 16. (A) The spins at different locations along the *x*-axis are aligned with *z* initially. The RF pulse is applied along the *x*-axis. **(B)** After the RF pulse has ended, the spins are all aligned parallel to the *y*-axis. **(C)** The application of the negative gradient lobe forces some spins to move faster and some slower. This results in dephasing. **(D)** The positive gradient lobe forces the previously fast moving

experiment. Therefore, we expect the top of the gradient echo to reflect T_2*-related signal losses. Compare this to the spin echo that reflects T_2, and you now have the tools for measuring both of these time constants. The T_1 time constant can be measured by either an inversion or saturation recovery pulse sequence.

IMAGING

So far, we have been able to acquire a signal from the patient that we have put into the static magnetic field. However, the signals we collect from the patient's head or arms or heart cannot be distinguished from one another. Rather, we have been acquiring with our antenna the net sum of all the signals that originate from the different tissues of the patient. When all is said and done, we have no means for distinguishing the exact origin of these signals. This is because we have not encoded in any particular way the magnetization in space; that is, we have not given the magnetization any unique characteristics based on where it is situated in space.

To localize the signal in 3D space, one has to provide three distinct processes that will provide a one-to-one correspondence between location and some other measurable characteristic of the tissue. For MR imaging, these three processes are slice selection, frequency encoding, and phase encoding. These processes will be described in the sections that follow. The Fourier transformation, which is essential for extracting spatial information from the encoded MR signal, will also be described. Note that, for illustration, the image that we will collect will be an axial one, that is, perpendicular to the long axis of the body. However, any 3D image orientation may be acquired with appropriate control of the scanner, which is a major advantage of MRI. For clinical scanners, the patient is introduced to the magnetic field B_0 such that the head-feet direction is parallel to B_0 and therefore along the z-axis. The typical gradient echo imaging pulse sequence is shown in Fig. 17; this is the sequence that will be used in the following sections to introduce the principles of imaging with MR. Note that this is not a complete gradient echo imaging sequence because some details have been omitted for the purpose of this basic presentation.

SLICE SELECTION

The first step in encoding the signal in space is slice selection. So far, we have been exciting with RF all the magnetization vectors in the body of the patient such that the vectors are rotated from the z-axis down to the y-axis (e.g., Fig. 16B); this is done irrespective of where these vectors are located. The goal with slice selection is not to excite all spins but rather only those spins within a particular plane (i.e., within a slice) of imaging interest. Such slices could be selected to go across the head, the heart, or any other tissue.

Within the slice of interest, we want the magnetization to be rotated down to the y-axis and eventually to produce a signal. In any other point in space, the magnetization should remain along the z-axis and therefore will not yield a signal. Slice selection is accomplished by applying a gradient field along the z-axis (Fig. 14C) at the same time that

---

Fig. 16. *(Continued)* spins to move slow and the previously slow moving spins to move fast. This results in rephasing. **(E)** When the positive gradient lobe is applied for the same time as the previous negative lobe then full rephasing occurs. The effects of the two gradient lobes cancel out. **(F)** The positive gradient lobe continues to be applied and further dephasing is observed.

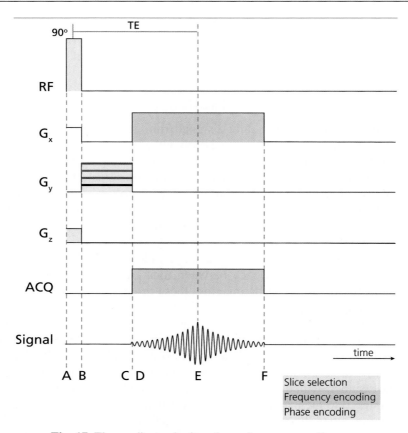

Fig. 17. The gradient echo imaging pulse sequence diagram.

the RF pulse is played out (Fig. 17, beige color). The gradient field along the z-axis causes spins at different planes parallel to the transverse plane to precess at different frequencies.

Only the spins in a plane where the precessional Larmor frequency v_0 is equal to the frequency v_1 of our RF pulse will respond to the RF pulse and be brought on the transverse plane. In other words, only the spins in the plane that is on-resonance with the RF pulse (Eq. 2) will produce a signal. Do not forget that we have full control of the RF pulse frequency, so we can select any such plane parallel to the xy-plane. How thick a plane we excite is set both by the gradient strength G_Z and the characteristics of the RF pulse. Without going into details, the stronger G_Z gets, the thinner the slice we can select.

In our imaging experiment, we have so far managed to localize in one dimension by allowing only magnetization from one particular slice along the z-axis to participate in signal formation. As a result, the signal we collect will be similar to the one seen in Fig. 7 but much smaller in size (or amplitude) because all the remaining slices that were excluded by slice selection no longer contribute to the signal acquired. We now need to encode the signal along the remaining two dimensions, x and y.

FREQUENCY ENCODING

If we apply a gradient pulse during the time we acquire the MR signal (Fig. 17, dark blue areas), we effectively encode the signal in space in a manner that we can exploit so that we can determine the signal's origin. A gradient pulse that is played out at the same

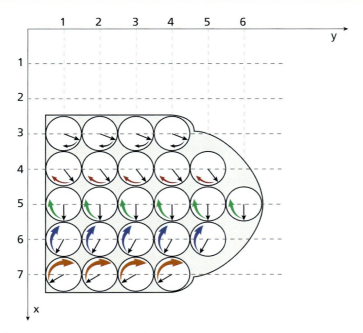

Fig. 18. A bird's eye view of the imaging slice: The application of a readout gradient along the *x*-axis forces the spins to precess at different frequencies according to their *x* position. Note that the *y* position of a spin plays no role in this process.

time as the acquisition window (i.e., during the time we "read out" the signal) is called a *readout gradient*. In fact, the gradient echo we introduced in Figs. 15 and 16 is an example of an MR signal that is acquired in the presence of a readout gradient applied along the *x*-axis (G_X). We can see that our imaging pulse sequence (Fig. 17) also acquires a gradient echo because the G_X gradient pulse is used in the same manner. The G_X readout gradient pulse is *frequency–encoding* the MR signal. We already know how the dephasing with a negative gradient pulse followed by rephasing with a positive gradient pulse creates a gradient echo, so there is no need to explain this further. Rather, the next paragraphs will focus on why the gradient echo contains spatial information and how that information is extracted.

Let us assume that we are imaging an object that resembles a slice of bread that lies on the transverse plane (Fig. 18). Note that this is a bird's eye view from the *z*-axis down to the *xy*-plane. The application of a readout gradient G_X (Fig. 17, time interval DF) forces the magnetization at different points of the *x*-axis to precess at different speeds (Fig. 18, speeds of black, red, green, blue, orange that are progressively higher). Therefore, the magnetization at different rows has now a unique characteristic, that is, a different precessional frequency that can be potentially used to localize the signal along the *x*-axis.

It is not difficult for us to see these different frequencies, which correspond to the rows in Fig. 18, because they are separately drawn. For instance (Fig. 19A, black trace), the vectors corresponding to the magnetization at *x* = 3 would form (as a result of their spinning) a sinusoidal wave with, for example, a rotational speed of 300 rotations per second (i.e., a "black" frequency of 300 Hz) and a signal intensity (i.e., amplitude) of 4 units because there are 4 "disks" with magnetization vectors in that row. Then, the

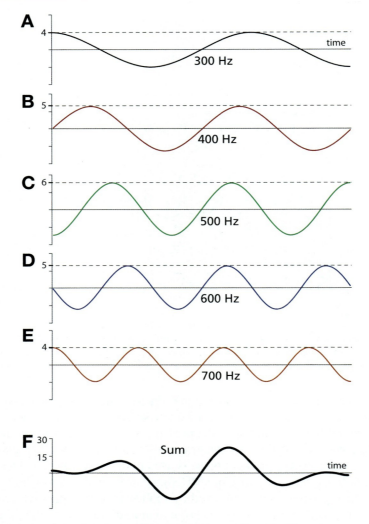

Fig. 19. The signals originating from the rows of spins in Fig. 18. The colors correspond 1-1 with those of Fig. 18. Spins along the x-axis that are further away from the isocenter emit a sinusoidal waveform that has a higher frequency (e.g. **E**). The sum of all sinusoids (**F**) is what we observe.

magnetization at $x = 4$ (Fig. 19B, red trace) would correspond to a faster rotating sine wave (red frequency, 400 Hz) with an amplitude of 5, the magnetization at $x = 5$ (Fig. 19C, green trace) to an even faster sine (green frequency, 500 Hz) with an amplitude of 6, at $x = 6$ (Fig. 19D, blue trace) to a sine with blue frequency of 600 Hz and amplitude of 5, and finally at $x = 7$ (Fig. 19E, orange trace) to a sine with orange frequency of 700 Hz and amplitude of 4. Note how the frequency of the sine becomes higher further away from zero (as expected because of the higher precessional speed caused by the progressively stronger field) and how the amplitude of the sine is modulated by how many disks of magnetization correspond to each row within our object.

Because the sinusoidal waveforms from the different locations are separately drawn in Fig. 19A–E, it is easy for us to see the different frequencies generated by the precessing magnetization vectors seen in Fig. 18. However, the picture becomes more

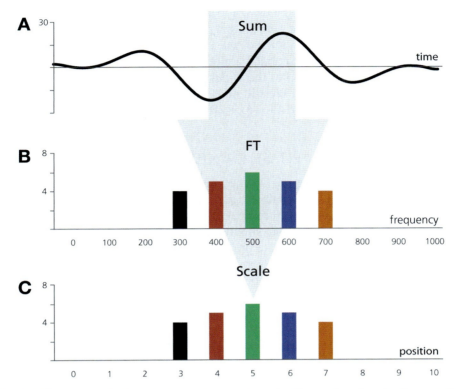

Fig. 20. (A) The sum of all sinusoidal waveforms originating from spins along various *x*-axis positions (Fig. 19F) contains the spatial information within it. **(B)** The Fourier transformation extracts the spectral information from the detected signal. Note that the *x*-axis represents frequencies in Hz. **(C)** Frequencies can be converted into position along the *x*-axis because the encoding strength of the readout gradient is known.

difficult to visualize if we take into account that we actually observe the sum of all these spinning vectors, that is, the sum of all the color sinusoids seen in Fig. 19A–E. In other words, we observe the net sum seen in Fig. 19F, and we are then asked if we can decipher that it contains all five waveforms seen in Fig. 19A–E. If we could do this, then we could pinpoint with certainty the origin of the signal along the *x*-axis.

Fortunately, a mathematical tool exists that can reconstruct the original signals from their sum. This tool is the *Fourier transformation*, and to us it will be just a black box that can take a signal (e.g., such as the gradient echo) and tell us what sinusoidal waveforms exist in it. In other words, the Fourier transformation can tell us what frequency (also known as spectral) components are contained within the signal.

In this case, the Fourier transformation would take the signal seen in Fig. 20A (which we copied for ease of visualization from Fig. 19F) and create from it Fig. 20B. In Fig. 20B, we see the frequencies of the sine waves that exist within our gradient echo. Notice that following the Fourier transformation the horizontal axis has changed into a "frequency" axis. It is therefore said that the Fourier transformation converts a signal from the time domain (Fig. 20A) to the frequency domain (Fig. 20B). Each bar in Fig. 20B corresponds to a frequency of one of the sinusoidal waveforms present within the gradient echo (Fig. 20A). Because we know that 300 Hz corresponds to a location at

$x = 3$ on the x-axis, 400 Hz corresponds to a location at $x = 4$ on the x-axis and so on, we can scale accordingly the frequency axis into a position axis (Fig. 20C). Notice that each of the bars shows the correct amplitude of the x-axis location it represents (Fig. 18).

Therefore, we have managed to obtain a plot that shows how many spins contributed to our signal at any given location of the x-axis. In other words, we have now a projection of our object onto the x-axis. We still need to find out how we can extract information along the last remaining axis, the y-axis. Then, our image of this slice of bread will be complete.

PHASE ENCODING

Because frequency encoding has worked nicely for determining where the signal originates from the x-axis, it is tempting to say that one also could use frequency encoding along the y-axis, and this way an image could be formed. Unfortunately, if we were to apply the same frequency encoding simultaneously along both the x- and y-axis, then we would only manage to differentiate our signal's position along a single axis that is tilted halfway between x and y. In other words, we could not separate along the two different axes the effect of frequency encoding. This makes sense because magnetization at $x = 3$ and at $y = 3$ will both precess at 300 Hz according to our previous example. Once added, there is no way to differentiate the two. Phase encoding is introduced to overcome this problem.

Phase encoding is based on the principle that information about the signal's point of origin on the y-axis can be represented by the phase (also known as the angle, measured in degrees) of the magnetization vector. Both in the one-pulse experiment (Fig. 8) and the gradient echo imaging pulse sequence (Fig. 15), right after the 90° RF pulse is applied along the x-axis, the magnetization lies along the y-axis. If we set the y–axis as our point of reference the y-axis, then all the magnetization vectors following the RF pulse have a phase (or angle) of 0° relative to it (Fig. 16B). If a short G_Y gradient pulse (along the y-axis) is played out immediately after the RF pulse but also before the acquisition begins (Fig. 17, e.g., green G_Y pulse, light blue shaded area), then the magnetization vectors will precess at different speeds according to their position on the y-axis for that short period of time.

As a result, at the end of the G_Y pulse the magnetization vectors will be at progressively larger angles relative to the y-axis (i.e., they will have acquired more phase) the further away from zero they are located (Fig. 21). (This is equivalent to having runners of different capabilities starting to run at the same time from the start of a circular track and observing where they are located at a particular point in time later. Instead of logging their performance by means of the distance they run, we log their performance by means of the arc they run, i.e., how much phase each runner acquired.) Note that after the end of the G_Y phase-encoding gradient pulse the magnetization vectors no longer precess at different speeds (Fig. 21). Information about their position onto the y-axis has been encoded onto their phase.

Because position on the y-axis has been encoded onto the phase of the magnetization at each location, one would expect that it would be easy to extract this information when we finally acquire the MR signal. Unfortunately, the Fourier transformation can be of no help with such a data set. The reason is obvious if one observes that when two vectors are added it is not possible to tell from their sum what the original vectors were. Figure 22 demonstrates this point: the sum of the two blue vectors as well as the sum of

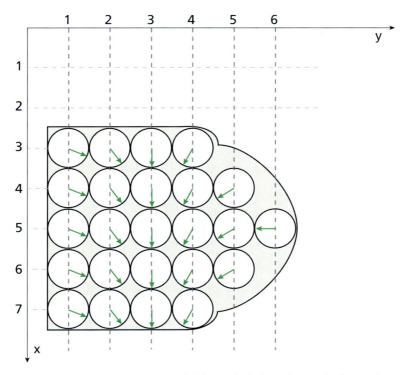

Fig. 21. The phase encoding gradient pulse, which is applied along the y-axis, forces the magnetization vectors to precess at different frequencies. At the end of the pulse the magnetization vectors precess with the same frequencies but have acquired phase proportional to their position along the y-axis.

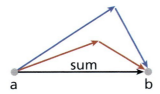

Fig. 22. Knowing the sum of two vectors cannot directly be used to find out which two vectors were added together. There is an infinite number of pairs of vectors that can yield the same sum.

the two red vectors both result in the same vector (black). In fact, one can think of an infinite number of two-vector combinations that can produce the same result. It is the equivalent to the futile attempt of trying to determine the exact path of a journey from its starting and ending points alone. The solution to unscrambling the y-axis position-encoded information from the phase of the magnetization vectors lies with converting this phase information into frequency information, which the Fourier transformation can deal with.

Let us consider the effects of the phase-encoding gradient pulse seen in Fig. 17 in more detail. Let us also assign some phase numbers for illustration purposes. At $y = 1$, there are five disks of magnetization vectors (Fig. 21), and we assume that for the black phase-encoding gradient pulse strength (Fig. 17, black G_Y phase-encoding waveform, light blue shaded area) the resulting phase accumulated is 10° (Fig. 23, $y = 1$, black

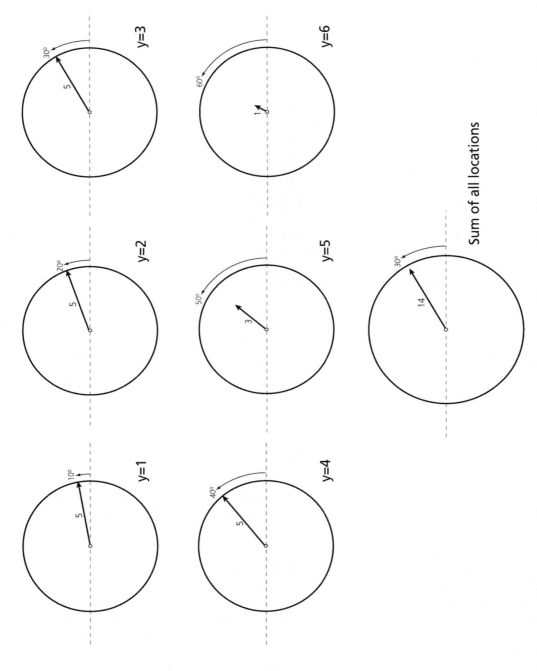

Fig. 23. The phase accumulated by magnetization (black arrows) of the imaged object (Fig. 21) at different positions of the *y*-axis is shown. This is the phase right after the black phase encoding gradient pulse (Fig. 17, interval BC) has been applied. The sum of all locations (black arrow, 14 units long with 30° phase) is what is observed by us.

24

arrow). Then, at $y = 2$, 20° of phase would have accumulated (Fig. 23, $y = 2$, black arrow); at $y = 3$, 30° of phase would have accumulated (Fig. 23, $y = 3$, black arrow); at $y = 4$, 40° of phase would have accumulated (Fig. 23, $y = 4$, black arrow); at $y = 5$, 50° of phase would have accumulated (Fig. 23, $y = 5$, black arrow); last, at $y = 6$, 60° of phase would have accumulated (Fig. 23, $y = 6$, black arrow). This is the direct result of the progressively stronger magnetic field that the spins are experiencing away from $y = 0$. Note that at locations $y = 5$ and $y = 6$ the length of the arrow is adjusted to represent intensity of 3 and 1 magnetization disks, respectively (*see* Fig. 21). In Fig. 23, you can also see the sum (calculated via trigonometry) of all these vectors from all locations, which is a vector of length 14 and phase of 30°.

If we now repeat the experiment seen in Fig. 17, but this time we use instead the red phase-encoding gradient strength (i.e., double what we had with black), then the results will appear in Fig. 24 (red arrows) without much surprise: the corresponding phase accumulations are double (20°, 40°, 60°, 80°, 100°, 120° at $y = 1, 2, 3, 4, 5, 6$, respectively) because the red gradient pulse was twice as strong as the black pulse of the previous experiment. We receive and record the sum of all vectors for the red experiment, which is 18 in length and sits at 59° (Fig. 24, sum, red arrow).

If we repeat the experiment for a third time with the green phase-encoding gradient pulse (Fig. 17), which is three times stronger than the black, then again without any surprise at $y = 1, 2, 3, 4, 5, 6$ we will have phase accumulation of 30°, 60°, 90°, 120°, 150°, 180°, respectively (Fig. 25, green arrows). The net sum of all vectors is computed to be 21 units of length at 87° (Fig. 25, sum, green arrow).

In a similar manner, repeating the experiment for a fourth time with the blue phase-encoding gradient pulse (four times stronger than the black) results in phases of 40°, 80°, 120°, 160°, 200°, 140° for locations $y = 1, 2, 3, 4, 5, 6$, respectively (Fig. 26, blue arrows). The net sum of all blue vectors from this experiment is 23 in length and sits at 115° (Fig. 26, sum, blue arrow).

So far, we have repeated the same experiment four times but with increasing phase-encoding gradient strengths (Fig. 17, black, red, green, blue G_Y) and have recorded the four different results (Figs. 23 black, 24 red, 25 green, and 26 blue). Let us consolidate these results into one figure (Fig. 27). At $y = 1$ (Fig. 27, $y = 1$), we see that these four experiments result in phase accumulation at a rate of 10° per experiment; at $y = 2$ (Fig. 27, $y = 2$), the four experiments result in phase accumulation at a rate of 20° per experiment; at $y = 3$ (Fig. 27, $y = 3$), the four experiments result in phase accumulation at a rate of 30° per experiment; at $y = 4$ (Fig. 27, $y = 4$), the four experiments result in phase accumulation at a rate of 40° per experiment; at $y = 5$ (Fig. 27, $y = 5$), the four experiments result in phase accumulation at a rate of 50° per experiment; last, at $y = 6$ (Fig. 27, $y = 6$), the four experiments result in phase accumulation at a rate of 60° per experiment.

By looking at Fig. 27, one realizes now that we are talking about how fast phase accumulates at any given location on the y-axis across our four experiments. In other words, we have a "speed" concept that has been introduced by repeating the experiment multiple times at increasing phase-encoding gradient strengths. This represents an increasing frequency of rotation at any given location across the experiments (Fig. 27, orange speed arrows). It may seem strange that we are now talking about rotational speed (i.e., frequency) across experiments instead of across time, but nonetheless it is the same concept. Do not forget that a spinning vector creates a sinusoidal waveform;

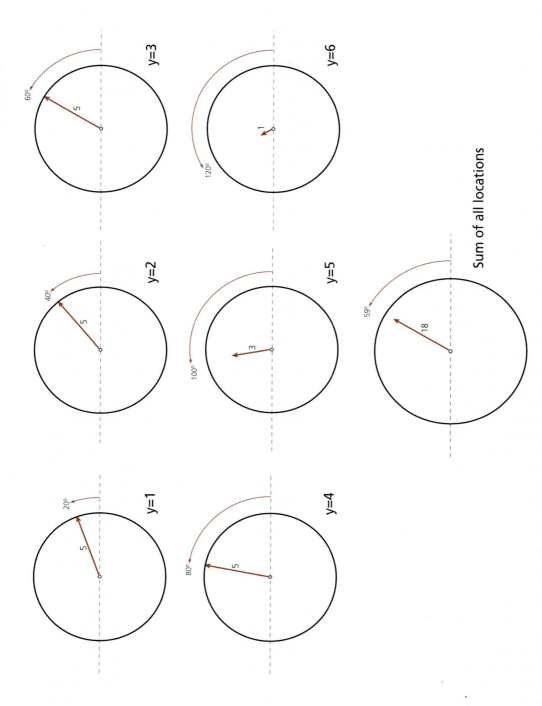

Fig. 24. The phase accumulated by magnetization (red arrows) of the imaged object (Fig. 21) at different positions of the *y*-axis is shown. This is the phase right after the red phase encoding gradient pulse (Fig. 17, interval BC) has been applied. The sum of all locations (red arrow, 18 units long with 59° phase) is what is observed by us.

26

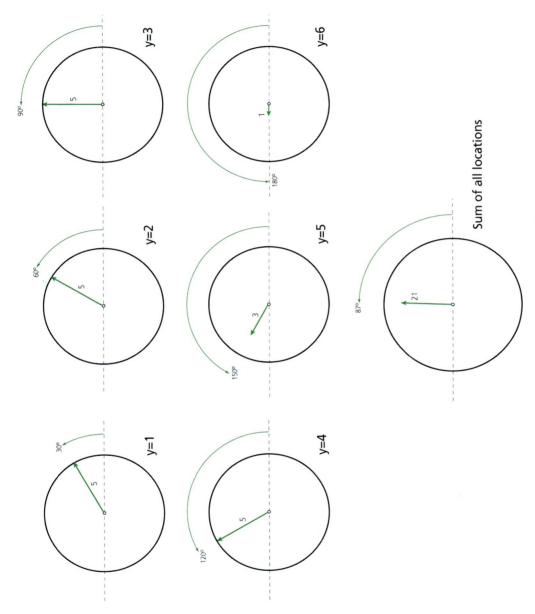

Fig. 25. The phase accumulated by magnetization (green arrows) of the imaged object (Fig. 21) at different positions of the *y*-axis is shown. This is the phase right after the green phase encoding gradient pulse (Fig. 17, interval BC) has been applied. The sum of all locations (green arrow, 21 units long with 87° phase) is what is observed by us.

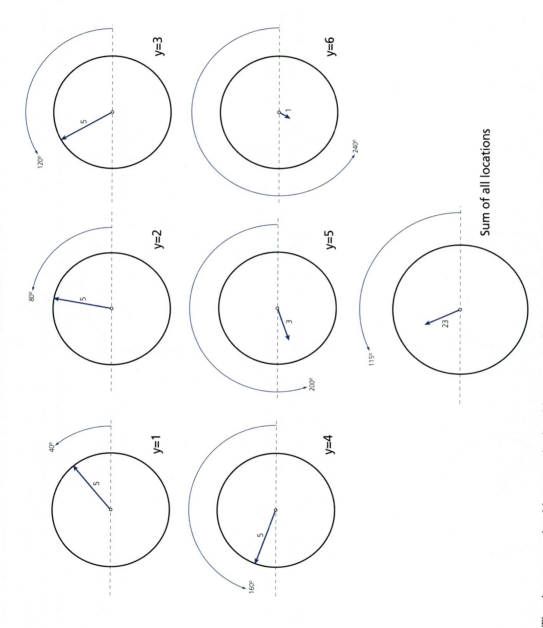

Fig. 26. The phase accumulated by magnetization (blue arrows) of the imaged object (Fig. 21) at different positions of the y-axis is shown. This is the phase right after the blue phase encoding gradient pulse (Fig. 17, interval BC) has been applied. The sum of all locations (blue arrow, 23 units long with 115° phase) is what is observed by us.

28

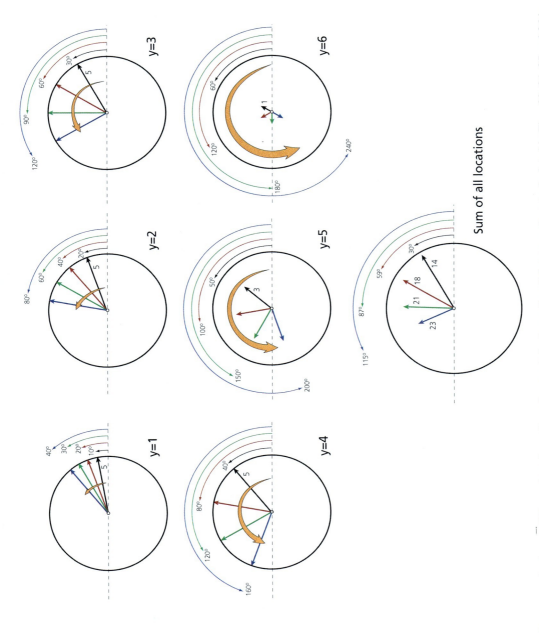

Fig. 27. The magnetization at different locations along the y-axis is shown for all four experiments depicted in Figs. 23, 24, 25 and 26 i.e. the black, red, green and blue magnetizations are shown. The different locations y = 1, 2, 3, 4, 5 and 6 exhibit 10°, 20°, 30°, 40°, 50°, and 60° phase accumulation per experiment respectively (orange "frequency" arrows). The "frequency" arrows represent each location and can be extracted by the Fourier transformation.

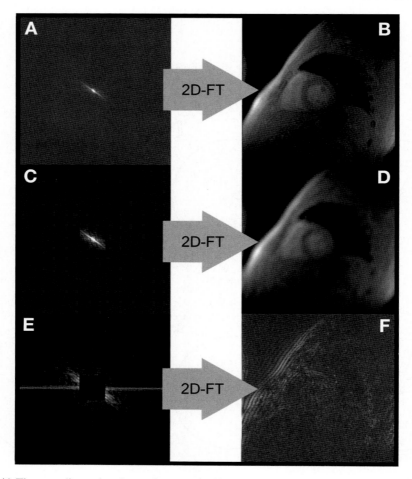

Fig. 28. (A) The two dimensional raw data matrix (*k*-space) holds in its rows the echoes from individual experiments executed with different phase encoding gradient steps. **(B)** A Fourier transformation of *k*-space (Fig. 28A) results in an image. **(C)** The center of *k*-space holds the bulk image contrast. **(D)** If only the center of *k*-space (Fig. 28C) is Fourier transformed then the image lacks detail. **(E)** The outer portions of *k*-space hold the details of the image. **(F)** If only the outer portions of *k*-space (Fig. 28E) are Fourier transformed then the image contains only the edges and detail of the object being imaged.

the faster it spins, the higher the frequency of the sinusoid. These spinning vectors, which have different rotational speeds across the four experiments, create sinusoidal waveforms of different frequencies that can provide information about location on the *y*-axis. Of course, we do not see the individual frequencies, but rather we observe the net sum (Fig. 27, sum of all locations) of these waveforms. In a similar way to that of frequency encoding (Figs. 19 and 20), the Fourier transformation can be used along the *y*-direction to unscramble these sinusoids and yield information regarding where magnetization vectors are located along the *y*-axis. This second Fourier transformation along the phase-encoding direction will provide us with the image of the slice of bread we placed in the magnet.

It is interesting to note that each of the four experiments provides us with a phase-encoded gradient echo, that is, one row of data. The data from multiple phase-encoded experiments (four in our example) are placed in a two-dimensional (2D) matrix (i.e., stacked into multiple rows). This matrix is called *k-space* (Fig. 28A), and its 2D Fourier transformation (2D-FT) results in an image (Fig. 28B) that we managed to extract from our patient by manipulating the different magnetic fields (B_1, G_X, G_Y, and G_Z) of the MR scanner.

The area around the center of *k*-space corresponds to the low spatial frequencies of the image. If only the area around the center of *k*-space (Fig. 28C) undergoes a Fourier transformation, then the resulting image will show bulk tissue contrast and will lack detail (Fig. 28D). On the other hand, if only the outer portions of *k*-space (Fig. 28E) are Fourier transformed, then the reconstructed image will depict only the edges and detail of the structures therein (Fig. 28F) (i.e., the high spatial frequency content).

An MR image can depict many different properties of the biological tissues that are imaged. For example, we can use the basic imaging principles in conjunction with a spin echo and acquire images that reflect the T_2 characteristics of the tissues. Or, we can use our imaging physics as we just described in conjunction with a gradient echo and long TE times to reflect the T_2* characteristics of the tissues. The possibilities are endless, and the remainder of this book introduces how these basic imaging principles are used to perform advanced cardiovascular MRI.

ACKNOWLEDGMENT

I give sincere thanks to Alan Hoofring for the artwork in this chapter.

2

Clinical Cardiac MRI Techniques

Leon Axel and Ruth Lim

CONTENTS

OVERVIEW
MAGNETIC RESONANCE IMAGING SAFETY
CARDIAC GATING
RESPIRATORY MOTION
IMAGE POSITIONING
BRIGHT BLOOD AND DARK BLOOD IMAGING
T_1 AND T_2 WEIGHTING
CINE IMAGING
PHASE CONTRAST IMAGING
CONTRAST ENHANCEMENT
REFERENCES

OVERVIEW

Cardiac magnetic resonance imaging (MRI) has many potential advantages over conventional cardiac imaging techniques. These include a lack of ionizing radiation, free choice of imaging planes, the capability for tissue characterization, qualitative and quantitative evaluation of the motion of both the blood and the myocardium, and assessment of regional perfusion. These capabilities have been realized through the implementation of many MRI techniques, which have many associated imaging options. Although this range of options to choose from when performing a cardiac MRI examination can be daunting, it provides a great deal of flexibility that can be used to tailor the examination to the patient and the particular clinical question to be addressed. Some of the current clinical indications for cardiac MRI are summarized in Table 1.

Optimal performance of a clinical cardiac MRI examination depends on appropriate choices of the imaging methods to be employed and of the corresponding values of the technical parameters of these methods. Although there are particular considerations involved in setting up different specific imaging methods, there are some considerations and tradeoffs that are common to almost all MRI methods.

In particular, there are tradeoffs to be considered related to the finite amount of time that is available for performing the examination because of both time pressure from clinical demand for use of the MRI system by other patients and the limited capacity of the patient to remain still within the system. In addition, if the patient is unstable, then the examination should be kept as short as possible, consistent with answering the clinical

From: *Contemporary Cardiology: Cardiovascular Magnetic Resonance Imaging*
Edited by: Raymond Y. Kwong © Humana Press Inc., Totowa, NJ

Table 1
Some Current Clinical Indications for Cardiac MRI

Masses	Anatomy, tissue characterization, vascularity
	Extent and characterization of masses (can identify fat)
Congenital heart disease	Anatomy, flow, function (no radiation)
	Connections, shunts, stenoses, surgical planning and follow-up
Cardiomyopathy	Anatomy, tissue characterization, function
	Hypertrophy (flow obstruction), fibrosis, inflammation
Ischemic heart disease	Anatomy, function, perfusion
	Ischemia, coronaries (limited), MI consequences such as scarring, dysfunction, pseudoaneurysm, aneurysm
Surgical/trauma follow-up	Anatomy, flow, enhancement
	Hematoma, infection, aneurysm, dehiscence, thrombosis, leak
Valve disease	Anatomy, flow, function
	Stenosis, regurgitation, masses, calcification (limited)
Pericardial disease	Anatomy, motion, enhancement
	Effusion, constriction (adhesions), compression, masses

question, because of the difficulty of fully monitoring and supporting patients inside the MRI system. The limited time available for data acquisition often leads to the need to choose between using that time for optimizing spatial resolution and sampling and optimizing temporal resolution. Optimizing spatial resolution in turn often comes at the cost of diminished signal-to-noise ratio (SNR), leading to another tradeoff to be considered.

A cardiac MRI examination typically consists of the acquisition a fairly standard set of images with common methods and in common orientations, supplemented with "optional" imaging that is particularly useful for the specific clinical condition in question. Ideally, the examination should be monitored by a physician, who can help choose these optional imaging methods as well as optimize the choice of imaging parameters. The physician can also modify the examination as needed to better evaluate any unexpected findings that may show up during the acquisition of the standard images.

A standard cardiac MRI examination will start with initial screening of the patient and setting up of cardiac gating (and possible intravenous access for contrast administration). This will be followed by MRI with initial quick "scout" localizing images and a stack of relatively rapid "survey" images through the chest (in one or more orientations) to obtain an initial overview of the heart and the associated intrathoracic anatomy. After identifying the location of the axes of the ventricles in three dimensions, basic static and cine images are acquired of the heart in standard short- and long-axis orientations, as well as various optional images, as indicated by the specific clinical questions.

In this chapter, we present a systematic approach to the performance of a clinical cardiac MRI examination, focusing on some of the associated technical considerations. Other chapters present more details on the imaging methods themselves and their applications to specific clinical conditions.

MAGNETIC RESONANCE IMAGING SAFETY

The single most important technical aspect of cardiac MRI is safety. Safety-related aspects of MRI include the possible effects of the powerful magnetic field of the MRI system on metal objects in or near the patient and possible heating produced by the strong radio-frequency (RF) field used in imaging, as well as potential claustrophobic sensations that can induced by the relatively restricted space around the patient inside the MRI system.

The magnetic fields inside the MRI system are typically on the order of 1.5 T, approximately 30,000 times stronger than the Earth's magnetic field. Just as the Earth's field produces a torque in magnetizable objects, like that which orients a compass needle to point north, magnetizable objects in the MRI system will experience a torque that tends to align them with the field of the system. Furthermore, near the entrance to the MRI system, where there is a strong gradient of the magnetic field strength, such objects will experience a strong attractive force into the magnet.

Although most surgically implanted metal objects, such as orthopedic bone implants, are made of only weakly magnetic metal alloys, many bits of metal traumatically introduced into the body (e.g., from industrial or battle injuries) may experience significant magnetic forces, which can produce discomfort or injury. A particular area of concern is the possibility of metallic fragments near the eye (e.g., from metal grinding or other industrial exposure), which could cause nerve damage and loss of vision if induced to move by the magnetic field. In addition, there are some medical metal implants that may experience significant magnetic forces on them, including some aneurysm clips and some of the early Starr-Edwards heart valves. There are published lists of medical devices that may be hazardous to bring into the MRI system (1). Many implanted cardiac pacemakers are sensitive to magnetic fields and may have their function altered by exposure to even a weak magnetic field, such as that in the vicinity of an MRI system.

Furthermore, many metallic objects in the normal uncontrolled medical environment, such as gas canisters, intravenous poles, or scissors, may be quite magnetizable and can cause injury to the patient (or damage to the MRI system) if they are inadvertently brought close to the system. The rapid change in the strength of these forces with distance from the magnet means that there may not be much warning as the objects are brought closer to the MRI system before they are abruptly "jerked" into the magnet.

To avoid these problems, all metal objects to be used in (or around) the MRI suite must first be carefully screened for magnetic risk, and all metal objects must be removed from both the patient and the medical personnel before they are allowed near the MRI system.

A different effect of the magnetic field is to cause the appearance of apparent changes in the electrocardiogram (ECG) caused by weak electric fields produced by the movement of the electrically conducting blood through the strong magnetic field. Although these electric fields are not harmful in themselves, they can interfere with the ability to monitor the patient's ECG while they are imaged.

The RF magnetic fields used in MRI can be on the order of tens of kilowatts, strong enough to induce currents that can cause heating sufficient to damage tissue if they are concentrated in a small area by "antenna" effects. Such antenna-like effects can be produced in loops of wire, such as the ECG monitoring leads used for cardiac gating or the thermistor leads in thermodilution catheters, and have caused burns in patients. To minimize the risk of such injury, any monitoring leads should be as short as possible, without any loops, and only ECG leads designed to be used with MRI (with distributed resistances to avoid concentrating any heating effects because of resistive losses at the contact with the skin) should be employed. If a patient has a pulmonary artery monitoring line in place, then it should be exchanged for one without electrical leads before placing the patient in an MRI system.

Another potential risk to patients with pacemakers or other implanted electronic devices is that the pulsed RF fields not only could damage the device or injure the tissue in which it is implanted, but also could possibly directly stimulate the tissue inappropriately. Again, there are published lists of implanted devices that may make it hazardous to undergo imaging. Even without such local antenna effects, the potentially harmful heating effects of the RF excitation pulses lead to limits on the corresponding specific absorption rate allowed in MRI.

Claustrophobia is another potential hazard of MRI, affecting on the order of 4% of patients. The confined space inside the MRI system can even bring out feelings of claustrophobia in some patients who do not expect them. The resultant tachycardia and tachypnea can make it difficult to get good images, even if the patient tries to go on with the examination despite feelings of claustrophobia. Fortunately, many patients who are initially reluctant to go into the system can be helped to relax sufficiently to be examined with suitable reassurance by the operator and physician; keeping the eyes closed (perhaps with the aid of a small towel or a "sleep mask") can also often help. However, in some cases, sedation (e.g., with an oral benzodiazepine) or even anesthesia can be necessary if the information sought from the MRI examination is really needed for clinical management.

CARDIAC GATING

Gating is an essential component of cardiac MRI to overcome blurring of images caused by myocardial contraction and flow effects from pulsatile blood. It allows accurate assessment of cardiac structure and function by coordinating image acquisitions with the cardiac cycle and the use of k-space segmentation to speed imaging. The most effective form of cardiac gating is electrocardiographic gating, by which imaging is triggered off the QRS complex of a three- or four-lead ECG. Segments of k-space data that make up a single image from MRI are obtained at the same point within the cardiac cycle over a series of sequential heartbeats, which serves to eliminate blurring caused by cardiac motion within a single image (Fig. 1) (2,3).

A satisfactory ECG trace must be obtained before scanning is commenced for optimal high-resolution diagnostic images, and time spent in achieving this is well rewarded in image quality. The skin may need to be shaved or cleaned to ensure that ECG electrodes are in good electrical contact with it. Lead placement is an important part of obtaining a diagnostic ECG trace, and this does not mirror standard diagnostic ECG positions for the limb leads. Leads should be closely spaced to minimize potentially interfering voltage differences between them when the patient is placed within the magnet, which can distort the ECG signal obtained. Optimal lead position also varies depending on the location, orientation, and size of each individual's heart. The goal is to obtain a well-defined and relatively high-amplitude QRS complex in which the R upstroke of ventricular depolarization is significantly larger than the T wave of the cardiac cycle, so that image triggering will occur consistently at the same point within the cycle. For safety reasons, the ECG leads should not be allowed to form loops, because of the risk of burns from the induction of a current by the strong RF power used in MRI.

Furthermore, care should be taken to recheck the ECG signal once the patient has entered the bore of the magnet as interference from voltages produced by the flow of the blood in the magnetic field (the magnetohydrodynamic effect) can distort the signal

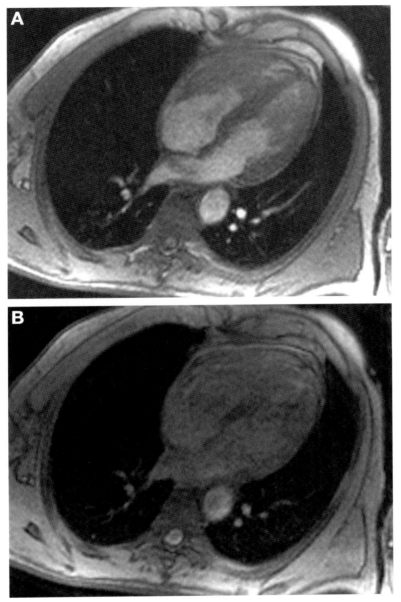

Fig. 1. Gradient echo FLASH image: (**A**) with cardiac gating; (**B**) without gating.

obtained (*see* Fig. 2), so that the R wave may no longer be clearly defined. This effect becomes more pronounced at higher field strengths as the weak physiologic ECG voltage (on the order of 1 mV or less) is forced to contend with proportionally stronger flow-induced voltages. Another potential source of interfering voltages in MRI is the magnetic gradient pulses used in imaging, which may induce voltages with amplitudes of 200–400 mV. The position of the ECG monitoring electrodes may need to be readjusted until an adequate trace is achieved.

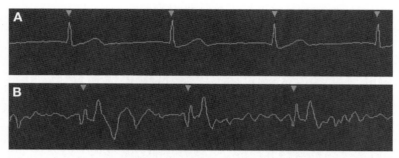

Fig. 2. ECG signal from (**A**) outside the bore of the magnet and (**B**) within the bore of the magnet, demonstrating distortion of the signal, with more prominent T waves.

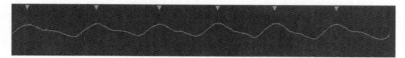

Fig. 3. Signal from the peripheral pulse, with demonstration of triggering with each pulse cycle.

Other problems that may be encountered with ECG gating in MRI are inappropriate triggering from voltage peaks produced by RF pulses during the examination and from flow potentials, as described previously. The current use of fiber-optic transmission of ECG signals significantly reduces artifacts from RF pulses, first described by Felblinger and colleagues in 1994 *(4)*. One way of overcoming inappropriate triggering is "vector-cardiography," first described in 1999 *(5)*; the QRS complex is identified not only by timing and magnitude but also in a "three-dimensional" voltage vector orientation by the monitoring equipment, such that any electrical signals with a different vector to the QRS complex will be ignored, even if they have a relatively larger magnitude.

Arrhythmias may lead to inadequate or inappropriate triggering if the imaging software does not recognize the R wave and can lead to image blurring and artifacts caused by inconsistent anatomical configuration of the heart if there is a substantial variation in the R–R interval. Increasing the number of averages obtained may help to improve images if an arrhythmia is present. If there is a significant cardiac arrhythmia, then an arrhythmia rejection setting can be selected in which cardiac cycles with R–R intervals that fall outside a range specified by the operator are not used for image acquisition. This will tend to increase overall acquisition time, which can be problematic in the setting of a breath-hold sequence. Low-voltage ECG traces may also lead to inadequate or inconsistent triggering.

Peripheral triggering, which can be obtained from MRI-compatible optical fingertip pulse monitors, provides a less-preferred but often adequate alternative if a satisfactory ECG signal cannot be obtained (Fig. 3). Images can be significantly more blurred because triggering off the peripheral pulse wave is delayed in relation to the R wave of the QRS complex.

Another theoretical alternative that has been described is "wireless" gating, by which periodic changes of the magnetic resonance (MR) signal from the beating heart during the cardiac cycle can be used as information to synchronize the MRI data acquisition for acquiring a crisp image without the need for electrodes and leads; however, this is not used in current clinical practice.

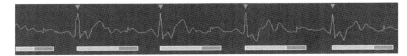

Fig. 4. Prospective ECG gating, with image acquisition commencing after triggering from the R wave and terminating before the end of each cardiac cycle.

Cardiac MR image acquisition can use either prospective gating, by which the QRS complex triggers data acquisition at the start of each cardiac cycle, typically over several cardiac cycles (*see* Fig. 4) *(6)*, or retrospective gating, by which there is continuous acquisition over several cardiac cycles, and postprocessing with suitable data interpolation leads to image reconstruction at selected time-points (phases) in the cardiac cycle, with the number of phases per cardiac cycle predetermined by the operator *(7)* based on the heart rate and the rate of data acquisition.

Prospective gating leads to better temporal resolution images; however, acquisition time may be longer. A portion at the end of each cardiac cycle is lost because data acquisition is generally interrupted near the end of diastole to await the onset of the next QRS complex, and the end portion of the cardiac cycle (usually 50–100 ms) is not sampled to allow for variation in length of each R–R interval. In addition, there may be an interval delay (trigger delay) between recognizing the R wave and commencing data acquisition. Also, as there is a period of the cardiac cycle when signal is not acquired, there is the tendency for tissues to recover magnetization during this period, which may cause the first image acquired after triggering to be brighter than the remaining images, which can be a disadvantage for cine images performed to assess ventricular wall motion. Dummy excitation pulses can be used during this period to prevent this magnetization recovery. Assessment of cardiac volumes and function is also affected by the method of ECG gating, with lower ejection fractions generally calculated with prospective vs retrospective ECG gating as portions of the cardiac cycle are not imaged *(8)*.

Retrospective gating leads to more temporal blurring because there is interpolation onto a set number of equally spaced phases for image reconstruction in each cardiac cycle, despite possible differences in the actual duration of each R–R interval. However, it is a more robust technique, with the advantages that it has more uniform signal intensity in time (because there is no interruption of the train of excitation pulses) and it can be used to image the whole cardiac cycle (because there is no need to stop image data acquisition before the end of diastole to wait for the next QRS detection). It is less sensitive to arrhythmias and is particularly useful for cine imaging, for which a smooth transition between cardiac cycles is preferable for assessing regional and global wall motion.

The *k*-space segmentation regarding cardiac MRI begins with the raw data (lines in "*k*-space"), or phase-encoding steps, which must be acquired to reconstruct a complete image. These can be grouped into segments, with one such segment, containing an operator-specified number of phase-encoding steps, treated as if they were all acquired at the same time, acquired every cardiac cycle. Such segments are acquired at approximately the same time-point in each consecutive cycle until sufficient raw data lines are obtained to reconstruct the image. Segments of raw data can be used to make either serial images at a single location over different phases of the cardiac cycle (single section, multiple phase), as with cine imaging for assessment of wall motion, or for multiple static images, with each obtained at a different phase in the cardiac cycle (multiple section, single phase), as is useful for assessment of myocardial scar tissue on delayed-enhancement images. With improving MR technology, stronger gradients have enabled faster imaging, and it is now possible to acquire multiple imaging sections over different phases of the cardiac cycle (multiple section, multiple phase) *(9)*.

For example, if a total of 256 phase-encoding steps are specified by the operator and there are 32 segments, then $256/32 = 8$ phase-encoding steps are acquired for images of a particular cardiac cycle phase over consecutive cardiac cycles. Each of the set of phase-encoding steps acquired within a segment is also known as a *view*, so that in the example, 8 views per segment would be obtained. If only 1 view for each image were acquired in each heartbeat (e.g., with a repetition time [TR] of 10 ms), then this would allow for the acquisition of more images per cardiac cycle and temporal resolution effectively equal to the TR. However, acquisition times needed to acquire 256 phase-encoding steps (at least 256 cardiac cycles) would be too long for breath-hold scanning, leading to blurring from respiratory motion. With an increase in the number of views per segment to 8, as in this example, temporal resolution would be eight times poorer (80 ms), but total acquisition time is decreased by a factor of 8 (32 cardiac cycles) with equivalent spatial resolution as more phase-encoding steps are completed within a heartbeat, and breath holding for the entire sequence becomes feasible.

As with many factors in MRI, there is a tradeoff between spatial and temporal resolution if overall acquisition time is to be kept as short as possible, which is vital for breath-holding sequences. Higher spatial resolution images will require more phase-encoding steps and subsequently a larger number of views per segment. This will lead to a decrease in temporal resolution as more time is taken to acquire each segment. As the R–R interval is finite, only a limited number of segments can be acquired with each cycle, and in the context of cine imaging, the number of cardiac phases that can be imaged will be decreased. To continue the example, using *k*-space segmentation of 8 views per segment, each segment will take 80 ms to acquire. If a patient has an R–R interval of 800 ms, then a maximum of $800/80 = 10$ phases can be acquired. In reality, fewer than 10 phases will be achievable because the last 50–100 ms of the cardiac cycle will be rejected to allow for differences between the lengths of each cycle. If more phases of the cardiac cycle are to be acquired in the same overall time, then the number of phase-encoding steps will need to be decreased, at the cost of spatial resolution.

Patient heart rate is also an important factor. In patients with slower heart rates, if the number of views per segment is kept low for high temporal resolution, acquisition times may extend beyond a reasonably achievable breath hold, as the same number of R–R intervals is still required to acquire enough data for an image. To keep total acquisition time low, the options in a bradycardic patient are either to increase the number of views obtained in each segment, at the cost of temporal resolution, or to decrease the number of views used to make up each image, decreasing spatial resolution or field of view. For higher heart rates, we can decrease the number of views per segment to achieve imaging of a comparable number of phases per cardiac cycle in a comparable total imaging time. Similarly, we can speed the process of acquiring data covering the heart by interleaving acquisitions at multiple levels, but at the cost of decreased temporal sampling or increased imaging (and breath-holding) time.

One method of improving the effective temporal resolution (or temporal sampling rate) in gated cardiac MR images is to use view sharing *(10)*. With this technique, views from one segment are combined with views from the next segment to artificially create a new, intermediate cardiac phase. For example, with single-section, multiple-phase imaging, if there are 10 segments in a cardiac cycle of 800 ms (disregarding time for arrhythmia rejection and triggering with prospective gating), each with 8 views per segment, with each view having a TR of 10 ms, then the sequence has a temporal resolution of $8 \times 10 = 80$ ms and 10 phases per cardiac cycle. Using view sharing, the last 4 views of 1 segment could be combined with the first 4 views of the next segment to create new intermediate phases between each existing phase. This would improve the nominal effective temporal resolution of the sequence, even though in reality the same number of views is acquired whether or not view sharing is used, and the true temporal resolution remains the same. However, the number of reconstructed phases within a cardiac cycle would be increased.

RESPIRATORY MOTION

Aside from cardiac motion, respiratory motion is another important cause of image blurring and "ghosting" artifact in the phase-encoding direction (Fig. 5). Respiratory motion is significant, with the most motion occurring in the craniocaudal direction, but there is also a degree of anterior-posterior and transverse motion of the diaphragm. This in turn changes the position and shape of the heart with respiratory phase, with motion of approximately 1 cm in the craniocaudal direction reported in the literature (11).

There are several ways of combating respiratory motion in clinical practice. The most widely used in standard cardiac sequences is breath holding by the patient during image acquisition. Although this can potentially eliminate respiratory motion, the length of each acquisition is limited by the individual's breath-holding capability, which in the elderly or debilitated may mean brief acquisition times of less than 10 seconds. Also, there may be variation in degree of breath holding with each breath, leading to changes in position of the heart and potential misregistration artifact if a series of contiguous images is acquired over sequential breath holds (12). There may even be variations in diaphragm position during a single breath hold. Imaging with breath holding at end-tidal expiration is one technique that can be used to reduce variability in diaphragm position between and within breath holds because it is a relatively reproducible condition (13). However, this practice may not be feasible in patients with limited respiratory reserve.

Alternatively, if the patient is unable to comply with breath-holding instructions, increasing the number of averages used to construct an image has been used to improve SNR and reduce respiratory motion artifacts (14). However, this increases overall scan time, and there are now more sophisticated methods of minimizing respiratory motion artifact that may be preferred.

Respiratory gating can be performed, with monitoring of respiratory motion during data acquisition. This can be implemented with either acquisition during a consistent part of the respiratory phase (typically the end-expiratory phase) or postprocessing of continuously acquired data, with rejection of data acquired outside a specified respiratory window. This may involve the use of a bellows, which is comprised of a strain gage physically wrapped around the patient's chest to monitor chest wall motion, which provides a crude reflection of respiratory motion.

A respiratory navigator provides an alternative method of gating that directly tracks diaphragmatic motion. This is based on the acquisition of signal from a column of

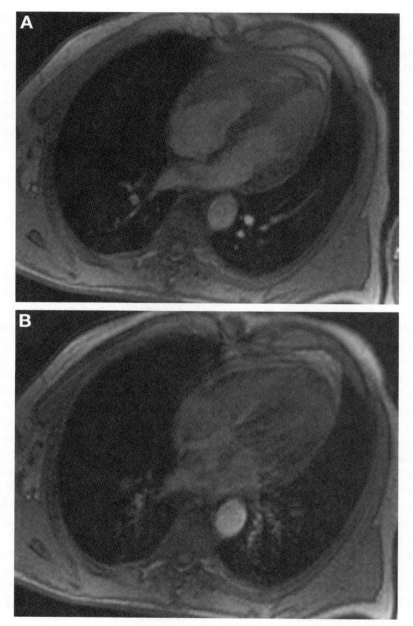

Fig. 5. (A) Breath-hold gradient echo FLASH image; **(B)** same image with free breathing.

material centered on the moving diaphragm, which is positioned so it is perpendicular to its interface with the lung and parallel to its direction of motion *(15)*. The column excitation is commonly achieved by the intersection of consecutive slice-selective planar excitations with intersecting 90° and 180° excitations.

Detecting the echoes obtained from the navigator column with a readout gradient oriented along the column provides an accurate depiction of the moving edge. Acquiring these navigator echoes during the imaging sequence allows for continuous monitoring of diaphragmatic motion during data acquisition. This information can then be used in one of two ways: (1) with the patient free breathing and with data acquisition triggered by a set navigator acceptance window; and (2) using a multiple breath-hold technique, with signal from the navigator column fed back to the patient so that the patient can hold his or her breath at the same diaphragmatic position every respiratory cycle. Although the second technique has potential advantages in decreasing acquisition time, in practice the need for patient training and reliance on breath-holding capabilities means that there is no effective gain in time over the free-breathing navigator technique (16).

With the free-breathing technique, little patient cooperation is required. The main disadvantage compared with breath holding is the overall increase in scan time, but for sequences for which acquisition time is beyond a breath hold (e.g., high-resolution coronary magnetic resonance angiography [MRA]), use of a navigator free-breathing technique is clearly advantageous. As with ECG gating, this may be retrospective or prospective, with data acquisition triggered only when the diaphragm position falls within a defined navigator acceptance window.

There are several important components when planning a navigator-dependent sequence. The first is appropriate positioning of the navigator column or columns as this will determine the amount of diaphragmatic motion detected. Sachs and colleagues reported better image quality with the use of three orthogonal navigator columns; however, this was at the expense of scan time (17).

Regardless of the number of navigator columns used, these must be positioned over a diaphragmatic edge where the edge will move along the column during the respiratory cycle. Columns are typically positioned to intersect the right dome of the diaphragm. Care must be taken to ensure that the columns (and the slice-selective excitations used to produce them) do not extend into a region of interest as signal loss from the navigator pulse excitation will interfere with visualization of affected tissue (Fig. 6). The column cross section should be small to improve edge detection of the diaphragm.

Once the column positions are set, a "scout" sequence of column excitations is performed to assess the patient's diaphragmatic excursion over a series of respirations, and a two-dimensional (2D) histogram can then be obtained to summarize the frequencies at which different levels of the patient's diaphragm are measured over time (Fig. 7). The navigator acceptance window is then selected based on the appearance of the histogram. The acceptance window is centered on the highest point of the diaphragm, which occurs at end expiration, when there is a short period of relative diaphragmatic immobility. The width of the acceptance window is typically on the order of 4–5 mm, with wider windows leading to improved scanning efficiency (with acceptance of a larger portion of the respiratory cycle) but with increased image blurring and vice versa for narrower windows.

One problem inherent in the free-breathing navigator technique is respiratory drift, by which diaphragmatic position may alter over time as a patient becomes more relaxed or agitated. This may cause the edge of the diaphragm to move progressively out of the navigator acceptance window with successive respirations, such that there is the potential for little or no triggering of data acquisition throughout the respiratory cycle. Again, as with many facets of MRI, there is a tradeoff between the narrowness of the acceptance window and overall acquisition time.

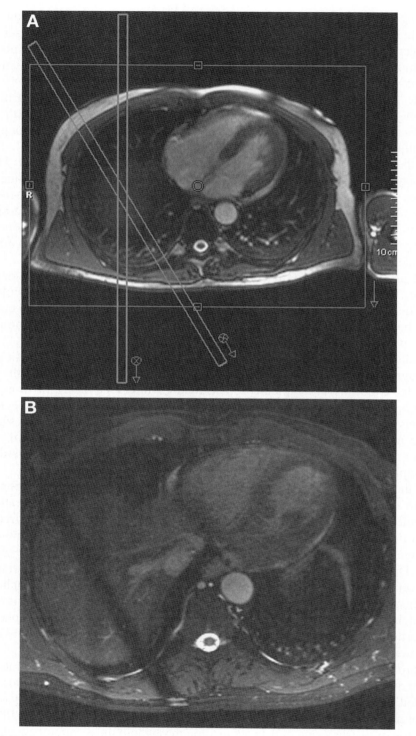

Fig. 6. (A) Navigator column placement (defined by the intersection of two separate columns) at the dome of the right hemidiaphragm; **(B)** loss of signal in the image at the sites from which navigator echoes are obtained.

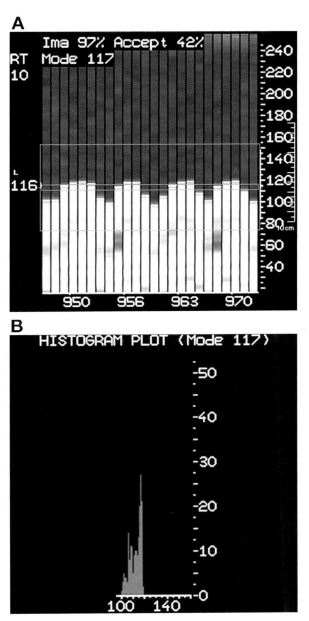

Fig. 7. (A) Graph depicting diaphragm position in the *y*-axis and time in the *x*-axis with use of a respiratory navigator; **(B)** histogram summarizing the frequency of diaphragm positions during a navigator-dependent sequence.

The application of correction factors in the navigator sequence may help to improve its accuracy and improve scan efficiency. Real-time prospective slice following attempts to correct for motion of the heart through tracking of the diaphragm. However, this is complicated by the different amounts of motion in different locations of the heart during the respiratory cycle, with relatively less motion occurring at the base of the heart compared with its inferior surface. Use of the slice-following technique allows the use of a wider acquisition window without significant loss of image quality and, with greater acceptance during each respiratory cycle, allows for faster overall scan time *(18)*. However, correction factors are specific to the individual and therefore may require an initial preparatory sequence to determine the degree of motion of a patient's heart at different respiratory phases *(19)*. Retrospective motion correction postprocessing techniques are now also being realized *(20)*.

Another form of respiratory gating that has been described is utilizing the ECG variations that can be encountered with each respiratory cycle to provide information about respiratory phase *(21)*. However, this is not used in current clinical practice.

IMAGE POSITIONING

Unlike standard views of the thorax in the axial, sagittal, or coronal planes, cardiac MR images are generally obtained along the long and short axes of the heart. The ability to obtain views in any orientation without the limitations imposed by finding an adequate window for insonation is one of the main strengths of MRI over echocardiography. Similar to echocardiography, views in the left ventricular (LV) short axis, horizontal and vertical long axes, and through the LV outflow tract are typically obtained in a routine cardiac MR study and allow assessment of cardiac chamber morphology and function. These views can be easily obtained with a knowledge of basic cardiac anatomy.

Multiplanar scout images are initially obtained to ensure that the heart and LV in particular are well centered within the imaging field of view for optimal visualization. From these images, a stack of breath-hold axial images can be obtained (Fig. 8). These form the basis for setting up images along the cardiac axes and provide an overview of the thorax in case of associated or incidental pathology. A vertical long-axis or two-chamber scout view can then be obtained by planning off a selected axial view depicting the left atrium, mitral valve, and LV and obtaining a single image perpendicular to this that passes through the estimated plane of the LV apex (Fig. 9A). From this two-chamber scout, a horizontal long-axis or four-chamber scout view that includes the LV axis can then be obtained, again by acquiring a similar image perpendicular to the two-chamber view that passes through the mitral valve, and the estimated position of the LV apex (Fig. 9B). A short stack of short-axis views can then be acquired orthogonal to both the two-chamber and four-chamber scout views at the level of the LV and right ventricular bases (Fig. 9C).

True two-chamber, four-chamber, three-chamber, and short-axis views of the heart can then be obtained from this series of planning images. A true four-chamber view can be acquired by planning an image perpendicular to a short-axis view through the ventricular bases, which is also perpendicular to the interventricular septum and is below the level of the aortic valve (Fig. 10A). A two-chamber view can be acquired by bisecting the mitral valve and the LV apex on the four-chamber view (Fig. 10B), and a three-chamber view can be acquired off a scout short-axis view that is parallel to the LV outflow tract (Fig. 10C).

Alternatively, two-, three-,and four-chamber views can be planned from a midventricular-level short-axis scout image, with scan planes centered on the center of the LV, with each scan plane separated from the other two by 60°. The two-chamber plane will pass parallel to the two points where the right ventricle meets the septum, the three-chamber view will be oriented 60° anticlockwise to this as viewed from the apex, and the four-chamber view will be oriented another 60° anticlockwise (Fig. 10E). True short-axis views can be

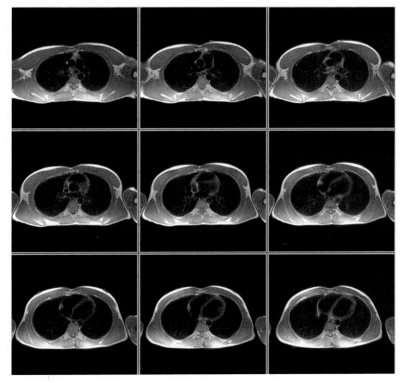

Fig. 8. Axial double-inversion recovery steady-state free-precession images for further image planning and overview of the chest.

obtained by planning these completely orthogonal to both true four- and two-chamber views (Fig. 10D). Various different imaging sequences, including cine imaging for assessment of cardiac motion and function or delayed contrast-enhanced images for assessment of myocardial scar tissue, can then be obtained using the same image positions. This is vital for correlating areas of structural and functional abnormality and allows for sequential comparisons for patients who undergo multiple studies during the course of their management.

Aside from selecting appropriate positioning of images along the orientation of the cardiac axes, care must be taken to select an appropriate field of view to balance the demands of adequate spatial resolution with acquisition time. The phase-encoding direction should be placed along the direction in the plane where the patient's diameter is shortest, which for most patients is in the anterior-posterior direction when obtaining sagittal or axial views. This allows a reduction in the number of phase-encoding steps, with a subsequent saving in scan time, which is particularly important for breath-hold sequences. However, if the number of phase-encoding steps is decreased too much, aliasing or "wrap" of structures outside the chosen field of view will occur in this direction. This could potentially obscure the region of interest (Fig. 11).

The orientation and position of the field of view are also important factors to consider to minimize aliasing. Orientation in the phase-encoding direction should try to parallel the orientation of the heart and anterior chest wall in planning images. Every effort should be made to have the field of view well centered, such that peripheral structures

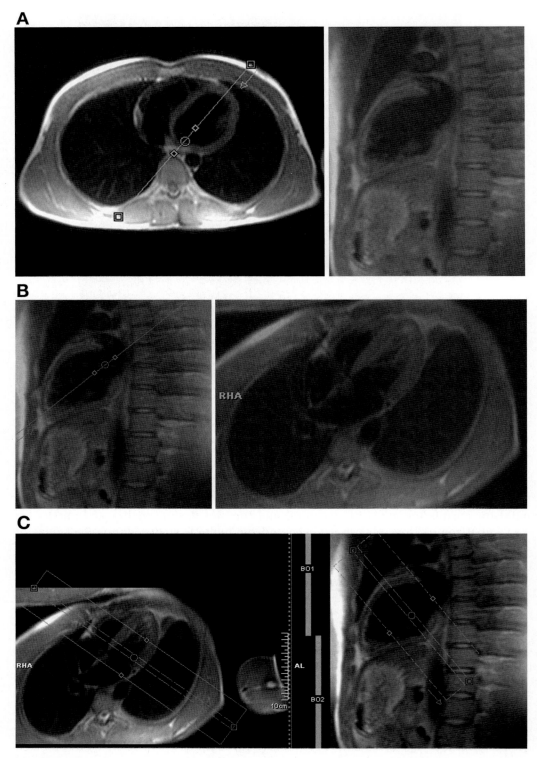

Fig. 9. Setup and acquired "scout" images to determine true cardiac axes: **(A)** near two-chamber scout; **(B)** near four-chamber scout; **(C)** short-axis image stack through the ventricular bases.

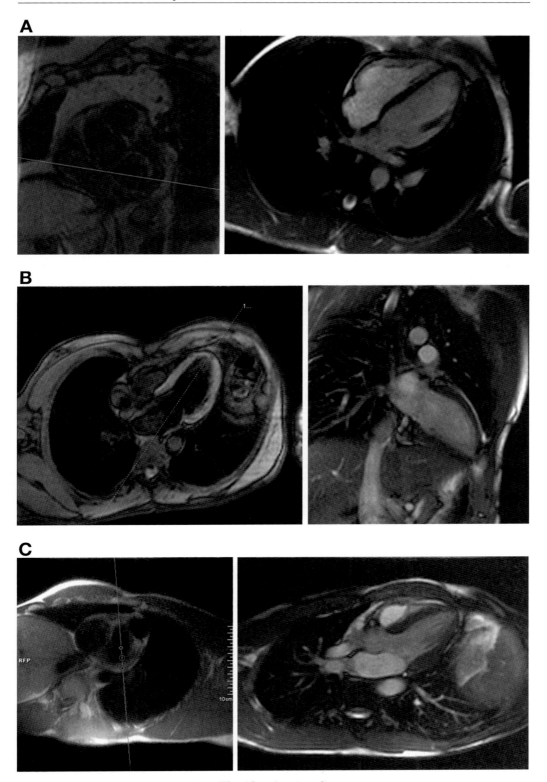

Fig. 10. *(Continued)*

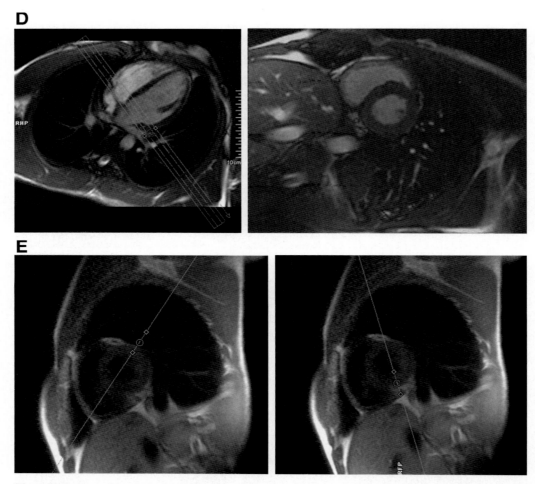

Fig. 10. Setup and images obtained along the true cardiac axes: **(A)** four chamber; **(B)** two chamber; **(C)** three chamber; **(D)** short axis; **(E)** alternate method of acquiring long-axis views from a midventricular short-axis scout view (setup for four chamber long axis on left and two chamber long axis on right).

remain within the prescribed region, preventing them from causing artifact from aliasing. This is particularly important in sequences for which parallel imaging is used, which are more sensitive to aliasing, and for which the artifact will appear in the center of the images obtained *(22)*.

Aside from the standard cardiac views described, there may be additional or alternative views required for specific indications. For example, cardiac MRI is commonly used if arrhythmogenic right ventricular dysplasia is suspected. Dedicated high-resolution images targeting the right ventricular wall are required if arrhythmogenic right ventricular dysplasia is to be identified or definitively excluded. Images should be obtained as perpendicular as possible to the right ventricular free wall as it is thin and not well visualized if obliquely intersecting views are acquired. These can be planned from scout sagittal images through the right ventricle (Fig. 12).

Another important indication for cardiac MRI is for the evaluation or follow-up of congenital heart disease. Supplementary views may commonly be required because of

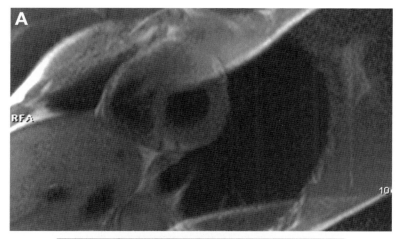

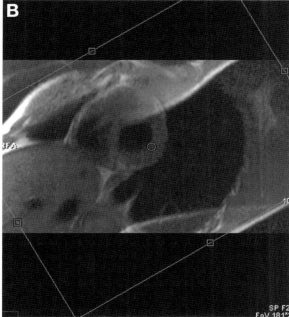

Fig. 11. *(Continued)*

atypical anatomy in these patients. For example, a view oriented appropriately to the interatrial septum may be useful in the assessment of atrial septal defect or patent foramen ovale. It is often important in congenital heart disease to evaluate the right ventricular outflow tract; this evaluation can be obtained by systematically acquiring orthogonal long-axis views beginning with a long-axis view through the right ventricle (Fig. 13).

Three-dimensional (3D) contrast-enhanced MRA is useful for the evaluation of the aorta and pulmonary arteries. It is also highly effective for the assessment of collateral vessels or shunts, with the use of rapid sequential time-resolved short echo time (TE) and low flip angle gradient echo imaging *(23)*. There is again a tradeoff between maximal anatomic coverage and minimal acquisition time, and this is an important consideration in choosing the plane of coverage of the 3D slab. If the aorta is the focus of the study, then

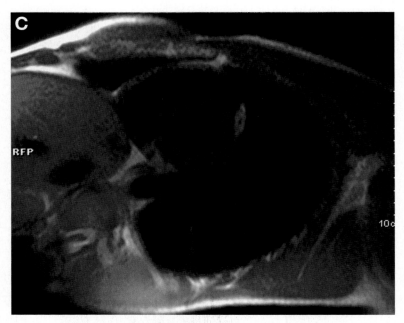

Fig. 11. (A) Aliasing with folding of chest wall into the region of interest; **(B)** angling the scan field of view to follow the chest wall to prevent peripheral structure aliasing; **(C)** corrected image from **(a)** after adjusting field of view.

an oblique sagittal plane parallel to the orientation of the aortic arch is recommended (Fig. 14). If the pulmonary arterial system requires assessment (e.g., in the evaluation of main or branch pulmonary artery stenosis), then a coronal plane will provide maximal anatomic coverage.

BRIGHT BLOOD AND DARK BLOOD IMAGING

A striking aspect of cardiac MRI is that blood can appear either bright or dark in the images, depending on how they were acquired. This is largely caused by the different effects of motion on the MR signal with different signal acquisition methods (including time-of-flight [TOF] and phase shift effects) *(24)*, although the distinctive relaxation times of blood can also play a role, particularly in steady-state free precession (SSFP) or contrast agent-enhanced imaging. These effects can be exploited to produce useful image contrast between the blood and the heart wall and can even provide qualitative or quantitative assessment of flow.

When imaging with rapid T_1-weighted gradient echo imaging (e.g., fast, low-angle shot [FLASH]), the blood can appear relatively bright compared to the adjacent stationary tissue. This is caused by the replacement between consecutive excitations of the partially magnetically saturated blood left in the slice being imaged from the last excitation, by more fully magnetized blood flowing into the slice from upstream (*see* Fig. 15). This more magnetized blood produces a stronger signal and appears relatively bright in the images as compared to the more stationary heart wall, which does not get replenishment of its magnetization; this has been called *flow-related enhancement*. Note that through-plane motion of the heart wall can actually produce a noticeable alteration of the signal from the heart wall itself during the cardiac cycle, although the

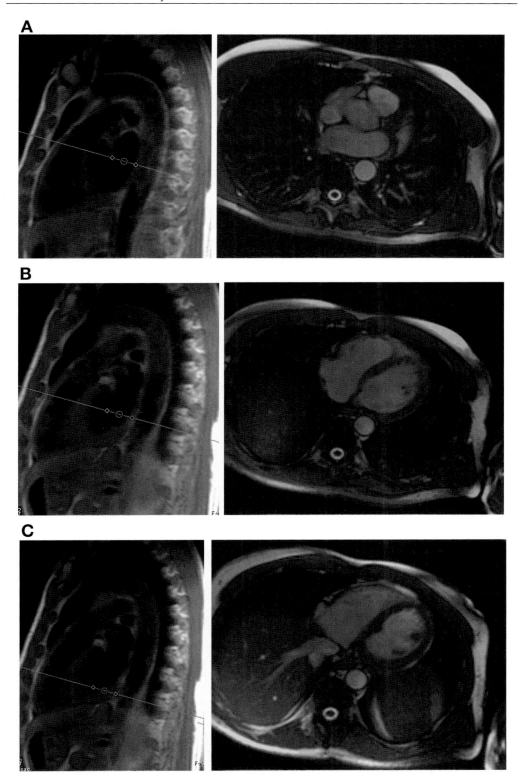

Fig. 12. *(Continued)*

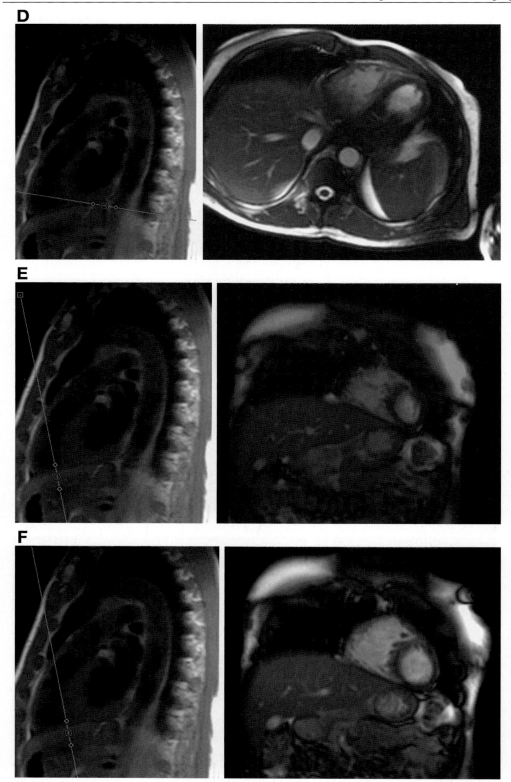

Fig. 12. (A)–(F) Examples of images perpendicular to the right ventricular wall and demonstrating their planning.

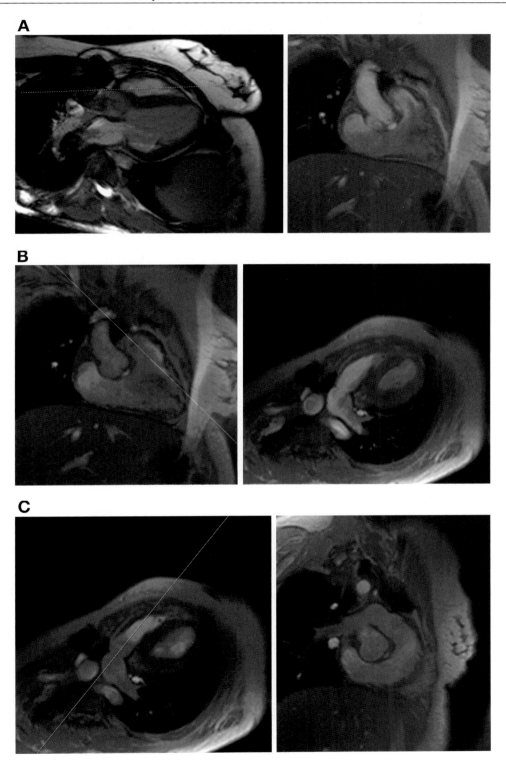

Fig. 13. (A) Image through the vertical long axis of the right ventricle; **(B)** orthogonal to image **(A)** bisecting the right ventricular outflow tract; **(C)** orthogonal to image **(D)** bisecting the right ventricular outflow tract and main pulmonary artery. Note that the patient has had banding of the main pulmonary artery because of mildly hypoplastic left ventricle.

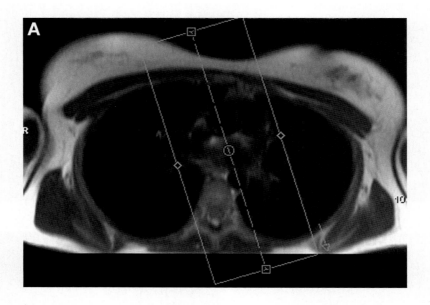

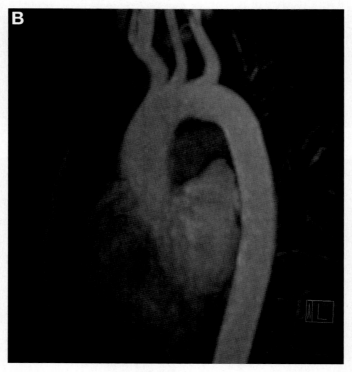

Fig. 14. *(Continued)*

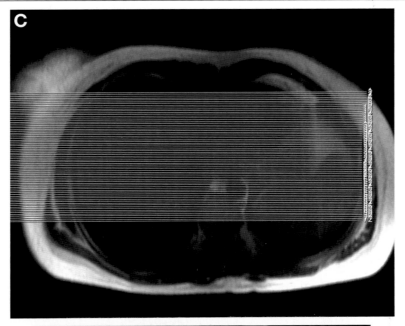

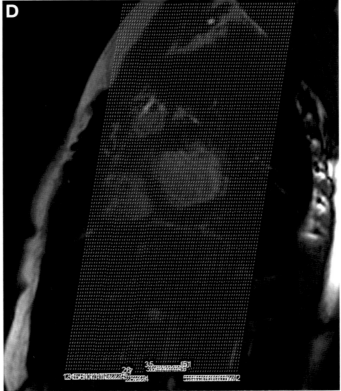

Fig. 14. *(Continued)*

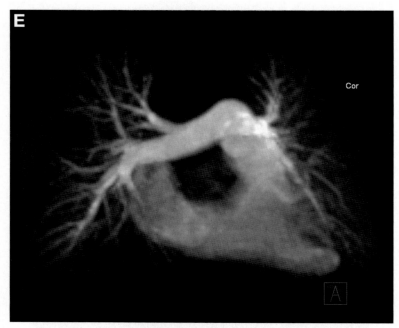

Fig. 14. (A) Oblique sagittal 3D field of view for MRA targeting the aortic arch, planned off an axial HASTE image; **(B)** subtracted maximal intensity projection (MIP) image obtained from the MRA slab depicted; **(C)** planning from true axial HASTE image for pulmonary MRA; **(D)** planning from sagittal HASTE image, demonstrating angle of planned images to obtain maximal coverage of the pulmonary arteries; **(E)** subtracted MIP image acquired in the pulmonary arterial phase (Obtained from planning images C and D).

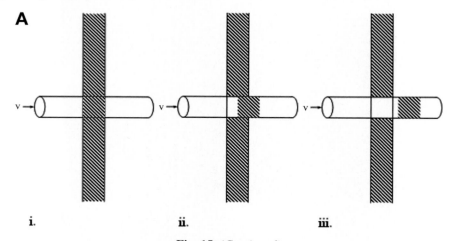

Fig. 15. *(Continued)*

relatively slower motion of the wall leads to less signal enhancement than that seen for the blood. Also note that when imaging a thick slab of tissue with gradient echo imaging techniques, the flow-related enhancement may only be apparent in blood vessels near the entrance side of the slab as the blood may get repeatedly excited (and thus partially saturated) as it flows deeper into the slab.

When imaging the heart with spin echoes produced by 90° and 180° spatially selective RF excitations, motion of the blood between the two excitations can lead to a

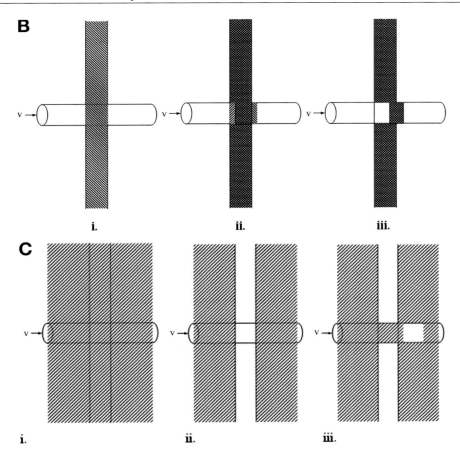

Fig. 15 (A) Time-of-flight (TOF) effects in gradient echo imaging. Residual partially saturated (reduced magnetization) spins left in imaged slice immediately after spatially selective excitation **(i)** are washed out of the slice by blood flow and replaced by more magnetized spins from upstream **(ii** and **iii)** prior to the next excitation, resulting in a brighter blood image. **(B)** TOF effects in spin echo imaging. Spins in imaged slice excited by initial spatially selective 90° excitation **(i)** may be partially washed out of the slice prior to the application of the spatially selective 180° refocusing excitation **(ii)**. Only those spins experiencing both excitations will contribute to the final spin echo **(iii)**, resulting in reduced signal from the blood. **(C)** TOF effects in double inversion-recovery dark blood imaging. Prior to imaging, a nonselective inversion excitation is applied to the whole volume **(i)**, followed immediately by a spatially selective reinversion excitation of the slice to be imaged **(ii)**, restoring its magnetization to the initial state. When imaging after an appropriate delay **(iii)**, the blood flowing into the slice will have approximately zero magnetization, resulting in a dark blood image.

decreased signal from blood as it needs to experience both RF pulses to produce the signal. This tendency to darkening of the blood in spin echo imaging, caused by motion, can be enhanced by adding extra pulses to decrease the magnetization of the inflowing blood. This black blood appearance can be readily achieved by applying two 180° pulses in rapid succession. The first one is nonselective to produce effective inversion of the magnetization of everything within the RF coil; the next is a selective 180° pulse centered at the location of the slice to be imaged effectively to restore the magnetization of the stationary tissues in the slice to their starting condition. If we then wait for the magnetization of the blood in the inverted regions to pass through a zero-magnetization state (on their way back toward their equilibrium magnetization state) before imaging, then those blood-filled structures in which blood that has been replaced by blood from outside the slice will appear black.

Motion of excited spins along magnetic field gradients, such as those used in MRI, can result in the signal from the moving spins acquiring a phase shift relative to the signal from adjacent stationary spins. Although the phase information is not directly displayed in conventional MRI, it can still affect the displayed magnitude. For example, if there is a strong spatial gradient of velocity (and its associated phase) in a given region, then there can be interference between the different phases and a resulting loss of the net local signal from the blood. In addition, if there is unsteady flow, as in turbulence associated with a jet, then the associated fluctuations in the signal phase can lead to a local loss of image intensity. Both of these effects can lead to darkening of the image of the blood in bright blood imaging of abnormal flows, such as those associated with stenoses.

When using SSFP imaging methods, the blood can produce a strong signal independent of its motion because of its relaxation time properties and thus appear bright in the MR images. In SSFP, rapidly repeated excitations produce an increased signal by setting up a condition in which the magnetization is refocused between each excitation; in blood (and other fluids), the high ratio of the T_2 to the T_1 relaxation times results in a strong signal. The phase of the resulting signal depends on the local field strength. However, when the local magnetic field strength varies with position such that the flowing blood is carried from an area with one phase into an area with the opposite phase, the steady state will be interrupted, and the resulting fluctuations in the blood signal can cause local signal loss and artifacts that can propagate into other areas of the image.

Another way that blood can appear bright in the image is caused by shortening of the T_1 relaxation time by injection of an MRI contrast agent, which will lead to increased signal in the presence of T_1 weighting in the imaging method. If a 3D volume is rapidly and repeatedly imaged after the injection of a bolus of contrast agent, then the blood vessels with high concentrations of the agent at the time of image acquisition will appear bright. If the image acquisition is fast enough, then the delay after the injection can be adjusted to have prominent enhancement of only a desired portion of the vascular tree (e.g., arteries vs veins or pulmonary vs systemic) (Fig. 16). Choosing the timing of this delay can be aided by acquiring a rapid series of sequential images of a representative vessel after the injection of a small test bolus of the agent, often called a *timing run* (Fig. 17). The bright vessel images in the imaged region can then be processed with a suitable computer program to produce a synthetic angiographic display of the vessels from any desired point of view (an MRA).

T_1 AND T_2 WEIGHTING

The relative contributions of the T_1 and T_2 relaxation times to the image contrast depend on the specific imaging method employed and the choice of the relevant imaging variable values, particularly the time between consecutive excitations (the repetition time, TR) and the time between the excitation and the detection of the signal as a gradient or spin echo (the echo time, TE).

In general, the shorter the TR, the less time there will be for recovery of the magnetization between excitations, so that regions with shorter T_1 values (e.g., fat or contrast-enhanced blood) will tend to appear relatively brighter (T_1 weighting). Similarly,

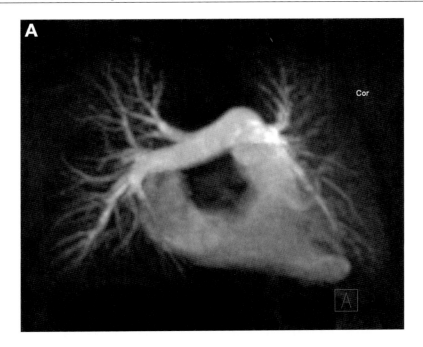

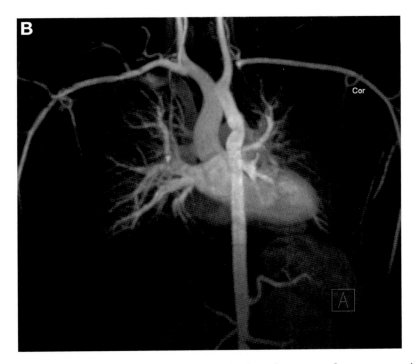

Fig. 16. Sequential images acquired after a single injection of contrast after an appropriate timing delay to obtain (**A**) a pulmonary arterial phase and (**B**) a systemic arterial phase. Note abnormal kinking of the proximal descending aorta in this patient status post–aortic coarctation repair. The left subclavian artery is also occluded from prior surgery.

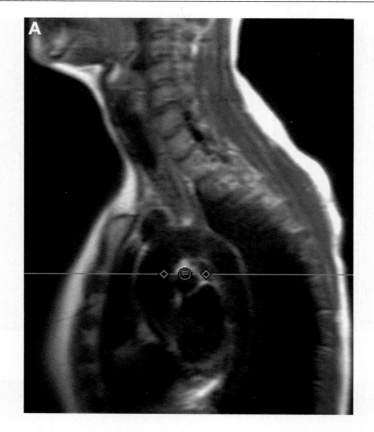

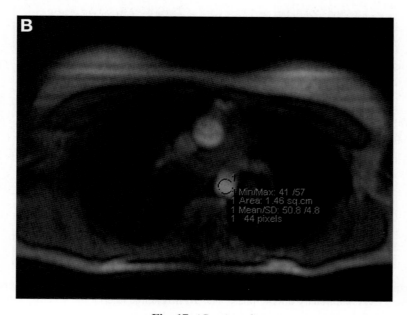

Fig. 17. *(Continued)*

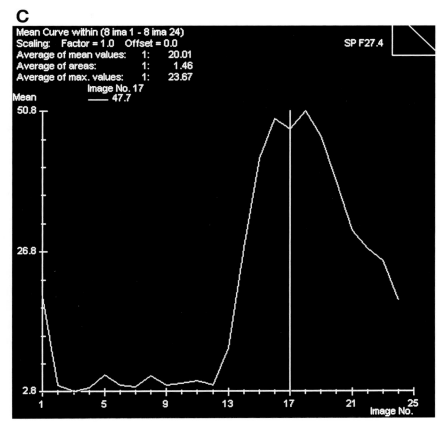

C

Mean Curve within (8 ima 1 - 8 ima 24)
Scaling: Factor = 1.0 Offset = 0.0   SP F27.4
Average of mean values: 1:   20.01
Average of areas: 1:   1.46
Average of max. values: 1:   23.67
              Image No. 17
Mean   ——— 47.7

Fig. 17. (A) Planning image for timing run single slice acquired sequentially after injection of a small amount of intravenous contrast; **(B)** example of image acquired during the timing run with region of interest placed over the descending aorta; **(C)** graphical depiction of signal intensity within the region of interest over time, allowing for selection of the appropriate timing delay when signal intensity within the thoracic aorta is maximal if a thoracic MRA is required.

the longer the TE, the more time there will be for decay of the signal before its detection, so that regions with longer T_2 values (e.g., fluid or edematous tissue) will tend to appear relatively brighter (T_2 weighting). In the case of imaging approaches employing a train of repeated spin echoes (generated with multiple 180° refocusing excitations after an initial 90° excitation), the effective TE is the time after the initial excitation when the imaging data near the center of k-space are acquired. If the heart rate is rapid, then it may be necessary to set up the T_2-weighted imaging sequence so that the excitations skip alternate heartbeats, and the potentially competing effects of T_1 weighting can be minimized.

Note that, in the case of gradient echo imaging, local magnetic field inhomogeneities (e.g., caused by local iron deposition) can lead to incomplete refocusing of the echo and resultant signal loss (T_2* weighting); this can cause darkening in images of hemochromatosis or in old hematomas. Also note that motion between initial excitation and refocusing pulses can lead to decreased signal in the spin echo imaging methods (as described for blood flow), so that pericardial effusions, for example, may not appear as bright as might be expected in T_2-weighted imaging.

The characteristic short T_1 value of fat leads to it tending to have a bright appearance in MRI. This can be helpful (e.g., in delineating the bright pericardial fat from the lower signal of the pericardium or the myocardium). If it is desired to suppress the signal from fat, then there are two approaches that can be used. In one approach, a short time inversion-recovery (STIR) sequence is used for imaging, with the inversion time kept short so that the recovering fat magnetization is approximately nulled (and it thus will appear dark) at the time of excitation for image data acquisition, and longer T_1 tissues will still have a significant amount of magnetization and will appear relatively brighter. Even though the magnetization of the other tissues with longer T_1 values will actually be negative, this will not affect their appearance in conventional MRI displays, which only display the magnitude of the local signal. Although this approach to fat suppression is fairly robust, it is not specific to fat as other regions with similar short T_1 values will also have their magnetization nulled by the inversion pulse.

A more specific approach to fat suppression is to use a frequency-selective saturation pulse tuned to the resonance frequency of the fat (which differs by about 3.5 parts per million from that of water) to null the magnetization of fat. When followed immediately by an excitation pulse for imaging data acquisition, this will result in effective nulling of the signal from fat. This is particularly useful for verifying the fat content of masses such as lipomas. However, note that, in the presence of magnetic field inhomogeneity, the local resonance frequency of fat will vary correspondingly, so that a frequency-selective pulse that effectively suppresses fat in one region may fail to do so in another or may even result in water saturation *(25)* (Fig. 18).

CINE IMAGING

The ability of MRI methods to synchronize the image data acquisition with the cardiac cycle (as described) permits reconstruction of high-quality movies (*cine imaging*) of the different phases of the cardiac cycle, even though the imaging data may be acquired over the course of multiple cardiac cycles. This is of course dependent on the cardiac cycles being reasonably consistent with each other, which may not be the case in the presence of cardiac arrhythmias.

Cine imaging can be readily implemented with gradient echo imaging (e.g., FLASH imaging); (*see* Fig. 19) this can be gated either retrospectively or prospectively. The blood in cardiac chambers and vessel lumens appears bright in cine gradient echo imaging because of the flow-related enhancement effects described. Note that the amount of this flow-related enhancement can depend on the orientation of the images: for short-axis cine imaging with gradient echoes, the flow is primarily perpendicular to the image plane, leading to a prominent and consistently bright image of the blood within the cardiac chambers and vessel lumens; with long-axis cine imaging, the presence of a significant component of within-plane flow can lead to less of a bright blood effect in the images. Also, note that through-plane motion of the heart wall itself may similarly lead to a noticeable amount of phasic variation in the apparent brightness of the myocardium.

The amount of saturation of the signal from the relatively stationary tissues caused by the repeated excitation pulses depends on both the strength of the pulses (the size of the flip angle) and the time between the pulses (TR). With increasing size of the flip angle in rapid gradient echo imaging, there is initially an increase in signal because more excitation is produced, but this is then offset by the greater saturation effects of further increases in the flip angle, leading to an optimum flip angle for maximum signal

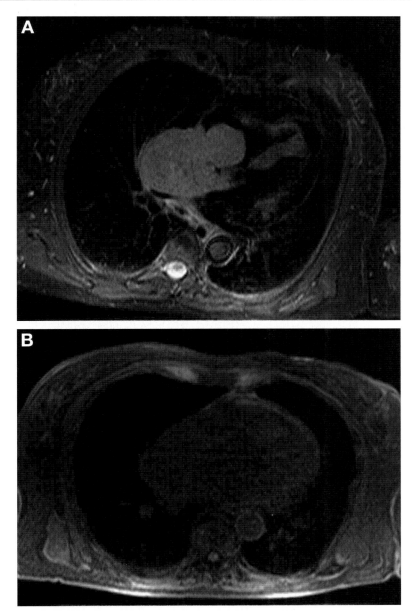

Fig. 18. (A) Short tau inversion recovery image; (B) non contrast frequency-selective fat-saturated 3D gradient echo T_1 weighted sequence demonstrating uneven suppression of the fat of the chest wall. Note the large bilobed mass within the right atrium, with extension through to the pericardium, caused by non-Hodgkin's lymphoma.

strength at given values of TR and T_1 (the Ernst angle). This signal dependence on flip angle has a fairly broad maximum; flip angles on the order of 25° or so generally work well for cine imaging with gradient echoes.

The TE is generally kept as short as possible in gradient echo cine imaging to keep the imaging as fast as possible. The signal from fat and water will evolve different phases between the time of their initial excitation and the time of their signal detection

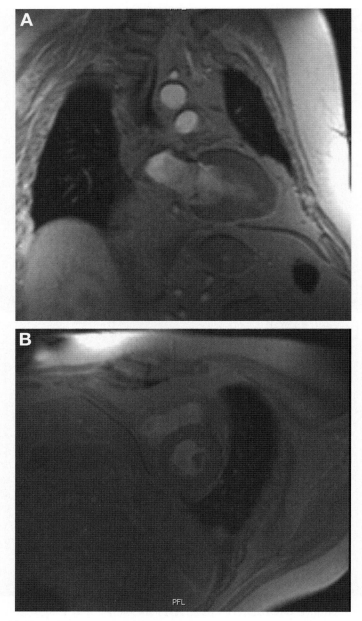

Fig. 19. FLASH images: (**A**) long-axis two-chamber and (**B**) short-axis views.

because of the difference in their resonance frequencies. Depending on the value of TE, fat and water may be in phase or out of phase in the final image, leading to corresponding different appearances of the interfaces between fat and water caused by volume averaging of their signals (e.g., at the boundaries of the epicardial fat with the epicardium or the pericardium), even though the phase itself is not directly displayed in the conventional MR images.

As the hardware of MRI systems has become faster and more stable, the use of SSFP imaging approaches for cine imaging has become more popular. As the achieving of a

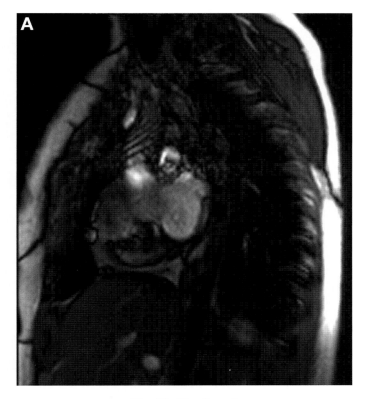

Fig. 20. *(Continued)*

steady state in SSFP relies on maintaining a continuous stream of excitation pulses, cine imaging with SSFP is used with retrospective gating only. The bright signal from blood in SSFP cine imaging depends on the relaxation times of blood rather than on its motion, leading to a more consistent bright blood appearance independent of image orientation or blood flow patterns. However, the interference with achieving the steady state when the blood is flowing in an inhomogeneous magnetic field (such as may be created by metal from surgical procedures, such as valve prostheses, or even from the patient themselves, particularly at high magnetic field strengths) can lead to significant image artifacts from the blood. In such cases, by adjusting the frequency of the RF transmitter, we may be able to minimize the artifacts (Fig. 20). Another limitation of SSFP imaging at higher magnetic fields is the associated heating (SAR) that the rapidly repeated excitation pulses it uses can create.

A useful variant of cine imaging for use with motion evaluation is to combine it with magnetization tagging, such as produced with spatial modulation of magnetization (SPAMM) *(26)* (Fig. 21). In tagged MRI, localized perturbations are created in the magnetization of the body, which appear in subsequent images as dark marks that move with the underlying tissue. Thus, we can follow the motion of otherwise indistinguishable portions of the heart wall (e.g., to permit direct observation of aspects of the motion such as circumferential or longitudinal shortening) that would otherwise be essentially invisible.

In tagged MRI, the persistence of the tags is limited by the T_1 relaxation time of the myocardium. The saturation effects of the imaging excitation pulses can also lead to

B

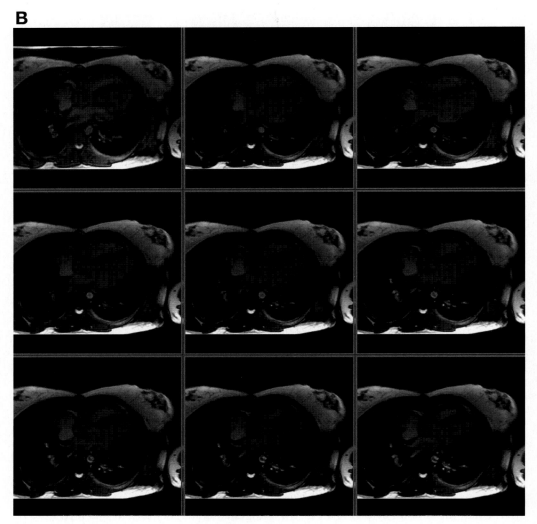

Fig. 20. (A) Artifact from magnetic field inhomogeneity in an SSFP sequence performed at 3 T; **(B)** frequency scout, with images obtained with small adjustments in the frequency of the RF transmitter to find the most suitable frequency.

fading of the tags, so that the excitation flip angle is generally decreased in tagged cine imaging to minimize the fading effects of the imaging on the tags. The longer T_1 relaxation times at higher field strengths tends to lead to better tag persistence at these fields.

PHASE CONTRAST IMAGING

Another useful variant of cine imaging is to use the motion-induced phase shifts that can arise in MRI described here to image the local velocities in vascular and cardiac structures directly (Fig. 22). In performing such phase contrast imaging of velocity, there are some choices that must be made by the operator.

First, as only one spatial component of velocity can be measured at a time, the component to be measured must be chosen. This is typically the component perpendicular to the imaging plane as this is most useful for flow volume calculations. Correspondingly,

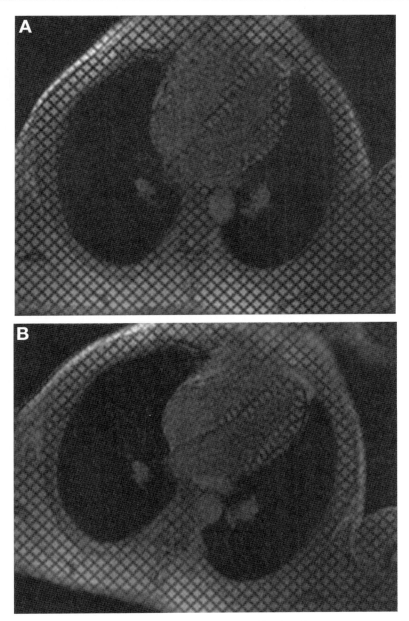

Fig. 21. Four-chamber view with magnetization tagging, allowing for more accurate depiction of wall motion during cine imaging: **(A)** in diastole; **(B)** in systole.

when studying volume flows, the imaging plane is optimally chosen to be perpendicular to the axis of the vessel lumen of interest. If measurements of more velocity components are desired, then this will require additional image acquisitions (and correspondingly more imaging time). Although the acquisition of multiple velocity components can be interleaved to improve spatial registration of the data, this cannot be used to reduce the imaging time except at the cost of reduced temporal or spatial resolution.

Another imaging parameter choice that must be made is the value of the velocity encoding value (venc). This is the velocity for which the corresponding phase shift

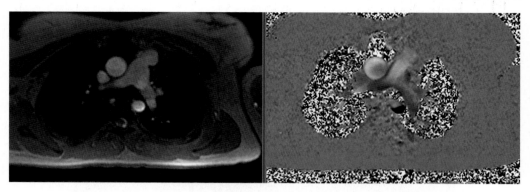

Fig. 22. (A) Magnitude (for anatomic correlation) and **(B)** phase contrast images, demonstrating through-plane flow through the ascending and descending aorta that is occurring in opposite directions. In-plane flow in the adjacent right pulmonary artery is also evident.

will be ±180°. Greater velocities, leading to greater phase shifts than this, will be indistinguishable (aliased) from velocities with smaller magnitudes and possibly opposite sign. Although a venc on the order of 150 cm/second should suffice for capturing most normal arterial flows, the higher velocities that can be found in abnormal flows (e.g., related to accelerations through areas of stenosis) can require the use of higher venc values. On the other hand, when studying slower flows, the use of lower values of venc can improve the accuracy of the measurements.

As with conventional cine imaging, there are compromises that must be made between the competing demands of spatial, temporal, and velocity resolution. If we are willing to restrict our spatial resolution or field of view, then we can potentially increase the temporal resolution enough to study pulse waves traveling along vessels or increase the imaging rate enough to follow the dynamic response of flows to transient perturbations such as respiratory maneuvers.

Although phase contrast imaging methods are primarily used to study the velocity of flowing blood, analogous to Doppler ultrasound (but without any limitations on the direction of the velocity measurement), they can also be used to study the velocity of the heart muscle (analogous to tissue Doppler studies). This can provide an alternative to tagged approaches for studying regional cardiac function. There are various relative advantages and disadvantages of these different approaches, and the methods for their application to clinical questions are still under development and evaluation.

CONTRAST ENHANCEMENT

As mentioned, the bolus injection of MRI contrast agents can be used to transiently increase the signal from the blood and of the signal from the regions to which they are delivered by the blood. The transient increase in brightness of blood vessels produced by a contrast agent bolus can be used for the production of 3D MRA images, and the transient increase in tissue brightness produced by a bolus can be used to assess the relative perfusion of the tissue. Slightly delayed imaging of the tissue after the bolus injection can be used to assess for inflammation or other sources of increased enhancement; longer delayed imaging of enhancement can be used to bring out areas of infarction or scarring.

In performing 3D MRA studies with contrast agents, there are typically several steps. First, we acquire scout volumetric images of the region we plan to image to check that

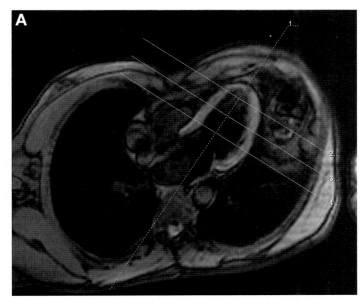

Fig. 23. *(Continued)*

the image position we have specified will cover the region we are interested in imaging without any interference by image aliasing of other regions outside it. The strong T_1 weighting of the imaging methods employed usually results in relatively poor SNR of these scout images prior to the injection of contrast agent.

As described, a timing run may be performed, with rapid sequence imaging of the target vessel after injection of a small test bolus of the contrast agent to find out how long the bolus will take to arrive after injection; this can be used in setting the delay between injection and the start of image data acquisition. Just prior to the acquisition of the contrast-enhanced images, a noncontrast image data set may be acquired for use in subtracting the baseline-unenhanced structures (assuming good spatial registration between the two data sets). The contrast dose for the MRA acquisition is adjusted for the patient's size, and the duration of the injection is adjusted to be suitable for the duration of the data acquisition. The contrast agent bolus injection is followed by injection of a bolus of normal saline to flush the remaining contrast agent out of the peripheral veins.

Acquisition of the dynamic contrast-enhanced data sets is typically performed in multiple passes to permit assessment of the sequential phases of the enhancement of different structures (e.g., pulmonary and systemic or arterial and venous) and allow for possible unexpected variations in the timing of the optimal enhancement phase of the structures of interest. After acquisition of the 3D enhanced images (and any optional subtraction of preenhancement images), the manufacturer-supplied image-processing programs are used to interactively explore the data sets and reconstruct MRA images of the structures of interest.

For MRI studies of perfusion, we again use initial scout images to make sure that the region of interest will be covered adequately (Fig. 23). Again, the SNR of these precontrast scout images will generally be relatively poor. In perfusion imaging, we typically try to acquire multiple images of the heart within each heartbeat, with the acquisitions interleaved at multiple locations within the heart. The number of locations that can be

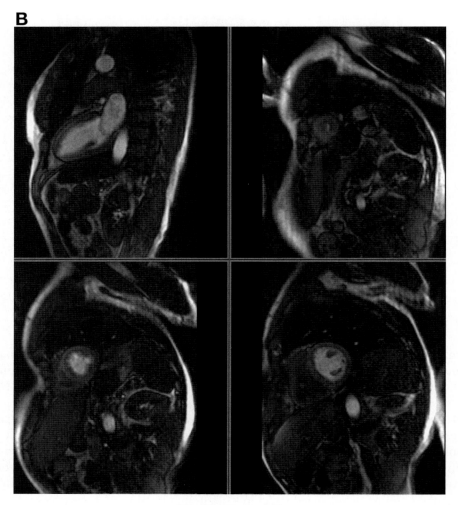

Fig. 23. *(Continued)*

monitored in this way will depend on the heart rate and the speed of the imaging. T_1 sensitization of the imaging to bring out the arrival of the contrast agent bolus is typically achieved by the application of a saturation pulse at the start of each image acquisition.

For quantitative studies of perfusion, it may be necessary to take extra steps to ensure accurate saturation throughout the region of interest *(27)*. The rate of the contrast bolus injection will be limited by the size and location of the intravenous cannula used for the injection but is typically on the order of 5 mL/second for 2 seconds; injecting for longer times does not yield much improvement in the level of tissue enhancement achieved. The contrast bolus is immediately followed by a saline bolus, as for MRA studies. The patient is instructed to hold his or her breath during the image acquisitions for as long as possible and then to breathe quietly to minimize the respiratory effects.

The early phase of enhancement of tissue after injection of a contrast bolus is related to the "vascularity" of the tissue and reflects a combination of the delivery of the contrast agent to the tissue by the blood flow, the fractional blood volume of the tissue, and the leakiness of the microcirculation permitting extravascular exchange of the contrast

C

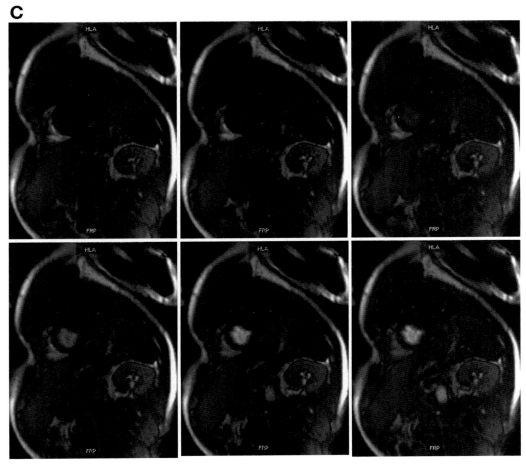

Fig. 23. (**A**) Planning image for first pass perfusion sequence; (**B**) selection of images acquired. In this example, three short-axis views and one long-axis two-chamber view are repeatedly obtained in rapid succession with the dynamic injection of intravenous gadolinium; (**C**) the sequence (a short-axis view) depicts initial blood pool phase followed by enhancement of the myocardium. Hypoperfusion of a segment of myocardium may indicate the presence of ischemia or infarction.

agent. For example, inflammation associated with infectious processes may show prominent early enhancement, as may vascular areas of tumors.

Imaging of the late phase of enhancement of tissue after injection of a contrast bolus (delayed enhancement) can be used to bring out areas of abnormal accumulation of contrast agent (e.g., caused by effective temporary "trapping" of the contrast agent in local areas of fibrosis, such as in healed infarcts). Such areas of accumulation of contrast agent in the myocardium can be made more prominent in the images by using inversion-recovery (IR) imaging to effectively null the signal from the normal myocardium, so that the shorter local T_1 times resulting from contrast agent accumulation (e.g., in areas of fibrosis) will result in corresponding brighter signals *(28)*.

In choosing the time for performing delayed enhancement imaging, there must be a long enough delay for the contrast agent largely to clear out of the normal myocardium; it must be short enough for there to still be sufficient contrast agent left in the abnormal region to show up in the images. A time on the order of 10–15 minutes after the injection

A

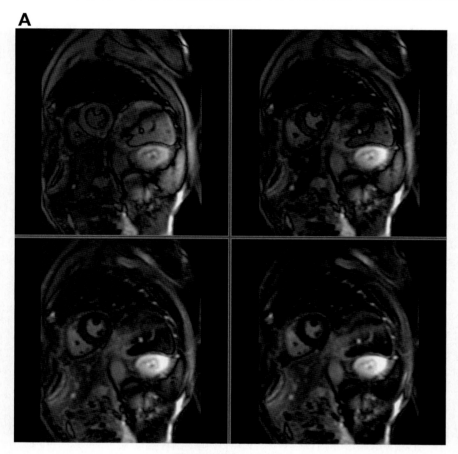

Fig. 24. *(Continued)*

of the contrast agent generally works well. The optimal inversion time to be used for nulling the signal from the normal myocardium will depend on the particular contrast dose and delay time used and on the physiology of the individual patient and must be empirically adjusted for each study.

One way to adjust this parameter is to perform a modified cine image with an inversion pulse at the start of the cardiac cycle (an inversion time or TI scout), so that each reconstructed cardiac phase corresponds to a different inversion time, and then to look for the time of the phase that best nulls the normal myocardium (Fig. 24). Note that the imaging itself will affect the effective T_1 recovery process, so that the best value to choose for the actual imaging inversion time may still need to be adjusted from this time. A modified IR imaging method that collects enough additional data to permit a phase-sensitive image reconstruction can reduce the need to choose the value of the IR time precisely to null the myocardium *(29)*.

An additional consideration in delayed enhancement imaging is the choice of whether to perform a rapid 3D (or stacked 2D) image acquisition, which can be repeated in different image orientations to best evaluate different portions of the myocardium, or to acquire serial 2D images, which can have better temporal and spatial resolution but at the cost of longer image acquisition times. A useful compromise is routinely to acquire the 3D image sets, adding acquisition of individual 2D images of any questionable areas.

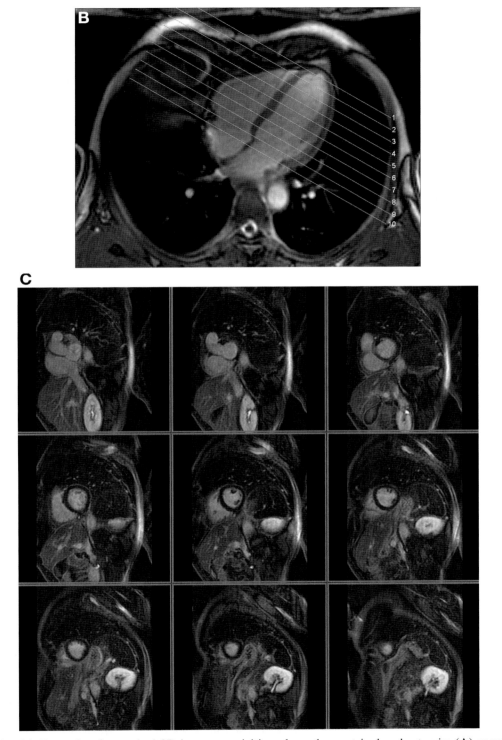

Fig. 24. Example of a stacked 2D image acquisition along the ventricular short axis: (**A**) scout sequence to determine optimal inversion time when normal myocardium is nulled. Such optimal inversion time is then used for imaging a parallel short-axis stack (**B**) to achieve maximal signal nulling of normal myocardium (**C**).

REFERENCES

1. Shellock FG. Reference manual for magnetic resonance safety. Los Angeles: Saunders; 2003.
2. Atkinson DJ, Edelman RR. Cineangiography of the heart in a single breath hold with a segmented turboFLASH sequence. Radiology 1991;178:357–360.
3. Edelman RR, Manning WJ, Burstein D, Paulin S. Coronary arteries: breath-hold MR angiography. Radiology 1991;181:641–643.
4. Felblinger J, Lehmann C, Boesch C. Electrocardiogram acquisition during MR examinations for patient monitoring and sequence triggering. Magn Reson Med 1994;32:523–529.
5. Fischer SE, Wickline SA, Lorenz CH. Novel real-time R-wave detection algorithm based on the vector-cardiogram for accurate gated magnetic resonance acquisitions. Magn Reson Med 1999;42:361–370.
6. Boxerman JL, Mosher TJ, McVeigh ER, Atalar E, Lima JA, Bluemke DA. Advanced MR imaging techniques for evaluation of the heart and great vessels. Radiographics 1998;18:543–564.
7. Lenz GW, Haacke EM, White RD. Retrospective gating: a review of technical aspects and future directions. Magn Reson Imaging 1989;7:445–455.
8. Sievers B, Addo M, Kirchberg S, et al. How much are atrial volumes and ejection fractions assessed by cardiac magnetic resonance imaging influenced by the ECG gating method? J Cardiovasc Magn Reson 2005;7:587–593.
9. Lee VS, Resnick D, Bundy JM, Simonetti OP, Lee P, Weinreb JC. Cardiac function: MR evaluation in one breath hold with real-time true fast imaging with steady-state precession. Radiology 2002;222:835–842.
10. Foo TK, Bernstein MA, Aisen AM, et al. Improved ejection fraction and flow velocity estimates with use of view sharing and uniform repetition time excitation with fast cardiac techniques. Radiology 1995;195:471–478.
11. Danias PG, Stuber M, Botnar RM, Kissinger KV, Edelman RR, Manning WJ. Relationship between motion of coronary arteries and diaphragm during free breathing: lessons from real-time MR imaging. AJR Am J Roentgenol 1999;172:1061–1065.
12. Holland AE, Goldfarb JW, Edelman RR. Diaphragmatic and cardiac motion during suspended breathing: preliminary experience and implications for breath-hold MR imaging. Radiology 1998;209:483–489.
13. Plathow C, Ley S, Zaporozhan J, et al. Assessment of reproducibility and stability of different breath-hold maneuvres by dynamic MRI: comparison between healthy adults and patients with pulmonary hypertension. Eur Radiol 2006;16:173–179.
14. Haacke EM, Patrick JL. Reducing motion artifacts in two-dimensional Fourier transform imaging. Magn Reson Imaging 1986;4:359–376.
15. Ehman RL, Felmlee JP. Adaptive technique for high-definition MR imaging of moving structures. Radiology 1989;173:255–263.
16. Taylor AM, Keegan J, Jhooti P, Gatehouse PD, Firmin DN, Pennell DJ. Differences between normal subjects and patients with coronary artery disease for three different MR coronary angiography respiratory suppression techniques. J Magn Reson Imaging 1999;9:786–793.
17. Sachs TS, Meyer CH, Pauly JM, Hu BS, Nishimura DG, Macovski A. The real-time interactive 3-D-DVA for robust coronary MRA. IEEE Trans Med Imaging 2000;19:73–79.
18. Danias PG, McConnell MV, Khasgiwala VC, Chuang ML, Edelman RR, Manning WJ. Prospective navigator correction of image position for coronary MR angiography. Radiology 1997;203:733–736.
19. Taylor AM, Keegan J, Jhooti P, Firmin DN, Pennell DJ. Calculation of a subject-specific adaptive motion-correction factor for improved real-time navigator echo-gated magnetic resonance coronary angiography. J Cardiovasc Magn Reson 1999;1:131–138.
20. Wang Y, Ehman RL. Retrospective adaptive motion correction for navigator-gated 3D coronary MR angiography. J Magn Reson Imaging 2000;11:208–214.
21. Felblinger J, Boesch C. Amplitude demodulation of the electrocardiogram signal (ECG) for respiration monitoring and compensation during MR examinations. Magn Reson Med 1997;38:129–136.
22. Goldfarb JW. The SENSE ghost: field-of-view restrictions for SENSE imaging. J Magn Reson Imaging 2004;20:1046–1051.
23. Finn JP, Baskaran V, Carr JC, et al. Thorax: low-dose contrast-enhanced three-dimensional MR angiography with subsecond temporal resolution—initial results. Radiology 2002;224:896–904.
24. Axel L. Blood flow effects in magnetic resonance imaging. AJR Am J Roentgenol 1984;143:1157–1166.
25. Axel L, Kolman L, Charafeddine R, Hwang SN, Stolpen AH. Origin of a signal intensity loss artifact in fat-saturation MR imaging. Radiology 2000;217:911–915.

26. Axel L, Montillo A, Kim D. Tagged magnetic resonance imaging of the heart: a survey. Med Image Anal 2005;9:376–393.
27. Kim D, Cernicanu A, Axel L. B(0) and B(1)-insensitive uniform T(1)-weighting for quantitative, first-pass myocardial perfusion magnetic resonance imaging. Magn Reson Med 2005;54:1423–1429.
28. Simonetti OP, Kim RJ, Fieno DS, et al. An improved MR imaging technique for the visualization of myocardial infarction. Radiology 2001;218:215–223.
29. Kellman P, Arai AE, McVeigh ER, Aletras AH. Phase-sensitive inversion recovery for detecting myocardial infarction using gadolinium-delayed hyperenhancement. Magn Reson Med 2002;47:372–383.

3   Anatomy of the Heart and Great Arteries

Lawrence M. Boxt and Martin J. Lipton

CONTENTS

INTRODUCTION

Magnetic resonance imaging (MRI) techniques produce high spatial, contrast, and temporal resolution image data for evaluation of cardiac and great vessel anatomy, regional tissue characterization, vascular blood flow, cardiac chamber filling and contraction, regional myocardial dynamics, and myocardial perfusion. MRI produces series of tomographic images of the heart and great arteries in arbitrary section, allowing tailoring of an examination to address a specific clinical problem or a systematic analysis of cardiac structure and physiological function. Recognition of a particular or general abnormality is based on recognition of variance between the instant image data at hand and the expected normal appearance of the heart and great arteries.

In this chapter, we describe the anatomy of the heart and great arteries as demonstrated on MRI. Anatomy as portrayed by MRI significantly differs from that observed in the dissection lab or operating room. On MRI, we view these structures in tomographic images. That is, rather than viewing the entire organ and its relationship with surrounding organs, we view the heart in slices. The analogy of echocardiographic imaging is quite appropriate for magnetic resonance (MR) examination of the heart. In other words, the MR scanner produces images of sections of the heart and great vessels that may be

From: *Contemporary Cardiology: Cardiovascular Magnetic Resonance Imaging*
Edited by: Raymond Y. Kwong © Humana Press Inc., Totowa, NJ

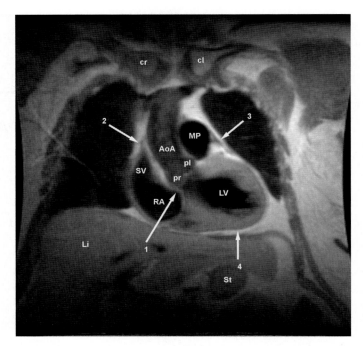

Fig. 1. Coronal double-inversion recovery image (from a 50-year-old woman) obtained through the right (cr) and left (cl) clavicular heads and posterior right (pr) and posterior left (pl) aortic sinuses of Valsalva. The subaortic interventricular septum includes the atrioventricular septum (arrow 1) between the right atrium (RA) and left ventricle (LV). The entry of the superior vena cava (SV) into the RA is posterior to the orifice of the right atrial appendage (not visualized). The pericardium attaches along the ascending aorta (AoA) on the right heart border (arrow 2) and on the pulmonary artery (arrow 3) on the left. The low signal pericardial space (arrow 4) continues along the diaphragmatic surface of the heart. The liver (Li) and stomach (St) are labeled.

interpreted to recognize normal structure, differentiate normal from abnormal, and begin the process of morphologic diagnosis.

MR diagnosis is based on visualization of a series of images, each obtained in prescribed or arbitrary anatomic section. By analysis of left-to-right, anterior-to-posterior, and superior-to-inferior relationships among adjacent structures, we create a three-dimensional image of these organs in our mind. By recognizing the variance between what we expect and what we see, we begin to acquire a sense of what is abnormal. Recognition of abnormality is based first on recognition of the normal.

It is the purpose of this chapter to describe the anatomy of the heart and great vessels and demonstrate the appearance of these structures on MR examination.

PERICARDIUM

The heart is contained within the middle mediastinum by the pericardium. The visceral pericardium is adherent to the ventricular myocardium and cannot be visually separated from the epicardial fat. The parietal pericardium may be identified as a paper-thin surface of high signal intensity surrounding the heart and great arteries (Figs. 1–3). On the left side of the heart, it attaches over the top of the main pulmonary

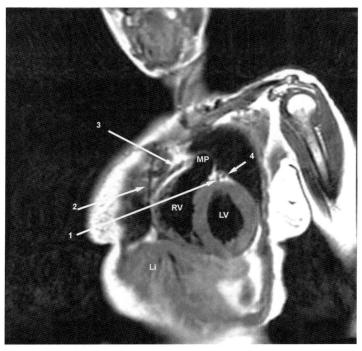

Fig. 2. Left anterior oblique (LAO) sagittal double-inversion recovery image from a 60-year-old woman. The anterior, trabeculated right ventricle (RV) lies immediately behind the right internal mammary artery (arrow 2). Notice how the pericardium (arrow 3) attaches on the top of the main pulmonary artery (MP). Embedded within the epicardial fat above the left ventricular (LV) myocardium, the anterior descending (arrow 1) and circumflex (arrow 4) coronary arteries have split from the left main coronary artery (not seen).

artery (PA). The ascending aorta is enveloped up to about the level of the azygos vein. Recesses (potential spaces) in the pericardium are typically found anterior to the ascending aorta and medial to the main PA (the anterior aortic recess), between the ascending aorta and transverse right PA (the superior pericardial recess), and around the entry of the pulmonary veins to the left atrium (LA). Visualization of the parietal pericardium depends on the presence and extent of low-density fatty deposition in the pericardial fat pad and middle mediastinum.

AORTA

The aorta is attached to the heart by the annulus fibrosis. The annulus supports the aortic valve and is part of a fibrous skeleton that supports the mitral and pulmonary valves as well. The aortic annulus lies nearly in the center of the heart, just oblique to the plane of the cardiac short axis (Figs. 1, 4, and 5). The thoracic aorta is divided into a series of segments. The bulbous aortae or bulbous portion of the aorta lies between the aortic annulus and the tubular portion of the aorta. Within this segment, the aorta is widest, measuring up to 3 cm within the aortic sinuses of Valsalva (Figs. 1 and 5–7).

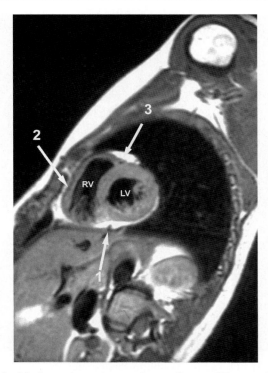

Fig. 3. Short-axis double-inversion recovery image from a 25-year-old man. Notice how fat surrounds the heart (arrows 1 and 3). Right ventricular (RV) free-wall myocardium can be separated from the pericardial fat by the pencil-thin pericardial space (arrow 2). The posterior descending coronary artery is seen in cross section as a signal void within the epicardial fat along the inferior aspect of the interventricular septum (arrow 1).

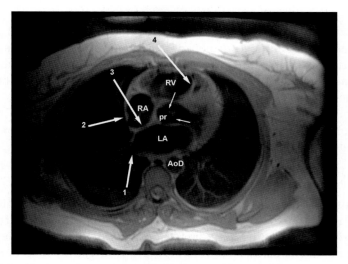

Fig. 4. Axial double-inversion recovery image from a 45-year-old woman. The right ventricle lies anteriorly. Myocardial trabeculation between the interventricular septum and right ventricular free wall (arrow 4) is identified. Within the sinus portion of the aorta, the posterior right aortic sinus of Valsalva (pr) and aortic valvular commissures (small arrows) are evident. The right (RA) and left (LA) atria are separated, at this level, by the secundum interatrial septum (arrow 3). The right lower lobe pulmonary vein (arrow 1) is just entering the LA.

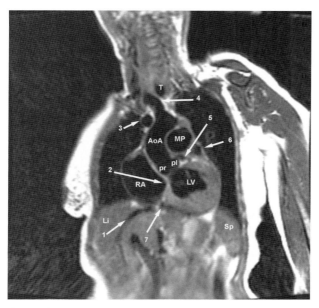

Fig. 5. Left anterior oblique (LAO) sagittal double-inversion recovery image (from a 60-year-old woman) through the sinus portion of the aorta. The left main and proximal left anterior descending coronary arteries (arrow 5) arise from the posterior left aortic sinus of Valsalva (pl). Immediately inferior to the posterior right is the atrioventricular septum (arrow 2), separating the right atrium (RA) from the left ventricle (LV). A hepatic vein (arrow 1) passes through the liver (Li) toward the diaphraphragmatic surface of the RA, lateral to coronary sinus (arrow 7), seen in cross section embedded within the fat of the inferior portion of the posterior atrioventricular ring. The liver (Li) and spleen (Sp) are labeled.

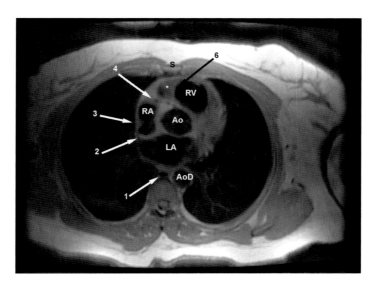

Fig. 6. Axial double-inversion recovery image from a 45-year-old woman. Within the aortic root (Ao), the origin and proximal course of the right coronary artery (arrow 4) is evident. The left atrium (LA) lies between the Ao and descending aorta (AoD). The right (RA) and left (LA) atrium are separated at this level by the sinus venosus portion of the interatrial septum (arrow 2). Along the lateral aspect of the RA, the high signal intensity crista terminalis (arrow 3) may be visualized. The right ventricle (RV) lies behind the sternum (S) and is again apparently segregated into two portions (*) by a myocardial trabeculation. The azygos vein (arrow 1) is labeled.

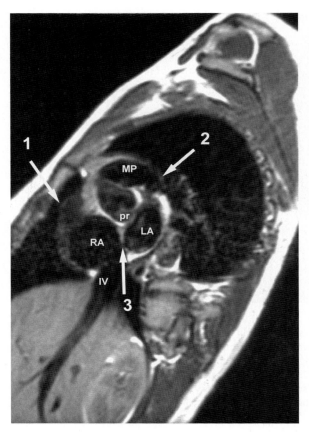

Fig. 7. Short-axis double-inversion recovery image from a 25-year-old man through the posterior right aortic sinus of Valsalva (pr). In this section, the right atrial appendage (arrow 1) lies directly anterior to the aorta, and the left atrial appendage (arrow 2) is at the same level as the distal main pulmonary artery (MP). Notice the relationship of the pr with the left (LA) and right (RA) atria and the superior interatrial septum (arrow 3). In this plane, the inferior vena cava (IV) is found entering the RA.

The width of the ascending aorta is less than 37 mm. The axis of the most proximal portion of the ascending aorta points slightly anteriorly and toward the right. As the aorta ascends, it continues to be directed slightly toward the right and anteriorly, displacing the superior vena cava (SV) toward the right. Thus, in coronal section, the right lateral wall of the ascending aorta gently curves toward the right, and in the sagittal section, it curves anteriorly (Figs. 1, 5, 6, and 8–16). The aorta returns to the midline by the level of the body of the second right costal cartilage. As the aorta continues its ascent, it curves dorsally and toward the left to form the aortic arch. Although the total length of the ascending aorta averages 5–5.5 cm, body habitus, diaphragm position, and chest conformation all have influence on its appearance.

The aortic arch lies almost entirely behind the manubrium of the sternum (Fig. 17). It is not contained within the pericardium. The plane of the aortic arch lies in an off-sagittal, left anterior oblique plane (Figs. 8 and 17). The origins of the three major aortic branches (the innominate, left common carotid, and left subclavian arteries) are slightly ventral to the vertex of the arch (Figs. 5 and 18–23).

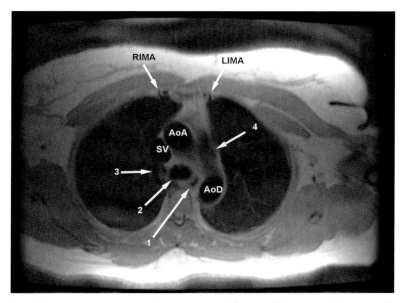

Fig. 8. Axial double-inversion recovery image from a 45-year-old woman. The ascending (AoA) and descending (AoD) aorta are identified. The top of the main pulmonary artery (arrow 4) is now coming into view. Both the right (RIMA) and left (LIMA) internal mammary arteries have reached the anterior chest wall just to the right and left of midline, respectively. At this level, the azygos vein (arrow 3) is passing over the right hilum to drain into the posterior aspect of the superior vena cava (SV). The trachea (arrow 2) and esophagus (arrow 1) are labeled.

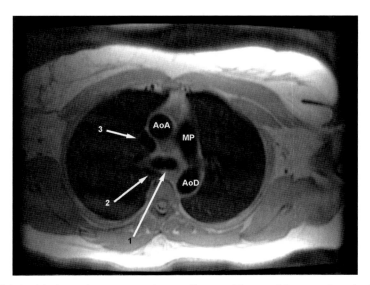

Fig. 9. Axial double-inversion recovery image (from a 45-year-old woman) at the level of the carina (arrow 1). The ascending (AoA) and descending (AoD) aorta are labeled. The body of the main pulmonary artery (MP) passes toward the AoD to become the left pulmonary artery. At this level, the azygos vein (arrow 2) can be seen moving toward the right to pass over the right hilum. The superior vena cava (arrow 3) lies toward the right and posterior to the AoA.

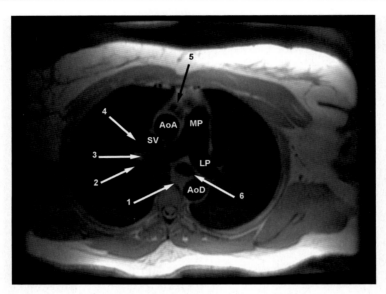

Fig. 10. Axial double-inversion recovery image (from a 45-year-old woman) at the level of the pulmonary artery bifurcation. The main (MP) pulmonary artery continues as the left (LP) pulmonary artery; the right pulmonary artery (arrow 3) passes behind the ascending aorta (AoA) and superior vena cava (SV) to the right hilum. Note that the right pulmonary artery is anterior to the right bronchus (arrow 2); the LP is just about to cross over the top of the left bronchus (arrow 6). The right upper lobe pulmonary vein (arrow 4) lies anterior to the right pulmonary artery. At this anatomic level, the ascending aorta (AoA) has become enveloped by the pericardium; an anterior pericardial space (arrow 5) is apparent.

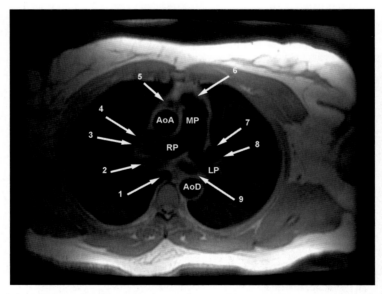

Fig. 11. Axial double-inversion recovery image from a 45-year-old woman. The superior aspect of the right ventricular outflow (arrow 6) is now apparent. The left pulmonary artery (LP) has crossed the left bronchus (arrow 9) to enter the left hilum. Note that the left upper lobe pulmonary vein (arrow 7) is anterior to the left upper lobe pulmonary artery (arrow 8). The right pulmonary artery (RP) lies anterior to the right bronchus (arrow 2). The right upper lobe pulmonary vein (arrow 4) lies anterior to the right upper lobe pulmonary artery (arrow 3). Immediately anterior to the ascending aorta (AoA) is the anterior pericardial space (arrow 5). The azygos vein (arrow 1) is labeled.

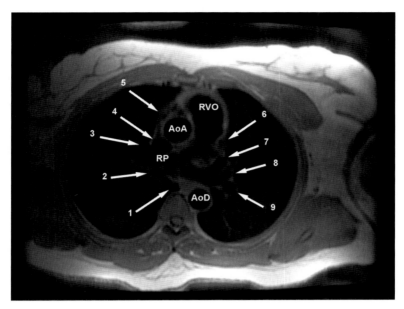

Fig. 12. Axial double-inversion recovery image from a 45-year-old woman. The left-sided right ventricular outflow (RVO) tract lies anterior to the ascending aorta (AoA). At this level, we begin to see the tip of the left (arrow 6) and the right (arrow 5) atrial appendages. The right atrial appendage lies anterior to the AoA. The left atrial appendage lies anterior to the left upper lobe pulmonary vein (arrow 7) and artery (arrow 8). The left pulmonary artery (arrow 9) lies anterior and to the left of the descending aorta (AoD). The right upper lobe pulmonary vein (arrow 3) lies adjacent to the superior vena cava (arrow 4) and anterior to the right pulmonary artery (RP). The RP lies anterior to the right bronchus (arrow 2). The azygos vein (arrow 1) is identified.

The innominate artery originates from the arch and takes a slightly rightward course anterior to the midline trachea before dividing into the right common carotid and right subclavian arteries. The left common carotid artery originates slightly dorsal and to the left of the innominate and dorsal and to the left of the trachea. The origin of the left subclavian artery is from the dorsal aspect of the aortic arch. It takes an almost vertical course from the aorta toward the thoracic outlet and then turns toward the left and pulmonary apex.

The aortic arch is usually left sided, mildly displacing the trachea toward the right (Figs. 17, 21, and 23). The diameter of the aortic arch in adults under 60 years of age is between 2.5 and 3.0 cm. Over the age of 60 years, 3.5 cm is within normal limits. The ligamentum arteriosum (the remnant of the ductus arteriosus) is attached to the inferior aspect of the arch, just beyond the origin of the left subclavian artery. The proximal descending thoracic aorta lies to the left of the spine (Fig. 8).

As it travels from cephalad to caudad in the posterior mediastinum, it comes to lie near the midline (Fig. 24). The descending thoracic aorta tapers from approximately 23 mm (at the level of T4) to about 20 mm (at the level of T12). The (usually) three bronchial arteries originate from the ventral aspect of the descending aorta, between the levels of T5 and T6. Paired intercostal arteries originate from the dorsal aspect of the aorta, between the 3rd and 11th intercostal spaces.

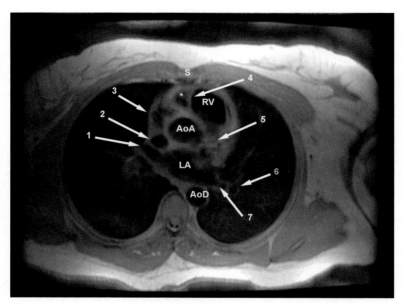

Fig. 13. Axial double-inversion recovery image from a 45-year-old woman. The left atrium (LA) lies between the proximal ascending aorta (AoA) and descending aorta (AoD). At this level, the proximal left anterior descending coronary artery (arrow 5) is visualized. The right upper lobe pulmonary vein (arrow 1) drains into the LA behind the superior vena cava (arrow 2); the left lower lobe vein (arrow 7) empties into the LA from anterior to the descending aorta (AoD). The left lower lobe pulmonary artery (arrow 6) lies lateral and anterior to the lower lobe vein. Note the trabecular appearance of the right atrial appendage (arrow 3) as it wraps around the anterior aspect of the AoA. The sinus portion of the right ventricle (RV) lies anteriorly, immediately behind the body of the sternum (S). A myocardial trabeculation (arrow 4) extends from the interventricular septum to the right ventricular free wall, apparently isolating a medial portion of the RV chamber (*).

SUPERIOR VENA CAVA

Immediately cephalad to the aortic arch, the left subclavian vein is joined by the left internal jugular vein to form the left innominate vein (Figs. 15 and 17). The left innominate vein crosses from left to right just anterior to the aortic arch and proximal innominate artery to join the confluence of the right subclavian and internal jugular veins, forming the SV, to the right of the aorta (Figs. 5, 16, 18, 19, and 22).

The SV passes behind the right sternal margin to enter the pericardium at the level of the second costal cartilage. The SV receives the azygous vein just above the right upper lobe bronchus (Figs. 9, 19–21, 25–28, 30). As the superior cava passes through the mediastinum to drain into the right atrium (RA), it passes from anterior to posterior to the ascending aorta, entering the RA at the level of the third costal cartilage. The SV drains into the RA just posterior to the orifice of the right atrial appendage (RAA) and slightly anterior to the entrance of the inferior vena cava (IVC; Figs. 12, 19, 23). The posterior wall of the SV as it enters the RA is the sinus venosus portion of the interatrial septum, and it separates the SV from the LA (Fig. 6).

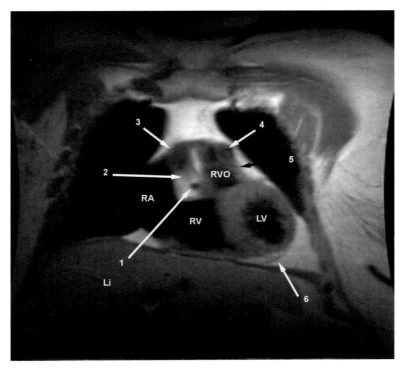

Fig. 14. Coronal double-inversion recovery image (from a 50-year-old woman) through the origin of the right coronary artery (arrow 1). Stil within the right atrium (RA) and right ventricle (RV), we visualize more of the left ventricle (LV). The superior and medialmost aspect of the right atrial appendage (arrow 3) lies anterior to the faintly visualized anterior aspect of the ascending aorta (arrow 2). The right ventricular outflow (RVO) extends posterior to the right ventricular sinus (RV), separated by the infundibulum. The pulmonary artery sinuses of Valsalva (arrow 4) are supported by the pulmonary valve (arrow 5). Inferoapical pericardium is marked (arrow 6).

RIGHT ATRIUM

The cavity of the RA is segregated into an anterior trabeculated portion and posterior smooth-walled portion by the crista terminalis, the remnant of the vein of the sinus venosus (Figs. 4, 6, 29, and 30). The lateral RA wall is thin; the distance between the cavity of the RA and the outer lateral border of the heart should be no greater than 3 mm. Increased thickening usually means a pericardial effusion or pericardial thickening. The RAA is a broad-based, triangular structure contained within the pericardium; it extends from about the middle of the heart obliquely around the ascending aorta (Figs. 12, 13, 16, 31, and 32). Collapsed when RA pressure and volume are normal, the pectinate muscles characteristically seen in the RA anterior to the crista terminalis tend to prevent its collapse. When enlarged, the pectinate muscles of the RAA appear as intracavitary filling defects, analogous to ventricular myocardial bundles in the right ventricle (RV; Fig. 10).

The coronary sinus extends from the confluence of the great cardiac vein, between the LA and left ventricle (LV) in the posterior atrioventricular (AV) ring, and then

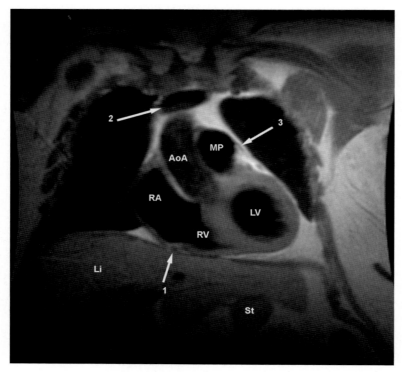

Fig. 15. Coronal double-inversion recovery image from a 50-year-old woman. The left innominate vein (arrow 2) passes from left to right and superior to inferior, cephalad to the top of the ascending aorta (AoA). The distal right coronary artery (arrow 1) is viewed in cross section as it passes into the underside of the anterior atrioventricular ring, between the right atrium (RA) and inflow portion of the right ventricle (RV). The pericardium on the left side of the heart (arrow 3) is seen attaching to the top of the main pulmonary artery (MP). In this normal individual, abdominal situs solitus is indicated by the right-sided liver (Li) and left-sided stomach (St).

passes beneath the LA to the diaphragmatic surface of the heart to drain into the RA medial and slightly superior to the entry of the IVC (Figs. 19–23, 25, and 33). The eustacian valve separates these two structures. The suprahepatic portion of the IVC usually receives the hepatic veins before draining into the heart. Occasionally, the hepatic veins drain directly into the floor of the RA.

The interatrial septum separates the LA from the RA (Figs. 4, 6, 7, 23, 25, and 31). It forms a curved surface, usually bowing toward the RA. Normal thinning in the region of the foramen ovale may be seen; this change in septal thickness is exaggerated in individuals with extra fat deposits around the heart and elsewhere. The RA should appear nearly the same size as the LA. Measurement of RA size is less difficult than estimation of RA volume. Nevertheless, RA enlargement is associated with clockwise cardiac rotation.

The tricuspid valve resides within the anterior AV ring, immediately subjacent to the right coronary artery. The plane of the valve annulus is nearly sagittal and may therefore be visualized in axial section. The septal and anterior leaflets appear as long filling

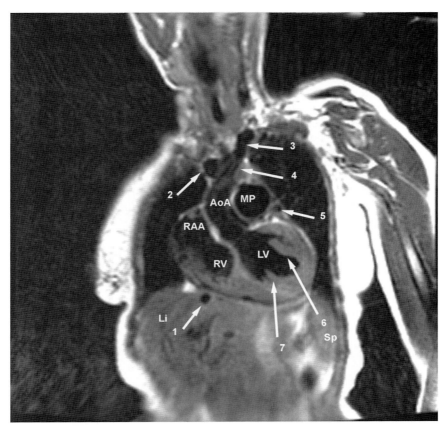

Fig. 16. Left anterior oblique (LAO) sagittal double-inversion recovery image (from a 60-year-old woman) through the ascending aorta (AoA). In this section, the right atrial appendage (RAA) is anterior to the AoA and superior to the inflow portion of the right ventricle (RV). Before joining the right innominate vein (arrow 2) to form the superior vena cava, the left innominate vein (arrow 3) passes anterior to the left common carotid artery (arrow 4). Inferior and toward the left from the main pulmonary artery (MP), the tip of the left atrial appendage (arrow 5) can be seen. Note the left ventricular papillary muscles (arrows 6 and 7). The spleen (Sp) and intrahepatic (Li) inferior vena cava (arrow 1) are noted.

defects attached to the AV ring and connected to the RV free wall and septum by fine chordae and papillary muscles of varying size.

RIGHT VENTRICLE

The RV resides immediately posterior to the sternum, more or less in the midline (Figs. 2–4, 6, 13, 24, 29–31). Unless hypertrophied, the RV free-wall myocardium is only about 2–3 mm in thickness and difficult to visualize. The shape of the RV can be surmised by visualizing the ventricle as the sum of the axial sections obtained during computed tomographic examination. From the level of the pulmonary valve, moving caudad, the shape of the ventricle changes. The RV outflow tract is round, surrounded by the ventricular infundibulum (Figs. 13 and 29), and lies to the patient's left. Moving in a caudad direction, the chamber increases in size, assuming a triangular shape; the

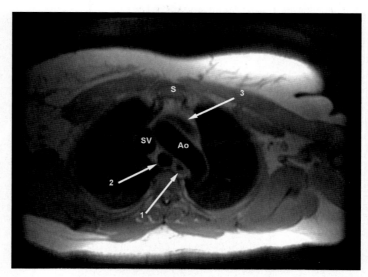

Fig. 17. Axial double-inversion recovery image from a 45-year-old woman. The aortic arch (Ao) runs anterior to posterior and right to left, passing anterior to the air-filled esophagus (arrow 1) and trachea (arrow 2). At this level, the left innominate vein (arrow 3) has not joined with the right innominate vein to form the superior vena cava (SV).

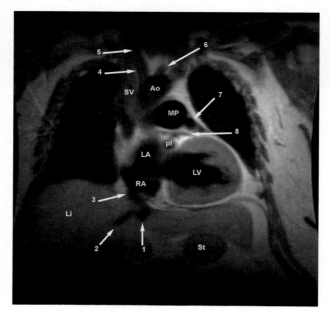

Fig. 18. Coronal double-inversion recovery image from a 50-year-old woman. A hepatic vein (arrow 2) approaches the intrahepatic inferior vena cava (arrow 1). The suprahepatic inferior vena cava (arrow 3) is seen entering the posterior aspect of the right atrium (RA). The left atrium (LA) lies cephalad, posterior and medial to the RA, communicating with the left ventricle (LV) across the mitral valve (not visualized). The left main coronary artery (arrow 8) is seen originating from the posterior left aortic sinus of Valsalva (pl). The superior vena cava (SV) is posterior to the ascending aorta (not visualized) and within the same tomographic plane as the aortic arch (Ao). The innominate (arrow 4), right common carotid (arrow 5), and origin of the left common carotid (arrow 6) arteries are visualized. The fingerlike left atrial appendage (arrow 7) is viewed in cross section, just inferior and to the left of the main pulmonary artery (MP).

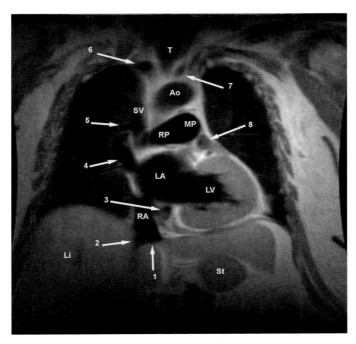

Fig. 19. Coronal double-inversion recovery image from a 50-year-old woman. A hepatic vein (arrow 2) drains into the suprahepatic inferior vena cava (arrow 1), which enters the right atrium (RA) medial and inferior to the coronary sinus (arrow 3). The coronary sinus (arrow 3) lies to the right of the fat in the posterior atrioventricular ring, beneath the left atrium (LA). The right upper lobe pulmonary vein (arrow 4) drains into the LA anterior to the right hilum. The azygos arch (arrow 5) can be seen draining to the posterior aspect of the superior vena cava (SV). The proximal-most right subclavian artery (arrow 6) can be seen immediately after its origin from the innominate artery. A segment of the left common carotid artery (arrow 7) lies to the left of the cervical trachea (T). The right pulmonary artery (RP) courses from superior to inferior and left to right along the roof of the LA to pass behind the SV. The body of the left atrial appendage (arrow 8) is contained by pericardium and lies just above the fat of the posterior atrioventricular ring.

base is formed by the AV ring and the apex at the intersection of the free wall and interventricular septum (Figs. 9 and 10).

The tricuspid valve is separated from the pulmonary valve by the infundibulum. The RV surface of the interventricular septum is irregular (Fig. 35). Although the septomarginal trabeculation may not always be identified, papillary muscles extending from it to the tricuspid valve leaflets are commonplace. Numerous muscle bundles extend from the interventricular septum across the RV chamber to the free wall (Figs. 2, 4, 6, and 13). The inferiormost of these is the moderator band, which carries the conducting bundle.

The interventricular septum normally bows toward the RV (Figs. 2 and 4), so that in short-axis reconstruction, the LV appears as a doughnut and the LV cavity as the hole (Figs. 3 and 36). The RV in short-axis section appears as an appendage to the LV, extending from slightly inferior to the inferiormost aspect of the interventricular septum, RV outflow tract, and pulmonary valve, which resides superior to the LV (Figs. 2, 3, 36, and 37).

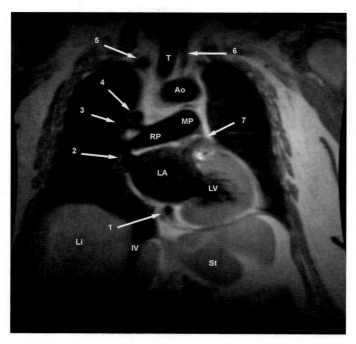

Fig. 20. Coronal double-inversion recovery image from a 50-year-old woman through the origin of the right upper lobe pulmonary artery (arrow 3). The right pulmonary artery continues the left-to-right and cephalad-to-caudad course along the roof of the left atrium (LA). The right upper lobe pulmonary vein (arrow 2) drains into the LA just anterior to the right pulmonary artery. The azygos arch (arrow 4) is seen in cross section as it passes over the right hilum. The proximal right subclavian artery (arrow 5) is viewed in cross section as it passes toward the right shoulder; the left common carotid artery (arrow 6) lies to the left of the trachea (T). The middle left heart border forming the left atrial appendage (arrow 7) is seen draining into the left atrium. The roof of the coronary sinus (arrow 1) is formed by the floor of the LA. The inferior left heart border is formed by the left ventricular (LV) myocardium. The liver (Li) and stomach (St) are labeled.

PULMONARY ARTERY

The pulmonary valve lies slightly out of the axial plane, so it may appear elongated in conventional axial acquisition (Figs. 7, 12, 14, and 37). The caliber of the main PA should be about the caliber of the ascending aorta at this anatomic level. The left PA is the extension of the main PA over the top of the LA (Figs. 3 and 29). When the PA crosses the left bronchus, it becomes the left PA (Figs. 11, 12, 21, 25, 26, and 38). The right PA originates from the underside of the main PA and passes along the roof of the LA posterior to the ascending aorta and SVC to enter the right hilum (Figs. 10–12, 19–23, and 27). The pericardium is reflected over the top of the main PA (Figs. 1 and 15).

PULMONARY VEINS

The upper lobe pulmonary veins lie anterior to their respective pulmonary arteries (Figs. 12, 19, and 21). As the left upper lobe vein courses inferiorly, it passes in front of the left PA and enters the LA immediately posterior to the orifice of the left atrial

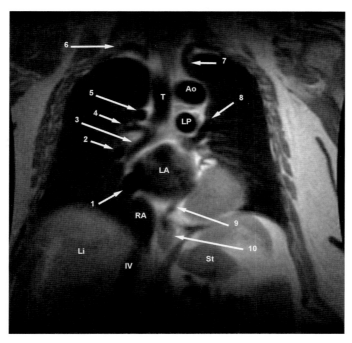

Fig. 21. Coronal double-inversion recovery image (from a 50-year-old woman) through the origin of the right bronchus (arrow 3) from the trachea (T). The aortic arch (Ao) lies to the left of the T. The course of the right (arrow 6) and left (arrow 7) subclavian arteries over their respective pulmonary apices is well seen. The left upper lobe pulmonary vein (arrow 8) drains to the left of the left pulmonary artery (LP) before it enters the left atrium (LA). The right lower lobe pulmonary vein (arrow 1) is seen draining to the inferior aspect of the LA. The right hilum is well demonstrated. The azygos arch (arrow 5) passes over the right upper lobe bronchus (arrow 4) at the level of the right bronchial origin. Incidentally, notice the short course from the tracheal bifurcation to the origin of the right upper lobe bronchus. The right hilar pulmonary artery (arrow 2) is not greater in caliber than its adjacent right bronchus. Embedded within the fat of the posterior atrioventricular ring, the coronary sinus (arrow 9) has not yet entered the right atrium (RA). Immediately proximal to the diaphragmatic hiatus, the distal esophagus (arrow 10) has not yet connected with the stomach (St). The liver (Li) and intrahepatic inferior vena cava (IV) are labeled.

appendage (LAA; Figs. 11, 12, 21, 22). The right upper lobe vein lies anterior to the right PA. It passes from anterior to posterior and inferiorly to enter the LA immediately posterior to the entrance of the SVC into the RA (Figs. 12, 13, 19, 20, 27, and 38). The left lower lobe pulmonary vein always courses in a caudad direction directly anterior to the descending thoracic aorta before entering the posterior left aspect of the LA (Figs. 13 and 28). The right lower lobe vein drains to the right posterior inferior aspect of the LA (Figs. 4, 21, and 29).

LEFT ATRIUM

The LA lies posterior, superior, and toward the left with respect to the RA (Figs. 4, 18, 19, 22, 23, and 27). The two atria share the interatrial septum, which forms an oblique surface between the two. The interatrial septum normally thins in the region of

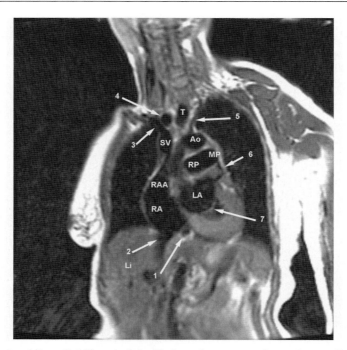

Fig. 22. Left anterior oblique (LAO) sagittal double-inversion recovery image from a 60-year-old woman. In this section, the proximal right pulmonary artery (RP) is seen arising from the main pulmonary artery (MP), passing inferiorly and toward the right, over the roof of the left atrium (LA). Immediately inferior to the MP, turbulence within the mouth of the left atrial appendage (arrow 6) is seen. At this same level, the mouth of the right atrial appendage (RAA) is viewed as well. Notice the left-to-right relation between the LA and the right atrium (RA). The coronary sinus (arrow 1) to the right of the fat of the posterior atrioventricular ring lies medial and slightly superior to the entry of the inferior vena cava (arrow 2) into the RA. The right innominate vein (arrow 3), which lies to the right of the innominate artery (arrow 4) has joined the left innominate vein (not viewed) to form the superior vena cava (SV). The origin and proximal portion of the left vertebral artery (arrow 5) is seen. The mitral valve (arrow 7) is labeled.

the foramen ovale. The LA is just about the same size as the RA. The inner surface of the LA is baldly smooth. The confluence of the left upper lobe pulmonary vein and orifice of the LAA is a redundant endothelium, which may appear thickened in its medial-most aspect. The LAA is long and fingerlike (Figs. 5, 16, 18, 19). Analogous to the RAA, it contains pectinate musculature. However, these myocardial trabeculations are always smaller in caliber than those of the RAA and almost never cross from one face of the appendage to the other. The LAA runs from caudad to cephalad, around the left aspect of the heart, below the level of the pulmonary valve.

The mitral valve lies within the posterior AV ring, immediately subjacent to the circumflex coronary artery (Figs. 22 and 32). Fibrous continuity between the anterior mitral leaflet and the aortic annulus is demonstrated on axial acquisition (Fig. 22).

LEFT VENTRICLE

The LV lies posterior and to the left with respect to the RV; the inflow of the LV lies to the left of the inflow to the RV (Figs. 4 and 30). The LV myocardium is nearly uniform in thickness (1 cm at end diastole) (Figs. 3 and 36). However, in axial acquisition,

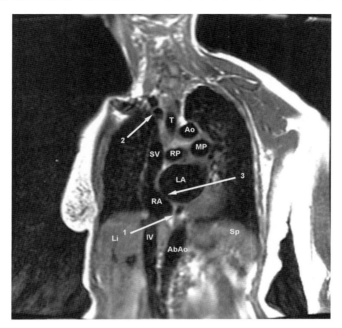

Fig. 23. Left anterior oblique (LAO) sagittal double-inversion recovery image from a 60-year-old woman. The secundum interatrial septum (arrow 3) separates the left (LA) from right (RA) atrium. Inferior to the LA, the coronary sinus (arrow 1) runs in the posterior atrioventricular ring, medial to the entry of the inferior vena cava (IV) into the RA. The superior vena cava (SV) lies in the same plane as the transverse right pulmonary artery (RP). Just to the right of the midline trachea (T), the origin of the right subclavian artery (arrow 2) is viewed in cross section. The abdominal aorta (AbAo) lies to the left of the intrahepatic (Li) IV.

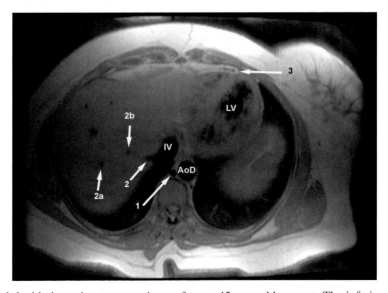

Fig. 24. Axial double-inversion recovery image from a 45-year-old woman. The inferior aspect of the left ventricular cavity (LV) is seen. Below the diaphragm, a right hepatic vein (arrow 2) is seen entering the inferior vena cava (IV). In addition, other segmental hepatic veins (arrows 2a and 2b) are viewed. Note the signal void of the pericardial space (arrow 3) sandwiched between the epicardial and pericardial fat layers. The azygos vein (arrow 1) and descending thoracic aorta (AoD) are labeled.

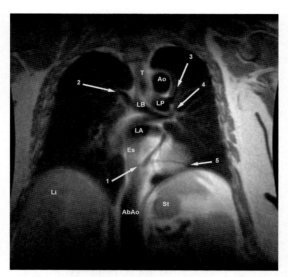

Fig. 25. Coronal double-inversion recovery image from a 50-year-old woman. The morphologic left lung is characterized by the passage of the left pulmonary artery (LP) over the left bronchus (LB). Notice the long course the LB takes before giving the left upper lobe bronchus (arrow 4). Arising from the LP, the left upper lobe pulmonary artery (arrow 3) courses parallel to the Ao. The trachea (T) lies to the right of the aortic arch (Ao). Passing obliquely within the high signal intensity fat of the posterior atrioventricular ring, the coronary sinus (arrow 1) is joined by an inferior cardiac vein (arrow 5) passing along the epicardium of the posterior left ventricular wall. Along the right border, the azygos arch (arrow 2) is seen curving from a paraspinal position laterally to begin to arch over the right hilum. The intermediate-intensity band formed by the anterior aspect of the esophagus (Es) shares the tomographic section containing the back wall of the left atrium (LA). Lumbar spine lordosis pushes the abdominal aorta (AbAo) anteriorly.

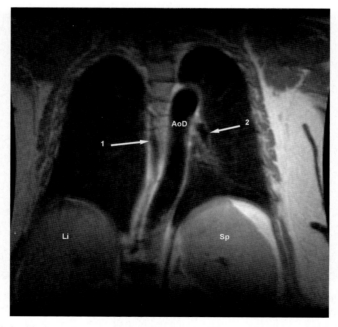

Fig. 26. Coronal double-inversion recovery image from a 50-year-old woman. This plane is posterior to the heart, which is not visualized. The liver (Li) and spleen (Sp) are labeled. The azygos vein (arrow 1) ascends just to the right of the descending thoracic aorta (AoD). In this tomographic plane, the distal left pulmonary artery (arrow 2) is seen.

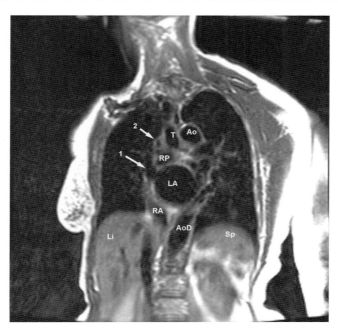

Fig. 27. Left anterior oblique (LAO) sagittal double-inversion recovery image from a 60-year-old woman. The left-sided aortic arch (Ao) displaces the trachea (T) to the right. The right upper lobe pulmonary vein (arrow 1) is seen draining into the left atrium (LA) immediately anterior to the right pulmonary artery (RP) passage over the LA toward the right hilum. Seen in cross section, the azygos vein (arrow 2) arches over the right hilum prior to drainage into the superior vena cava (not seen). The right heart border-forming right atrium (RA) lies inferior and toward the right with respect to the LA and lower descending thoracic aorta (AoD). The liver (Li) and spleen (Sp) are labeled.

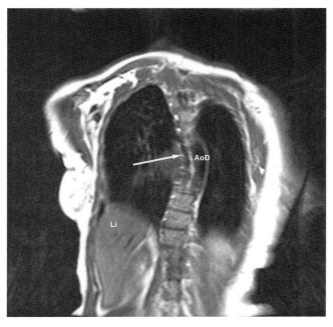

Fig. 28. Left anterior oblique (LAO) sagittal double-inversion recovery image from a 60-year-old woman. The azygos vein (arrow) ascends just to the right of the descending thoracic aorta (AoD).

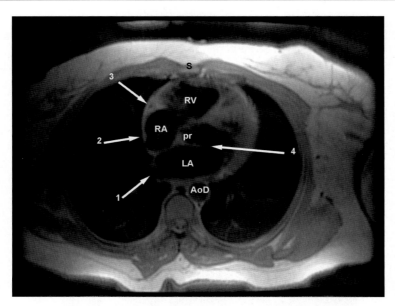

Fig. 29. Axial double-inversion recovery image from a 45-year-old woman. The anterior right ventricle (RV) lies behind the sternum (S). The right coronary artery can be seen in cross section, traveling within the fat of the anterior atrioventricular ring (arrow 3). The crista terminalis (arrow 2) is seen as a high signal intensity object along the lateral wall of the right atrium (RA). The right lower lobe pulmonary vein is seen entering the left atrium (LA). Notice how the anterior mitral leaflet (arrow 4) is continuous with the aortic annulus and posterior right aortic sinus of Valsalva (pr). The descending aorta (AoD) is labeled.

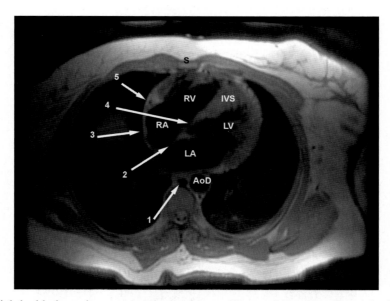

Fig. 30. Axial double-inversion recovery image from a 45-year-old woman. The right (RV) and left (LV) ventricles share the interventricular septum. The anterior aspect of the septum is muscular (IVS). The posterior aspect of the septum contains the membranous portion (arrow 4) immediately inferior to the aortic valve. At this level, the primum interatrial septum (arrow 2) forms the medial aspect of the interatrial septum between the right (RA) and left (LA) atria. The crista terminalis (arrow 3), right coronary artery in cross section (arrow 5), azygos vein (arrow 1), and sternum (S) are labeled.

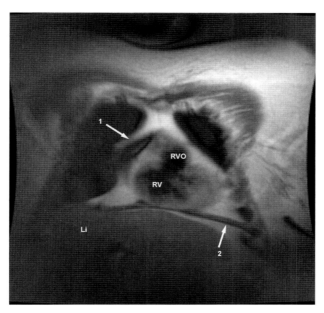

Fig. 31. Coronal double-inversion recovery image (from a 50-year-old woman) obtained immediately posterior to the sternum. The sinus (RV) and outflow (RVO) portions of the right ventricle occupy the retrosternal space. The anterior tip of the triangular-shaped right atrial appendage (arrow 1) is not heart border forming. A small portion of the left diaphragm (arrow 2) is seen. The liver (Li) is labeled.

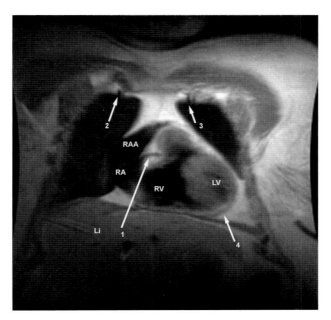

Fig. 32. Coronal double-inversion recovery image from a 50-year-old woman. The cavity of the right heart border forming right atrium (RA), the broad-based and triangular-shaped right atrial appendage (RAA), and the inflow portion of the right ventricle (RV) occupy the anterior of the heart. Here, only a small portion of the left ventricular (LV) cavity is visualized. The pericardial space (arrow 4) just inferior to the cardiac apex is characterized by low-signal fluid and pericardium separating high-signal fat. The right coronary artery (arrow 1) is seen passing toward the right within the fat of the right atrioventricular ring. The right (arrow 2) and left (arrow 3) internal mammary arteries are visualized passing over the thoracic apices toward the anterior chest wall.

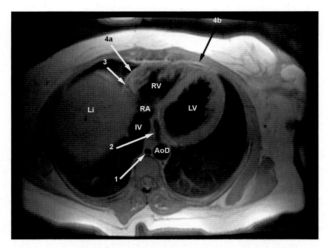

Fig. 33. Axial double-inversion recovery image from a 45-year-old woman. The signal of the right hemidiaphragm and liver (Li) fill most of the right chest. The right (RV) and left (LV) ventricles are separated by the muscular interventricular septum. At this level, the right coronary artery (arrow 3) has turned along the inferior aspect of the anterior atrioventricular ring. The coronary sinus (arrow 2) runs to the right of the fat of the posterior atrioventricular ring, beneath the left atrium (not visualized) and immediately medial to the LV. The inferior vena cava (IV) has passed through the Li and is just entering the posterior aspect of the RA. Note the pencil-thin signal void of the pericardial space (arrows 4a and 4b) between the high signal of the epicardial and pericardial fat. The azygos vein (arrow 1) is labeled.

the posterior LV wall may appear thicker than the septal or apical myocardium (or vice versa) (Fig. 30) because it has been cut obliquely with respect to its internal axis.

Although some trabecular myocardial filling defects may be identified within the ventricular cavity, the LV is characterized by its smooth walls and two large papillary muscles (Figs. 16 and 36). These always originate from the posterior wall of the ventricle. The plane of the interventricular septum is directed anterior to the coronal plane and inferiorly toward the left hip. It normally bows toward the RV (Figs. 2, 3, 15, 30, 32, and 38). The aortic valve shares the fibrous trigone of the heart and is, as described, in continuity with the anterior mitral leaflet (Figs. 1, 5, 7, 29, and 34).

The posterior AV ring also contains the coronary sinus (Figs. 5, 19–23, 25, 27, and 33). This vein lies anterior to the circumflex artery and passes around the ring between the LA and LV to run beneath the LA prior to its drainage into the RA. Before entering the RA, it receives other venous tributaries, which run along the epicardial surface of the heart.

CORONARY ARTERIES

The aortic valve divides the aortic bulb into the three sinuses of Valsalva, named by their anatomic location. The anterior aortic sinus lies anteriorly between the RAA and RV outflow (Figs. 35, 39, and 40). There are two posterior sinuses. The posterior right sinus is the inferiormost sinus, lying above the AV septum and between the right and left atria (Figs. 1, 4, 5, 7, 29, 34, and 41). This is also referred to as the non-coronary sinus; it does not provide an origin for a coronary artery. The posterior left sinus is the most superior in position, lying directly anterior to the LA (Figs. 1, 5, 18, 34, and 40B).

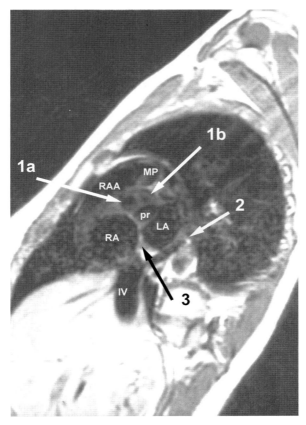

Fig. 34. Short-axis double-inversion recovery image (from a 25-year-old man) through the aortic valve. The anterior (arrow 1a), posterior left (arrow 1b), and posterior right (pr) aortic sinuses of Valsalva are labeled. The coronary sinus (arrow 2) passes beneath the left atrium (LA) within the posterior atrioventricular ring toward the right atrium (RA). The right atrial appendage (RAA) lies anterior to the aortic root. The suprahepatic inferior vena cava (IV) drains into the posterior aspect of the RA lateral to the drainage of the coronary sinus. Fatty infiltration of the interatrial septum (arrow 3) enhances its appearance.

The coronary arteries originate from the aorta, immediately above the sinuses and below the sinotubular ridge, a transition in caliber between the sinuses and the tubular portion of the aorta. The left main coronary artery originates from the posterior left sinus. It usually arises from the upper third of the sinus and takes a slightly cephalad and left-ward course toward the epicardium. It then dips below the LAA and heads back toward the posterior AV ring to become the circumflex artery (Figs. 5, 18, 39B, and 40C). The circumflex artery passes through the posterior AV ring, giving marginal branches along the posterior wall of the LV (Figs. 2, 39B, 39C, 40A, and 40B). Prior to the passage of the left main artery beneath the LAA, the left anterior descending artery arises from the left main. The left anterior descending artery passes behind the RV outflow and along the top of the interventricular septum toward the cardiac apex (Figs. 2, 13, 18, 39A, and 39B).

The right coronary artery originates from the upper portion of the anterior sinus of Valsalva. It takes an abrupt turn toward the right, beneath the RAA, to enter the epicardial fat of the anterior AV ring. It then passes within the ring, between the bodies of the RA

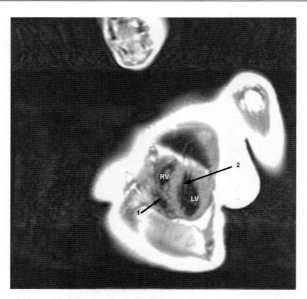

Fig. 35. Left anterior oblique (LAO) sagittal double-inversion recovery image from a 60-year-old woman. The anterior right ventricle (RV) and posterior left ventricle (LV) both share the interventricular septum. Notice how the RV side of the septum (arrow 1) is markedly trabeculated, and the LV side (arrow 2) is relatively smooth.

and RV, toward the cardiac crux, the intersection of the AV rings and interventricular septum, along the diaphragmatic surface of the heart (Figs. 6, 32, 39C, and 40).

The posterior descending artery perfuses the inferior interventricular septum and may act as an important collateral bed in patients with atherosclerotic heart disease. In 85% of individuals, the posterior descending artery arises from the distal right coronary artery; this is called a *right dominant circulation* (Fig. 45).

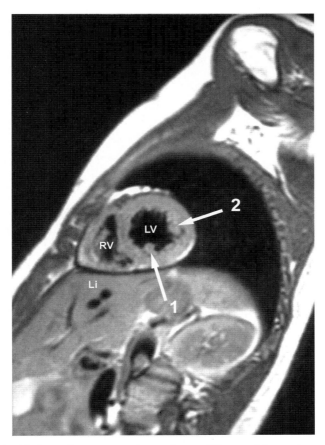

Fig. 36. Short-axis double-inversion recovery image from a 25-year-old man through the base of the left ventricular (LV) papillary muscles (arrows 1 and 2). Notice how the right ventricular (RV) chamber extends slightly inferior to the LV chamber. The liver (Li) is labeled.

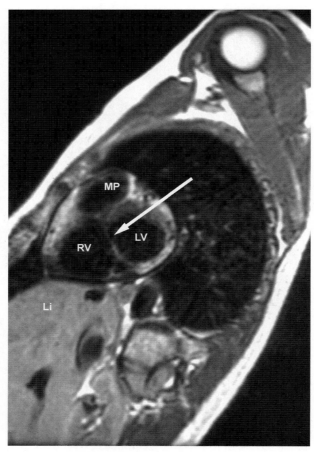

Fig. 37. Short-axis double-inversion recovery image from a 25-year-old man through the posterior interventricular septum (arrow). The main pulmonary artery begins to course from the top of the right ventricle (RV) over the top of the left ventricle (LV).

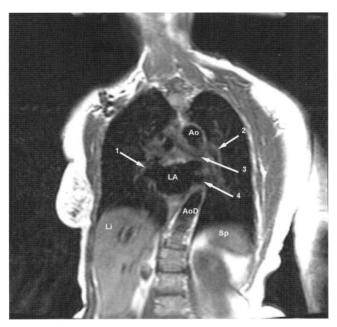

Fig. 38. Left anterior oblique (LAO) sagittal double-inversion recovery image (from a 60-year-old woman) through the distal aortic arch (Ao) and posterior aspect of the left atrium (LA). The right upper lobe pulmonary vein (arrow 1) is seen draining into the LA. The left pulmonary artery (arrow 2) lies superior and posterior to the distal left bronchus (arrow 3). The left lower lobe pulmonary vein (arrow 4) drains into the LA immediately anterior to the descending aorta (AoD), which has not yet entered the abdomen. Liver (Li) and spleen (Sp) are labeled.

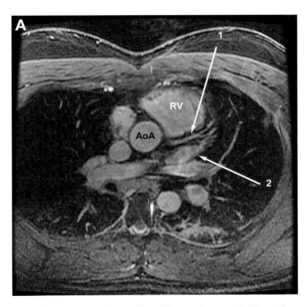

Fig. 39. Axial fat-saturated, contrast-enhanced gradient echo acquisitions from a 45-year-old woman. **(A)** Anterior descending coronary artery (arrow 1) passes along the top of the interventricular septum between the right ventricle (RV) and left atrial appendage (arrow 2). The ascending aorta (AoA) is labeled. **(B)** Image obtained 3 mm inferior to **(A)**. The origins of the left anterior descending (arrow 2) and circumflex (arrow 4) coronary arteries from the left main artery (arrow 1) are visualized. The

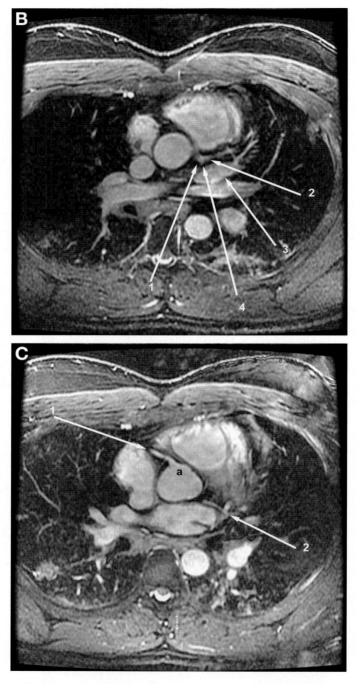

Fig. 39. *(Continued)* circumflex is cut off as it moves out of plane, inferior to the left atrial appendage (arrow 4). **(C)** Image obtained 3 mm inferior to **(B)**. The proximal circumflex artery (arrow 2) passes beneath the left atrial appendage to enter the posterior atrioventricular ring. At this level, the origin and proximal right coronary artery (arrow 1) are seen arising from the anterior aortic sinus of Valsalva (a).

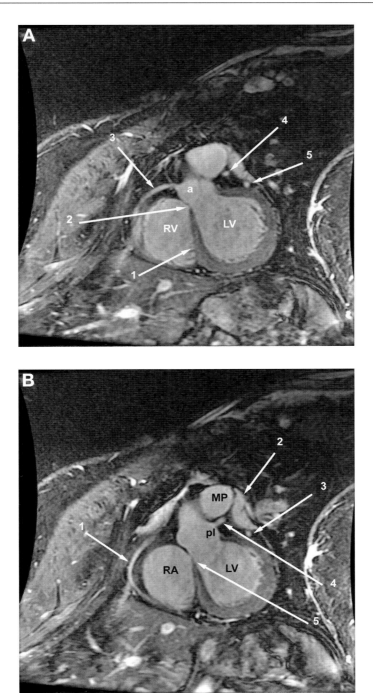

Fig. 40. *(Continued)*

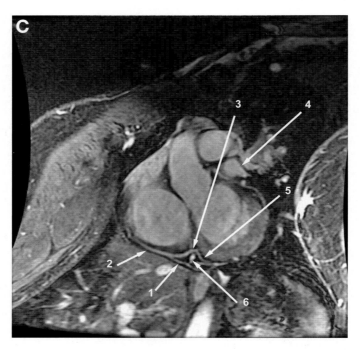

Fig. 40. Left anterior oblique (LAO) sagittal fat-saturated, contrast-enhanced gradient echo acquisitions from the patient in Fig. 39. **(A)** After the right coronary artery (arrow 1) originates from the anterior aortic sinus of Valsalva (a), it passes into the signal void of the fat within the anterior atrioventricular ring. The membranous (arrow 2) and muscular (arrow 1) interventricular septum separates the right (RV) from left (LV) ventricles. Portions of the distal left main (arrow 4) and proximal circumflex (arrow 5) arteries are labeled. **(B)**. Left anterior oblique (LAO) sagittal fat-saturated, contrast-enhanced gradient echo acquisition 4 mm to the left of Fig. 40A. The midright coronary artery (arrow 1) passes through the saturated fat of the anterior atrioventricular ring. Originating from the posterior left aortic sinus of Valsalva (pl), the left main coronary artery (arrow 4) passes behind the main pulmonary artery (MP) toward the left atrial appendage (arrow 2). The proximal circumflex artery (arrow) is seen beneath the left atrial appendage. The atrioventricular septum (arrow 5) separates the left ventricle (LV) from the medial portion of the right atrium (RA). **(C)**. Left anterior oblique (LAO) sagittal fat-saturated, contrast-enhanced gradient echo acquisition 4 mm to the left of Fig. 40B. The distal right coronary artery (arrow 2) is seen passing around the inferior aspect of the anterior atrioventricular ring. In the posterior aspect of the ring, the distal right coronary artery (arrow 3) passes over the coronary sinus (arrow 6) and continues in the posterior atrioventricular ring as the posterior left ventricular branch (arrow 5). Immediately prior to passing over the coronary sinus, the posterior descending artery (arrow 1) arises. The left atrial appendage (arrow 4) is marked.

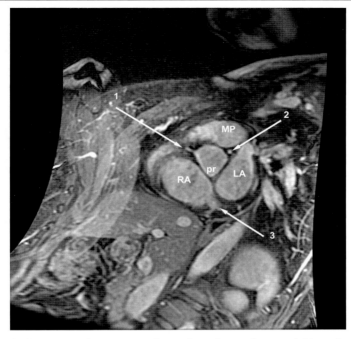

Fig. 41. Short-axis fat-saturated, contrast-enhanced gradient echo acquisitions from the patient in Fig. 39. In this section through the aortic root, the origin of the right coronary artery (arrow 1) is seen entering the anterior atrioventricular ring. Note the relationship among the posterior right aortic sinus of Valsalva (pr), the left atrium (LA), and right atrium (RA). The proximal left main coronary artery (arrow 2) is seen behind the proximal main pulmonary artery (MP). The coronary sinus (arrow 3) is seen entering the posterior aspect of the RA.

4

Normal Left and Right Ventricular Volume and Function

Ralf Wassmuth and Jeanette Schulz-Menger

CONTENTS

In patients with heart disease, quantification of left ventricular (LV) function and mass is important for prognosis *(1,2)*. Cardiac magnetic resonance imaging (MRI) measurements of LV function have already been helpful in the prognostic assessment of patients *(3)*.

SEQUENCES

The standard approach to measure LV volume and function includes steady-state free precession (SSFP) gradient echo sequences *(4)*, with one slice acquired during a breath hold of about 10–15 heartbeats. During each cardiac cycle, a portion of the data is recorded and later fused to form an averaged movie of ventricular contraction. Unlike echocardiography, MRI for clinical application is currently not a real-time technique. The SSFP gradient echo sequences (also known as TrueFisp, FIESTA, or balanced FFE) have replaced earlier versions of spoiled gradient echo sequences, exceeding

From: *Contemporary Cardiology: Cardiovascular Magnetic Resonance Imaging*
Edited by: Raymond Y. Kwong © Humana Press Inc., Totowa, NJ

them in contrast to noise *(5,6)*, endocardial border detection *(7)*, and temporal resolution. Spoiled gradient echo sequences are only used in case of high turbulences when SSFP might result in too many artifacts.

Both fat and fluid appear bright on SSFP images; therefore, the differentiation of epicardial fat and pericardial fluid can sometimes be difficult. Additional T_2-weighted images, delineating fluid as bright signal, might help. Alternatively, more technically demanding ways in differentiating fat from water have been proposed *(8)*. Cine loops might even be acquired after contrast administration, although this will diminish the excellent contrast between bright blood and dark myocardium. Increasing the flip angle can compensate for this effect to a certain extent.

FAST IMAGING

Various techniques are already in use to shorten scan time, including view sharing and parallel imaging. By these methods, more than one slice can be acquired per breath hold. However, compared to standard SSFP, view-sharing SSFP results in underestimation of end-diastolic volume (EDV) and stroke volume, that is, lower ejection fraction (EF) *(9)*. This diastolic underestimation was even more evident using parallel imaging for LV coverage in a single breath hold *(10)*.

However, a single study of 12 volunteers and 8 patients comparing view-sharing SSFP with a temporal resolution of only 91 ms with standard SSFP found no differences in LV size and EF *(11)*. Hunold et al. compared two different ways of parallel imaging for LV cine loops and found more signal to noise and fewer artifacts in GRAPPA *(12)* compared to mSENSE *(13)*. Wintersperger et al. compared single-breath hold acquisition of the whole ventricle using GRAPPA at a temporal resolution of 48 ms with standard segmented single-slice SSFP technique and found no difference in semiautomatically derived LV measurements *(14)*. Other experimental approaches for real-time cine imaging also include radial *(15)* or spiral SSFP *(16,17)*.

POSITIONING

Cardiac imaging requires the precise and reproducible angulation of the imaging planes along the cardiac axes. Therefore, a double-oblique orientation has to be established. The long axis of the heart usually deviates about 40° left from a true sagittal axis and 40° downward from the axial plane. It is important to ensure that the long axis obtained truly hits the apex as any deviation will result in major foreshortening of all further measurements. Most centers use fast scout images for axial slices through the heart, followed by a vertical long axis through the apex and the middle of the mitral valve. Based on this, the true long axis can be acquired. A stack of short-axis slices aligns rectangular to the true long axis parallel to the mitral valve plane.

ELECTROCARDIOGRAM TRIGGER

Apart from performing near-real-time acquisition, most imaging techniques require a robust electrocardiogram (ECG) trigger to run properly *(18)*. Vector ECG has been found less vulnerable to artifacts from the magnetic field *(19,20)*. Alternatively, a pulse trigger can be used for cine imaging. Retrospective triggering is the method of choice as it includes late diastole for better coverage of atrial filling *(21)*. Prospective triggering underestimates true EDV and EF *(10,21,22)*. Considerable variations in the R–R interval and arrhythmias can compromise image quality; however, many patients with atrial fibrillation but sufficient rate control can be scanned with good results.

RESOLUTION

The product of repetition time and numbers of *k*-space lines acquired determines the temporal resolution in cine imaging. With lower temporal resolution, it is less likely to correctly determine true systole; therefore, EF will be underestimated. Decreasing spatial resolution also results in underestimation of EF because of partial volume effect, but to a smaller extent. Typical spatial resolution in a routine scan using SSFP sequences is about 1.5 mm/pixel. This will result in about 5 pixels across the ventricular wall given a wall thickness of 10 mm. We recommend a high temporal resolution of 45 ms or less with a spatial resolution of 1.5 mm/pixel *(23)*.

SLICE ORIENTATION AND COVERAGE

Full coverage of the LV with contiguous short-axis slices is the standard approach for quantification. It does not require any geometrical assumptions and represents complete volumetric coverage. Using fast, low-angle shot gradient echo sequences in infarct patients, Cottin et al. demonstrated that the effect of a 10-mm gap in the short-axis stack on LV EDV and EF measurement was still lower than interobserver variability *(24)*.

However, the definition of the most basal slice with its impact on EDV and EF poses a problem for reproducibility *(25)*. To shorten scan time but ensure reproducibility, Messroghli et al. proposed a "three-out-of-five" approach for assessment of regional function, prescribing five short-axis slices but obtaining only three of them *(26)*.

Alternatively, a radial long-axis approach with 8–10 slices has been advocated for better delineation of the mitral valve plane *(27)*. Interestingly, the long-axis approach resulted in lower variability than the standard short-axis stack for LV volume but not for mass.

Multiplanar volumetric measurements surpass biplanar measurements in accuracy and reproducibility regardless of whether echo or MRI is concerned *(28)*. Still, for most routine studies regarding normal or close to normal ventricles in a high-throughput setting, we consider the acquisition of one short-axis plus three long-axis loops sufficient for assessment of LV size and systolic function.

Friedrich et al. compared biplanar long-axis with multiple short-axis measurements and found good overall agreement between two-dimensional and three-dimensional measurements, although EF was overestimated by biplanar long-axis measurements. Biplanar long-axis measurements were less sensitive to detect LV dilation *(29)*. If dilation or considerable remodeling is present or high reproducibility for follow-up is required, then we prefer the more comprehensive approaches described.

MEASUREMENTS AND EVALUATION

All major hardware vendors deliver dedicated evaluation software for ventricular function analysis. Platform-independent software is also commercially available. Manual tracking of the endocardial and epicardial contours to measure volumes and mass is still the standard approach. It contributes less to variability than planning of the slice position itself *(30)*. For most routine studies regarding normal or close-to-normal ventricles, we consider quantification of two or three long-axis loops sufficient for analysis. This can be done in a few minutes. For grossly abnormal hearts or for precise follow-up, a stack of short-axis images is required. In this case, manual analysis is time consuming. Therefore, more approaches for automatic or semiautomatic contour detection are under investigation but not yet in routine application *(31)*.

Francois et al. compared manual, automatic, and semiautomatic segmentation of LV mass in animals that were sacrificed for ex vivo measurements *(32,33)*. Manual contours were closer to the ex vivo standard than automatic contours, with the latter overestimating the true volume. Not excluding the papillary muscles from the ventricular volume contributes to the problem. We recommend to include endocardial trabeculae and papillary muscles into myocardial mass in short axis as they are hard to differentiate from the wall in systole *(34,35)*. Papavassiliu et al. argued against this approach but for inclusion of the trabeculae in the LV volume because of better reproducibility *(36)*. However, accuracy was not assessed in this study. Large portions of the myocardial wall have a trabecular structure. Even if it looks uniform on conventional magnetic resonance (MR) images, autopsy studies and experimental high-resolution MRI *(37)* reveal the trabecular structure of myocardium. We regard the neglect of trabeculations as an unnecessary oversimplification for the sake of reproducibility sacrificing accuracy. Improving spatial resolution in future MRI will reveal even more trabeculae. There is consensus that, in long-axis measurements, the papillary muscle should be excluded from the wall to avoid overestimation of ventricular mass *(27,29)*.

In short-axis evaluation, the most basal slice has to be defined in a consistent manner. Including or excluding the basal slice will introduce a large variation in EDV *(38)*. The ventricular myocardium in the most basal slice often looks like a horseshoe instead of a completely closed ring. It has been proposed to include a slice if 50% *(39)* or 75% *(27)* of the myocardial ring is visible. Care has to be taken to start with a corresponding basal systolic slice. Because of the longitudinal shortening of the heart, the number of systolic slices will often be one or two less than in diastole.

NORMAL VALUES

Several sets of normal values have been published for cardiac MRI. However, the normal values for SSFP-derived images *(40,41)* differ from those for the earlier gradient echo images *(38,42,43)*. With higher temporal resolution, there is less blurring, and walls therefore appear thinner. LV mass is smaller and LV volume is larger in animals *(32)* and humans *(40)*. Normal values are not absolute numbers but should be indexed to body size.

There is uncertainty whether to normalize for height or body surface area. We recommend normalization for height as this is genetically determined, whereas adjustment for body surface area benefits the obese *(43)*. Alternatively, the fat-free body mass has to be estimated in a cumbersome way *(44)*. Professional athletes have to be evaluated separately as they often show results outside the normal range for the general population, including a mildly increased LV EDV and mildly decreased EF *(45)*.

WALL STRESS

Wall stress is the product of intracavity pressure and size over wall thickness. Dilated, thinned ventricles suffer from increased end-systolic wall stress. Changes in wall stress may be a sensitive early marker for slowly deteriorating LV function. The wall stress can be estimated using LV EDV and systolic blood pressure as a surrogate for LV pressure. Several groups measured regional wall stress using MRI before and after intervention *(46,47)*.

RIGHT VENTRICLE

In contrast to echocardiography and ventriculography, MRI offers full insight into right ventricular (RV) anatomy and function in any orientation. Its complex anatomy, smaller wall thickness, and abundance of trabecular structures have precluded easy quantification like that available for the LV. Reproducibility is therefore lower than for the LV *(48)*.

There is still no consensus about the optimal slice orientation in RV imaging. The published literature predominantly favors short-axis imaging *(42,49,50)* as this is often available anyway for LV measurements. Including the trabeculae into RV myocardial mass, Shors et al. could demonstrate excellent agreement between in vivo canine short-axis SSFP measurements and autopsy *(33)*. However, LV short axis does not equal RV short axis *(39)*. Moreover, it may be difficult to define the proximal and distal end of the RV, that is, the tricuspid valve plane and the infundibulum. At least the tricuspid valve plane is better defined in long-axis or axial slices.

In evaluation of small regional wall motion abnormalities like in arrhythmogenic right ventricular cardiomyopathy, a reduced slice thickness compared to the LV standard might be preferred. Alfakih et al. compared short-axis and axial orientation and found a higher reproducibility for axial slices *(51)*. Arrhythmogenic right ventricular cardiomyopathy protocols proposed the combination of axial and sagittal cine imaging *(52)*. Even in normal volunteers, RV contraction patterns might appear abnormal to the inexperienced investigator; therefore, regional wall motion abnormalities should be interpreted with great caution *(53)*.

LEFT ATRIUM

In diastolic dysfunction, left atrial (LA) size increases as a result of ventricular resistance to filling. Therefore, LA volume has been prognostically important after myocardial infarction *(54,55)* and in dilated cardiomyopathy *(56)*. A comprehensive study of a patient with heart failure should therefore include a quantitative measurement at least of the LA. The traditional way of measuring LA size in a single plane by echo m-mode is limited in accuracy and reproducibility and should be replaced by multiplane or volumetric measurements *(57–59)*. Volumetric stacks of four-chamber view loops *(60–62)* and biplanar *(63)* and short-axis orientation have been proposed for MRI measurements of LA volume.

DIASTOLIC FUNCTION

Compared to echocardiography, MRI currently has limited temporal resolution. Therefore, diastolic function has not been in the focus of MRI research in recent years. Chapter 19 gives an overview about new promising concepts.

COMPARISON TO OTHER MODALITIES

MRI has been extensively validated against the traditional imaging modalites as well as against animal models and autopsy studies *(32)*. It has been accepted as the gold standard for LV mass. The excellent reproducibility of MRI measurements *(30)* results in fewer patients required to detect true differences in LV parameters compared to echocardiography *(64)*. Therefore, MRI is the method of choice to conduct scientific studies of changes in LV parameters as the sample size decreases significantly *(65,66)*. In a multicenter trial, MRI reproducibility was somewhat lower, possibly related to specific problems in one of the reading centers *(67)*.

In large clinical trials, LV function has often been assessed with echo or other traditional imaging methods. For example, the implementation of an internal defibrillator has been recommended for patients after myocardial infarction with an EF below 30% based on echo, radionuclide imaging, or X-ray angiography *(68)*. The resulting numbers for EF might not necessarily translate 1:1 into short-axis-derived MRI results.

OUTLOOK

The heart failure epidemic *(69,70)* will ensure continuous demand for noninvasive assessment of cardiac function. Future technical improvements in MRI will allow image acquisition for the whole ventricle in a single breath hold. With increasing temporal resolution, assessment of diastolic function *(71,72)* and flow-derived estimation of intracardiac pressure will be feasible *(73)*. For further reading regarding MRI assessment of LV function, see recent reviews in the literature *(39,74,75)*. Compared to other imaging modalities, MRI not only assesses wall motion and function but also has the sweeping ability to characterize tissue *(76)*.

REFERENCES

1. Raymond I, Mehlsen J, Pedersen F, Dimsits J, Jacobsen J, Hildebrandt PR. The prognosis of impaired left ventricular systolic function and heart failure in a middle-aged and elderly population in an urban population segment of Copenhagen. Eur J Heart Fail 2004;6:653–661.
2. Solomon SD, Zelenkofske S, McMurray JJ, et al. Sudden death in patients with myocardial infarction and left ventricular dysfunction, heart failure, or both. N Engl J Med 2005;352:2581–2588.
3. Hundley WG, Morgan TM, Neagle CM, Hamilton CA, Rerkpattanapipat P, Link KM. Magnetic resonance imaging determination of cardiac prognosis. Circulation 2002;106:2328–2333.
4. Plein S, Smith WH, Ridgway JP, et al. Measurements of left ventricular dimensions using real-time acquisition in cardiac magnetic resonance imaging: comparison with conventional gradient echo imaging. Magma 2001;13:101–108.
5. Carr JC, Simonetti O, Bundy J, Li D, Pereles S, Finn JP. Cine MR angiography of the heart with segmented true fast imaging with steady-state precession. Radiology 2001;219:828–834.
6. Barkhausen J, Ruehm SG, Goyen M, Buck T, Laub G, Debatin JF. MR evaluation of ventricular function: true fast imaging with steady-state precession vs fast low-angle shot cine MR imaging: feasibility study. Radiology 2001;219:264–269.
7. Thiele H, Nagel E, Paetsch I, et al. Functional cardiac MR imaging with steady-state free precession (SSFP) significantly improves endocardial border delineation without contrast agents. J Magn Reson Imaging 2001;14:362–367.
8. Reeder SB, Markl M, Yu H, Hellinger JC, Herfkens RJ, Pelc NJ. Cardiac CINE imaging with IDEAL water-fat separation and steady-state free precession. J Magn Reson Imaging 2005;22:44–52.
9. Barkhausen J, Goyen M, Ruhm SG, Eggebrecht H, Debatin JF, Ladd ME. Assessment of ventricular function with single breath-hold real-time steady-state free precession cine MR imaging. AJR Am J Roentgenol 2002;178:731–735.
10. Kunz RP, Oellig F, Krummenauer F, et al. Assessment of left ventricular function by breath-hold cine MR imaging: comparison of different steady-state free precession sequences. J Magn Reson Imaging 2005;21:140–148.
11. Lee VS, Resnick D, Bundy JM, Simonetti OP, Lee P, Weinreb JC. Cardiac function: MR evaluation in one breath hold with real-time true fast imaging with steady-state precession. Radiology 2002;222: 835–842.

12. Griswold MA, Jakob PM, Heidemann RM, et al. Generalized autocalibrating partially parallel acquisitions (GRAPPA). Magn Reson Med 2002;47:1202–1210.

13. Hunold P, Maderwald S, Ladd ME, Jellus V, Barkhausen J. Parallel acquisition techniques in cardiac cine magnetic resonance imaging using TrueFISP sequences: comparison of image quality and artifacts. J Magn Reson Imaging 2004;20:506–511.

14. Wintersperger BJ, Nikolaou K, Dietrich O, et al. Single breath-hold real-time cine MR imaging: improved temporal resolution using generalized autocalibrating partially parallel acquisition (GRAPPA) algorithm. Eur Radiol 2003;13:1931–1936.

15. Kuhl HP, Spuentrup E, Wall A, et al. Assessment of myocardial function with interactive non-breath-hold real-time MR imaging: comparison with echocardiography and breath-hold Cine MR imaging. Radiology 2004;231:198–207.

16. Nayak KS, Hargreaves BA, Hu BS, Nishimura DG, Pauly JM, Meyer CH. Spiral balanced steady-state free precession cardiac imaging. Magn Reson Med 2005;53:1468–1473.

17. Narayan G, Nayak K, Pauly J, Hu B. Single-breathhold, four-dimensional, quantitative assessment of LV and RV function using triggered, real-time, steady-state free precession MRI in heart failure patients. J Magn Reson Imaging 2005;22:59–66.

18. Gatehouse PD, Firmin DN. The cardiovascular magnetic resonance machine: hardware and software requirements. Herz 2000;25:317–330.

19. Fischer SE, Wickline SA, Lorenz CH. Novel real-time R-wave detection algorithm based on the vector-cardiogram for accurate gated magnetic resonance acquisitions. Magn Reson Med 1999;42:361–370.

20. Chia JM, Fischer SE, Wickline SA, Lorenz CH. Performance of QRS detection for cardiac magnetic resonance imaging with a novel vectorcardiographic triggering method. J Magn Reson Imaging 2000;12:678–688.

21. Feinstein JA, Epstein FH, Arai AE, et al. Using cardiac phase to order reconstruction (CAPTOR): a method to improve diastolic images. J Magn Reson Imaging 1997;7:794–798.

22. Sievers B, Addo M, Kirchberg S, et al. Impact of the ECG gating method on ventricular volumes and ejection fractions assessed by cardiovascular magnetic resonance imaging. J Cardiovasc Magn Reson 2005;7:441–446.

23. Miller S, Simonetti OP, Carr J, Kramer U, Finn JP. MR Imaging of the heart with cine true fast imaging with steady-state precession: influence of spatial and temporal resolutions on left ventricular functional parameters. Radiology 2002;223:263–269.

24. Cottin Y, Touzery C, Guy F, et al. MR imaging of the heart in patients after myocardial infarction: effect of increasing intersection gap on measurements of left ventricular volume, ejection fraction, and wall thickness. Radiology 1999;213:513–520.

25. Marcus JT, Gotte MJ, DeWaal LK, et al. The influence of through-plane motion on left ventricular volumes measured by magnetic resonance imaging: implications for image acquisition and analysis. J Cardiovasc Magn Reson 1999;1:1–6.

26. Messroghli DR, Bainbridge GJ, Alfakih K, et al. Assessment of regional left ventricular function: accuracy and reproducibility of positioning standard short-axis sections in cardiac MR imaging. Radiology 2005;235:229–236.

27. Bloomer TN, Plein S, Radjenovic A, et al. Cine MRI using steady state free precession in the radial long axis orientation is a fast accurate method for obtaining volumetric data of the left ventricle. J Magn Reson Imaging 2001;14:685–692.

28. Chuang ML, Hibberd MG, Salton CJ, et al. Importance of imaging method over imaging modality in noninvasive determination of left ventricular volumes and ejection fraction: assessment by two- and three-dimensional echocardiography and magnetic resonance imaging. J Am Coll Cardiol 2000;35:477–484.

29. Friedrich MG, Schulz-Menger J, Strohm O, Dick AJ, Dietz R. The diagnostic impact of 2D- vs 3D- left ventricular volumetry by MRI in patients with suspected heart failure. Magma 2000;11:16–19.

30. Danilouchkine MG, Westenberg JJ, de Roos A, Reiber JH, Lelieveldt BP. Operator induced variability in cardiovascular MR: left ventricular measurements and their reproducibility. J Cardiovasc Magn Reson 2005;7:447–457.

31. Angelie E, de Koning PJ, Danilouchkine MG, et al. Optimizing the automatic segmentation of the left ventricle in magnetic resonance images. Med Phys 2005;32:369–375.

32. Francois CJ, Fieno DS, Shors SM, Finn JP. Left ventricular mass: manual and automatic segmentation of true FISP and FLASH cine MR images in dogs and pigs. Radiology 2004;230:389–395.

33. Shors SM, Fung CW, Francois CJ, Finn JP, Fieno DS. Accurate quantification of right ventricular mass at MR imaging by using cine true fast imaging with steady-state precession: study in dogs. Radiology 2004;230:383–388.

34. Marcus JT, Kuijer JPA, Goette MJW, Heethaar RM, Van Rossum AC. Left ventricular mass measured by magnetic resonance imaging: effect of endocardial trabeculae on the observed wall thickness. J Cardiovasc Magn Reson 2000;2:301–302.

35. Thiele H, Paetsch I, Schnackenburg B, et al. Improved accuracy of quantitative assessment of left ventricular volume and ejection fraction by geometric models with steady-state free precession. J Cardiovasc Magn Reson 2002;4:327–339.

36. Papavassiliu T, Kuhl HP, Schroder M, et al. Effect of endocardial trabeculae on left ventricular measurements and measurement reproducibility at cardiovascular MR imaging. Radiology 2005; 236:57–64.

37. Peters DC, Ennis DB, McVeigh ER. High-resolution MRI of cardiac function with projection reconstruction and steady-state free precession. Magn Reson Med 2002;48:82–88.

38. Marcus JT, DeWaal LK, Gotte MJ, van der Geest RJ, Heethaar RM, Van Rossum AC. MRI-derived left ventricular function parameters and mass in healthy young adults: relation with gender and body size. Int J Card Imaging 1999;15:411–419.

39. Alfakih K, Reid S, Jones T, Sivananthan M. Assessment of ventricular function and mass by cardiac magnetic resonance imaging. Eur Radiol 2004;14:1813–1822.

40. Alfakih K, Plein S, Thiele H, Jones T, Ridgway JP, Sivananthan MU. Normal human left and right ventricular dimensions for MRI as assessed by turbo gradient echo and steady-state free precession imaging sequences. J Magn Reson Imaging 2003;17:323–329.

41. Grebe O, Kestler HA, Merkle N, et al. Assessment of left ventricular function with steady-state-free-precession magnetic resonance imaging. Reference values and a comparison to left ventriculography. Z Kardiol 2004;93:686–695.

42. Lorenz CH, Walker ES, Morgan VL, Klein SS, Graham TP Jr. Normal human right and left ventricular mass, systolic function, and gender differences by cine magnetic resonance imaging. J Cardiovasc Magn Reson 1999;1:7–21.

43. Salton CJ, Chuang ML, O'Donnell CJ, et al. Gender differences and normal left ventricular anatomy in an adult population free of hypertension. A cardiovascular magnetic resonance study of the Framingham Heart Study Offspring cohort. J Am Coll Cardiol 2002;39:1055–1060.

44. Whalley GA, Doughty RN, Gamble GD, et al. Association of fat-free mass and training status with left ventricular size and mass in endurance-trained athletes. J Am Coll Cardiol 2004;44:892–896.

45. Abergel E, Chatellier G, Hagege AA, et al. Serial left ventricular adaptations in world-class professional cyclists: implications for disease screening and follow-up. J Am Coll Cardiol 2004;44:144–149.

46. Delepine S, Furber AP, Beygui F, et al. 3-D MRI assessment of regional left ventricular systolic wall stress in patients with reperfused MI. Am J Physiol Heart Circ Physiol 2003;284:H1190–H1197.

47. Setser RM, White RD, Sturm B, et al. Noninvasive assessment of cardiac mechanics and clinical outcome after partial left ventriculectomy. Ann Thorac Surg 2003;76:1576–1585; discussion 1585–1586.

48. Grothues F, Moon JC, Bellenger NG, Smith GS, Klein HU, Pennell DJ. Interstudy reproducibility of right ventricular volumes, function, and mass with cardiovascular magnetic resonance. Am Heart J 2004;147:218–223.

49. Rominger MB, Bachmann GF, Pabst W, Rau WS. Right ventricular volumes and ejection fraction with fast cine MR imaging in breath-hold technique: applicability, normal values from 52 volunteers, and evaluation of 325 adult cardiac patients. J Magn Reson Imaging 1999;10:908–918.

50. Sandstede J, Lipke C, Beer M, et al. Age- and gender-specific differences in left and right ventricular cardiac function and mass determined by cine magnetic resonance imaging. Eur Radiol 2000;10:438–442.

51. Alfakih K, Plein S, Bloomer T, Jones T, Ridgway J, Sivananthan M. Comparison of right ventricular volume measurements between axial and short axis orientation using steady-state free precession magnetic resonance imaging. J Magn Reson Imaging 2003;18:25–32.

52. Tandri H, Friedrich MG, Calkins H, Bluemke DA. MRI of arrhythmogenic right ventricular cardiomyopathy/dysplasia. J Cardiovasc Magn Reson 2004;6:557–563.

53. Sievers B, Addo M, Franken U, Trappe HJ. Right ventricular wall motion abnormalities found in healthy subjects by cardiovascular magnetic resonance imaging and characterized with a new segmental model. J Cardiovasc Magn Reson 2004;6:601–608.

54. Moller JE, Hillis GS, Oh JK, et al. Left atrial volume: a powerful predictor of survival after acute myocardial infarction. Circulation 2003;107:2207–2212.

55. Beinart R, Boyko V, Schwammenthal E, et al. Long-term prognostic significance of left atrial volume in acute myocardial infarction. J Am Coll Cardiol 2004;44:327–334.

56. Rossi A, Cicoira M, Zanolla L, et al. Determinants and prognostic value of left atrial volume in patients with dilated cardiomyopathy. J Am Coll Cardiol 2002;40:1425.

57. Lester SJ, Ryan EW, Schiller NB, Foster E. Best method in clinical practice and in research studies to determine left atrial size. Am J Cardiol 1999;84:829–832.

58. Pritchett AM, Jacobsen SJ, Mahoney DW, Rodeheffer RJ, Bailey KR, Redfield MM. Left atrial volume as an index of left atrial size: a population-based study. J Am Coll Cardiol 2003;41:1036–1043.

59. Tsang TS, Barnes ME, Gersh BJ, et al. Prediction of risk for first age-related cardiovascular events in an elderly population: the incremental value of echocardiography. J Am Coll Cardiol 2003;42:1199–1205.

60. Jarvinen VM, Kupari MM, Poutanen VP, Hekali PE. A simplified method for the determination of left atrial size and function using cine magnetic resonance imaging. Magn Reson Imaging 1996;14:215–226.

61. Poutanen T, Ikonen A, Vainio P, Jokinen E, Tikanoja T. Left atrial volume assessed by transthoracic three dimensional echocardiography and magnetic resonance imaging: dynamic changes during the heart cycle in children. Heart 2000;83:537–542.

62. Hauser TH, McClennen S, Katsimaglis G, Josephson ME, Manning WJ, Yeon SB. Assessment of left atrial volume by contrast enhanced magnetic resonance angiography. J Cardiovasc Magn Reson 2004;6:491–497.

63. Ingkanisorn WP, Arai AE. Left atrial volume assessment by cardiac magnetic resonance. J Cardiac Magnetic Resonance 2005;7:274–275.

64. Grothues F, Smith GC, Moon JC, et al. Comparison of interstudy reproducibility of cardiovascular magnetic resonance with two-dimensional echocardiography in normal subjects and in patients with heart failure or left ventricular hypertrophy. Am J Cardiol 2002;90:29–34.

65. Bellenger NG, Davies LC, Francis JM, Coats AJ, Pennell DJ. Reduction in sample size for studies of remodeling in heart failure by the use of cardiovascular magnetic resonance. J Cardiovasc Magn Reson 2000;2:271–278.

66. Strohm O, Schulz-Menger J, Pilz B, Osterziel KJ, Dietz R, Friedrich MG. Measurement of left ventricular dimensions and function in patients with dilated cardiomyopathy. J Magn Reson Imaging 2001;13:367–371.

67. Hoffmann R, von Bardeleben S, ten Cate F, et al. Assessment of systolic left ventricular function: a multi-centre comparison of cineventriculography, cardiac magnetic resonance imaging, unenhanced and contrast-enhanced echocardiography. Eur Heart J 2005;26:607–616.

68. Moss AJ, Zareba W, Hall WJ, et al. Prophylactic implantation of a defibrillator in patients with myocardial infarction and reduced ejection fraction. N Engl J Med 2002;346:877–883.

69. Redfield MM. Heart failure—an epidemic of uncertain proportions. N Engl J Med 2002;347:1442–1444.

70. Bleumink GS, Knetsch AM, Sturkenboom MC, et al. Quantifying the heart failure epidemic: prevalence, incidence rate, lifetime risk and prognosis of heart failure. The Rotterdam Study. Eur Heart J 2004;25:1614–1619.

71. Paelinck BP, de Roos A, Bax JJ, et al. Feasibility of tissue magnetic resonance imaging: a pilot study in comparison with tissue Doppler imaging and invasive measurement. J Am Coll Cardiol 2005;45:1109–1116.

72. Zwanenburg JJ, Gotte MJ, Kuijer JP, et al. Regional timing of myocardial shortening is related to prestretch from atrial contraction: assessment by high temporal resolution MRI tagging in humans. Am J Physiol Heart Circ Physiol 2005;288:H787–H794.

73. Thompson RB, McVeigh ER. Fast measurement of intracardiac pressure differences with 2D breath-hold phase-contrast MRI. Magn Reson Med 2003;49:1056–1066.

74. Pujadas S, Reddy GP, Weber O, Lee JJ, Higgins CB. MR imaging assessment of cardiac function. J Magn Reson Imaging 2004;19:789–799.

75. Pons-Llado G. Assessment of cardiac function by CMR. Eur Radiol 2005;15(suppl 2):B23–B32.

76. Fuster V, Kim RJ. Frontiers in cardiovascular magnetic resonance. Circulation 2005;112:135–144.

5

Quantitative MRI Techniques in Regional Myocardial Function

Anthony H. Aletras and Han Wen

CONTENTS

INTRODUCTION

Magnetic resonance imaging (MRI) not only depicts anatomical details, but can be sensitized to the movement and deformation of soft tissues such as the muscle of the heart and can provide measurements of tissue motion at high resolution. A particularly useful class of methods for assessing the contractile function of the myocardial wall is displacement imaging. Magnetic resonance (MR) displacement imaging measures the change of position of tissue elements over a period of time starting from a reference time-point. In concept, it is similar to tracking the three-dimensional (3D) movement of implanted radio-opaque markers in cine fluoroscopy, but instead of using extraneous markers, controlled modulations of various aspects of tissue proton magnetization are utilized as noninvasive markers. Advances in phase modulation techniques allow all pixels of an image to be tracked simultaneously and therefore give high-density measurements of tissue motion.

In evaluating regional cardiac function, displacement fields are the basis for computing functional maps of myocardial strain, strain rates, and torsion. Strain represents local

From: *Contemporary Cardiology: Cardiovascular Magnetic Resonance Imaging*
Edited by: Raymond Y. Kwong © Humana Press Inc., Totowa, NJ

deformation and is often calculated from the differences in displacement vectors of adjacent pixels. Torsion and twist of the ventricle generally refer to the rotation of the ventricular wall around its longitudinal axis, and torsion maps are obtained by calculating the rotation of individual pixels.

The first displacement-imaging methods were formulated in 1988 and utilized modulation of the image intensity *(1,2)*. Specifically, radial and linear grids of low signal intensity were created by nulling the magnetization in those locations, which are called *tags*. Tags persist for a period comparable to the T_1 relaxation time and move with the underlying tissue. The displacement vectors of tag intersect points can be quantified by directly identifying their positions in the magnitude images.

Besides image intensity, the phase of the MRI signal can be modulated to allow tracking of individual pixels *(3–5)*. A distinct advantage of phase-based methods is the ability to measure the displacement vector of each pixel. A prerequisite is that the phase value of the spins should be preserved over durations comparable to the cardiac cycle, which is met with the stimulated-echo mode of image acquisition. Such methods are called displacement encoding with stimulated echo (DENSE) *(6,7)*.

In 1998, it became clear that magnitude-modulated, or tagged, images can be processed efficiently by analyzing the concurrent phase modulation of one of the spectral peaks in *k*-space using a method called harmonic phase (HARP) analysis *(8,9)*. Soon, there was a convergence of phase and intensity modulation methods that resulted in the realization that the phase-based approach is effective for displacement imaging in terms of both resolution and automated image processing. Several optimizations for stimulated-echo imaging soon followed, which resulted in artifact-free displacement maps at high spatial and temporal resolution in the human heart *(10–13)*.

The following sections describe the principles of displacement imaging with intensity and phase modulations, technical optimizations in image acquisition, and automated image processing. In the discussion of basic MRI physics in Chapter 1, we avoided as much as possible the introduction of mathematical equations and formulas but focused more on the principles underlying image formation. The state-of-the-art methods introduced here require some rudimentary mathematical approaches, but we minimize our reliance on these. Rather, we focus on the processes the equations represent and how they can be used to enhance our understanding of MRI techniques applied to measuring regional myocardial contractile function.

A REVIEW OF GRADIENT PULSES

Chapter 1 discusses that the magnetization vector, which eventually is encoded in 3D space to create images, is usually observed within the rotating frame of reference. In other words, we choose to focus on the effects of the dynamic fields such as the radio-frequency (RF) pulse B_1 and the gradients G_X, G_Y, and G_Z. We also saw that the application of a gradient pulse along a particular axis (*x*, *y*, or *z*) forces the magnetization on the *xy*-plane to spin faster or slower (i.e., at different frequencies) depending on where the magnetization lies along that axis. The further away from the center of the magnet (i.e., the isocenter), the faster or slower the net magnetization spins. As an example, if a G_Y gradient is applied along the *y*-axis, then the *xy*-plane magnetization at a location *y* will spin at

$$\gamma_0 = \gamma G_Y y \tag{1}$$

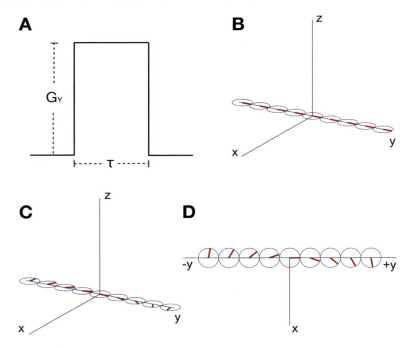

Fig. 1. (A) A rectangular gradient pulse with amplitude (i.e., strength) of G_Y and duration τ. **(B)** Transverse magnetization at different locations along the y-axis prior to applying the gradient pulse; all aligned with the y-axis. **(C)** After the gradient pulse is applied, the transverse magnetization along the y-axis has accumulated different amounts of phase. **(D)** A "bird's eye" 2D view of the transverse magnetization as seen from the top of the z-axis shows that phase linearly accumulates with respect to y.

where γ is the gyromagnetic ratio. Note in Eq. 1 that the frequency of spinning (also known as *precession*) γ_0 is linearly related to the location y where the magnetization lies. As a result of these different spinning frequencies, we expect to have accumulated a different amount of phase φ (i.e., different angle) depending on the location as time passes. This is similar to cars starting from the same point and moving with different speeds; we expect them to be at different locations as time passes. As discussed in the phase-encoding section of Chapter 1, magnetization further away from the isocenter will accumulate more phase. The relationship is also linear, that is,

$$\varphi = \gamma G_Y y \tau \qquad (2)$$

where τ is the duration of the G_Y gradient pulse. Because we assume that the gradient pulse is rectangular in shape for this simple example, the amplitude G_Y of the pulse times its duration τ represents the area A_Y under the pulse (Fig. 1A). So, Eq. 2 is simplified to

$$\varphi = \gamma A_Y y \qquad (3)$$

Equation 3 says that the amount of phase φ accumulated by magnetization located at a distance y from the isocenter is proportional to the distance y and the area A_Y of the gradient pulse that is applied along the y-axis. Figure 1B shows the magnetization before the application of the gradient pulse for $y = -8, -6, \ldots, 0, \ldots, 6, 8$ cm along the y-axis. Figure 1C shows the resulting phase accumulations at the same locations along the y-axis after the gradient pulse of Fig. 1A is played out. Given an applied

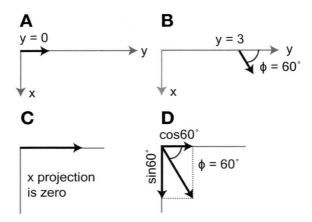

Fig. 2. (A) Following the gradient pulse, the transverse magnetization at $y = 0$ is aligned with the y-axis. **(B)** Following the gradient pulse, the transverse magnetization at $y = 3$ is no longer aligned with the y-axis but rather has accumulated 60° of phase. **(C)** The magnetization at $y = 0$ (Fig. 1A) has a maximal projection onto the y-axis and a zero projection onto the x-axis. **(D)** The magnetization at $y = 3$ (Fig. 1B) has a cos(60°) projection onto the y-axis and a sin(60°) projection onto the x-axis.

gradient area A_Y, note that there is a one-to-one correspondence between location y and accumulated phase φ. Figure 1D shows the same information as Fig. 1C except that this is a bird's eye view of the xy-plane.

Before we subjected the magnetization to the G_Y gradient pulse, all the magnetization was aligned with the y-axis (Fig. 1B). There was no magnetization along the x-axis in this experiment up to that point in time. Something interesting happens after the gradient pulse is applied: magnetization along the x-axis is formed. Let us see why this happens by taking a look at how magnetization that has acquired phase projects onto the x- and y-axes. For example (Fig. 2A), according to Eq. 3, the magnetization at $y = 0$ will accumulate zero phase ($\varphi = 0$) and, because it is aligned with the y-axis, will have a maximal projection onto the y-axis and a zero x-axis projection (Fig. 2C). On the other hand (Fig. 2B), the magnetization at $y = 3$ has accumulated some phase (e.g., 60°) and as such has projections on both the x- and y-axes (Fig. 2D).

From trigonometry (Fig. 2D), we observe that the projection onto the y-axis is given by $\cos(\varphi)$ and the projection onto the x-axis by $\sin(\varphi)$. This is true for all locations, and therefore we can calculate for any location y (via Eq. 3) the accumulated phase φ and from this phase the amount of magnetization projected onto the x- and y-axes for that particular location. The value of this fact will become evident.

Before finishing with this review of gradient pulses and the phase they impart onto the magnetization, it is important to remember that only when the spins are on the xy-plane do they accumulate phase. Whenever the magnetization is along the z-axis, it is protected from any gradient fields, and no phase accumulation occurs.

A BRIEF NOTE ON RADIO-FREQUENCY PULSES

Although the ensuing discussion on RF pulses seems a bit out of place, the following concept is needed for this chapter. Simply stated, an RF pulse has the ability to affect only magnetization that is perpendicular to it; any magnetization aligned with the RF pulse does not respond to i.e., RF pulse. For example (Fig. 3A), if magnetization M is

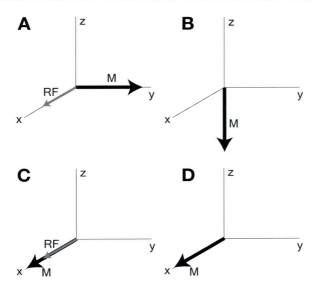

Fig. 3. (A) A 90° RF pulse applied perpendicular to the magnetization M. **(B)** Since the RF pulse is perpendicular to the magnetization M, the magnetization precesses about the RF pulse and ends up along the $-z$-axis. **(C)** A 90° RF pulse applied along the axis of the magnetization M. **(D)** Since the RF pulse is aligned with the magnetization M, the magnetization remains along its original axis and is not perturbed by the RF pulse.

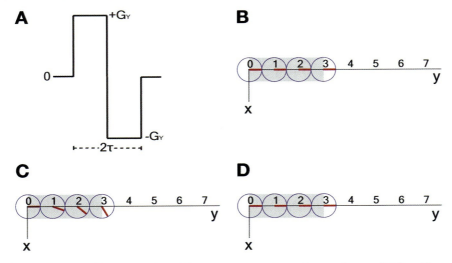

Fig. 4. (A) A bilobe gradient pulse. Each lobe has duration of τ and opposite amplitude with respect to the other lobe. **(B)** An object (gray area) and the magnetization within the object at different y locations before the bilobe pulse is applied. **(C)** After the positive lobe the magnetization at each location within the object acquires phase proportional to y. **(D)** The negative lobe takes away as much phase from each location as the phase given by the positive pulse since the object has not moved.

along the y-axis and a 90° RF pulse is applied along the x-axis, then the magnetization will precess (or spin) about the magnetic field of the RF pulse (on the yz-plane) to move to the $-z$-axis (Fig. 3B). However, if the magnetization M is along the x-axis at the time when the same RF pulse is applied (Fig. 3C), then it will remain along the x-axis (Fig. 3D) because it is aligned with the RF pulse.

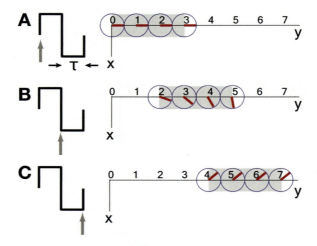

Fig. 5. (A) Before the bilobe gradient pulse is applied the magnetization within the object (gray area) is aligned with the y-axis at all locations. **(B)** After the first positive lobe has finished, the object (moving at a constant speed of 20 m/second) has moved two centimeters to the right. Phase within the object has accumulated as described in the text. **(C)** At the end of the second negative lobe the object has moved an additional two centimeters to the right and its phase is uniform. This phase is proportional to the distance the object has traveled as described in the text.

PHASE CONTRAST VELOCITY IMAGING AND THE BI-LOBE GRADIENT PULSE

The easiest way to map motion, with the intent of extracting information on regional myocardial contractile function, is via the application of a bilobe gradient pulse (Fig. 4A). This bi-lobe pulse consists of two side-by-side gradient pulses that are identical in every respect except for their polarity. Let us see how this works. Assume once more that the net magnetization of an object to be imaged has been brought on the xy-plane and aligned with the y-axis (i.e., right after excitation with a 90° RF pulse has occurred).

Let us take a look at the easiest case and assume also that the 3-cm long object to be imaged (Fig. 4B, gray area) is not moving at all. The application of the first (positive) half of the bi-lobe will result in the object's magnetization to accumulate phase depending on the magnetization's location y (Fig. 4C); the further away from zero, the more phase accumulates. Then, the application of the negative half of the bi-lobe pulse will take away from every location within the object the exact same amount of phase that was just imparted by the positive half (Fig. 4D). This is true only because the object to be imaged has not moved at all, and therefore the phase imparted by the first positive half can be perfectly undone by the second negative half.

For example, if the magnetization at $y = 3$ accumulated 60° of phase in the first half, then it will accumulate –60° in the second half because it has not moved and is still at $y = 3$ while the second half is applied. The net phase at the end of the bi-lobe gradient pulse for the magnetization at $y = 3$ is zero (Fig. 4D). For the magnetization at $y = 2$, the positive lobe will impart 40° phase, and the negative imparts –40° phase. Therefore, the net phase is zero at $y = 2$ (Fig. 4D). It is easy to show that this is true for any location within the object if the object remains stationary throughout the entire application of the bi-lobe gradient pulse. The zero phase in the image tells us that the object moved with zero velocity, that is, it did not move at all.

PC velocity phase

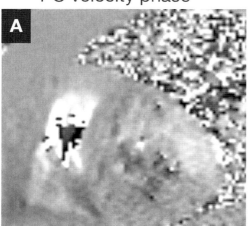

PC velocity magnitude

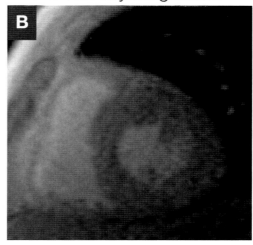

Fig. 6. (A) Phase contrast (PC) velocity phase image. The intensity of each pixel corresponds to the velocity of the velocity of the tissue at that location. **(B)** The magnitude image from the PC velocity scan contains no velocity information but rather anatomical information.

Now let us consider that our object is not stationary but rather is moving along the y-axis. Again, for simplicity's sake, we assume that the object is 3-cm long, and its left-most end is at $y = 0$ (Fig. 5A) at the beginning of the bi-lobe gradient pulse. We also assume that the object will move a total of 4 cm to the right by the time this bi-lobe pulse ends. The bi-lobe interval τ (Fig. 4A) is assumed to be 1/1000 second, and our object is moving at a constant speed of 20 m/second.

Let us focus on the object's leftmost end. During the bi-lobe's positive half, this magnetization will move from $y = 0$ to $y = 2$ (Fig. 5B). Because this is motion at a constant speed, the magnetization will accumulate phase as if it were located on the average at $y = 1$ (i.e., the average of $y = 0$ and $y = 2$). If we use the same phase accumulation numbers from the static phantom example, we expect the leftmost end of our object to have accumulated 20° by the end of the positive half of the bi-lobe (Fig. 5B). During the negative half of the bi-lobe, the left end of the object will move from $y = 2$ to $y = 4$. On the average, it will accumulate phase as if it were located at $y = 3$, that is, –60°. The net phase is +20° – 60° = –40° (Fig. 5C).

We can do the same for the rightmost end of the object, which will move from $y = 3$ to $y = 5$ during the positive half of the pulse, thus accumulating phase of 80° because on the average it was located at $y = 4$ (Fig. 5B). During the negative half of the pulse, the rightmost end of the object will move from $y = 5$ to $y = 7$, therefore accumulating phase of –120°. The net phase of the rightmost end is +80° –120° = –40° (Fig. 5C); that is, it is the same as that of the leftmost end of the object. This can be shown to be true for all the locations in-between the two ends. So, every part of our object carries a phase of –40° at the end of the bi-lobe gradient pulse application. It can also be shown that if it was moving at half the speed (i.e., 10 m/second), then the entire object would have accumulated half the phase (i.e., –20°); if at twice the speed, then the phase would have been –80°; and so on. In other words, the phase the object carries reflects its speed along the axis of the gradient pulse, in this case the y-axis because a G_Y bi-lobe was applied.

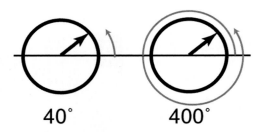

Fig. 7. A magnetization vector that has accumulated phase of 40° and a magnetization vector that has accumulated phase of 360° + 40° = 400° cannot be distinguished from one another.

The equation that governs the relationship between the velocity υ of an object and the observed accumulated phase φ is

$$\varphi = \gamma A_Y \upsilon \tau \qquad (4)$$

or as it is most commonly written

$$\varphi = \gamma m_Y \upsilon \qquad (5)$$

where m_Y is the first-order moment (i.e., area A_Y times the duration τ) of the bi-lobe gradient.

A typical phase contrast (PC) velocity phase image with encoding along the y-axis is seen in Fig. 6A. The brightness of each pixel in the image corresponds to the phase of the magnetization at that point in space and therefore to the velocity of that piece of tissue. Note that stationary tissues are represented by gray; the fastest moving tissues are either black or white depending on the direction of motion. The corresponding magnitude image shown in Fig. 6B ignores the phase information and represents only tissue T_1 and T_2^* properties; that is, it represents the length (or magnitude) of the magnetization vector at that point in space.

It is interesting to note that when it comes to phase we can only detect one cycle of 360°. Phase accumulation of 400° by a fast-moving object, for example, could be interpreted as either 400° or 40° because the magnetization would complete one cycle and end up at 40° (Fig. 7). Phase aliasing occurs in this case, and we can no longer tell these two cases apart. This uncertainty is unacceptable because it can lead to gross underestimation of motion. We therefore keep the gradient moments at levels that allow only ±180° of phase acquisition. This allows for both positive and negative motions to be accurately measured. The encoding velocity υ_{enc} is the velocity that causes 180° phase to be detected. This is the parameter the technologist sets at the MRI scanner. One wants to be conservative and always prescribe a slightly larger υ_{enc} than the maximum velocity expected in the image.

The bi-lobe gradient pulse is not the only reason why spins accumulate phase. In theory, two PC velocity-encoded images with different υ_{enc} can be subtracted to suppress other sources of phase shifts. In practice, however, these other sources cannot totally be ignored. In particular, when slow velocities are measured, large gradient first-order moments need to be used, thus resulting in systematic phase error from eddy currents induced in the magnet's cryostat by the gradient pulsing. This systematic phase error degrades the measurements from the myocardium, which moves relatively slowly (<30 cm/second). Because the phase error is consistent, time averaging

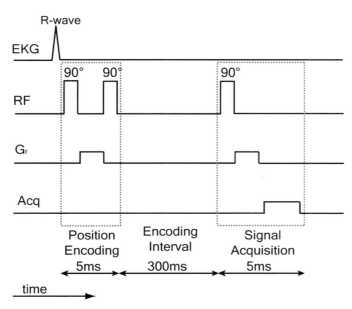

Fig. 8. The stimulated acquisition mode (STEAM) pulse sequence diagram.

of data does not help reduce it. Better actively shielded gradients in the future may reduce eddy currents and allow the use of PC velocity imaging in routine functional cardiac exams.

With current magnet hardware, the development of methods other than PC velocity imaging to assess myocardial motion and contractility (i.e., strain) became important. Interestingly, all these other methods utilize stimulated echoes. Therefore, before describing these methods, we introduce the theory behind stimulated echoes.

STIMULATED ECHOES

Position Encoding

We have seen that gradient echoes (GEs) are generated by gradient pulses, and spin echoes are formed following 180° RF pulses. Stimulated echoes are the third type of echoes in MRI. The stimulated-echo acquisition mode (STEAM) pulse sequence to generate stimulated echoes is depicted in Fig. 8. The basic concept is simple: position encode the entire heart just before systole begins, wait for the heart to move to a new location (e.g., end-systole), collect a short-axis or long-axis image at the new location, and use the previously encoded position information to generate myocardial motion data. Note that Fig. 8 does not show the gradient imaging pulses for the sake of simplicity, and that it is not drawn to scale. In this section, we describe the first part of the STEAM sequence, which deals with position encoding and magnetization storage along the z-axis.

For myocardial motion measurements, the STEAM pulse sequence is played out right after the detection of the QRS complex of the EKG (Fig. 8). Because of the electromechanical coupling delay in the heart, even before the heart starts to contract the first 90° RF pulse (applied along the x-axis) brings all the magnetization from the

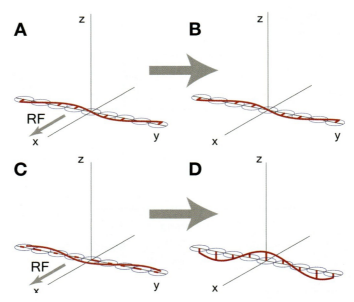

Fig. 9. By applying a G_Y gradient, the transverse magnetization on the y-axis acquires phase and therefore now has both x- and y-axis projections. **(A)** The sine projections of the transverse magnetization are aligned with the x-axis. **(B)** A 90° RF pulse along the x-axis has no effect on these sine x-axis components since it is aligned with them. **(C)** The cosine projections of the transverse magnetization are aligned with the y-axis. **(D)** The 90° RF pulse along the x-axis rotates these cosine y-axis components onto the longitudinal z-axis.

z-axis down on the y-axis. Then, a gradient pulse (e.g., G_Y) is applied, and position encoding is achieved because phase is accumulated according to the spins' position on the y-axis as we discussed earlier. Therefore, at the beginning of systole, if the spin is located at y_1, then phase φ_1 will accumulate according to Eq. 3 as follows:

$$\varphi_1 = \gamma A_Y y_1 \tag{6}$$

Next, the second 90° RF pulse tips the position-encoded magnetization along $-z$. By doing so, it is guaranteed that the encoded magnetization is protected from the decay processes of the transverse plane (i.e., T_2^*, which is on the order of 25 ms in the heart) and only experiences T_1 decay, which occurs along the z-axis. Because the T_1 of myocardium is about 850 ms and the average heartbeat is of the same order, a large portion of the signal will remember the position-encoding process throughout the cardiac cycle. In other words, the magnetization carries with it a phase label, with which it was stamped even before myocardial contraction started. This phase label stamp can be used later in the cardiac cycle to extract motion/displacement information. However, along with this benefit, storing the position-encoded magnetization along $-z$ also has repercussions.

As discussed in the review of gradient pulses, the application of the position-encoding gradient G_Y rotates magnetization vectors that were initially aligned with the y-axis away from the y-axis depending on the magnetization's distance from the isocenter. This creates magnetization components (also known as projections) along the x-axis as well (*see* example in Fig. 2). As seen, the x-axis holds the $\sin(\varphi)$ (Fig. 9A) projection, and the y-axis holds

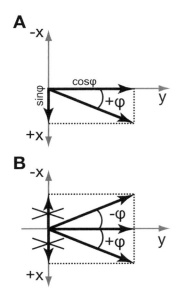

Fig. 10. (A) When both components ($\sin\varphi$ and $\cos\varphi$) are present then a vector is uniquely identified as having phase of φ. **(B)** When the $\sin\varphi$ component of a vector with phase φ is lost then it is no longer possible to distinguish it from a vector with phase $-\varphi$ i.e., from its complex conjugate.

the $\cos(\varphi)$ projection (Fig. 9C) of the magnetization. The second RF pulse is applied along the same direction as the first RF pulse (i.e., along x), and therefore it is aligned with the $\sin(\varphi)$ (x-axis) components and is perpendicular to the $\cos(\varphi)$ (y-axis) components. Recall from our prior discussion on RF pulses (Fig. 3) that only the $\cos(\varphi)$ components of the magnetization will respond to the RF pulse and will be stored along the z-axis (Fig. 9D); the $\sin(\varphi)$ components will not respond in any way and will remain on the xy-plane (Fig. 9B). With the gradient strengths used for typical stimulated echo experiments, half of the magnetization is contained in the $\sin(\varphi)$ (x-axis) components, which decay rapidly on the xy-plane because of T_2^*. Therefore, 50% of the signal is irreversibly lost at this stage, and it is the penalty for generating stimulated echoes.

Storing the position-encoded magnetization along the z-axis and losing the $\sin(\varphi)$ (x-axis) components has one more consequence. Each magnetization vector is uniquely defined by its x-axis and y-axis components; that is, one and only one magnetization vector can be created by combining these components (Fig. 10A). If the $\sin(\varphi)$ components are lost, as is the case with stimulated echoes, then an uncertainty arises regarding the polarity of the vector. We can no longer tell if the magnetization vector that corresponds to the $\cos(\varphi)$ component has a phase of $+\varphi$ or $-\varphi$ (Fig. 10B). Both these vectors have the same $\cos(\varphi)$ but opposite $\sin(\varphi)$; however, $\sin(\varphi)$ and the information it holds has been lost. This is equivalent to introducing the magnetization vector with phase $-\varphi$ in our signal and is usually referred to as introducing the complex conjugate. It will be shown in later sections that, this can be exploited to create tagged images or can be a source of artifacts in DENSE images.

Position encoding and storing of the magnetization with STEAM occurs within 10 ms after the QRS complex is detected. Therefore, the entire process is completed before myocardial motion occurs.

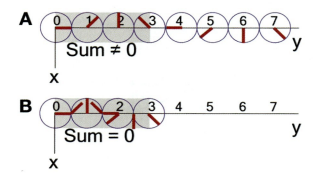

Fig. 11. (A) Prior to systolic contraction the tissue within the voxel (gray area) contains magnetization that constructively adds to create a detectable signal. **(B)** Following systolic contraction the voxel (gray area) contains its original tissue as well as neighboring tissue. In this case the magnetization from these two types of tissue adds destructively and zero signal can be detected i.e., signal loss due to intravoxel dephasing has occurred.

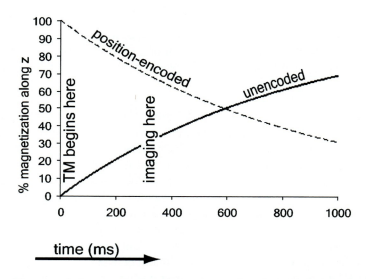

Fig. 12. The position-encoded magnetization that was created at time = 0 forgets the position encoding as time goes by according to T1 decay. At time = 0 there is no unencoded magnetization; however, gradually such unencoded magnetization (FID) appears according to T1 recovery.

The Encoding Interval TM

The next step in the STEAM pulse sequence is simply to wait for a period of time (encoding interval, also known as mixing time [TM]; Fig. 8). This is the time period for which we wish to measure the motion/displacement of the myocardium. During this period of time, several interesting events occur.

The most obvious thing that happens is that, because of myocardial contraction, the heart moves to a new position, carrying with it the phase label that will be used later to extract motion data. However, this motion is not only translational: the myocardium undergoes torsion and contraction to eject blood out of the ventricles. This deformation (also known as strain) changes the shape of the position-encoded tissue locally and can result in signal loss because of intravoxel dephasing when the time comes to acquire the signal.

Figure 11A shows myocardium that has just been position encoded and one of the voxels (also known as a 3D pixel) of our image (shaded area). The three magnetization vectors within this voxel have different phases but overall are constructively adding to produce a signal. As systole occurs, the tissue shortens and changes its shape (Fig. 11B). As a result of contraction, position-encoded magnetization from neighboring locations enters into the voxel. If enough contraction occurs such that the position-encoded magnetization within our voxel spans phases of 360° (i.e., a full cycle), then these vectors add in a destructive manner, and the net signal observed from the voxel becomes zero (Fig. 11B). This dephasing of the magnetization because of contraction within a voxel can create undesired signal loss or be used for measuring myocardial strain, discussed in Intravoxel Dephasing Imaging. Intravoxel dephasing because of blood motion is also responsible for the effective obliteration of signal arising from within the ventricular cavity, resulting in black blood contrast with STEAM.

During the encoding interval (Fig. 8), the position-encoded magnetization, which has been stored along the z-axis, decays exponentially according to T_1 (Fig. 12, position encoding occurred at time = 0 ms). This means that, as time goes by, more and more of the encoded magnetization "forgets" that the encoding took place. As discussed, it is fortunate that T_1 is long enough so that a large portion of the position-encoded magnetization is still available for imaging later in the cardiac cycle (signal is acquired at time = 300 ms).

Also as a result of T_1 relaxation during the encoding interval, magnetization that has no "memory" of the position-encoding process recovers from zero along the positive z-axis (Fig. 12). This magnetization pool carries no phase information with respect to position and is commonly referred to as the FID (free-induction decay), or 0th harmonic for reasons that will become apparent. The FID component is usually undesirable because it carries no information with respect to motion.

Last, as we discussed, during the encoding interval magnetization that remains on the xy-plane decays rapidly with a T_2^* exponential rate constant (approximately 35 ms). If in certain applications the encoding interval needs to be shorter than 105 ms ($3T_2^*$), then crusher gradient pulses can be employed to further suppress its amplitude.

Signal Acquisition

The last part of the STEAM pulse sequence (Fig. 8) deals with acquiring a displacement-encoded signal, that is, a signal that reflects the motion incurred by the contracting myocardium during the encoding interval. The heart has now moved to its new position (e.g., end-systole) at the end of the encoding interval TM and a third 90° RF pulse recalls from $-z$ onto the xy-plane the position-encoded magnetization. A gradient pulse G_Y is applied prior to acquiring the signal. This pulse has identical amplitude and duration as the position-encoding gradient pulse that was applied at the beginning of the STEAM pulse sequence. This second pulse cancels out the effect of the position-encoding first gradient for stationary tissue (e.g., akinetic myocardium). For any tissue that has moved during the TM interval, this cancellation is not possible, and residual phase remains. As we discuss in the DENSE section, this phase reflects tissue displacement over the TM period in a similar manner as the phase in PC velocity encoding represents velocity. The bulk cancellation of the two gradient pulses results in the formation of a stimulated echo.

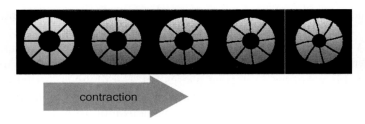

Fig. 13. The original tagging method proposed crushing the signal in selected radial bands perpendicular to the imaged slice. The resulting signal voids were then tracked over time to track myocardial motion.

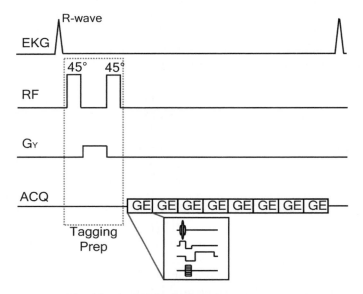

Fig. 14. The SPAMM tagging pulse sequence diagram.

MYOCARDIAL TAGGING

Zerhouni et al. *(1)* presented the concept of "tagging" for the purpose of quantifying regional myocardial function. In principle, multiple images corresponding to different cardiac phases were arranged together in a video loop so that a short-axis view of the beating heart could be displayed. The myocardium was tagged by creating radial dark bands through the heart at the beginning of the cardiac cycle and imaging them with the aforementioned video loop as they moved with the heart (Fig. 13). One can think of these dark bands as coarse virtual ultrasonic crystals that follow the myocardium as it contracts. These bands are in fact areas where the magnetization was purposefully destroyed so it did not contribute to the signal of the video loop images. This drop in signal, which occurs within slices perpendicular to the imaged slice, lasts as long as T_1, which is enough to follow myocardial motion for most of the cardiac cycle.

An alternative tagging method was introduced by Axel et al. *(2,14)*: Spatial Modulation of Magnetization (SPAMM). This new method has been in use since as a valuable research tool and is based on stimulated echoes. Again, the idea is based on creating "signal voids" at the beginning of the cardiac cycle and monitoring them afterward, as they move along

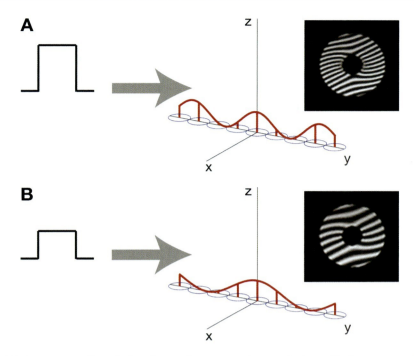

Fig. 15. (A) A strong gradient during the tagging preparation results in rapid phase accumulation along locations of the y-axis, a rapidly changing cosine and, as a result, closely spaced tags. **(B)** A weak gradient during the tagging preparation results in slower phase accumulation along locations of the y-axis, a slowly changing cosine and, as a result, tags that are not as closely spaced as the ones in A).

with the tissue, by means of a series of gradient (GE) echo images acquired at different cardiac phases (video loop). The basic components of the SPAMM tagging pulse sequence within one heartbeat are seen in Fig. 14.

Recalling our discussion on generating stimulated echoes, note that the first part of SPAMM is almost identical with the first part of the STEAM pulse sequence (Fig. 8). The idea once more is to position encode the magnetization and store it along the z-axis. Also, recall from our discussion that as we store the position-encoded magnetization, we lose the x-axis magnetization components (Fig. 9B). The y-axis magnetization that is stored corresponds to the $\cos(\varphi)$ projections of the magnetization, which has acquired different amounts of phase φ along the y-axis. Therefore, by definition, different locations on the y-axis have different amounts of signal stored according to a cosine function; in other words, the stored magnetization with SPAMM is spatially modulated by a cosine (Fig. 15A). How fast the cosine is changing along the y-axis depends on how fast phase accumulates along that direction, which in turn depends on the strength of the position-encoding gradient pulse (Fig. 15B). The "mountain tops" of the cosine function will eventually yield high signal in the image, and the "valleys" will represent areas of dark bands in the image. Therefore, the strength of position-encoding gradient controls the tag spacing in the image.

Note that there is a major difference between the stored magnetization in Fig. 15A and that shown in Fig. 9D: the magnetization in Fig. 15A is all positive; that in Fig. 9C is symmetrically set about $z = 0$, and it has both positive and negative values. For SPAMM, we will reconstruct conventional magnitude images that strip off the sign and phase of the magnetization but preserve the length of the magnetization vector only. Therefore, it

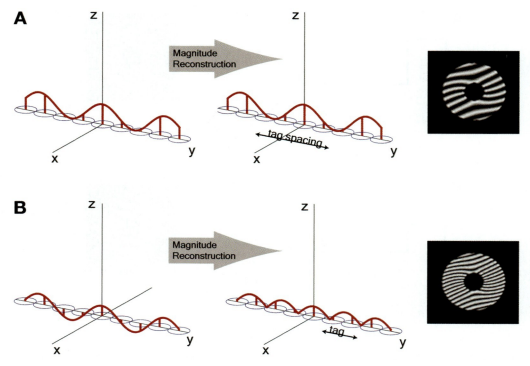

Fig. 16. (A) SPAMM with 45° RF pulses during the tagging preparation results in magnetization that is positive at all *y* locations. Magnitude reconstruction, which strips the sign of the magnetization, does not alter the tag spacing. **(B)** SPAMM with 90° RF pulses during the tagging preparation results in magnetization that is positive at some *y* locations and negative at others. Magnitude reconstruction, which strips the sign of the magnetization, results in undesirable altered tag spacing.

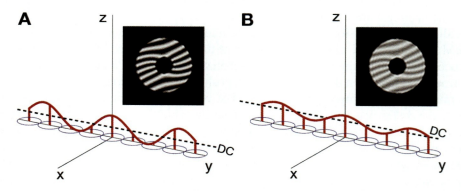

Fig. 17. (A) SPAMM with 45° RF pulses during the tagging preparation results in a DC offset such that the position encoded magnetization (i.e., the cosine pattern) is all positive right after the preparation is applied. **(B)** At a time point later, the unencoded DC offset grows due to T1 recovery and the position encoded cosine shrinks due to T1 decay. This results in tag fading over time.

is important to have only positive stored magnetization (Fig. 16A) so that the valleys of the sine will correspond to zero signal (i.e., dark bands). Otherwise, the cosine will lose its sign during magnitude image reconstruction, the negative values will be converted into positive ones, and the cosine will appear to have a different tag spacing (Fig. 16B).

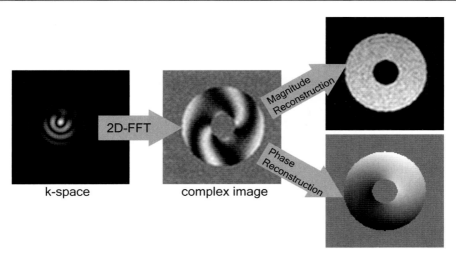

Fig. 18. The complex raw 2D data collected from an imaging experiment (i.e., k-space) is Fourier transformed to produce a complex image (i.e. an image that contains information about the magnetizations's amplitude and phase). If magnitude reconstruction is performed then a magnitude image is obtained. With phase reconstruction, the phase of the magnetization is visualized.

Unless other methods that can handle such data sets are applied *(15,16)*, this is undesirable. This is why with SPAMM (Fig. 14) 45° RF pulses are used to prepare the magnetization instead of the 90° pulses used with STEAM (Fig. 8). This way, part of the magnetization is never position encoded with the 45° pulses and acts as an offset (Direct Component (DC) offset) for the cosine to ride on it so it does not have negative values.

The positive-only cosine (Fig. 17A) is the sum of a conventional STEAM-like cosine and this DC offset (Fig. 17A, dashed line) generated by the 45° RF tag preparation pulses in SPAMM. Note that this DC component carries no position information but rather facilitates the extraction of meaningful position-encoded information from the cosine. After the SPAMM position encoding is completed, T_1 relaxation occurs as with STEAM as time passes. The cosine position-encoded magnetization will decay exponentially (Fig. 12), and the tags will fade as a result (i.e., the cosine will shrink) (Fig. 17B). Also, T_1 recovery will result in more unencoded magnetization to relax along the z-axis, therefore adding to the existing unencoded DC component of the SPAMM images (i.e., the DC offset will become larger) (Fig. 17B). As a result, the tag valleys will no longer be at zero, therefore making the analysis of SPAMM images more cumbersome. Methods have been introduced to suppress the DC component in SPAMM imaging *(15,16)*. Eventually, because of T_1 relaxation, the position-encoded cosine will become zero, and the unencoded DC component will become maximal; that is, the tags will no longer exist in the acquired images.

Once a video loop with tag lines is obtained, the tags are usually tracked with automated or semiautomated software packages to record their motion over the cardiac cycle. Because the tag spacing (about 5 mm) is on the order of the myocardial wall thickness, only a few of these measurements can be made within the imaged slice. Therefore, these measurements are commonly interpolated parametrically within a model of the heart (usually an ellipsoid) and processed to yield local strain (also called deformation) measurements that show if the myocardium is contracting locally *(17,18)*.

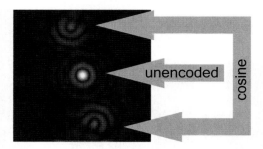

Fig. 19. Typical *k*-space encountered with a SPAMM tagging acquisition. The center peak corresponds to the unencoded magnetization (DC offset). The two outer peaks correspond to the cosine position encoded magnetization.

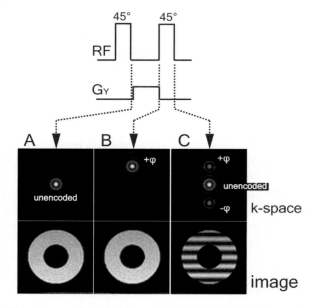

Fig. 20. Demonstration of how *k*-space and images would look like if data had been acquired at different time points of the SPAMM tagging preparation. **(A)** Following the first RF pulse all magnetization is position-unencoded. **(B)** The position encoding gradient encodes transverse magnetization and simply shifts *k*-space. A portion of the magnetization is still along the *z*-axis and remains unencoded. **(C)** As the magnetization gets stored along the *z*-axis *k*-space contains three peaks and tagging signal voids appear in the image.

SPATIAL MODULATION OF MAGNETIZATION TAGGING AND *k*-SPACE

Although SPAMM tagging can be explained by focusing on the cosine spatial modulation generated during the position-encoding part of the pulse sequence (Figs. 8, 16, 17), there are merits to looking at the same process from a *k*-space rather than an image perspective. This description helps with the introduction of the remaining techniques in this chapter and also enhances our understanding of stimulated echoes and their uses.

We introduced in Chapter 1 the concept of *k*-space. To recap, *k*-space contains the raw data we acquire with an imaging pulse sequence (Fig. 18). When Fourier

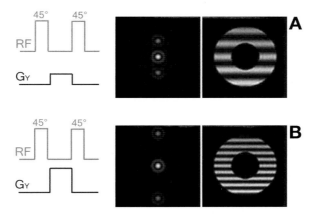

Fig. 21. (A) A weak encoding gradient during the SPAMM tagging preparation results in peaks that are relatively close to each other and, as a result, tags that are not close to each other. (Compare to Fig. 16A) **(B)** A stronger encoding gradient during the SPAMM tagging preparation results in peaks that are further apart from each other and, as a result, reduced tag that spacing. (Compare to Fig. 16B)

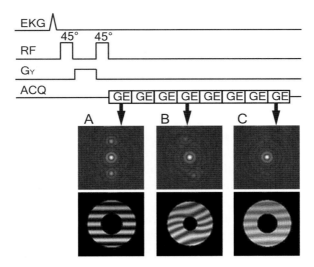

Fig. 22. (A) Prior to systolic contraction (i.e., right after the SPAMM tagging preparation) the three *k*-space peaks result in optimal tag definition and no tag deformation. **(B)** At end-systole the position-encoded outer *k*-space peaks have decayed and the center unencoded peak has grown resulting in tag fading. The tags reflect myocardial contraction. **(C)** At the end of the cardiac cycle the outer position-encoded peaks have further decayed and the center peak further grown. As a result, the tags in the image have faded even more. Since the heart has returned to its initial position at the end of the cardiac cycle no contraction is observed relative to the beginning of the cardiac cycle.

transformed in two dimensions, *k*-space yields the desired complex image. If the magnitude is reconstructed, then we get a magnitude image (e.g., an image that is T_1 weighted). If the phase is extracted by the reconstruction software, then we get a phase image (e.g., a PC-velocity encoded image). Note that most of the signal in *k*-space is concentrated at its center, which corresponds to bulk contrast in the resulting image. The outer edges of *k*-space have less energy and correspond to the small details in the image (i.e., edge definition).

The application of the SPAMM position-encoding preparation (Fig. 14) yields a slightly different k-space (Fig. 19) from that of a conventional image (Fig. 18): instead of having one bright peak, there are three peaks with SPAMM. Without going into mathematical details, the center peak corresponds to the unencoded magnetization, that is, the DC offset we saw in Fig. 17. The two outer peaks correspond to the cosine position-encoded magnetization. These three peaks arise as a result of the position-encoding gradient pulse and the way this magnetization is stored along the z-axis.

With the SPAMM tagging preparation (Fig. 20), right after the first RF pulse there is only unencoded magnetization, and therefore k-space would look normal (Fig. 20A). The position-encoding gradient pulse shifts this peak away from the center (Fig. 20B); the stronger the gradient, the more it shifts. Storing the magnetization along the z-axis creates the phase uncertainty we discussed with STEAM (Fig. 10), that is, the introduction of the complex conjugate with phase $-\varphi$ as a result of losing the x-axis projections. In k-space, this appears as a new peak that is a mirror image of the existing peak, located symmetrically about the center of k-space (Fig. 20C). One can think of this process as taking a copy of the k-space with the one peak, flipping it like a burger, and adding it to the unflipped one. Because the magnetization was not all position encoded (see discussion of 45° vs 90° RF pulses), these two encoded peaks are added to yet another k-space, which is not shifted away from the center because this magnetization never experienced the position-encoding gradient (Fig. 20C). This happens as the magnetization is stored along $-z$. It is the interaction of these three k-space peaks that produces the tagging pattern in SPAMM. Think of it as interference between the three k-space peaks that produces the cosine tagging pattern in the images. None of these peaks alone would create the familiar tagging pattern. Note also in Fig. 20C that the tags are not yet deformed because the myocardium has not contracted yet.

Figure 21 shows two gradient pulses of different strengths applied during the tag preparation period for creating tagging patterns and their corresponding k-spaces. Note that the stronger the gradient, the further shifted are the position-encoded peaks, and the closer the tag-spacing is. This is because the interference between the peaks occurs at the outer edges of k-space.

Figure 22 shows k-space as it evolves because of T_1 relaxation. Note that right after the preparation has finished the relevant contribution of the three peaks results in well-defined dark bands (Fig. 22A). By end-systole (Fig. 22B), the position-encoded peak and its mirror image have decayed, and the center unencoded peak rises, therefore resulting in tag fading. At the end of the heartbeat (Fig. 22C), the center unencoded peak dominates, and little tagging is left in the image (compare Fig. 22 to Fig. 17).

In conclusion, the tagging lines seen in SPAMM images are created by interactions between k-space peaks. The tag spacing as well as the tag fading over time can be visualized both in the image and by looking at the relevant k-space peaks. These observations prove useful in the next sections, particularly in describing HARP imaging.

DISPLACEMENT ENCODING WITH STIMULATED ECHOES

We discussed that a systematic phase error is added to the phase in PC velocity imaging. This has been a limiting factor in measuring myocardial motion with this method. There are two ways one could potentially devise to improve the quality of phase measurements. One would be to minimize the systematic phase error by improving the hardware of the MRI scanner, in particular its gradient coil characteristics. However, such

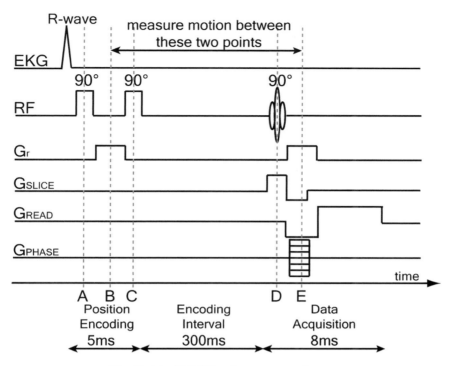

Fig. 23. The DENSE pulse sequence diagram.

improvements are expensive and usually compromise other specifications of the scanner, such as the space available for the patient. The other is to measure, instead of velocities, the displacement of the myocardial tissue over a longer period of time such that the systematic error becomes a smaller portion of the overall measurement.

DENSE relies on this second approach by utilizing the STEAM pulse sequence for the sole purpose of measuring displacement and strain *(6,7)*. Displacement by definition is the change of position over a period of time. Knowledge of displacement also enables us to reliably track material points in 3D space over time, which is a necessary step in observing temporal behavior of functional measures such as strain.

The DENSE pulse sequence is shown in Fig. 23. Motion encoding occurs in general along any direction r (where r can be any one of the x-, y-, or z-directions). DENSE utilizes the phase information of the STEAM pulse sequence to measure myocardial motion. As soon as the R-wave of the EKG is detected, the spins are tipped onto the xy-plane (Fig. 23A), and the entire heart is position encoded by a gradient pulse G_r (Fig. 23B). As with STEAM, if the tissue of interest is at location r_1 at the time when the position-encoding gradient pulse G_r is applied, then according to Eq. 6, the tissue would be position encoded by accumulating phase φ_1 of

$$\varphi_1 = \gamma A_y r_1 \tag{7}$$

Then, the encoded magnetization is stored along $-z$ by the second RF pulse (Fig. 23C), where it is protected from T_2^* decay. Note that this carries the consequences we talked about when describing STEAM (i.e., loss of 50% of signal, generation of complex conjugate k-space peak). At the time-point in the cardiac cycle where we want to measure

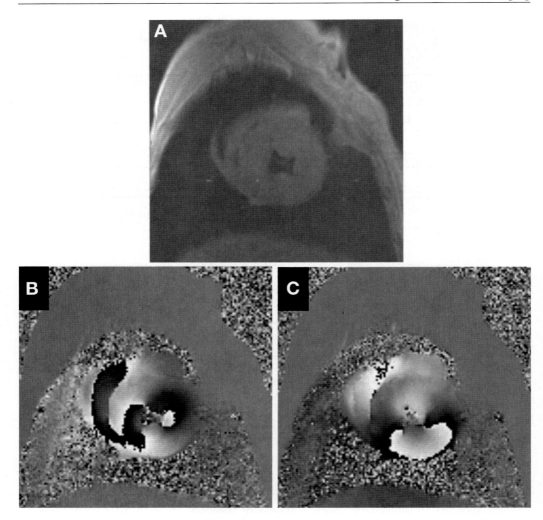

Fig. 24. (A) The magnitude DENSE image contains only anatomical information. **(B)** This phase image contains data with respect to motion along the *x*-axis. **(C)** This phase image contains data with respect to motion along the *y*-axis.

displacement relative to the R-wave (e.g. end-systole), a third RF pulse (Fig. 23D) recalls the position-encoded magnetization onto the *xy*-plane as part of an imaging sequence, which involves slice selection, frequency, and phase encoding. However, prior to acquiring the stimulated echo with the imaging sequence, a pulse identical to the position-encoding gradient pulse G_r is played out (Fig. 23E). If the tissue of the slice to be imaged is now at a new location r_2, then it would accumulate phase φ_2 of

$$\varphi_2 = \gamma A_y r_2 \tag{8}$$

The total phase φ_{TOTAL} that the tissue would accumulate would be $\varphi_2 - \varphi_1$ rather than the sum of the phases. The reason is that the second and third RF 90° pulse have changed the sign of φ_1 because they act collectively as an 180° pulse. This is similar to what we saw with spin echoes. Therefore, phase will reflect myocardial motion according to the following equation:

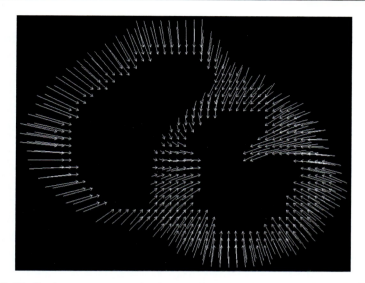

Fig. 25. 2D displacement arrow plot derived from the phase maps shown in Fig. 24.

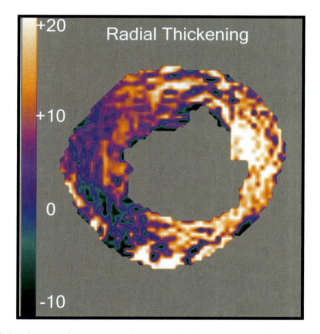

Fig. 26. Radial thickening strain computed automatically from the displacement plot of Fig. 25. White zones correspond to normally contracting myocardium and black zones show contractile abnormalities.

$$\varphi_{TOTAL} = \gamma A_y \delta \tag{9}$$

where δ is the distance $r_2 - r_1$ that the tissue moved. In other words, the tissue is displacement encoded because the phase of each myocardial pixel in the DENSE image is proportional to the displacement δ the tissue within of that pixel.

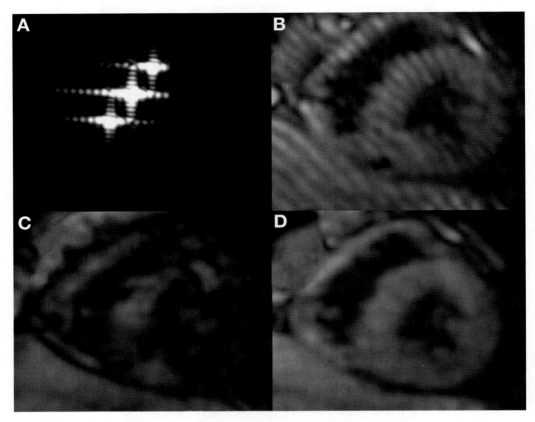

Fig. 27. (A) Unwanted DC and complex conjugate *k*-space peaks during a DENSE experiment. **(B)** The interaction of the three *k*-space peaks results in tagging artifacts. **(C)** Stronger position encoding gradients can reduce the tagging artifacts at the expense of signal losses due to intravoxel dephasing. **(D)** Tag-free DENSE images without intravoxel dephasing losses can be acquired with weak position encoding gradients by suppressing the DC and complex conjugate *k*-space peaks via inversion pulses or RF phase cycling.

A typical DENSE magnitude image is shown in Fig. 24A and provides no motion information. A DENSE phase image is shown in Fig. 24B. This particular phase image shows motion along the *x*-axis. Note that, because of regional contraction, the myocardium shows values other than gray, which reflects zero motion. In contrast, the chest wall, which is stationary, appears gray. For 2D in-plane motion measurements, another DENSE phase map with encoding along the *y*-axis was acquired (Fig. 24C).

The combination of the two phase maps yields a displacement plot (Fig. 25) in which each arrowtail corresponds to the position of a pixel at the beginning of systole and each arrowhead to the final position at end-systole. Because each pixel carries its own displacement information, there are numerous measurements made within the myocardium. This is different from SPAMM tagging, for which one has to rely on few tag lines across the myocardial wall to extract motion data. Also, with DENSE, data processing is automated and rapid without need of data modeling.

Strain computed from DENSE displacement images is usually provided along the circumferential and radial directions. These strain maps show how much a portion of the myocardium shortened in the circumferential direction and how much it thickened along the radial direction as a result of local contractile action. Normally, contracting myocardium (Fig. 26) should exhibit strain of about 20% along both directions (white part of the scale), and abnormal myocardium would exhibit reduced strain (black part of the scale).

For DENSE images to be artifact free, it is imperative that only one peak in k-space is sampled, and that there is no interaction with other k-space peaks. However, DENSE is based on STEAM; therefore, the DC and complex conjugate peaks also exist. We saw that the interaction of the three k-space peaks (Fig. 27A) results in tag lines in the image (Fig. 27B). Although this is desirable in SPAMM tagging, it is highly undesirable in DENSE because it causes dark areas where the phase cannot be measured, and therefore no motion measurements can be made.

The tag line artifact in DENSE can be suppressed by using a strong position-encoding gradient, which shifts the unwanted two peaks out of k-space. This produces tag-free DENSE phase images (Fig. 27C). However, because of the strong gradients used, intravoxel dephasing (Fig. 11) causes signal losses in areas where there is a lot of local myocardial contraction.

Two alternatives to using strong gradients for suppressing the unwanted k-space peaks were proposed early on with the inception of DENSE *(10)*. These are the use of an inversion pulse and RF phase cycling and have been shown to produce quality DENSE images (Fig. 27D) without local signal losses *(11–13)*. Combinations of these methods have been shown to work well with Sensitivity Encoding (SENSE) acceleration *(19)* and navigator techniques *(20)* to bring DENSE closer to routine clinical applications.

DENSE is capable of acquiring one *(11)* or more cardiac phases *(20,21)* of displacement measurements. Each approach has its own pros and cons. It is important to realize that once the magnetization is position encoded at the beginning of the cardiac cycle it becomes a valuable commodity. In fact, storing the encoded magnetization along the z-axis costs 50% in signal, and T_1 decay causes additional signal loss as time goes by. The position-encoded magnetization also decays as part of the image formation process, and once used up one has to wait until the next heartbeat when the process begins anew.

If multiple images are to be formed at different cardiac phases, then the position-encoded magnetization has to be divided among those images. This results in images with lower signal-to-noise ratio (SNR). In other words, the displacement measurements become noisier and less reliable. Spatial and temporal smoothing *(22)* can be employed to lessen the effect. Also, methods have been proposed that combine the DENSE-encoded stimulated echo with its complex conjugate for improving the SNR *(23)*. However, overall strain measurements obtained from such multiphase methods are of lower resolution and noisier unless longer acquisitions are used *(20)*.

An alternative is to sacrifice temporal resolution and collect only one image with high resolution and high SNR at end-systole *(12)*. Such images possess enough SNR so that they can be further accelerated, and data collection can be within a reasonable breath hold for patient scans *(19)*. The final choice between multiphase and single-phase DENSE should be made depending on the specific application.

For obtaining serial displacement measurements over time, there are two modes of DENSE: cine and tissue-tracking modes. In cine mode, a single displacement encoding unit at the beginning of the cardiac cycle is followed by a series of image acquisition units, each unit corresponding to a measurement at a point in time. The image acquisition unit can be one of a few types, including GE and fully balanced steady-state

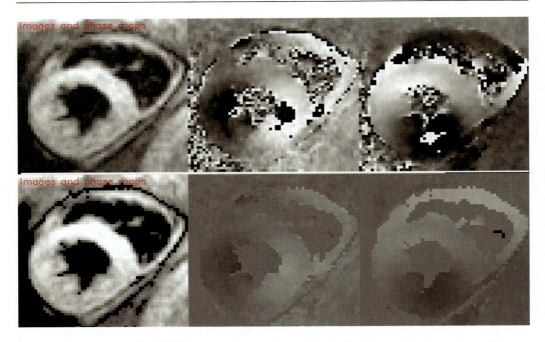

Fig. 28. The top row of DENSE images shows phase noise in the left ventricular cavity and lungs. Also, phase wrapping can be seen within the myocardium. The bottom row shows that the phase maps, after automatic data processing, are phase unwrapped and that a mask properly identifying myocardial tissue has been placed.

free precession (SSFP) readouts. These readout methods refer to different ways in which the encoded magnetization is divided and imaged over serial time-points. The GE readout is less affected by off-resonance effects from either main field heterogeneity or chemical shift, and therefore suitable for both normal and high-field scanners. It is, however, less efficient in the use of encoded magnetization because the portion used by each readout unit is discarded. The fully balanced SSFP readout is efficient in the use of the encoded magnetization because each readout unit refocuses the magnetization for subsequent use. However, it is affected by off-resonance effects and less suited for high-field scanners.

In tissue-tracking mode, the image acquisition occurs at a fixed time during the cardiac cycle; the displacement-encoding step is performed at a series of time-points. Image acquisition can again take different forms, including GE or fully balanced SSFP. A train of echoes is acquired after each encoding step, which improves both imaging speed and efficiency in the utilization of the encoded magnetization. The acquisition period may span up to 100 ms and is usually placed in a period of minimal motion, such as end-systole or end-diastole.

Each of the two modes of multiphase DENSE imaging has its advantages. Cine mode imaging is often faster when a large number of time-points are needed, but the encoded magnetization is shared among these time-points and the resolution or SNR of the images can be limited. Tissue-tracking mode generally takes longer when many time-points are needed but results in better resolution or higher SNR.

A principle distinction between the two modes concerns tracking material points in the 3D space. In cine mode, the displacement field is measured in Eulerian coordinates,

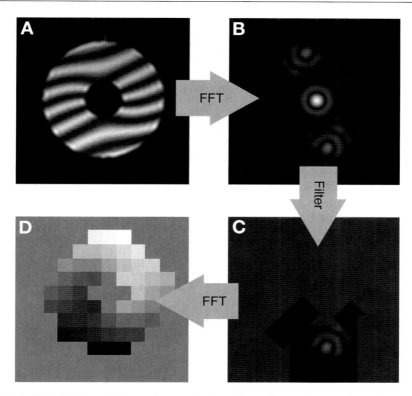

Fig. 29. (A) A SPAMM tagged image from which motion information needs to be extracted. **(B)** HARP processing starts with inverse Fourier transforming the tagged image. Three peaks are observed after the Fourier transform. **(C)** One of the two position-encoded harmonics is preserved via a filter. **(D)** A Fourier transformation yields a tag-less phase image from which motion data can be extracted directly.

meaning that the displacement vectors of a fixed grid are measured for all time-points, and the same grid point represents different material points over time. In tissue-tracking mode, the displacement field is measured in Lagrangian coordinates, for which the images are acquired at the same position and time, and the encoding step occurs at different times. Therefore, in tissue tracking, the same pixel corresponds to the same material point for all times. Under certain assumptions, it is feasible to follow material points using cine mode data by grid interpolation. However, in the case of significant through-slice motion and a small number of slices, this interpolation procedure may introduce some errors. Use of 3D material-point tracking is one of the considerations when choosing a particular multiphase DENSE implementation.

Data processing in phase-modulated displacement imaging includes several well-defined steps: the reconstruction of complex images, the conversion of the phase data into displacement fields, and calculations of functional maps (such as strain and torsion) from the displacement fields. For routine evaluation of cardiac function in the clinical environment, automation of image processing is an indispensable step for maintaining accuracy and uniformity of the diagnoses.

A technical challenge in automation is the removal of unwanted areas such as the ventricular cavities and the lung spaces. Fortunately, the high resolution of phase-modulated displacement data facilitates this process. In bulk elastic tissue such as the myocardial wall, material displacement should vary smoothly both in space and in time. These criteria are effective in removing unwanted pixels in the displacement data because pixels outside bulk tissue tend to have either drastic motion, such as that in the ventricular cavities, or noisy phase values, such as in the lung spaces around the heart. In Fig. 28, automatic image masking and phase unwrapping of DENSE data prior to the calculation of strain images are illustrated.

HARMONIC TAG PROCESSING

As discussed, one of the challenges in processing SPAMM-tagged images has been the automated tag detection by software packages. The fading of the tags in diastole and discontinuities caused by intravoxel dephasing make this a difficult task. Osman et al. *(9)* approached SPAMM tag tracking from a telecommunications theory perspective and came to the conclusion that the deformation of the tag lines can be extracted by the process shown in Fig. 29. First, they inverse Fourier transformed the tagged image (Fig. 29A) to extract its "harmonics" (Fig. 29B). Then, a filter was applied to extract the first harmonic while suppressing the others (Fig. 29C). Then, a Fourier transform was used to produce a phase image devoid of tag lines (Fig. 29D), which was subsequently interrogated to extract motion information.

Given the discussion of STEAM and DENSE, it is easy to understand how HARP processing works without resorting to telecommunications theory. We can identify the harmonics depicted in Fig. 29B as the raw k-space of a STEAM experiment with the three relevant peaks. In HARP, the processing starts from tagged images, and this is why the inverse Fourier transform is needed to produce the original k-space data. We already know that, in the k-space depicted in Fig. 29B, one of the two outer peaks (first harmonics) carries the motion information. The other outer peak is the complex conjugate, which carries the exact same information but with the opposite sign, as we saw with STEAM and DENSE. The center peak is the DC and carries no displacement information. We know that we should not allow these peaks to interact to avoid tag line artifacts in the phase maps. Therefore, we now understand why HARP tag processing isolates the first harmonic and filters out the remaining k-space peaks (Fig. 29C). We see how the last Fourier transform produces a phase image where each pixel carries displacement information similar to DENSE.

An appeal of HARP analysis is that it can be applied without any modifications to the tagging SPAMM pulse sequence and other tagging sequences. However, there is also a tradeoff. When the HARP filter is applied to select one of the first harmonic peaks, the effective area of sampled k-space is narrowed, and correspondingly the resulting images have lower resolution. In fact, the pixel size in HARP phase maps is equal to the tag spacing of the original tagged image. Interpolation can be used to increase the apparent resolution of HARP analysis results; however, the underlying information is the same as that of conventional tagging analysis. HARP also adopted the methods of spectral peak selection and suppression used in DENSE to overcome the resolution limits.

INTRAVOXEL DEPHASING IMAGING OF CONTRACTION WITH STRAIN-ENCODED MRI

We have seen how intravoxel dephasing has been mostly a nuisance in DENSE, for which signal drop in areas of increased contraction was observed. This required new

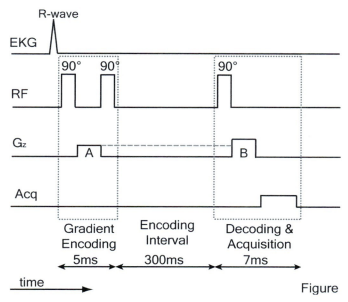

Fig. 30. The SENC pulse sequence diagram.

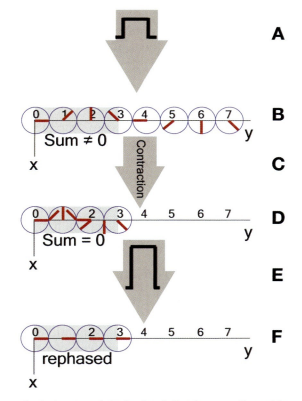

Fig. 31. Contraction results in intravoxel dephasing following encoding with a position encoding gradient. A stronger gradient pulse can be used prior to the readout to rephase the magnetization within a voxel.

approaches in terms of suppressing the interfering peaks in k-space so that the strength of the position-encoding gradient pulse could be lowered *(10)* and intravoxel dephasing eliminated. However, it was recognized from the beginning that intravoxel dephasing could provide a measure of deformation by itself *(7)*. Osman et al. *(24)* presented SENC, which is based on utilizing intravoxel dephasing with stimulated echoes to image strain across the imaging slice.

The basic concept of the SENC pulse sequence is shown in Fig. 30. The basic STEAM pulse sequence is modified to unbalance the position-encoding gradient pulse (Fig. 30A) and its counterpart during the image readout (Fig. 30B). Let us see how this works. We have seen (Fig. 11) that when the phases of the tissue depicted by a pixel in the image complete a full cycle (360°) as a result of contraction, then intravoxel dephasing occurs, and the signal within that pixel becomes zero.

Here is another way to think about it. A given gradient pulse (Fig. 31A) causes a distribution of phases within a pixel (Fig. 31B, gray area) because the pixel occupies some length along the gradient's direction. For this example, we chose the gradient such that only 180° degrees of phase are accumulated within the pixel. Therefore, some intravoxel dephasing occurs, but signal is still available. If the heart contracts (Fig. 31C) enough so that tissue from the neighboring pixel moves into our pixel, then dephasing to a full 360° degrees occurs (Fig. 31D). Note that because double as much phase has accumulated in our pixel because of contraction, the "correct" gradient for canceling this phase with STEAM would be a gradient of double the strength (Fig. 31E), which would create a doubly dense phase distribution compared to the original encoding gradient of Fig. 31A. Therefore, this doubly strong gradient would successfully cancel out the phase (Fig. 31F). A crude way to think of it in terms of the gradient pulses A and B of Fig. 30 is

$$\varphi_A + \varphi_{CONTRACTION} = \varphi_B \qquad (10)$$

Because one cannot assume if the myocardium is going to contract or expand within a given pixel, with SENC two or three experiments are done by unbalancing the second gradient pulse both in a positive and in a negative direction, and the images are combined.

Like many other techniques in MRI, SENC is a way of translating a usually unwanted phenomenon such as intravoxel dephasing into useful information about tissue deformation. Also, because it is based on signal losses, it does not require the reconstruction of phase images, but rather the magnitude images are used, therefore shortening the image reconstruction further. A weakness of SENC is that it is limited to strain in one direction and does not provide information about global movement such as torsion.

EPILOGUE

Displacement imaging with DENSE is a relatively new idea in MRI and enables quantitative assessment of regional function in the heart. In concept, it is the same as cine fluoroscopy using radio-opaque markers and sonomicrometry using implanted ultrasonic crystals. However, it is a major improvement over the invasive techniques, and with the development of pixel-by-pixel measurements provides high-density data over the whole heart. Displacement imaging in the heart began with intensity tagging and experienced a period of rapid development using phase tagging. With better knowledge of how to modulate the phase and intensity of MRI signal for the purpose of measuring motion, there has been a convergence of the various techniques and a unified understanding of the different spin labeling, image acquisition, and analysis methods. Besides direct measurements of the displacement field, it has also been shown that SENC can be used to indicate compression or expansion of the slice thickness and therefore the strain component perpendicular to the slice plane.

When compared with other imaging modalities, including echocardiography and multidetector computed tomography, cardiac MRI is a true 3D modality with unparalleled soft tissue contrast and image resolution. To translate the superior image quality into more accurate assessment of cardiac function, it is necessary to go beyond visual inspection of the images to detailed and quantitative results using automated image analysis. MRI displacement imaging and particularly phase-tagging techniques are quantitative by nature and fulfill this role.

ACKNOWLEDGMENT

We give sincere thanks to Carolina Fayos for the artwork in this chapter. Support was provided by the Intramural Research Program of the National Institutes of Health.

REFERENCES

1. Zerhouni EA, Parish DM, Rogers WJ, Yang A, Shapiro EP. Human heart: tagging with MR imaging—a method for noninvasive assessment of myocardial motion. Radiology 1988;169:59–63.
2. Axel L, Dougherty L. MR imaging of motion with spatial modulation of magnetization. Radiology 1989;171:841–845.
3. Callaghan PT, Eccles CD, Xia Y. NMR microscopy of dynamic displacements—k-space and q-space imaging. J Phys E-Sci Instrum 1988;21:820–822.
4. Reese TG, Wedeen VJ, Weisskoff RM. Measuring diffusion in the presence of material strain. J Magn Reson B 1996;112:253–258.
5. Chenevert TL, Skovoroda AR, O'Donnell M, Emelianov SY. Elasticity reconstructive imaging by means of stimulated echo MRI. Magn Reson Med 1998;39:482–490.
6. Aletras AH, Ding S, Balaban RS, Wen H. Displacement encoding in cardiac functional MRI. Proc Intl Soc Magn Reson Med April 1998:281.
7. Aletras AH, Ding S, Balaban RS, Wen H. DENSE: displacement encoding with stimulated echoes in cardiac functional MRI. J Magn Reson 1999;137:247–252.
8. Osman NF, Prince JL. Direct calculation of 2D components of myocardial strain using sinusoidal MR tagging. Proc SPIE Med Imag Conf July 1998:142–152.
9. Osman NF, Kerwin WS, McVeigh ER, Prince JL. Cardiac motion tracking using CINE harmonic phase (HARP) magnetic resonance imaging. Magn Reson Med 1999;42:1048–1060.
10. Aletras AH, Wen H. Methods and apparatus for mapping internal and bulk motion of an object with phase labeling in magnetic resonance imaging. International Application Published Under the Patent Cooperation Treaty. US Government 65185/00[773421], 1–38. 9-9-2004. Australia. 8-5-1999 2001;WO 01/11380 A2:10/12/2001.
11. Aletras AH, Arai AE. meta-DENSE complex acquisition for reduced intravoxel dephasing. J Magn Reson 2004;169:246–249.
12. Aletras AH, Wen H. Mixed echo train acquisition displacement encoding with stimulated echoes: an optimized DENSE method for in vivo functional imaging of the human heart. Magn Reson Med 2001;46:523–534.
13. Epstein FH, Gilson WD. Displacement-encoded cardiac MRI using cosine and sine modulation to eliminate (CANSEL) artifact-generating echoes. Magn Reson Med 2004;52:774–781.
14. Axel L, Dougherty L. Heart wall motion: improved method of spatial modulation of magnetization for MR imaging. Radiology 1989;172:349–350.
15. Fischer SE, McKinnon GC, Maier SE, Boesiger P. Improved myocardial tagging contrast. Magn Reson Med 1993;30:191–200.
16. Aletras AH, Freidlin RZ, Navon G, Arai AE. AIR-SPAMM: alternative inversion recovery spatial modulation of magnetization for myocardial tagging. J Magn Reson 2004;166:236–245.

17. Bazille A, Guttman MA, McVeigh ER, Zerhouni EA. Impact of semiautomated vs manual image segmentation errors on myocardial strain calculation by magnetic resonance tagging. Invest Radiol 1994;29:427–433.
18. McVeigh ER, Atalar E. Cardiac tagging with breath-hold cine MRI. Magn Reson Med 1992;28:318–327.
19. Aletras AH, Ingkanisorn WP, Mancini C, Arai AE. DENSE with SENSE. J Magn Reson 2005;176: 99–106.
20. Pai VM, Wen H. Developing a navigator-guided approach to non-breathhold multiphase cardiac strain maps using DENSE. Soc Card Magn Reson 2003:386.
21. Kim D, Gilson WD, Kramer CM, Epstein FH. High-resolution myocardial tissue tracking with breathhold cine DENSE. Soc Card Magn Reson 2003;411.
22. Spottiswoode BS, Zhong X, Meintjes EM, Mayosi BM, Epstein FH. Improved myocardial tissue tracking and strain accuracy in cine-DENSE using temporal fitting. Proc Intl Soc Magn Reson Med 2005:778.
23. Kim D, Epstein FH, Gilson WD, Axel L. Increasing the signal-to-noise ratio in DENSE MRI by combining displacement-encoded echoes. Magn Reson Med 2004;52:188–192.
24. Osman NF. Detecting stiff masses using strain-encoded (SENC) imaging. Magn Reson Med 2003; 49:605–608.

6 Clinical Applications of CMR Techniques for Assessment of Regional Ventricular Function

Victor A. Ferrari and Kevin J. Duffy

CONTENTS

INTRODUCTION

Cardiovascular magnetic resonance (CMR) allows for a highly accurate description of segmental wall motion and quantitation of contractile function. The excellent contrast between the endocardium and blood pool improves measurement of wall thickness, end-diastolic and end-systolic volumes, and left ventricular (LV) ejection fraction. Other noninvasive imaging modalities such as echocardiography assume a uniform LV geometry when calculating these global parameters. Errors caused by these assumptions are magnified when the LV shape is deformed, such as in dilated cardiomyopathy or after a myocardial infarction (MI). Because CMR acquires images in a tomographic set of planes, no assumptions regarding LV geometry are made. Not only does CMR produce more accurate global measurements, but also regional function can be precisely quantitated. The purpose of this chapter is to describe the clinical applications of these techniques for assessment of segmental right ventricular (RV) and LV function.

From: *Contemporary Cardiology: Cardiovascular Magnetic Resonance Imaging*
Edited by: Raymond Y. Kwong © Humana Press Inc., Totowa, NJ

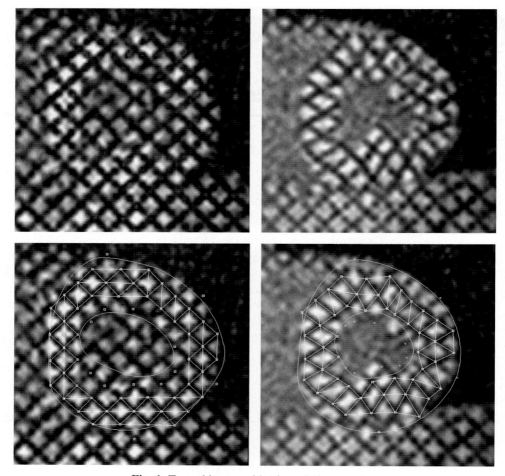

Fig. 1. Tagged image with triangulation overlay.

A unique aspect of CMR is its ability to measure intramural myocardial function, which had been possible only with implanted ultrasound crystals or radio-opaque beads. These approaches use alterations in magnetization to affect tissue signals or to measure the myocardial velocities in a quantitative manner (*see* Chapter 5 for the technical details of these methods).

One technique, known as tissue tagging, uses a grid of alternating stripes (formed by selectively unexcited protons or water molecules) to produce intramyocardial fiducial markers that are tracked via computer to create triangular finite elements that aid in calculating local function (Fig. 1). Previous work *(1,2)* demonstrated the complex regional relationship between transmural function and location within the heart. Software algorithms track the stripe or tag intersections and use these points in a manner similar to implanted markers. An approach known as homogeneous strain analysis converts one-dimensional stretches to two- (2D) or three-dimensional (3D) strain values. The advantage of the multidimensional analysis is that measurements may be made at any geographic location in the myocardium from base to apex or within the walls (between endocardium and epicardium).

ASSESSMENT OF REGIONAL LEFT VENTRICULAR FUNCTION

Weiss et al. *(3)* developed a method for quantification and mapping of regional wall thickening throughout the LV as an index of regional ischemia by utilizing the 3D geometry to calculate the perpendicular wall thickness of a 3D volume element of tissue. This 3D volume element provides a better discrimination of ischemic from nonischemic zones in a canine model of acute ischemia.

The accurate assessment of regional LV function has been improved greatly with myocardial tissue tagging, in which electronic markers persist through end-systole, allowing tracking of areas of interest while the heart moves and rotates through the cardiac cycle. Lima et al. *(4)* showed in an animal model that CMR with tissue tagging allows accurate assessment of systolic wall thickening, with good correlation to invasive methods using sonomicrometers. The strongest correlation between magnetic resonance imaging (MRI) and percentage systolic wall thickening by sonomicrometer crystals is achieved by using the 3D volume element approach by accounting for obliquity between the image plane and the LV wall.

Several studies have proven the value of assessing regional LV function in a multiplanar manner. Using myocardial tagging in a radial orientation, Azhari, Denisova, and colleagues demonstrated that endocardial dysfunction was the best discriminant of ischemia *(5,6)*. Scott et al. *(7)* studied myocardial displacement, radial thickening, and circumferential shortening by tagged CMR in normal subjects at baseline and during infusion of dobutamine. Dobutamine infusion resulted in a uniform increase in all measured parameters from baseline up to 10-µg/kg/minute infusion without further increase at higher doses. Therefore, the normal response to dobutamine involves a plateau in function after the 10-µg/kg/minute dose partly because of achievement of maximum inotropy, but also due to a decrease in preload (Fig. 2).

DETECTION OF MYOCARDIAL ISCHEMIA

The analysis of wall motion abnormalities with dobutamine stress echocardiography is an established method for detection of myocardial ischemia. CMR has been combined with stress modalities for the evaluation of coronary artery disease. Sayad et al. *(8,9)* described quantitation of LV wall thickening using CMR with myocardial tagging in 10 patients with segmental wall abnormalities at rest. Each subject underwent CMR scanning at baseline, after dobutamine infusion up to 10 µg/kg/minute, and 4–8 weeks after revascularization. Using CMR with tagging, resting end-diastolic and end-systolic wall thicknesses in abnormal segments at rest were compared with those measured at peak dobutamine and again after revascularization. It was found that end-systolic wall thickness after low-dose dobutamine infusion predicted improvement in segmental function after revascularization. Alternatively, segments with a resting end-systolic wall thickness of less than 7 mm did not improve after revascularization. Thus, dobutamine CMR (DMRI) with tagging techniques predicted viability in myocardial segments with resting wall motion abnormalities.

A major advantage of CMR is its ability to obtain images in patients regardless of the quality of their echo windows, body habitus, or the presence of lung disease. Hundley et al. *(10)* studied 153 patients with poor acoustic windows referred for CMR examination to evaluate for inducible myocardial ischemia. Intravenous dobutamine (peak dose 40 µg/kg/minute) and atropine (if necessary) were used to achieve a target

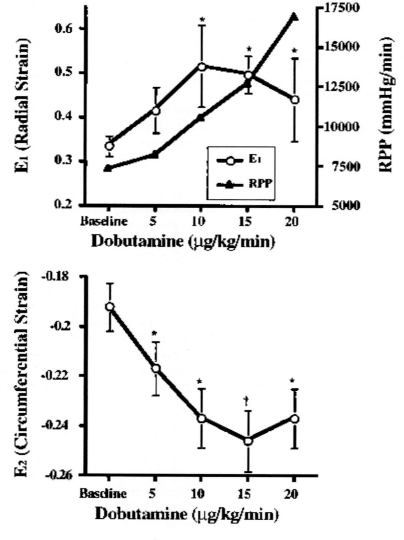

Fig. 2. Line graphs of strain versus dobutamine infusion rate. Top, radial strain (E1) increases from baseline to 10 µg/kg/minute infusion but reaches a plateau, whereas rate-pressure product (RPP) continues to rise. Bottom, circumferential strain (E2) increases (becomes more negative) from baseline to 10 µg/kg/minute and also peaks. Reproduced from Scott et al. [Scott 1999] with permission of the American Journal of Cardiology.

heart rate of greater than 85% of the maximum predicted heart rate. Fast cine imaging and display to assess LV wall thickening throughout the stress test were used. The sensitivity for detecting coronary artery narrowing of more than 50% ranged from 75% for one-vessel disease to 92% when three-vessel or left main disease was present, with a specificity of 83%. In the 103 patients with a negative DMRI examination, the cardiovascular occurrence-free survival rate was 97%, confirming the predictive capability of this technique.

Nagel et al. *(11)* performed a DMRI study in 208 consecutive patients with suspected coronary artery disease using high-dose dobutamine (up to 40 μg/kg/minute) as compared to dobutamine stress echocardiography (DSE). Overall, DMRI quality was better than DSE (good or very good in 82 vs 51%). DMRI was superior in terms of sensitivity (which increased from 74.3 to 86.2%) and specificity (from 69.8 to 85.7%) compared with DSE.

The benefits of DMRI over DSE included fewer errors caused by observer bias, quality of the imaging window, and better endocardial and epicardial definition, which allows more accurate quantitation of regional function. New 2D methods are becoming available to track rapid and complex motion in ischemia *(12)*, which may permit earlier detection of ischemia.

INFARCTION

CMR is also an especially good tool for the detection and quantification of MI. Infarction is a heterogeneous process that can affect predominantly the endocardium or can be more transmural. An MI can result in multiple patchy areas of necrosis surrounded by viable myocardium. The size of the infarction varies depending on the size of the occluded artery, the location within the artery (e.g., proximal vs distal), and the capacity of the collateral circulation. Assessment of the extent of an infarction is essential for both diagnostic and prognostic purposes. Two methods of focus here are direct functional assessment (e.g., regional wall motion) in conjunction with perfusion assessment.

CMR with tissue tagging can highlight differences in regional abnormalities of myocardial function in great detail, quantitatively assessing regional cardiac function. Strain analysis can highlight areas of infarction and assess the effects of infarction on the noninfarcted regions of the ventricle. CMR techniques *(13)* have demonstrated that circumferential and longitudinal strains are decreased not only in the infarcted areas but also in the remote zones in patients with reperfused anteroapical infarction. This study also showed increases in the radius of curvature of the ventricular walls in both the infarcted and remote zones. Together, these findings imply an increase in wall stress in regions distant from large infarctions that results in globally decreased function, which may lead to a more global post-MI chronic cardiomyopathy (Fig. 3).

A similar study *(14)* using tagged CMR and 2D finite-element analysis early after anteroapical infarction clearly demonstrated decreased wall strain and reorientation of the short-axis vector of myocardial contraction away from the centroid of the LV. Early after infarction, remote zone hyperfunction was seen, indicating a possible compensatory increase in function remote from the infarcted area. Average short- and long-axis strain values decreased to approximately 25% of normal in infarcted regions. The authors suggested that CMR could be a useful technique to predict whether patients with large infarctions will undergo unfavorable ventricular remodeling based on noninvasive wall strain information. A third study *(15)* demonstrated similar findings of decreased strains with nonradial direction of contraction not only in anteroapical MI, but also in infarcts of all coronary distributions.

CMR also provides information on corresponding regional perfusion abnormalities in infarcted myocardium. Enhancement of the CMR signal occurs with the administration of a gadolinium-containing contrast agent. Perfusion or enhancement CMR is performed by injecting a bolus of Gd contrast agent and observing the bolus as it passes from the LV blood cavity into the myocardium and beyond. First-pass and late images (steady state, 45–50 cardiac cycles) are acquired. One-dimensional circumferential

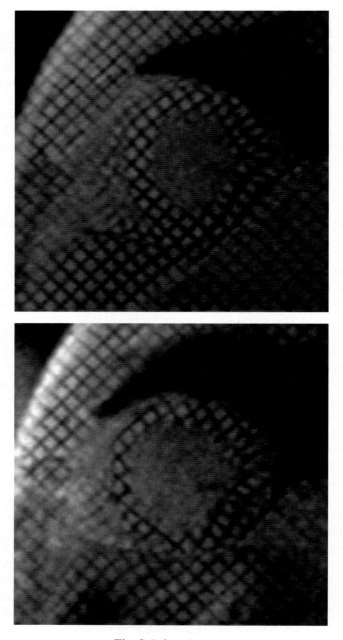

Fig. 3. Infarct images.

shortening was measured in the remote and infarcted regions, including all enhancement patterns, at week 1 and week 7 post-MI. Myocardium with a hypoenhanced signal intensity on first-pass imaging regardless of the delayed contrast pattern showed limited recovery of function by 7 weeks post-MI and probably reflects predominantly infarcted myocardium. Alternatively, myocardial segments that demonstrate delayed

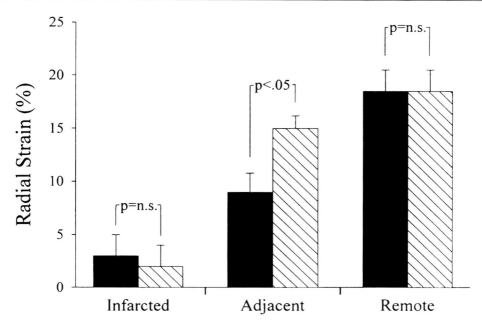

Fig. 4. Bar graphs of radial strain in dogs with high (>35%, solid bar) and low (<35%, hatched bar) amounts of MO within infarcted myocardium. Reproduced from Gerber et al. [Gerber 2000] with permission of Circulation.

hyperenhancement without initial hypoenhancement display significant late functional recovery and are likely composed of predominantly viable myocardium.

Microvascular obstruction (MO) is an important predictor of unfavorable remodeling after MI by preventing adequate healing early after MI. This phenomenon is also referred to as a *no-reflow territory* as seen after angioplasty of acute infarctions fails to return adequate flow to a vessel. The etiology appears to be necrosis of capillary beds or formation of thrombus or sludge in the capillaries within the infarct zone. Because CMR can evaluate both function and perfusion, this single test can assess the extent of MO and its effect on regional and global function using Gd contrast agent imaging. Infarcted myocardium demonstrates hyperenhancement late after contrast is injected (15 minutes). MO regions have hypoenhancement within a few minutes of injection.

A canine infarct model *(16)* has been used to explore this relationship. Animals with a greater extent of MO had a significantly greater risk of developing unfavorable remodeling within 10 days of infarction as assessed by CMR functional imaging. Figure 4 shows the differences in regional radial strain (similar to wall thickening) for large (>35% of infarct volume) vs small (<35% infarct volume) degrees of MO.

Myocardial strains decreased significantly in the infarct regions, and the greater the area of MO within the infarction, the greater the decrease in myocardial strain. Strains were decreased not only in infarcted areas but also in regions adjacent to the infarct with normal perfusion. Therefore, techniques that assess functional or perfusion parameters alone would lead to incomplete characterization of infarcted and viable zones. Combined techniques are likely to improve our diagnostic and prognostic abilities.

Large areas of MO within an infarction are also predictive of cardiovascular complications in a human population *(17)*. MO by CMR was a more powerful

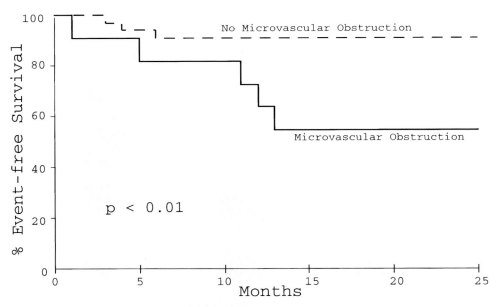

Fig. 5. Microvascular Obstruction and Event-Free Survival. Event-Free Survival is defined as a lack of cardiovascular death, reinfarction, congestive heart failure, or stroke. Reproduced from Wu et al. [Wu 1998] with permission of Circulation.

predictor of post-MI cardiovascular complications (death, reinfarction, congestive heart failure, embolic stroke, and unstable angina) than patency of the infarct-related artery, even controlling infarct size. Of the 11 patients with MO present on CMR scanning, 45% developed at least one complication vs only 9% of those without MO ($p < 0.02$), resulting in an odds ratio of 5.7 for patients with MO (Fig. 5). These studies concluded that determination of extent of MO has incremental prognostic information above and beyond identifying the infarct size alone.

VIABILITY

Assessment of viability is important in the management of ischemic heart disease because revascularization of dysfunctional but viable myocardium can improve function and survival. Traditionally, viability can be assessed through the evaluation of mechanical function (dobutamine echocardiography) or perfusion and metabolism (single photon emission computed tomography and positron emission tomography). More recently, CMR has been similarly developed to also evaluate mechanical function (dobutamine CMR with or without tagging) or perfusion and metabolism (contrast CMR and spectroscopic analysis).

Low-dose dobutamine echocardiography is an established method for the detection of viability. With low doses of dobutamine, the mechanical function of viable myocardium improves, and nonviable myocardium remains severely hypokinetic or akinetic. As with dobutamine echocardiography, DMRI can similarly detect increased function in dysfunctional but viable myocardium. When compared to positron emission tomography, DMRI correlates well, with a sensitivity of 88% and a specificity of 87% *(18)*.

DMRI can be used to accurately predict recovery of function after recent myocardial infarction. Dendale et al. compared low-dose dobutamine echocardiography with low-dose DMRI in 37 patients with recent myocardial infarction *(19)*. Both dobutamine echocardiography and CMR were performed within 4–12 days of admission. Viability was assessed qualitatively by visually evaluating which segments had increased contractility with dobutamine infusion. Echocardiography was then performed within 3–6 months of infarction to see if functional improvement occurred. CMR correctly predicted recovery of function in 79% of patients, similar to echocardiography (83%). Thus, both dobutamine echocardiography and CMR are useful tools for predicting recovery of function after infarction.

Myocardial tagging can be added to DMRI to make a more quantitative assessment of mechanical function. Sayad et al. described quantitation of LV wall thickening using CMR with myocardial tagging in 10 patients with segmental wall abnormalities at rest *(9)*. Each subject underwent CMR scanning at baseline, after dobutamine infusion up to 10 µg/kg/minute, and 4–8 weeks after revascularization. Using CMR with tagging, resting end-diastolic and end-systolic wall thicknesses in abnormal segments at rest were compared with those measured at peak dobutamine and again after revascularization. It was found that end-systolic wall thickness after low-dose dobutamine infusion predicted improvement in segmental function after revascularization. Alternatively, segments with a resting end-systolic wall thickness of less than 7 mm did not improve after revascularization. Thus, DMRI with tagging techniques predicted viability in myocardial segments with resting wall motion abnormalities.

DMRI with myocardial tagging can also be used in the setting of revascularized acute MI to predict recovery of function. Geskin et al. performed tagged dobutamine CMR studies in 20 patients within an average of 4 days after infarction with revascularization *(20)*. At approximately 8 weeks, a CMR without dobutamine was performed to assess for recovery of function. Those patients with a normal intramyocardial circumferential segment shortening on the initial study had greater recovery of function on the follow-up CMR.

HYPERTROPHIC CARDIOMYOPATHY

Hypertrophic cardiomyopathy (HCM), an autosomal dominant genetic disease caused by a defect in one of a number of genes of the sarcomere, is characterized by left ventricular hypertrophy (LVH) and myofibrillar disarray. There are many morphological variants, and frequently the pattern of hypertrophy is asymmetrical. Histologically, patients often have patchy areas of fibrosis, which may be visualized as areas of delayed hyperenhancement on CMR viability imaging *(21)*. Although ejection fraction is frequently normal or increased with HCM, force–length relationships are reduced, indicating decreased myocardial contractile function.

To further characterize contractile function in HCM, Young et al. *(22)* performed a homogeneous strain analysis on bidirectionally (2D spatial modulation of magnetization [SPAMM]-) tagged CMR images from 7 patients with HCM and 12 normal volunteers (Fig. 6). A 3D finite-element model was used to associate the short-axis and long-axis data. On a regional level, strain analysis revealed that circumferential shortening was reduced in the entire septum and most other regions in the HCM patients when compared to the normal controls. Although contractile function was reduced, LV torsion in the HCM group was increased by approximately 5°.

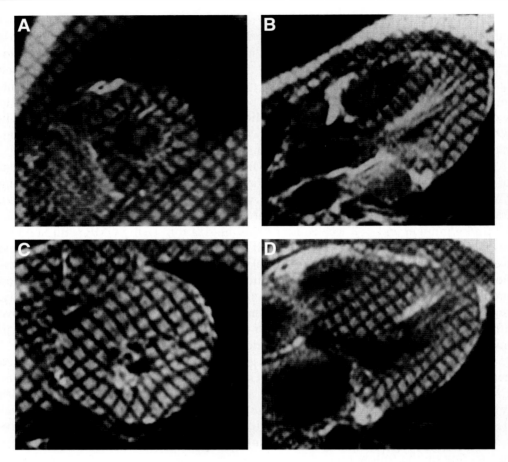

Fig. 6. (**A** and **B**) End-systolic short and long axis images of normal patient. (**C** and **D**) End-systolic short and long axis images of patient with hypertrophic cardiomyopathy. Segmental shortening is reduced in all walls except the lateral free wall. Reproduced from Kramer et al. [Kramer 1994] with permission of Circulation.

Similarly, Kramer et al. *(23)* found prominent regional heterogeneity in cardiac function in 10 HCM patients with a predominant pattern of asymmetric septal hypertrophy vs normal subjects. The 2D SPAMM-tagged short-axis CMR images were acquired at four levels from base to apex. Percentage circumferential shortening was compared at three transmural levels (endocardial, midwall, and epicardial) in four different regions around the short axis as well as from base to apex. Although circumferential shortening was less in the septal, inferior, and anterior walls, it was not significantly different in the lateral wall. At all short-axis levels, circumferential shortening was decreased in HCM, and longitudinal shortening was markedly reduced at the basal septum.

Not surprisingly, diastolic function is also abnormal in HCM. Ennis et al. *(24)* studied 8 patients with HCM and found that, in addition to decreased systolic strain, regional diastolic strain was reduced. The patients had decreased early diastolic strain rates, indicative of a prolonged early filling phase. The strain rate was then seen to increase during middiastole, signifying a continued slow filling phase and abnormal relaxation throughout diastole.

On many levels, HCM appears to be a heterogeneous process, with regional variability in the degree of wall thickness, the pattern of delayed enhancement, and reduced contractile function.

HYPERTENSIVE LEFT VENTRICULAR HYPERTROPHY

Patients often develop concentric LVH as a result of disorders associated with elevated afterload, such as systemic hypertension or aortic stenosis. As with HCM, compensatory hypertrophy may also lead to contractile dysfunction. In assessing global function with echocardiography, LVH patients typically have abnormal diastolic function early in their course with preserved systolic function. If afterload is not appropriately reduced by either antihypertensive medications (in hypertension) or aortic valve replacement (in aortic stenosis), then systolic dysfunction may eventually occur as well.

Palmon et al. *(25)* studied 30 patients with hypertension and concentric LVH using SPAMM tagging to more accurately quantitate regional contractile function. Circumferential and longitudinal shortening were depressed by approximately 5–10% when compared to normal volunteers. Unlike the normal volunteers, patients with hypertensive LVH had regional variability, with the greatest circumferential shortening occurring in the lateral wall and the least shortening occurring inferiorly.

Patients enrolled in the MESA (Multi-Ethnic Study of Atherosclerosis) study with concentric LVH and preserved systolic function were evaluated with CMR. Rosen et al. *(26)* analyzed tagged CMR studies in 441 such patients with the HARP (harmonic phase) analysis method and found that, as with previous smaller trials, LV systolic strain was decreased. This reduction in strain had regional variability, with a more pronounced effect in the left anterior descending coronary distribution.

In another analysis of the MESA patients, Edvardsen et al. *(27)* studied 218 patients with concentric LVH. In this study, although there was no difference in systolic strain between the LVH patients and the normal controls, there was a noticeable difference in diastolic function, with the LVH patients having significantly reduced regional diastolic strain rates, signifying a more prolonged and slower diastolic relaxation.

VALVULAR HEART DISEASE AND ITS EFFECT ON MYOCARDIAL FUNCTION

Although the heart valves may be evaluated by CMR through direct visualization of the leaflets and assessment of regurgitation through evaluation of regurgitant jets, valvular heart disease can also be assessed by evaluating its adverse effects on atrial and ventricular function through abnormal loading conditions.

In the pressure-overloaded state of severe aortic stenosis, there are contractile abnormalities such as with hypertensive heart disease. Stuber et al. studied *(28)* 12 patients with aortic stenosis, 11 world-championship athletes with physiological hypertrophy, and 11 normal volunteers. In the patients with aortic stenosis, torsion was significantly increased and diastole was delayed, as indicated by a late peak diastolic untwisting. In the athletes, despite their increased wall thickness, there were no abnormalities in systolic or diastolic function. In a further study of aortic stenosis, Nagel et al. *(29)* evaluated 13 patients with severe aortic stenosis and compared them to 11 healthy subjects. Similar results were obtained, with the maximal systolic torsion increased in the patients with aortic stenosis (from 8° to 14°) and the diastolic untwisting was delayed and prolonged.

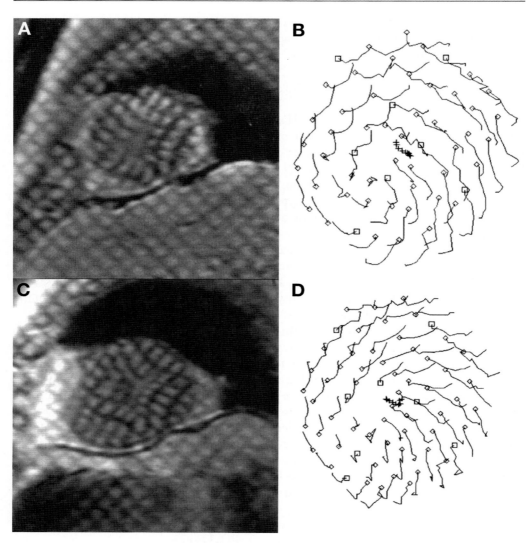

Fig. 7. 75 year old man with aortic stenosis. **(A)** End-systolic apical short axis tagged image before surgery. **(B)** Associated tagged intersection movement from end-diastole to end-systole. **(C)** End-systolic apical short axis tagged image three months after surgery. **(D)** Associated tagged intersection movement from end-diastole to end-systole. Reproduced from Sandstede et al. [Sandstede 2002] with permission of the American Journal of Roentgenology.

The abnormal pathologic changes associated with the high afterload state of aortic stenosis can actually be reversed, as demonstrated by Sandstede et al. *(30)* in their study of 12 patients with aortic stenosis who underwent aortic valve replacement (Fig. 7). Compared with 8 healthy volunteers, the patients with aortic stenosis prior to valve replacement had significantly higher torsion (25° compared to 14°). At 1 year after surgery, the apical torsion had normalized to 16°.

Aortic regurgitation, caused by the increased volume load on the LV, leads to LV dilatation and eccentric hypertrophy. Optimal timing for surgery can be difficult to determine as patients may remain relatively asymptomatic even as their LV becomes markedly abnormal. Ideally, aortic valve replacement should occur before permanent damage to the LV ensues. The quantification of regional LV function using tagged CMR could potentially detect subtle changes in myocardial function, which could herald the need to replace the aortic valve prior to the development of irreversible LV dysfunction.

Ungacta et al. *(31)* studied 6 patients with chronic severe aortic insufficiency by performing 2D tagged imaging before and after aortic valve replacement. Prior to surgery, when compared to normal controls, there was no difference in various contractile parameters such as global circumferential shortening or radial thickening. The patients with aortic insufficiency were again imaged approximately 5 months after surgery. When compared to their preoperative images, there also was no significant difference in overall circumferential shortening or radial thickening despite a decrease in LV volume and a return to a more normal ventricular geometry. On a regional basis, however, posterior wall strain was reduced.

Cupps et al. *(32)* studied LV wall stress in 19 patients with severe aortic regurgitation and compared the results to 19 normal controls. Using finite-element analysis to assess regional wall stress based on approximations of LV end-systolic pressure from carotid waveforms, wall stress was greater in all regions in the aortic insufficiency group, with global wall stress calculated to be 60% higher than in normal subjects. With further study, it is possible that wall stress could be used as a parameter in the difficult decision-making process of timing of aortic valve replacement.

Severe mitral regurgitation can result in abnormal myocardial contractile function, despite having normal global parameters such as ejection fraction. Mankad et al. *(33)* studied regional strain in 7 patients with severe mitral regurgitation before surgery and again approximately 8 weeks after surgery. Prior to surgery, maximum strain (similar to radial thickening) was increased compared to normals and became even greater after surgery. Prior to surgery, minimum strain (comparable to circumferential shortening) was decreased compared to normals, and it further declined after surgery.

PERICARDIAL DISEASE

The pericardium can be well visualized with CMR, despite having an average thickness of 1.5–2 mm *(34)*. CMR can be used to diagnose abnormalities of the pericardium itself as well as further delineate adjacent structures such as intrapericardial or extrinsic masses.

CMR can be especially useful in evaluating the pericardium in certain clinical conditions for which the diagnosis may not be definitively made using other tools. Differentiating between constrictive pericarditis and restrictive cardiomyopathy can often be difficult; CMR adds additional information in these cases. In addition to more clearly defining the anatomic structure of the pericardium through standard cine CMR imaging, tagged CMR allows the interpreter to discern whether the pericardium is adhered to the heart *(35)*. In normal hearts, the pericardium and the underlying heart move independently, where the underlying myocardium twists and the overlying pericardium does not (a relative "sliding" motion of the visceral and parietal pericardium). This can be visualized by using 1D or 2D tagged CMR; at end-diastole, the tag lines cross both the pericardium and myocardium, and with systole—in normals—the visceral pericardial/myocardial tags move together and become displaced relative to the parietal pericardium and its tags. In cases of constriction, because the parietal pericardium is often adhered to the underlying visceral pericardium/myocardium, no sliding motion occurs, and the parietal pericardial

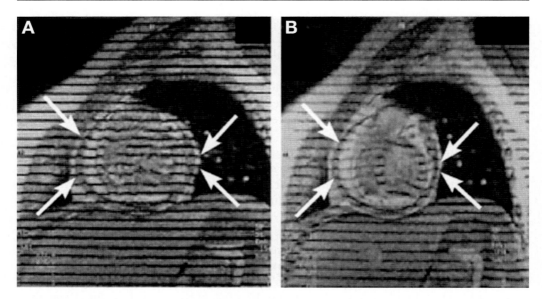

Fig. 8. Patient with constrictive pericarditis. (**A**) End-diastole. (**B**) End-systole. Due to the adherence of the pericardium to the myocardium, there is no shearing of tag lines at the interface between the two surfaces. Reproduced from [Kojima 1999] with permission of the New England Journal of Medicine.

tags remain aligned, and move and deform with, the visceral pericardium/myocardium and the associated tag lines (Fig. 8). It is important to remember that constriction is a complex diagnosis, and that the presence of pericardial adhesion(s) alone is not pathognomonic for the diagnosis. However, CMR can aid surgical planning by depicting the extent of adhesions or thickened pericardium and indicating to the surgeon whether cardiopulmonary bypass may be necessary to achieve a satisfactory pericardiectomy.

RIGHT VENTRICULAR FUNCTION

The ability to assess global and regional RV function accurately is valuable in the study of diseases affecting the RV, such as pulmonary hypertension, congenital heart disease, and arrhythmogenic RV dysplasia/cardiomyopathy (ARVD/C).

Because of the complex shape of the RV and its position in the near field, echocardiography is limited in obtaining an accurate assessment of RV size, shape, and function. Therefore, a tomographic approach with CMR or computed tomography may be used to acquire global RV parameters such as volumes and ejection fraction.

Like global function, regional function of the RV is similarly difficult to quantitate because of its complex geometry and its very thin wall, which makes strain analysis more challenging. For the LV, a 2D tag grid can be used to track intersection points within the myocardial wall; however, the RV is too thin for this to be practical. Instead, investigators have used either 1D tags, or bidirectional tags with tracking of the intersection of the tag lines with the midwall of the RV, rather than tracking intersection points of grid lines.

Young et al. *(36)* described a method of quantifying the 3D deformation of the RV. They acquired 1D tagged images of the RV in three orthogonal planes (Fig. 9). For each plane, they tracked the intersections between the tag lines and the RV midwall and created a finite-element model for representing the deformation. Using these models, they were able to characterize the motion of the RV free wall in both a normal patient and a patient with RV hypertrophy (RVH). In the normal patient, contraction occurred primarily tangential to the wall surface, with a component of sliding motion from the base of the heart toward the RV apex. This sliding phenomenon as well as ventricular torsion were visibly decreased in the patient with RVH. In addition, strain calculations were performed that revealed decreased maximum contraction in the patient with RVH.

Young et al.'s analytic technique (36) was subsequently applied by Fayad et al. (37) to 10 normal patients and 7 with chronic pulmonary hypertension to further characterize RV function. In normal patients, RV regional shortening was not uniform; RV short-axis shortening increased from the RV outflow tract to the RV apex, whereas long-axis shortening was more complex. In the patients with pulmonary hypertension, both short- and long-axis regional shortening were decreased, most prominently in the RV outflow tract and the basal septum.

Normal regional RV function was further characterized by Klein et al. (38). They evaluated 16 normal patients by performing 2D-grid tagged CMR. Through tracking the intersection points of the grid lines with the RV wall, they calculated the percentage segmental shortening and noticed a similar increasing gradient in segmental shortening from RV base to apex.

Tandri et al. (39) performed qualitative assessment of regional RV function in 20 patients with idiopathic RV outflow tract (RVOT) tachycardia. Black blood, double-inversion recovery CMR was performed in these patients and compared to 20 controls. Patients with RVOT tachycardia were found to have visually indistinguishable images from the controls. On quantitative analysis, global and regional parameters were also similar. Because RVOT tachycardia does not reveal structural abnormalities, the authors felt that these results argue against the hypothesis that RVOT may be an early form of ARVD/C.

Bomma et al. (40) studied global and regional RV and LV function in 14 patients with ARVD/C. Double-inversion recovery and gradient echo images were obtained in several short-axis sections through the heart. In patients with ARVD/C, global RV systolic function was reduced, and RV volumes were increased. Both of these findings were more pronounced toward the base of the RV.

Tagging methods may play an important role in future applications to congenital heart disease, for which a more quantitative approach to assessment of ventricular function could permit more precise titration of medications or choice of surgical approaches based on long-term functional measures (41).

NEW METHODS

While tagging provides valuable information on regional myocardial motion, it is limited by temporal as well as spatial resolution. Since the distance between tags is an important component of the strain measurements, the technique is only useful in areas of myocardium where one or more tags can be placed. Two- and three-dimensional acquisition and analysis methods have been developed to provide some independence from these problems, however, only limited success has been achieved to date. Nonetheless, investigators continue to refine these tools (42,43) for use with current pulse sequences and scanners.

In 1999, Aletras, Wen and colleagues developed a technique to improve the spatial and temporal resolution of a conventional phase contrast velocity encoding myocardial motion method for use with more rapid pulse sequences. It had the advantages of both

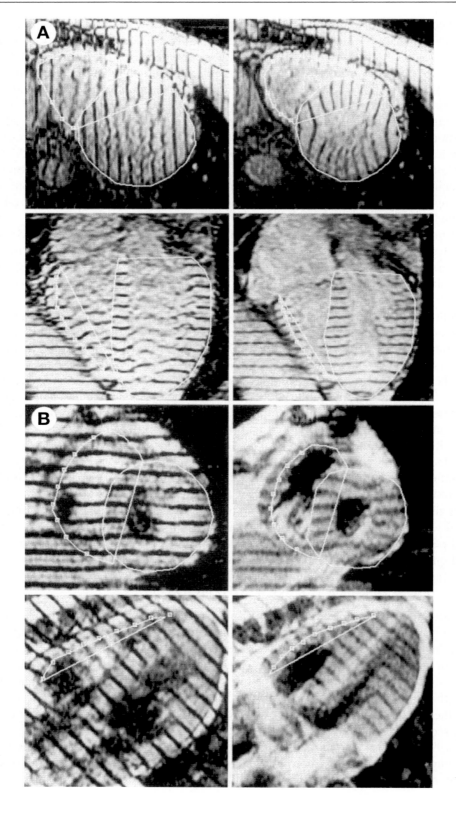

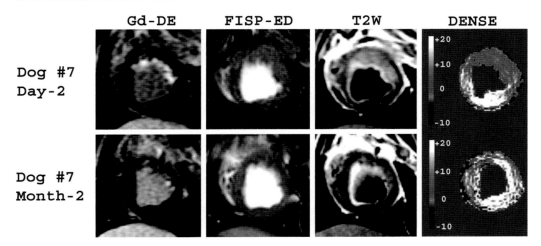

Fig. 10. The T2-weighted (T2w) image in the top row (Day 2 post-MI) show a hyperintense area (representing edema/area at risk) that is nearly transmural, while the infarcted area was only subendocardial, as seen using a gadolinium delayed enhancement technique (Gd-DE). The T2w hyperintense zone corresponded well to the hypokinetic zone on the DENSE systolic strain maps in the right column (radial thickening). Two months post-MI (bottom row), the T2W abnormality was nearly completely resolved and systolic strain had normalized (color scale = −10% to +20% strain). Normal strain is in the orange to white zone; blue-green represents severely hypokinetic to dyskinetic segments. (Reproduced from Aletras AH et al. with permission from Circulation).

tagging and phase velocity mapping sequences since it can measure larger displacements over longer time periods with greater spatial resolution. They called the method DENSE (for displacement encoding via stimulated echoes), and it has rapidly evolved as a very versatile imaging tool. Several refinements have increased its capabilities and eliminated certain artifacts that were inherent to the methodology *(44–48)*. A full review of the physics of this technique is available in Chapter 5.

Recent work by Gilson et al. *(49)* has demonstrated the power of this technique, even when applied to hearts as small as one-tenth the size of a human heart. In a mouse model of infarction, all regions of the LV were analyzable using DENSE, and strain measurements were possible regardless of slice location or wall thickness.

When combined with T2-weighted imaging to assess for myocardial edema following ischemia/reperfusion injury, DENSE permits a full assessment of not only the area at risk, but the degree and extent of myocardial salvage *(50)*. Translation to human studies is now possible to quantitatively study therapies to limit infarction size and the success of reperfusion strategies with a noninvasive technique. This combined technique provides a powerful new tool for one of the most critical fields of investigation in cardiovascular disease.

Fig. 9. *(Opposite page)* Tagged short-axis images showing RV midwall contours, LV epicardial contours, and RV contour-tag intersections. **(A)** Normal subject. **(B)** RVH patient. Left, end diastole; right, end systole. Upper, short-axis images; lower, long axis images. Reproduced from Young et al. [Young 1996] with permission of the American Journal of Physiology.

CONCLUSIONS

CMR methods are powerful tools for noninvasive assessment of regional RV and LV function. As modern cardiovascular care involves more difficult decision making, the need exists for a greater understanding of the complex 3D contractile patterns of the RV and LV. An integrated knowledge of the effects of through-plane motion, torsional displacement, and strain measurements independent of incident ultrasound beam angle are only a few of the advances that modern CMR techniques have provided. The clinical applications for these methods continue to expand. Evaluation of cardiomyopathies, myocardial viability, ventricular remodeling, and assessment of patients for resynchronization therapy are examples of disorders for which CMR has elucidated a new understanding of the mechanisms underlying these processes. More rapid acquisition and analysis methods, some of which are nearing clinical use, will further expand the clinical utility of these tools.

REFERENCES

1. Clark NR, Reichek N, Bergey P, et al. Circumferential myocardial shortening in the normal human left ventricle. Assessment by magnetic resonance imaging using spatial modulation of magnetization. Circulation 1991;84:67–74.
2. Young AA, Imai H, Chang CN, Axel L. Two-dimensional left ventricular deformation during systole using magnetic resonance imaging with spatial modulation of magnetization [erratum appears in Circulation 1994;90:1584]. Circulation 1994;89:740–752.
3. Weiss JL, Shapiro EP, Buchalter MB, Beyar R. Magnetic resonance imaging as a noninvasive standard for the quantitative evaluation of left ventricular mass, ischemia, and infarction. Ann N Y Acad Sci 1990;601:95–106.
4. Lima JA, Jeremy R, Guier W, et al. Accurate systolic wall thickening by nuclear magnetic resonance imaging with tissue tagging: correlation with sonomicrometers in normal and ischemic myocardium. J Am Coll Cardiol 1993;21:1741–1751.
5. Azhari H, Weiss JL, Rogers WJ, Siu CO, Shapiro EP. A noninvasive comparative study of myocardial strains in ischemic canine hearts using tagged MRI in 3-D. Am J Physiol 1995;268:H1918–H1926.
6. Denisova O, Shapiro EP, Weiss JL, Azhari H. Localization of ischemia in canine hearts using tagged rotated long axis MR images, endocardial surface stretch and wall thickening. Magn Reson Imaging 1997;15:1037–1043.
7. Scott CH, Sutton MS, Gusani N, et al. Effect of dobutamine on regional left ventricular function measured by tagged magnetic resonance imaging in normal subjects. Am J Cardiol 1999;83:412–417.
8. Sayad DE, Willett DL, Bridges WH, et al. Noninvasive quantitation of left ventricular wall thickening using cine magnetic resonance imaging with myocardial tagging. Am J Cardiol 1995;76:985–989.
9. Sayad DE, Willett DL, Hundley WG, Grayburn PA, Peshock RM. Dobutamine magnetic resonance imaging with myocardial tagging quantitatively predicts improvement in regional function after revascularization. Am J Cardiol 1998;82:1149–1151, A10.
10. Hundley WG, Hamilton CA, Thomas MS, et al. Utility of fast cine magnetic resonance imaging and display for the detection of myocardial ischemia in patients not well suited for second harmonic stress echocardiography. Circulation 1999;100:1697–1702.
11. Nagel E, Lehmkuhl HB, Bocksch W, et al. Noninvasive diagnosis of ischemia-induced wall motion abnormalities with the use of high-dose dobutamine stress MRI: comparison with dobutamine stress echocardiography. Circulation 1999;99:763–770.
12. Scott CH, Duffy KJ, Ivey BS, et al. Tagged magnetic resonance imaging can quantify regional functional variation during dobutamine stress in subjects with coronary stenoses. J Am Coll Cardiol 2000;35:453A.
13. Bogaert J, Bosmans H, Maes A, Suetens P, Marchal G, Rademakers FE. Remote myocardial dysfunction after acute anterior myocardial infarction: impact of left ventricular shape on regional function: a magnetic resonance myocardial tagging study. J Am Coll Cardiol 2000;35:1525–1534.
14. Marcus JT, Gotte MJ, Van Rossum AC, et al. Myocardial function in infarcted and remote regions early after infarction in man: assessment by magnetic resonance tagging and strain analysis. Magn Reson Med 1997;38:803–810.

15. Gotte MJ, van Rossum AC, Marcus JT, Kuijer JP, Axel L, Visser CA. Recognition of infarct localization by specific changes in intramural myocardial mechanics. Am Heart J 1999;138:1038–1045.

16. Gerber BL, Rochitte CE, Melin JA, et al. Microvascular obstruction and left ventricular remodeling early after acute myocardial infarction. Circulation 2000;101:2734–2741.

17. Wu KC, Zerhouni EA, Judd RM, et al. Prognostic significance of microvascular obstruction by magnetic resonance imaging in patients with acute myocardial infarction. Circulation 1998;97:765–772.

18. Baer FM, Voth E, Schneider CA, Theissen P, Schicha H, Sechtem U. Comparison of low-dose dobutamine-gradient-echo magnetic resonance imaging and positron emission tomography with [18F]fluorodeoxyglucose in patients with chronic coronary artery disease. A functional and morphological approach to the detection of residual myocardial viability. Circulation 1995;91:1006–1015.

19. Dendale PA, Franken PR, Waldman GJ, et al. Low-dosage dobutamine magnetic resonance imaging as an alternative to echocardiography in the detection of viable myocardium after acute infarction. Am Heart J 1995;130:134–140.

20. Geskin G, Kramer CM, Rogers WJ, et al. Quantitative assessment of myocardial viability after infarction by dobutamine magnetic resonance tagging. Circulation 1998;98:217–223.

21. Choudhury L, Mahrholdt H, Wagner A, et al. Myocardial scarring in asymptomatic or mildly symptomatic patients with hypertrophic cardiomyopathy. J Am Coll Cardiol 2002;40:2156–2164.

22. Young AA, Kramer CM, Ferrari VA, Axel L, Reichek N. Three-dimensional left ventricular deformation in hypertrophic cardiomyopathy. Circulation 1994;90:854–867.

23. Kramer CM, Reichek N, Ferrari VA, Theobald T, Dawson J, Axel L. Regional heterogeneity of function in hypertrophic cardiomyopathy. Circulation 1994;90:186–194.

24. Ennis DB, Epstein FH, Kellman P, Fananapazir L, McVeigh ER, Arai AE. Assessment of regional systolic and diastolic dysfunction in familial hypertrophic cardiomyopathy using MR tagging. Magn Reson Med 2003;50:638–642.

25. Palmon LC, Reichek N, Yeon SB, et al. Intramural myocardial shortening in hypertensive left ventricular hypertrophy with normal pump function. Circulation 1994;89:122–131.

26. Rosen BD, Edvardsen T, Lai S, et al. Left ventricular concentric remodeling is associated with decreased global and regional systolic function: the Multi-Ethnic Study of Atherosclerosis. Circulation 2005;112:984–991.

27. Edvardsen T, Rosen BD, Pan L, et al. Regional diastolic dysfunction in individuals with left ventricular hypertrophy measured by tagged magnetic resonance imaging—the Multi-Ethnic Study of Atherosclerosis (MESA). Am Heart J 2006;151:109–114.

28. Stuber M, Scheidegger MB, Fischer SE, et al. Alterations in the local myocardial motion pattern in patients suffering from pressure overload due to aortic stenosis. Circulation 1999;100:361–368.

29. Nagel E, Stuber M, Burkhard B, et al. Cardiac rotation and relaxation in patients with aortic valve stenosis. Eur Heart J 2000;21:582–589.

30. Sandstede JJW, Johnson T, Harre K, et al. Cardiac systolic rotation and contraction before and after valve replacement for aortic stenosis: a myocardial tagging study using MR imaging. AJR Am J Roentgenol 2002;178:953–958.

31. Ungacta FF, Davila-Roman VG, Moulton MJ, et al. MRI-radiofrequency tissue tagging in patients with aortic insufficiency before and after operation. Ann Thorac Surg 1998;65:943–950.

32. Cupps BP, Moustakidis P, Pomerantz BJ, et al. Severe aortic insufficiency and normal systolic function: determining regional left ventricular wall stress by finite-element analysis. Ann Thorac Surg 2003;76:668–675; discussion 675.

33. Mankad R, McCreery CJ, Rogers WJ Jr, et al. Regional myocardial strain before and after mitral valve repair for severe mitral regurgitation. J Cardiovasc Magn Reson 2001;3:257–266.

34. Bogaert J, Maes A, Van De WF, et al. Functional recovery of subepicardial myocardial tissue in transmural myocardial infarction after successful reperfusion: an important contribution to the improvement of regional and global left ventricular function. Circulation 1999;99:36–43.

35. Kojima S, Yamada N, Goto Y. Diagnosis of constrictive pericarditis by tagged cine magnetic resonance imaging. N Engl J Med 1999;341:373–374.

36. Young AA, Fayad ZA, Axel L. Right ventricular midwall surface motion and deformation using magnetic resonance tagging. Am J Physiol 1996;271:H2677–H2688.

37. Fayad ZA, Ferrari VA, Kraitchman DL, et al. Right ventricular regional function using MR tagging: normals versus chronic pulmonary hypertension. Magn Reson Med 1998;39:116–123.

38. Klein SS, Graham TP Jr, Lorenz CH. Noninvasive delineation of normal right ventricular contractile motion with magnetic resonance imaging myocardial tagging. Ann Biomed Eng 1998;26:756–763.

39. Tandri H, Bluemke DA, Ferrari VA, et al. Findings on magnetic resonance imaging of idiopathic right ventricular outflow tachycardia. Am J Cardiol 2004;94:1441–1445.
40. Bomma C, Dalal D, Tandri H, et al. Regional differences in systolic and diastolic function in arrhythmogenic right ventricular dysplasia/cardiomyopathy using magnetic resonance imaging. Am J Cardiol 2005;95:1507–1511.
41. Menteer J, Weinberg PM, Fogel MA. Quantifying regional right ventricular function in tetralogy of Fallot. J Cardiovasc Magn Reson 2005;7:753–761.
42. Qian Z, Metaxas DN, Axel L. Boosting and non-parametric based tracking of tagged MRI cardiac boundaries. Med Image Comput Comput Assist Interv Int Conf Med Image Comput Comput Assist Interv 2006;9(Pt 1):636–644.
43. Abd-Elmoniem KZ, Osman NF, Prince JL, Stuber M. Three-dimensional magnetic resonance myocardial motion tracking from a single image plane. Magn Reson Med 2007;58:92–102.
44. Aletras AH, Ding S, Balaban RS, Wen H. DENSE: Displacement encoding with stimulated echoes in cardiac functional MRI. Journal of Magnetic Resonance 1999;137:247–252.
45. Aletras AH, Balaban RS, Wen H. High resolution strain analysis of the human heart with fast-DENSE. Journal of Magnetic Resonance 1999;140:41–57.
46. Aletras AH, Wen H. Mixed echo train acquisition displacement encoding with stimulated echoes: An optimized DENSE method for in-vivo functional imaging of the human heart. Magn Reson Med 2001;46:523–534.
47. Epstein FH, Gilson WD. Displacement-encoded cardiac MRI using cosine and sine modulation to eliminate (CANSEL) artifact-generating echoes. Magn Reson Med 2004;52:774–781.
48. Kim D, Epstein FH, Gilson WD, Axel L. Increasing the signal-to-noise ratio in DENSE MRI by combining displacement-encoded echoes. Magn Reson Med 2004;52:188–192.
49. Gilson WD, Yang Z, French BA, Epstein FH. Measurement of myocardial mechanics in mice before and after infarction using multislice displacement-encoded MRI with 3D motion encoding. Am J Physiol Heart Circ Physiol 2005;288:H1491–1497.
50. Aletras AH, Tilak GS, Natanzon A, Hsu L-Y, Gonzalez FM, Hoyt RF, Arai AE. Retrospective determination of the area at risk for reperfused acute myocardial infarction with T2-weighted cardiac magnetic resonance imaging: Histopathological and DENSE functional validations. Circulation 2006;113:1865–1870.

7

Techniques for MR Myocardial Perfusion Imaging

Michael Jerosch-Herold

INTRODUCTION

Outside the field of magnetic resonance imaging (MRI), most techniques for myocardial perfusion imaging rely on the direct detection of injected tracers. Examples are tracers that emit γ-rays for single photon emission tomography or tracers that scatter ultrasound waves, such as injected gas-filled bubbles. With MRI, blood-borne contrast agents can be used to assess myocardial perfusion. The presence of the contrast agent in tissue is detected through the effects of the contrast agent on the signal from ^{1}H nuclei.

Because of the complexity and richness of the MRI technique, it is worthwhile to revisit in this chapter some fundamental concepts behind the application of MRI to myocardial perfusion imaging. This is an area of active research, and a basic understanding of the techniques and approaches is of value to any investigator wishing to learn about the application of magnetic resonance (MR) for myocardial perfusion imaging. The highly encouraging results published to date on the application of MR perfusion

From: *Contemporary Cardiology: Cardiovascular Magnetic Resonance Imaging*
Edited by: Raymond Y. Kwong © Humana Press Inc., Totowa, NJ

imaging for the detection of coronary disease (1) make it worthwhile to invest time and effort in understanding MR myocardial perfusion imaging and how it could be further optimized by new approaches currently under exploration.

With ^{1}H MRI, one detects the signal from water and other molecules with ^{1}H nuclei. A paramagnetic contrast agent can be used to alter the relaxation properties of ^{1}H nuclei in its vicinity. The detection of the transit of the contrast agent therefore relies on the use of MR pulse sequences that are sensitive to particular relaxation properties, either the transverse or the longitudinal relaxation with characteristic time constants T_2 and T_1, respectively.

The choice between T_1-weighted or T_2-weighted imaging methods is partly dictated by the physiological characteristics of the organ or tissue type studied. For the heart, the application of T_1-weighted imaging has proven to be most advantageous for several reasons, including the relatively large vascular volume in the heart, the difficulty of achieving good field homogeneity in the proximity of the lung space (which adversely affects T_2*-weighted imaging), and the general property that T_2-weighted techniques are more sensitive to motion than their T_1-weighted counterparts.

I will first review the use of MR contrast agents for perfusion imaging and the MR pulse sequence techniques most commonly employed for myocardial perfusion imaging. A discussion of novel technical developments such as parallel imaging and reduced-field-of-view imaging with unaliasing of overlaps is meant to show where the field is heading. The rapid introduction of MRI systems operating at field strengths of 3 T or higher merits consideration of the particular advantages and adjustments at higher field strengths. Last but not least, the close interaction between image acquisition techniques and postprocessing benefits from a discussion of efficient methods for arterial input sampling and the interpretation of contrast enhancement in the presence of water exchange.

PULSE SEQUENCE TECHNIQUES

T_1 is the relaxation time constant that characterizes the return of the longitudinal magnetization component to its equilibrium state after rotating the magnetization away from the direction of the static magnetic field (B_0). For example, one can apply an inversion pulse (180° pulse) so that the magnetization points in a direction opposite to the magnetic field after the 180° pulse. The rate at which the magnetization realigns with B_0 is characterized by T_1.

The transit of an MR contrast agent, such as Gd-DTPA (gadolinium diethylenetriamine pentaacetic acid), shortens both T_1 and also the relaxation time constant T_2*, which characterizes the decay of the MR signal (or transverse magnetization component) after a radio-frequency excitation. Signal intensity (SI) changes produced by shortening T_1 or T_2* proceed in opposite directions: a T_1-weighted pulse sequence results in an increase of SI during transit of the contrast agent, and a T_2*-weighted sequence will produce a loss of SI.

It is advantageous for perfusion imaging to maximize sensitivity to one of the two relaxation properties, T_1 or T_2*, at the expense of the other. Figure 1A shows images acquired in a patient during the first pass of a contrast agent bolus (0.03 mmol/kg body weight of Gd-DTPA) with a T_1-weighted imaging technique. Contrast enhancement is highest in the ventricular cavities, typically by a factor of 4–5 compared to myocardium when extracellular contrast agents are used. The curves in Fig. 1B show how the SI

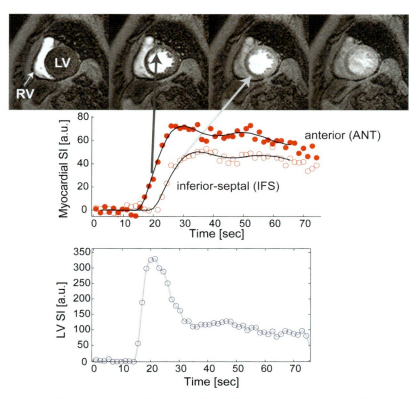

Fig. 1. The top row shows a subset of images collected in a patient during the first pass of an intravenously injected bolus of Gd-DTPA contrast (0.03 mmol/kg) on a 3-T scanner with a parallel imaging acceleration factor of 1.8. Contrast enhancement is first observed in the right ventricular (RV) cavity, then in the left ventricular (LV) cavity, and is followed by myocardial contrast enhancement. This particular patient had a perfusion deficit in the inferior septum. Two signal intensity curves are shown in graph (**B**), which give the average signal intensity in an anterior and inferior septal myocardial sector in each acquired image. The SI curve for the inferior septal sector shows delayed contrast uptake, with a slower rate of enhancement and lower peak enhancement than in the anterior sector.

changes during the course of the contrast transit in myocardial regions and in the left ventricular (LV) blood pool.

Although it has proven feasible to rapidly quantify T_1 to capture the transit of a contrast agent bolus through the heart *(2)*, it is more time efficient to use MRI pulse sequences that render the signal sensitive to T_1 without necessarily allowing a quantification of T_1. Quantifying T_1 implies that the magnetization recovery after an inversion pulse is sampled for 10–15 different inversion times (TI). In many instances, the relaxation recovery is well described by an exponential function and has the form

$$M_z = M_0 = \left[1 - \alpha \cdot \exp\left(-\frac{t}{T_1} \right) \right],$$

where M_0 is the equilibrium magnetization, t is the time elapsed after inversion (TI), and α is used here to describe the degree of magnetization inversion, with $\alpha = 2$ for a

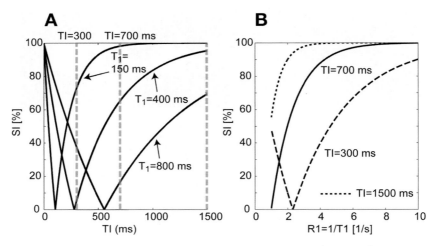

Fig. 2. The recovery of the longitudinal magnetization after inversion by a 180° inversion pulse follows in general an exponential relationship with a characteristic time constant T_1. In magnitude images, the information about the sign of the longitudinal magnetization component is not available, and the negative part of the inversion recovery curve is folded over, giving rise to the V-shaped curves of signal intensity vs inversion time (TI) shown in (**A**) for T_1 time constants of 150, 400, and 800 ms. For T_1-weighted imaging of contrast enhancement, one fixes TI and follows the SI changes brought about by transit of a contrast agent. The graph in (**B**) shows the signal intensity changes for a range of $R_1 = 1/T_1$ values for three different TI values, denoted in (**A**) by vertical dashed gray lines. For long TI values, the signal intensity reaches its equilibrium value at lower R_1 values than if TI is chosen to be short.

180° inversion pulse. When the inversion recovery (IR) is read out from magnitude images, one looses the information about the sign or phase of M_z.

For a T_1-weighted imaging technique, it is sufficient to sample the signal for a single TI. The concept is illustrated in Fig. 2, with the effective TI set by the time interval between inversion pulse and the readout of the low spatial frequencies. With properly chosen TI, a T_1-weighted signal increases when a contrast agent shortens T_1. Although the T_1 rate constant $(1/T_1)$ in blood is linearly proportional to the concentration of contrast agent, a similar, approximately linear relationship between SI and R_1 (or tracer concentration) can only be achieved over a limited range of concentrations with T_1-weighted imaging.

We consider here first the case of gradient echo imaging in the form of fast, low-angle shot (FLASH) acquisitions. The basic steps of slice-selective creation of transverse magnetization with a small flip angle radio-frequency pulse, phase encoding of the transverse magnetization, creation of a gradient echo, and readout of this echo can be carried out within a relatively short repetition time (TR), on the order of a few milliseconds. The time for a complete image acquisition with 100 phase encodings is on the order of 200 ms. For heart rates of up to 100 beats per minute, image acquisition times on the order of 150–250 ms are adequate to freeze cardiac motion. For T_1 weighting of the signal, one should use a pulse sequence with short echo time (TE) and short TR, and spoiling of the transverse magnetization after readout of each gradient echo.

An effective means of rendering the MRI signal sensitive to T_1 consists of applying a magnetization preparation pulse before the FLASH readout, with the image acquisition rapid enough compared to T_1 so that the effects of the magnetization preparation persist through most of the image readout. Applying the magnetization preparation before each phase encoding step would prove too time consuming for perfusion imaging.

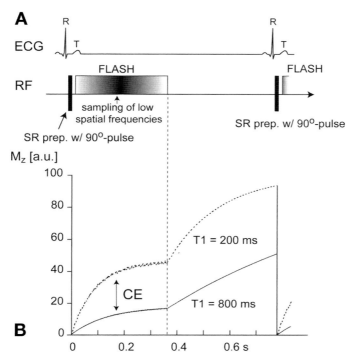

Fig. 3. The diagram in **(A)** for an ECG-triggered pulse sequence illustrates the timing of the saturation-recovery magnetization (SR) preparation right before the fast, low-angle, single-shot (FLASH) image read-out. In this example the phase-encodings sample high spatial frequencies near the beginning and end of the FLASH acquisition, and low spatial frequency encodings, which define image contrast, are performed in the middle of the FLASH acquisition. The diagram in **(B)** shows the evolution of the longitudinal magnetization after a saturation recovery (SR) magnetization preparation, followed by a fast gradient echo readout and a period of undisturbed relaxation recovery. The rapid application of radio-frequency pulses during the image readout alters the shape of the relaxation-recovery, giving rise to a shorter effective T_1 relaxation time constant than for the undisturbed relaxation recovery. With a linear phase-encoding order, the overall image contrast, set by the timing for reading out low spatial frequencies (low k-space), corresponds approximately to the signal acquired in the middle of the image acquisition. The vertical line labeled CE shows the differences in signal for $T_1 = 200$ ms and $T_1 = 800$ ms at this midpoint of the image readout. An advantage of the SR preparation is independence of contrast enhancement (CE), from the duration of the period of undisturbed relaxation or the heart rate, as the longitudinal magnetization is reset to zero before each image readout.

Figure 3A shows a simplified pulse sequence diagram for a turboFLASH or turbo fast field echo technique that uses a saturation recovery (SR) magnetization preparation *(3)*, followed by rapid readout of the image. Saturation of the longitudinal magnetization before the FLASH readout is done by application of a 90° radio-frequency pulse or composite radio-frequency pulses with a net flip angle of 90°, followed by dephasing (also called spoiling) of the transverse magnetization with gradient pulses. After saturation of the longitudinal magnetization, the FLASH image is read out during the recovery of the longitudinal magnetization. The evolution of the longitudinal magnetization component over one heart cycle is shown in the graph of Fig. 3B. A generalization of this sequence to a multislice perfusion imaging sequence is shown in Fig. 4.

With an IR preparation, one has in principle twice the dynamic range of signal recovery compared to SR. The larger dynamic range should allow a finer differentiation between

Multi-slice SR-prepared perfusion imaging

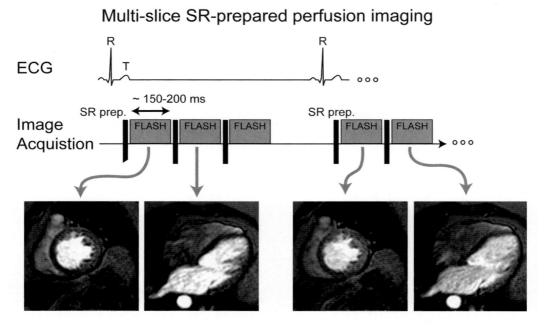

Fig. 4. The pulse sequence technique illustrated in Fig. 3 can easily be generalized to a multislice technique, as shown in this diagram. The saturation recovery (SR) preparation generally does only take 10–15 ms and can therefore be repeated for each slice, although it should preferably be slice nonselective to avoid alteration of the T_1 contrast in the blood pool caused by inflow of "unprepared" spins. The image readout, chosen in the above diagram to be a fast low-angle single-shot (FLASH) acquisition, can be replaced by different image readout modules, such as echo planar acquisitions or spiral acquisitions. Nevertheless, the FLASH readout is one of the more robust approaches, allowing application over a relatively wide range of magnetic field strengths. Of note in the FLASH images in the bottom row is the absence of any banding artifacts despite intersecting slice planes, which is a benefit of the SR preparation repeated for each slice.

different grades of myocardial contrast enhancement. As MR images normally only provide information about the magnitude of the signal, the usable dynamic range is effectively halved, but it is feasible to null the myocardial SI with an IR preparation on precontrast images, so that the appearance of contrast agent is more pronounced than with an SR preparation.

For the SR preparation, the delay between preparation and the FLASH readout is as short as feasible for optimal T_1 weighting. For an IR, one needs to have a longer delay (TI) between inversion pulse and FLASH readout so that the myocardial signal is close to null before contrast administration. Figure 5 shows a comparison of the dependence of the FLASH signal on R_1 for three FLASH sequence variants: without a magnetization preparation, and with SR and IR preparations.

The SI was expressed as percentage of the SI observed under the hypothetical condition that the TR is long compared to T_1 (TR $\rightarrow \infty$), with the other parameters (TE, flip angle) unchanged. The lowest R_1 value in the graph (≈ 1.1 s^{-1}) corresponds roughly to the "native" T_1 values of blood and myocardium, that is, before any administration of a contrast agent. With a bolus of approximately 0.1 mmol Gd-DTPA per kilogram of body weight, R_1 can peak at values as high as 10–15 s^{-1} in the ventricular blood pool *(4)*. Over the range of R_1 values from approximately 1 s^{-1} to 10 s^{-1}, the FLASH readout

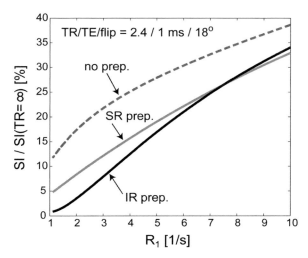

Fig. 5. The signal intensity measured with a fast gradient echo readout (TR/TE/flip = 2.4/1 ms/18°; 80 phase-encoding steps with linear ordering) was simulated for a range of R_1 values and for three different acquisition schemes with a saturation recovery (SR) preparation, an inversion recovery (IR) preparation, and without any magnetization preparation before the FLASH readout. The range of R_1 values corresponds roughly to R_1 changes in the LV cavity that occur with the transit of a bolus of Gd-DTPA contrast at a dosage of 0.05 mmol/kg body weight. The IR preparation gives the largest dynamic range for the SI changes, and the dynamic range is smallest when no magnetization preparation is used; in the latter case, the relation between SI and R_1 also deviates markedly from a linear relationship.

with IR preparation shows the largest dynamic range for SI changes, followed by the FLASH readout with SR preparation, and finally the FLASH readout without any magnetization preparation. The precontrast signal is lowest with the IR preparation, leading to high contrast enhancement, defined as percentage SI increase during transit of a contrast bolus relative to the precontrast signal. Visual perceptibility increases with the grey-scale dynamic range, and percent contrast enhancement has been used as a metric to assess perceptibility of contrast enhancement in perfusion studies.

In terms of linearity of SI vs R_1, the SR shows a deviation from linearity of less than 10–15%. With the IR preparation, the SI-vs-R_1 relation can show higher nonlinearity if the TI is not tuned to the expected range of R_1 changes, including a change from convex shape for higher R_1 values to concave shape for lower R_1 values. Near the bottom of the concave portion of the curve, the SI changes are relatively smaller compared to higher R_1 values, which can lead to an underestimation of contrast uptake. If the TI is chosen too short, then the curve ceases to be monotonically increasing with R_1 and instead has a V shape for low R_1 values, but in practice it may be difficult to notice this in perfusion studies.

The confounding effect of a V-shaped relationship between signal magnitude and R_1 is well known from imaging delayed contrast hyperenhancement in the heart, and this could in principle be avoided by phase-sensitive detection *(5)*. The saturation of the SI with increasing R_1 can only be avoided by using low contrast agent dosages and adjusting TI to tune the contrast enhancement to the range of R_1 values covered during contrast bolus passage.

Use of magnetization inversion as preparation for T_1 sensitization may require some creative rearrangement of the pulse sequence components to achieve longer TIs. With an inversion preparation, the optimal time between inversion and acquisition of the central k-space lines, which determines the overall image contrast, may require a delay of approximately 100–300 ms between magnetization preparation and image acquisition. Instead of an idle period, one can use the delay to acquire an image for another slice in which the magnetization was already prepared by a previous inversion pulse *(6)*. This slice-selective magnetization preparation scheme can suffer from through-plane motion (e.g., with rapid respiratory motion).

Although saturation of the magnetization reduces the T_1 sensitivity compared to an inversion pulse, it has the distinct advantage that the T_1 weighting is independent of any previous manipulations of the magnetization—the longitudinal magnetization component is always nulled by the SR preparation. Myocardial perfusion imaging is generally electrocardiogram (ECG) gated, which results in a T_1-sensitive signal that is dependent on the heart rate, and random fluctuations of the SI are introduced by heart rate irregularities. This type of heart rate-dependent fluctuations can be overcome by applying a magnetization saturation preparation after each R-wave, followed by readout of the image *(3)*. As shown in Fig. 3, the magnetization does not fully recover between applications of the magnetization preparation for normal heart rates because T_1 is of the same order as the duration of the cardiac cycle.

To summarize, it may be easiest to see localized deficits in relative contrast enhancement when images are acquired with an IR preparation compared to an SR preparation or absence of magnetization preparation. SR preparations have some distinct advantages, such as independence of contrast enhancement from heart rate and a rather favorable monotonic, nearly linear increase of SI with R_1 over the range of 1 to approximately 5 s^{-1}. Use of the SR preparation also lends itself well to use in multislice perfusion imaging *(7)*. Lack of a magnetization preparation results in relatively poorer contrast enhancement compared to use of an IR or SR magnetization preparation.

PERFUSION IMAGING WITH STEADY-STATE FREE PRECESSION

During gradient echo imaging, the gradient pulses applied for phase encoding and during gradient echo readout result in a position-dependent phase of the transverse magnetization, which can be reset by applying additional gradient pulses to reestablish phase coherence before the next radio-frequency pulse. Balancing the areas under the positive and negative gradient waveform lobes during each repetition interval (TR) combined with phase cycling of the radio-frequency excitation pulses (flip angle α) results in a steady state without spoiling of transverse magnetization. Most important, one overcomes the limitation of the Ernst angle and can use much higher flip angles α than feasible with spoiled gradient echo imaging to achieve a higher signal-to-noise ratio. A preparation consisting of a radio-frequency pulse with flip angle $-\alpha/2$ preceding by TR/2 the subsequent string of $\pm\alpha$ pulses with repetition time = TR for the image acquisition helps to attain the steady state more efficiently. Fast imaging with steady-state precession (FISP) produces a signal with weighting proportional to T_2/T_1 at a fixed flip angle: the steady-state free precession (SSFP) signal increases with T_2 and with $1/T_1$. It is therefore feasible to use SSFP for T_1-weighted imaging of contrast enhancement.

SSFP imaging can be combined with a magnetization preparation (preceding the $\alpha/2$ preparation) to accentuate the T_1 weighting for myocardial perfusion imaging *(8,9)*. The IR during the SSFP readout can be described as a monoexponential recovery *(10)*, but the apparent time constants of the magnetization recovery do not correspond to the true T_1 values, in particular at higher flip angles and when the T_2/T_1 ratio deviates significantly from 1 *(11)*. The measured T_1 is also a function of any off-resonance shift, which can result from field inhomogeneities, chemical shifts (e.g., fat-to-water shift), eddy currents, and so on.

Establishing a SSFP with FISP techniques works only within a relatively narrow frequency band centered at the Larmor frequency, and therefore any field inhomogeneities give rise to banding artifacts, which are observed at frequency shifts Δv, where the phase shift over a period TR equals TR $\times \Delta v = 1$. With TRs on the order of 2–3 ms, the SSFP technique works relatively well at 1.5 T.

SSFP perfusion imaging when used with an IR preparation for perfusion imaging yields higher contrast to noise than the spoiled gradient echo equivalent. A SR-prepared SSFP variant has also been applied for perfusion studies, although image quality was judged by some investigators to be inferior to the IR-prepared version for single-slice perfusion imaging *(8)*. For multislice perfusion imaging, the SR-prepared version nevertheless appears to be preferable *(12)*. With the SSFP techniques, the appearance of subendocardial black "banding" artifacts during wash-in of contrast into the LV cavity are more frequently observed than with spoiled gradient echo imaging. The SSFP technique is also more sensitive to motion and flow and should therefore be applied with care at heart rates above 100 beats per minute.

ULTRAFAST IMAGING TECHNIQUES

Besides the rather simple and robust approach of gradient echo imaging, there are faster methods, such as echo-planar imaging (EPI) *(13)* and spiral imaging, which can be used for very fast image acquisition in dynamic studies. With single-shot (two-dimensional, 2D) EPI, all phase encodings are performed during the decay of the signal excited by a slice-selective radio-frequency pulse. Instead of acquiring only a single line of data points in the spatial frequency space (*k*-space) after each radio-frequency excitation, as is done with conventional gradient echo imaging, one samples the spatial frequency space along a whole set of parallel lines. The effective echo time (TE) of the pulse sequence which determines the T_2^* weighting is now set by the time between the radio-frequency excitation and the acquisition of the data points corresponding to the phase encodings sampling low spatial frequencies.

By its very nature, EPI or spiral imaging does not allow TEs as short as feasible with gradient echo imaging (e.g., turboFLASH). For T_1-weighted imaging, the TE should be kept as short as feasible, or a spin-echo is used for the echo-planar readout *(14)*. The acquisition of T_1-weighted images can be split into multiple shots to reduce the effective TE and minimize artifacts from motion and field inhomogeneities *(15)*. During each shot, a subset of phase encodings is acquired with a train of 3–8 gradient echoes. These so-called hybrid EPI techniques have been successfully applied for myocardial perfusion imaging at lower field strengths and yield a higher signal-to-noise ratio than FLASH techniques *(16)*.

PARALLEL IMAGING FOR PERFUSION MAGNETIC RESONANCE IMAGING

So-called parallel imaging techniques *(17,18)* offer an attractive method for speeding up the image acquisition, which is more or less independent of the pulse sequence technique used. Parallel imaging refers to the simultaneous use of multiple coils and

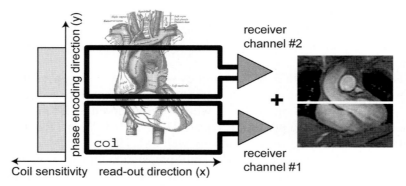

Fig. 6. A simplified scheme for parallel imaging is shown in this conceptual illustration with the assumption that the sensitivity profiles of two coil elements in a linear array do not overlap. The field of view in the phase-encoding direction can be halved, and two images for this reduced field of view are acquired over separate receiver channels. The two images can be combined into an image for a full field of view. In the more general case that the coil sensitivity profiles do overlap, a full-field-of-view image can still be reconstructed by determining the coil sensitivity profiles and using this information to eliminate fold-over. Parallel imaging algorithms can either be applied to the images (e.g., SENSE) or to the spatial frequency data (e.g., SMASH).

receiver channels to reduce the number of phase-encoding steps while preserving spatial resolution. The spatial sensitivity profiles of the coils are taken into account to substitute phase-encoding steps with appropriate linear combinations of the signals acquired through different pairs of coils and receiver channels.

For the sake of simplicity, one can consider the case when the sensitivity profiles of two coils are box shaped and do not overlap, as shown in Fig. 6. In this limiting case, one coil element could be arranged to image the heart from the base to the midventricle, and the second element picks up signal only from the midventricle to the apex. The phase-encoding direction should be chosen to fall in the direction from base to apex to take advantage of the coil sensitivity variation in that direction. The field of view in the phase-encoding direction can be halved and the number of phase-encoding steps reduced from N_p to $N_p/2$, and two images can be acquired in parallel. With a single coil, halving the field of view will cause a fold-over or aliasing artifact, but by acquiring two images with separate coils and receiver channels the fold-over is avoided in a trivial manner when the sensitivity profiles of the coils do not overlap. An image for the full field of view can be reconstructed by juxtaposition of the two images, each for one-half of the full FOV in this idealized example. The spatial resolution remains unchanged compared to an acquisition for the full field of view with N_p phase encodings. The image acquisition is sped up by a factor of two in this simple example ($R = 2$).

In the more general case of multiple coil elements with overlapping sensitivity profiles, the reconstruction will involve a linear combination of data acquired in parallel with multiple coil/receiver channels and a solution of the resulting system of linear equations. The algorithms can operate on the sensitivity-encoded images calculated for the individual coil elements (SENSE) *(18,19)* or on the spatial frequency data acquired with the coil elements (simultaneous acquisition of spatial harmonics, SMASH) *(17)*.

The higher image acquisition speed is achieved with parallel imaging at the price of a reduced signal-to-noise ratio, which drops at least by a factor equal to the square root of the speed-up factor $(\sim\sqrt{R})$. As myocardial perfusion imaging is noticeably limited by the attainable signal-to-noise ratio (S:N), the advantages of parallel imaging methods are tempered by any further reductions in S:N. In practical terms, speed-up factors higher than times two or three should be avoided for myocardial perfusion imaging with current coil array and receiver technology. The speed-up can also alter somewhat the contrast properties (T_1 weighting) because, without any other changes in the sequence parameters, the speed-up through parallel imaging reduces the time between magnetization preparation and the acquisition of the central k-space lines if a linear phase-encoding order is used.

TRADEOFFS BETWEEN TEMPORAL AND SPATIAL SAMPLING

Dynamic studies of contrast enhancement involve spatial sampling for the acquisition of each image and temporal sampling to detect SI changes at each spatial location. For myocardial perfusion imaging, the temporal sampling frequency should equal the heart rate. The image acquisition is repeated for every R–R interval in an ECG-gated acquisition. With this temporal resolution, the duration of myocardial contrast enhancement during the first pass of the contrast bolus will be sampled about 5–10 times at baseline and less often during maximal hyperemia, when blood flow in normal healthy human volunteers is approximately four times higher compared to baseline. As shown by Kroll et al., temporal sampling should be maximized, even at the expense of the signal-to-noise ratio, to optimize the quantitative assessment of myocardial perfusion (20). With multislice 2D acquisitions of 200 ms per slice, contrast enhancement can be sampled in three to five slices at baseline and two or three slices during hyperemia. With a temporal resolution equal in duration to a heart beat, it is generally not feasible to image the entire heart without resorting to parallel imaging techniques or other methods that allow a reduction of the image acquisition time.

It is possible to adjust temporal sampling methods to reduce the spatial sampling requirements. Without any other adjustments, a halving of the field of view would speed up the image acquisition by a factor of two but also cause aliasing. Madore et al. described an elegant framework, called UNaliasing by Fourier encoding the OverLaps using the temporal dimension unaliasing by fourier-encoding the overlaps using the temporal dimension (UNFOLD), for separating spatially aliased from nonaliased image components in dynamic studies (21–23). Essentially, the approach involves an alternation between two sets of interleaved phase encodings for successive image acquisitions, which results in a modulation of the aliased image components; unaliased image components are not modulated. The aliased image components can be removed by filtering of the temporal frequency spectrum at each pixel location.

A simplified version of such an approach is shown in Fig. 7. This approach assumes that there is no contrast enhancement in the aliased portion of the image and that the highest temporal frequency of contrast enhancement is lower than the frequency at which the aliased image components are modulated. The UNFOLD approach has been applied by Di Bella in myocardial perfusion studies (24) and was found to work well if the patient holds her or his breath as respiratory motion interferes with UNFOLD.

An elegant play on the ideas of UNFOLD was introduced for multislice imaging with multiband radio-frequency pulses to demonstrate that controlled aliasing in parallel imaging results in higher acceleration (CAIPIRINHA) for multislice imaging (25). The CAIPIRINHA technique, like UNFOLD, applies a phase modulation scheme to

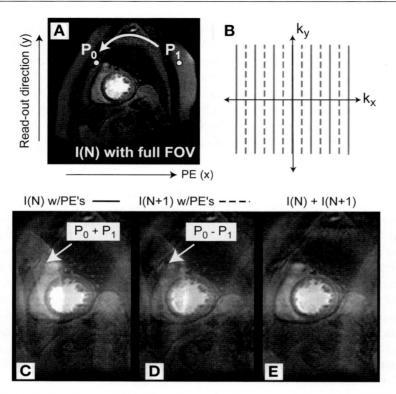

Fig. 7. Unaliasing by Fourier encoding the overlaps using the temporal dimension (UNFOLD) can be applied in dynamic studies by interleaving the phase encodings for acquisition of consecutive images. The interleaved phase encodings are shown as solid and dashed lines in (**A**). The full-field-of-view image in (**B**) was acquired by performing all phase encodings (dashed and solid lines) for the image acquisition; the consecutive images in (**C**) and (**D**) were acquired with only one subset of the phase encodings, which means that the field of view in the phase-encoding direction is halved, giving rise to fold-over artifacts. The relative shift of the phase encodings means that the fold-over artifacts are modulated in this case by a factor of ±1 for the fold-over on the left and ± for the fold-over on the right. This temporal modulation can be used to eliminate the fold-over by temporal filtering. To illustrate the basic concept, the image in (**E**) was obtained as a complex sum of the images from (**C**) and (**D**), which eliminates the fold-over artifact on the left of the image.

untangle image aliasing from simultaneously excited slices, in this case by phase cycling of the radio-frequency pulses. The 2D imaging techniques, compared to three-dimensional imaging, will always be most suitable for freezing cardiac motion in perfusion studies. Techniques like CAIPIRINHA and UNFOLD may bring about the necessary accelerations to allow multislice 2D imaging of the entire heart within a single heartbeat.

ARTERIAL INPUT SAMPLING

For a quantitative assessment of myocardial perfusion, one should take into consideration the characteristics of the contrast agent injection, preferably performed by the bolus method. The kinetics of the transit of the contrast bolus through the LV cavity determines the rate of myocardial contrast enhancement. The myocardial contrast enhancement can be modeled as linear response to the arterial input of contrast. For the quantification of myocardial perfusion, one therefore needs to measure both the myocardial response and the arterial input *(26)*.

Sampling of the arterial input is mostly performed in the LV cavity simply because the cavity is always visible on views used for myocardial perfusion imaging, whether short- or long-axis views. In our experience, it is best to sample the arterial input in the LV near the base of the heart, that is, close to the aortic outflow, and during diastole to minimize inflow-effects. In the LV cavity, the contrast enhancement is an order of magnitude higher than in myocardium. Any saturation of the signal enhancement at higher contrast agent concentrations is most likely to be observed in the blood pool and with an intravenous injection, first in the right ventricle and then in the LV cavity. Sampling the arterial input with some fidelity should entail that signal saturation is avoided, for example, by using low contrast agent dosages on the order of 0.03–0.04 mmol/kg body weight with fast gradient echo sequences (e.g., TR/TE/flip ~2 ms/1 ms/15–20° at 1.5 T). Using low contrast dosages decreases the myocardial contrast enhancement, and peak contrast to noise is in many respects the limiting factor in myocardial perfusion studies. Therefore, new approaches are sought to combine accurate arterial input sampling with optimal myocardial contrast enhancement.

Because of the relatively large dimensions of the cavity compared to the LV wall thickness, it is in principle feasible to acquire images at low spatial resolution to sample the arterial input. Acquisition of low-resolution images for the sole purpose of sampling the arterial input allows one to adjust the contrast sensitivity to the relatively higher concentration of contrast agent in the blood pool compared to the myocardium *(27,28)*. Figure 2B shows that, for an undisturbed relaxation recovery, the SI saturates first with increasing R_1 for longer TIs.

Approximately the same type of relationship holds when an image is acquired during the IR by using an image readout with low flip angle excitation pulses. This indicates that, for sampling of the arterial input, the T_1 weighting can be adjusted to avoid saturation of the signal intensity by acquiring images with relatively short effective delays (TIs) between magnetization preparation and image acquisition. If the arterial input is sampled with low spatial resolution, then the time penalty for acquiring additional images of the arterial input with optimal settings for T_1 weighting is within acceptable limits and approximately 60–100 ms.

A novel variation on this theme was proposed by Köstler et al. for radial imaging *(29)*. In radial imaging, low spatial frequencies are oversampled because the center of the spatial frequency space is traversed during each radial trajectory. One can exploit this to calculate low-resolution images, sufficient to depict the LV cavity, for multiple delays (TIs) after the initial magnetization preparation (e.g., a saturation pulse).

It should be mentioned that whatever magnetization preparation is used for T_1 weighting, it should at least, for the purpose of sampling the arterial input, be non-slice selective to avoid that blood flow (e.g., in the ventricular cavity) sweeps the prepared magnetization out of the slice during the image readout, which would undo the effects of the magnetization preparation. Also, for the myocardium, a non-slice-selective magnetization preparation renders the SI more insensitive to through-plane motion.

As an alternative for arterial input sampling, Christian and colleagues introduced a dual bolus injection technique *(30)*. A small contrast dosage and a several-fold higher contrast dosage are injected consecutively so that the contrast enhancement in the LV cavity and in the myocardium can be sampled separately under optimal conditions.

With the assumption of hemodynamic stability and by using equal injection volumes but different contrast agent dilutions, it is possible to use a scaled replica of the arterial input in the LV cavity, measured with the lower dosage bolus injection, to analyze the contrast enhancement in the myocardium observed with a later higher contrast agent dosage injection. Recirculation of contrast after the first injection should be negligible when the second bolus is injected, which is easily attained by using widely different dilution ratios for the two injections (e.g., equivalent to 0.005 mmol/kg and 0.1 mmol/kg of Gd-DTPA), even if both injections are performed within 20–30 seconds of each other.

PRACTICAL RECOMMENDATIONS

The experience of investigators in this field is slowly leading to some consensus on the technical requirements for myocardial perfusion imaging to maintain acceptable quality and reliability. Table 1 summarizes what are arguably settings that establish a good starting point for perfusion studies with fast, multislice T_1-weighted gradient echo techniques.

The adjustment of the protocol parameters for a myocardial perfusion study can proceed by following these steps:

1. Adjust the field of view to avoid fold-over artifacts and choose the phase-encoding direction to allow a rectangular field of view. The resolution in the readout direction should be approximately 1.5 mm, and resolution in the phase-encoding direction should not be less than 60% of the readout resolution.
2. Adjust the duration of the acquisition window to 80–90% of the R–R duration, depending on how regular the heart beat is. One may have to reset the number of slices to one or two. If the quality of the ECG trace is not acceptable, then switch trigger source to pulse oximeter or perform untriggered acquisition.
3. Maximize the number of slices that can be imaged within duration of acquisition window to allow for maximum coverage of the heart. Use remaining "idle" time within the acquisition window to increase resolution in the phase-encoding direction or reduce the speed-up factor for parallel imaging acquisitions to improve the signal-to-noise ratio. If the number of slices that fit in the acquisition window is unacceptably low, then one should go back and increase the speed-up factor for parallel imaging, increase the receiver bandwidth (i.e., decrease TE and TR), decrease the number of phase encodings, or use a combination of these measures.

The adjustments listed in Steps 1–3 are often made in an iterative fashion.

During the rapid contrast enhancement in the ventricular cavities, one sometimes observes transient artifacts at the endocardial border in the form of a black "rim" or thin black band from signal cancellation. There are multiple potential causes for such artifacts: the very abrupt SI change at the endocardial border, combined with a finite number of encoding steps in a direction perpendicular to the sharp intensity drop-off, causes so-called ringing artifacts that may manifest themselves as a thin black band next to the endocardial border. The difference in magnetic susceptibilities of blood loaded with contrast agent and myocardial tissue before uptake of contrast agent can produce signal loss at the interface between the blood pool and myocardial tissue because of partial volume effects. Finally, the acquisition of the phase encodings during recovery of the magnetization after a magnetization preparation pulse and the resulting modulation of the phase encodings by this magnetization recovery can pro-

Table 1

Parameter	Setting	Considerations
Spatial resolution	<2.5 mm in-plane resolution	Dark rim artifacts more prominent with poor resolution in phase-encoding direction
Temporal resolution	Equal to R–R duration	Period of myocardial contrast enhancement is relatively brief and most sensitive to blood flow level
Slice thickness	<10 mm	Thin slices (<6 mm) often give unacceptable signal to noise, and through-plane motion renders it meaningless to use very thin slices
Parallel imaging	Speed-up factor of 2 or less	Higher speed-up factors may substantially degrade the images
Flip angle	15–20° for fast gradient echo imaging	Assume here a TR/TE on the order of 2 and 1 ms, respectively; It is helpful to estimate the Ernst angle for the particular combination of TR and TE
Echo time (TE)	As short as feasible; ~1–2 ms recommended	Dark rim, or susceptibility artifacts, and motion artifacts at high heart rates, are more likely with longer echo times
Receiver Bandwidth	400–800 Hz/pixel for fast GRE	Bandwidth settings depend very much on choice of coil and characteristics of front-end receiver
T_1 weighting	Saturation recovery preparation	Inversion recovery gives stronger T_1 weighting but renders signal susceptible to heart rate variations
Contrast administration	Bolus injection, preferably with power injector at 3–5 mL/second for 0.5 mmol/mL dilution of Gd-DTPA	A slow infusion of contrast will lead to a loss of sensitivity for assessing blood flow, although it may be indirectly assessed then with the Kety-Schmidt method
Through-plane motion correction	Initial breath holding or navigator technique for slice tracking	In most cases, patient can only hold breath during initial contrast enhancement; navigator tracking is method of choice if slice position can be adjusted in real time

duce artifacts perpendicular to the phase-encoding direction. The dark rim at the endo-cardial border can be misinterpreted as a subendocardial perfusion defect. Increasing the spatial resolution by increasing the number of phase encodings often reduces the prominence of the dark rim artifacts. Image artifacts related to magnetic susceptibility are attenuated by minimizing the TE and, if echo trains are used, by reducing the echo train length.

MYOCARDIAL PERFUSION IMAGING AT HIGH MAGNETIC FIELD STRENGTHS

Magnetic field strengths higher than 1.5 T can be both a blessing and a bane for myocardial perfusion imaging. Use of higher field strengths results in a stronger signal than at lower field strengths; furthermore, T_1 time constants for myocardium increase with field strength, providing a wider dynamic range for contrast-induced T_1 changes. Unfortunately, techniques such as gradient echo imaging with SSFP do not work as well at high field strengths, as at 1.5 T, potentially depriving one of using a significant advance in MR sequence techniques. As perfusion pulse sequence optimization depends on the field strength, one can not easily compare the same technique with fixed parameters across different field strengths. But at least for gradient echo-imaging without SSFP, higher field strength does bring clear advantages.

SIGNAL ANALYSIS AND POSTPROCESSING

With ^{1}H MRI the presence of contrast agent is deduced from the reduction of the ^{1}H relaxation time constants and the increase of the ^{1}H signal if the signal is predominantly T_1 weighted. Water is a freely diffusible tracer, and although the contrast agent may be confined to the intravascular or extracellular space, the ^{1}H nuclei interacting with the paramagnetic contrast agent complexes may move back and forth between spaces permeated by contrast agent and inaccessible to contrast agent, respectively. This process is generally referred to as water exchange and, if ignored, leads to an overestimate of the distribution volume for the contrast agent—water carries the effect of the contrast agent to spaces inaccessible to the contrast agent itself.

The process of water exchange on T_1 measurements was carefully investigated a few decades ago, but the repercussions of the theory of water exchange on perfusion MRI have often been ignored, with some notable exceptions. In particular, Li et al. developed a comprehensive theory that wed the theory of water exchange with the Kety-Schmidt model *(31)*.

The effects of water exchange can be considered at the stage of the pulse sequence optimization or during postprocessing of the data. For the former, the work of Donahue *(32–34)* has made an important contribution by showing that the effects of water exchange can be minimized by driving the magnetization recovery through rapid application of radio-frequency pulses with a sufficiently high flip angle, as is done with rapid gradient echo imaging, with spoiling of the gradient echoes. Alternatively, one can incorporate the effects of water exchange into the tracer kinetic analysis, as shown by Li and colleagues *(31,35)*. The choice depends in part on the goals of the study: if determination of the lifetime of water in the vascular and interstitial spaces is of interest, then one would want to maximize the sensitivity to water exchange by adjustment of the pulse sequence parameters and incorporate the theory of water exchange in the analysis. For example, for higher flip angles, the sensitivity to water exchange is reduced *(34)*. One may want to minimize the effects of water exchange on the observed contrast enhancement if the focus is on quantifying perfusion only.

SPIN-LABELING TECHNIQUES IN THE HEART

Water can be used in perfusion studies as an endogenous contrast agent. To do this requires alteration of the state of ^{1}H nuclei with sharp spatial definition and observing the flux of these prepared ^{1}H nuclei into adjacent tissue (36–38). The experiments are typically run in a difference mode to subtract the background signal from stationary ^{1}H nuclei. Alteration of the state of ^{1}H nuclei typically consists of applying a spatially selective inversion pulse. The same acquisition is then repeated with a non-slice-selective inversion pulse, and the difference signal is proportional to the number of ^{1}H nuclei that have moved into or out of the slice imaged. The slice should be thin enough so that a detectable change of the magnetization can result from ^{1}H flux within less than a time on the order of T_1, with T_1 being the "lifetime" of the altered magnetization state.

The spin-labeling technique does not appear to be mature enough yet for routine clinical application, in part because some significant questions remain. Spin labeling depends on a relatively accurate direct or indirect quantification of T_1 differences because the inflow of labeled spins produces a relatively small change of T_1 that is proportional to the blood flow (39).

Interestingly, the errors for estimating myocardial blood flow with either contrast-enhanced techniques or spin-labeling have a reciprocal dependence on the level of blood flow. Previous studies have shown that the confidence bands for estimating blood flow increase in proportion to blood flow or the perfusion reserve (8). With spin labeling, the accuracy of estimating blood flow increases with blood flow because the proportion of labeled spins entering a slice is directly proportional to flow (39). It was therefore fortuitous that some of the first validation studies of the spin-labeling technique were made in rodents, for which myocardial blood flows even at baseline are three to five times higher than in humans.

OUTLOOK

Significant advances have been made in the technical development of myocardial perfusion imaging with MR. This exposition has focused on some tried and robust approaches while also offering an outlook on promising new developments, which may finally allow coverage of the entire heart with adequate temporal resolution. Exciting new prospects are appearing on the horizon, such as the use of hyperpolarized tracers, which have already been evaluated for renal (40) and cerebral (41) perfusion studies. Although it may be premature to include a discussion of perfusion imaging with hyperpolarized tracers in this overview, one should nonetheless acknowledge the enormous further improvements this may bring about. It is therefore fair to say that, with MRI, much room is left to exhaust the full potential of myocardial perfusion imaging, but at the same time the currently available techniques are already more than adequate for clinical studies.

ACKNOWLEDGMENTS

The author gratefully acknowledges support from NIH/NHBLI and from the Whitaker Foundation.

REFERENCES

1. Wilke NM, Jerosch-Herold M, Zenovich A, Stillman AE. Magnetic resonance first-pass myocardial perfusion imaging: clinical validation and future applications. J Magn Reson Imaging 1999;10:676–685.
2. Chen Z, Prato FS, McKenzie CA. T_1 fast acquisition relaxation mapping (T_1-FARM): an optimised reconstruction. IEEE Trans Med Imaging 1998;17:155–160.
3. Tsekos NV, Zhang Y, Merkle H, et al. Fast anatomical imaging of the heart and assessment of myocardial perfusion with arrhythmia insensitive magnetization preparation. Magn Reson Med 1995;34:530–536.
4. Bellamy DD, Pereira RS, McKenzie CA, et al. Gd-DTPA bolus tracking in the myocardium using T_1 fast acquisition relaxation mapping (T_1 FARM). Magn Reson Med 2001;46:555–564.
5. Mai VM, Chen Q, Bankier AA, et al. Imaging pulmonary blood flow and perfusion using phase-sensitive selective inversion recovery. Magn Reson Med 2000;43:793–795.
6. Slavin GS, Wolff SD, Gupta SN, Foo TK. First-pass myocardial perfusion MR imaging with interleaved notched saturation: feasibility study. Radiology 2001;219:258–263.
7. Wilke N, Jerosch-Herold M, Wang Y, et al. Myocardial perfusion reserve: assessment with multisection, quantitative, first-pass MR imaging. Radiology 1997;204:373–384.
8. Klocke FJ, Simonetti OP, Judd RM, et al. Limits of detection of regional differences in vasodilated flow in viable myocardium by first-pass magnetic resonance perfusion imaging. Circulation 2001; 104:2412–2416.
9. Chiu CW, So NM, Lam WW, Chan KY, Sanderson JE. Combined first-pass perfusion and viability study at MR imaging in patients with non-ST segment-elevation acute coronary syndromes: feasibility study. Radiology 2003;226:717–722.
10. Scheffler K, Hennig J. T_1 quantification with inversion recovery TrueFISP. Magn Reson Med 2001; 45:720–723.
11. Schmitt P, Griswold MA, Jakob PM, et al. Inversion recovery TrueFISP: quantification of T(1), T(2), and spin density. Magn Reson Med 2004;51:661–667.
12. Hunold P, Maderwald S, Eggebrecht H, Vogt FM, Barkhausen J. Steady-state free precession sequences in myocardial first-pass perfusion MR imaging: comparison with TurboFLASH imaging. Eur Radiol 2004;14:409–416.
13. Edelman RR, Li W. Contrast-enhanced echo-planar MR imaging of myocardial perfusion: preliminary study in humans. Radiology 1994;190:771–777.
14. Panting J, Gatehouse P, Yang G, et al. Echo-planar magnetic resonance myocardial perfusion imaging: parametric map analysis and comparison with thallium SPECT. J Magn Reson Imaging 2001;13: 192–200.
15. Epstein FH, London JF, Peters DC, et al. Multislice first-pass cardiac perfusion MRI: validation in a model of myocardial infarction. Magn Reson Med 2002;47:482–491.
16. Elkington AG, Gatehouse PD, Cannell TM, et al. Comparison of hybrid echo-planar imaging and FLASH myocardial perfusion cardiovascular MR imaging. Radiology 2005;235:237–243.
17. Sodickson DK, Manning WJ. Simultaneous acquisition of spatial harmonics (SMASH): fast imaging with radiofrequency coil arrays. Magn Reson Med 1997;38:591–603.
18. Pruessmann KP, Weiger M, Scheidegger MB, Boesiger P. SENSE: sensitivity encoding for fast MRI. Magn Reson Med 1999;42:952–962.
19. Pruessmann KP, Weiger M, Boesiger P. Sensitivity encoded cardiac MRI. J Cardiovasc Magn Reson 2001;3:1–9.
20. Kroll K, Wilke N, Jerosch-Herold M, et al. Accuracy of modeling of regional myocardial flows from residue functions of an intravascular indicator. Am J Physiol (Heart Circ Physiol) 1996;40: H1643–H1655.
21. Madore B. Using UNFOLD to remove artifacts in parallel imaging and in partial-Fourier imaging. Magn Reson Med 2002;48:493–501.
22. Madore B. UNFOLD-SENSE: a parallel MRI method with self-calibration and artifact suppression. Magn Reson Med 2004;52:310–320.
23. Madore B, Glover GH, Pelc NJ. Unaliasing by Fourier-encoding the overlaps using the temporal dimension (UNFOLD), applied to cardiac imaging and fMRI. Magn Reson Med 1999;42:813–828.
24. Di Bella EV, Wu YJ, Alexander AL, Parker DL, Green D, McGann CJ. Comparison of temporal filtering methods for dynamic contrast MRI myocardial perfusion studies. Magn Reson Med 2003;49: 895–902.
25. Breuer FA, Blaimer M, Heidemann RM, Mueller MF, Griswold MA, Jakob PM. Controlled aliasing in parallel imaging results in higher acceleration (CAIPIRINHA) for multi-slice imaging. Magn Reson Med 2005;53:684–691.

26. Jerosch-Herold M, Seethamraju RT, Swingen CM, Wilke NM, Stillman AE. Analysis of myocardial perfusion MRI. J Magn Reson Imaging 2004;19:758–770.

27. Gatehouse PD, Elkington AG, Ablitt NA, Yang GZ, Pennell DJ, Firmin DN. Accurate assessment of the arterial input function during high-dose myocardial perfusion cardiovascular magnetic resonance. J Magn Reson Imaging 2004;20:39–45.

28. Kim D, Cernicanu A, Axel L. Multi-Slice, First-pass myocardial perfusion MRI with undistorted arterial input function and higher myocardial enhancement at 3 T. Paper presented at: Scientific Sessions of the International Society of Magnetic Resonance in Medicine (ISMRM); May 11, 2005; Miami Beach, FL.

29. Köstler H, Ritter C, Baunach D, et al. Determination of the arterial input function in high dose radial myocardial perfusion imaging. Paper presented at: Scientific Sessions of the International Society of Magnetic Resonance in Medicine (ISMRM); May 11, 2005; Miami Beach, FL.

30. Christian TF, Rettmann DW, Aletras AH, et al. Absolute myocardial perfusion in canines measured by using dual-bolus first-pass MR imaging. Radiology 2004;232:677–684.

31. Li X, Huang W, Yankeelov TE, Tudorica A, Rooney WD, Springer CS Jr. Shutter-speed analysis of contrast reagent bolus-tracking data: preliminary observations in benign and malignant breast disease. Magn Reson Med 2005;53:724–729.

32. Donahue KM, Burstein D. Proton exchange rates in myocardial tissue with Gd-DTPA administration. New York: 1993. Proceedings of the 1993 conference of the Society of Magnetic Resonance in Medicine (SMRM), Berkeley, CA. Conference location was New York, NY.

33. Donahue KM, Weisskoff RM, Burstein D. Water diffusion and exchange as they influence contrast enhancement. J Magn Reson Imaging 1997;7:102–110.

34. Donahue KM, Weisskoff RM, Chesler DA, et al. Improving MR quantification of regional blood volume with intravascular T_1 contrast agents: accuracy, precision, and water exchange. Magn Reson Med 1996;36:858–867.

35. Landis CS, Li X, Telang FW, et al. Determination of the MRI contrast agent concentration time course in vivo following bolus injection: effect of equilibrium transcytolemmal water exchange. Magn Reson Med 2000;44:563–574.

36. Wacker CM, Fidler F, Dueren C, et al. Quantitative assessment of myocardial perfusion with a spin-labeling technique: preliminary results in patients with coronary artery disease. J Magn Reson Imaging 2003;18:555–560.

37. Waller C, Kahler E, Hiller KH, et al. Myocardial perfusion and intracapillary blood volume in rats at rest and with coronary dilatation: MR imaging in vivo with use of a spin-labeling technique. Radiology 2000;215:189–197.

38. Reeder SB, Atalay MK, McVeigh ER, Zerhouni EA, Forder JR. Quantitative cardiac perfusion: a noninvasive spin-labeling method that exploits coronary vessel geometry. Radiology 1996;200:177–184.

39. Zhang H, Shea SM, Park V, et al. Accurate myocardial T_1 measurements: toward quantification of myocardial blood flow with arterial spin labeling. Magn Reson Med 2005;53:1135–1142.

40. Johansson E, Olsson LE, Mansson S, et al. Perfusion assessment with bolus differentiation: a technique applicable to hyperpolarized tracers. Magn Reson Med 2004;52:1043–1051.

41. Johansson E, Mansson S, Wirestam R, et al. Cerebral perfusion assessment by bolus tracking using hyperpolarized [13]C. Magn Reson Med 2004;51:464–472.

8 Techniques in the Assessment of Cardiovascular Blood Flow and Velocity

Michael Markl

CONTENTS

INTRODUCTION

Magnetic resonance imaging (MRI) has been increasingly recognized for its role in the diagnosis, treatment planning, and clinical management of patients with cardiovascular disease and has several important advantages over alternative imaging modalities, including electrocardiogram (ECG) synchronized and direct three-dimensional (3D) volumetric imaging unrestricted by imaging depth. In addition, the intrinsic sensitivity of MRI to flow, motion, and diffusion offers the unique possibility to acquire spatially registered functional information simultaneously with the morphological data within a single experiment *(1–13,16–19,31,36,38)*. As a result, flow-sensitive MRI techniques, also known as phase contrast (PC) MRI, provide noninvasive methods for the accurate and quantitative assessment of blood flow or tissue motion. Characterizations of the dynamic components of blood flow and cardiovascular function provide insight into normal and pathological physiology and have made considerable progress *(14,15,20–29,35,55)*.

BASIC CONCEPTS: VELOCITY ENCODING

Most magnetic resonance (MR) sequences demonstrate more or less significant sensitivity to flow and motion, which can lead to artifacts in many applications. The intrinsic motion sensitivity of MRI, however, not only can be used to image vessels as

From: *Contemporary Cardiology: Cardiovascular Magnetic Resonance Imaging*
Edited by: Raymond Y. Kwong © Humana Press Inc., Totowa, NJ

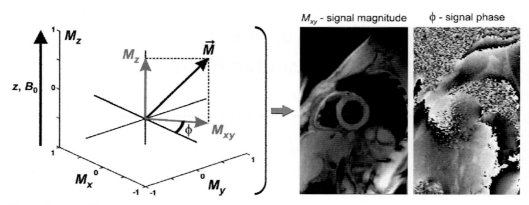

Fig. 1. Longitudinal (M_z) and transverse (M_{xy}) components of spin magnetization in blood or tissue generating the complex MR signal (left). Magnitude and phase images can be derived from the length and orientation of the transverse magnetization component (right). In combination with appropriate encoding gradients, phase images are motion sensitive and can be used to directly measure the local velocities of moving spins on a pixel-to-pixel basis.

in PC MR angiography but also to quantify blood flow and motion of tissue. Based on the observation that the local spin magnetization is a vector quantity (*see* also Fig. 1), phase images can be extracted from the measured MR signal in addition to magnitude data typically reconstructed after data acquisition.

Using appropriate velocity-encoding gradients, flow- or motion-dependent phase effects can be used to measure two data sets with different velocity-dependent signal phase at otherwise identical acquisition parameters. Subtraction of the two resulting phase images allows the quantitative assessment of the velocities of the underlying flow or motion *(18)*. If the motion of the tissue under investigation does not change fast with respect to the temporal resolution of data acquisition, the corresponding velocities can be approximated to be constant during the measurement of a single time frame. Based on these approximations, velocity encoding is usually performed using bipolar gradients as depicted in Fig. 2 and Fig. 4, which do not lead to any phase encoding of stationary spins. Moving spins, however, will experience a linear velocity-dependent phase change that is proportional to not only the blood flow velocity itself but also the amplitude and timing of the gradient. Adjusting gradient duration or gradient strength therefore permits the flexible adjustment of velocity-induced phase shifts and thus the control of the velocity sensitivity (*venc*) of a flow measurement by the user.

Note that only velocity components along the direction of the bipolar flow-encoding gradient contribute to the phase of the MR signal such that only a single velocity direction can be encoded with an individual measurement. In addition, background phase effects caused by susceptibility of field inhomogeneity can not be refocused using bipolar gradients.

To filter out such phase effects in a typical PC experiment, two measurements with different flow sensitivities (e.g., bipolar gradients of inverted polarity as in Fig. 2) are thus necessary to isolate the velocity-encoded phase shifts and encode flow or motion along a single direction. Subtraction of phase images from two such measurements

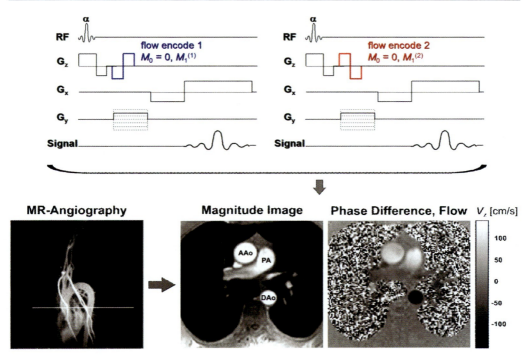

Fig. 2. (Top) Gradient echo pulse sequences for one-directional velocity encoding along the slice direction using bipolar gradients with opposite polarity. See appendix at the end of this chapter for the definition and discussion of gradient moments M_0 and M_1 used for flow encoding. (Bottom) Resulting through-plane measurement of blood flow velocities in the ascending (AAo) and descending (DAo) aorta and the pulmonary artery (PA). The gray scale values in the phase difference image (right) correspond to systolic blood flow velocities normal to the image plane. Note the enhanced velocity noise in regions of low signal (lungs) in the magnitude images. The temporal evolution of the phase contrast images with through-plane velocity encoding and additional velocity noise filtering is also depicted in supplemental Movie 1.

results in phase difference images in which each pixel value is directly proportional to the underlying blood flow velocity (*see* also Fig. 2). A more detailed discussion of MR signal properties and velocity encoding is given in this chapter's appendix.

PC MRI also requires knowledge of the magnitude of the velocities that are to be imaged. For too high velocities, the velocity-dependent phase shift can exceed $\pm\pi$, and aliasing occurs. Velocity sensitivity *(venc)* is thus defined as the velocity that produces a phase shift of π radians and is determined by the difference of the gradients used for velocity encoding. Consequently, the highest velocity, which is expected, has to be used to define the velocity encoding to avoid unintentional phase wrapping *(45)*. Figure 3 shows an example of a through-plane flow measurement with blood flow velocities in the descending aorta exceeding the user-selected *venc*. The resulting velocity aliasing can clearly be identified as bright signal (arrow), falsely indicating reversed flow velocities in a region with otherwise negative flow velocities.

As for all MRI techniques, PC velocity images suffer from noise that can lead to errors in the acquired velocities. It can be shown that the noise in the velocity-encoded images, defined as the standard deviation σ_ϕ of the phase differences in a homogeneous

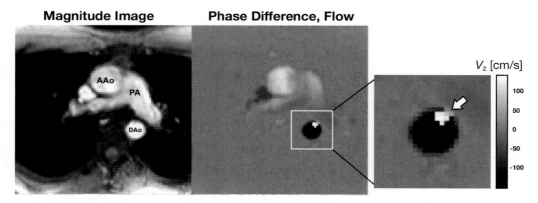

Fig. 3. (Top) Typical appearance of velocity aliasing in through plane-encoded blood flow velocities measurements in the ascending (AAo) and descending (DAo) aorta and the pulmonary artery (PA). Regions in the DAo with systolic blood flow velocities exceeding the predefined velocity sensitivity (*venc*) lead to misencoding of blood flow and a phase wraparound in the phase difference images (right, white arrow). Lower blood flow velocities in the ascending aorta (i.e., < *venc*) results in unaliased and more homogeneous depiction of through-plane flow.

region with no flow or motion, is inversely related to the signal-to-noise ratio (SNR) in the corresponding magnitude images ($\sigma_\phi \sim 1/SNR$) *(36,46)*. Noise in the velocities derived from the phase difference data can therefore be estimated by

$$\sigma_n = \frac{\sqrt{2}}{\pi} \frac{venc}{SNR}.$$

For a given SNR, the velocity noise is thus determined by the user-selected velocity sensitivity (*venc*), resulting in a trade-off between the minimum detectable velocity due to noise and the maximum velocity that can be detected without aliasing. For optimal noise performance, the *venc* should therefore always be selected as small as possible.

METHODS AND IMPLEMENTATION

Several velocity-encoding strategies exist and have been reported in the literature, including echo time (TE) or gradient moment optimized implementations *(18,20–21)*.

A possible alternative is provided by so-called flow compensation techniques that permit the acquisition of a reference scan with vanishing velocity-dependent signal phase. Here, gradient switching schemes are chosen such that, in addition to static spins, all velocity-induced phase shifts are refocused at TE. These schemes can be analytically calculated and designed for all three spatial encoding directions. Usually, first-order motion compensation is sufficient for acquisition of artifact-free images.

Velocity encoding is then performed by a second scan with added bipolar gradients but otherwise identical parameters (*see* Fig. 4). As a result, the reference scan generates background phase images only while the second motion sensitive scan is used to define velocity sensitivity (*venc*) and encode blood flow velocities. An advantage over other methods is related to reduced pulsatile flow artifacts in the reference images. However, in comparison to standard pulse sequences, additional gradients are necessary, which may lead to increased echo and repetition times.

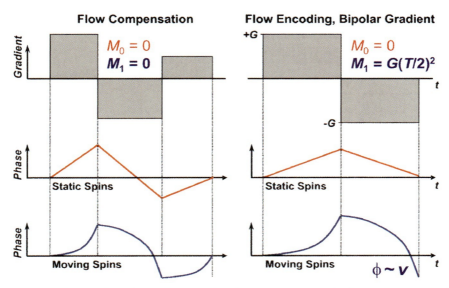

Fig. 4. Schematic illustration of velocity encoding for phase contrast MRI. Application of a bipolar gradient (right) results in an MR signal phase directly proportional to the local flow or object motion; static tissue is fully refocused. Subtraction from a reference scan with flow compensation eliminates background effects and permits direct quantification of flow and tissue motion. See appendix at the end of this chapter for the definition and discussion of gradient moments M_0 and M_1 used for flow encoding.

Because velocity sensitization can only be achieved in one direction per experiment, at least four independent measurements (reference scan and three motion-sensitive measurements in x-, y-, and z-directions) have to be performed to gain a 3D velocity data set with isotropic flow or motion sensitivity.

The first-order approximation (constant velocities) typically used for PC MRI is only valid if the involved velocities do not change significantly with respect to the temporal resolution (i.e., TE) of the pulse sequence *(58,62,74)*. To ensure that the velocities of moving spins can be assumed to be constant while data corresponding to a certain time frame is received, the most widely used techniques for PC data acquisition are therefore based on fast radio-frequency (RF)-spoiled gradient echo-based sequences.

To synchronize PC measurements with periodic tissue motion or pulsatile flow, data acquisition is typically gated to the cardiac cycle, and time-resolved (cine) anatomical images are collected to depict the dynamics of tissue motion and blood flow during the cardiac cycle *(19,25–29,33,39,50,55,70)*.

To accomplish this task, the measurement has to be repeated over a number of ECG cycles to gain a sequence of images representing different phases of cardiac motion. Those ECG-gated cine images are acquired using k-space segmented scan procedures usually based on gradient echo or segmented echo-planar imaging pulse sequences.

For PC velocity mapping, bipolar gradients have to be introduced at appropriate positions, and several sets of cine images have to be acquired because multiple scans with different first-gradient moment scans are needed to derive blood or tissue velocities from

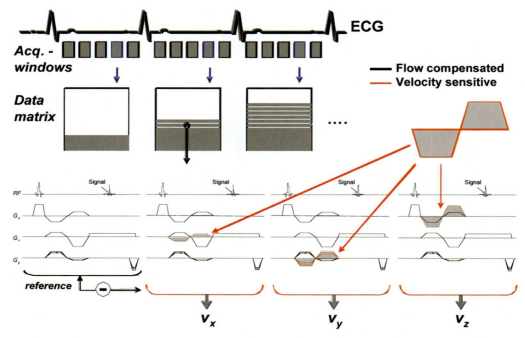

Fig. 5. Example of cardiac-gated *k*-space segmented cine phase contrast MRI for three-directional velocity encoding. For each *k*-space line, a flow-compensated reference scan and three motion-sensitive scans (added bipolar gradients) are acquired in an interleaved manner. Measurements are synchronized with the ECG cycle. The temporal resolution and total scan time can be flexibly adjusted by the number of velocity-sensitive acquisitions and *k*-space segments.

the data. Thus, for each slice or 3D slab under investigation, successive acquisitions have to be performed for reference scan and up to three motion-sensitized acquisitions to derive one- to three-directional velocity fields from the data. To minimize artifacts in phase difference images related to subject motion, interleaved velocity encoding is often performed, for which the different flow encodes are kept as close together as possible in time. To enhance scan efficiency, flow compensation and encoding gradients are usually integrated into the imaging gradients (*see* Fig. 5).

Measurements are most often performed during breath holding; the *k*-space segmentation factor, i.e. number of acquired *k*–space lines during one cardiac cycle for each time frame, can be used to trade off spatial and temporal resolution and total acquisition time.

For high temporal and spatial resolution scans or acquisition of multiple slices or entire 3D volumes, single breath hold periods are no longer sufficient to collect the required data, and respiration control such as navigator gating or triggering by mechanical bellows has to be introduced into the imaging sequence.

Temporal and spatial resolution of the PC cine images can be further increased by the use of view-sharing techniques for data acquisitions. Here, central parts of *k*-space are updated more frequently if compared to outer regions of the raw data matrix. Several applications of this technique have already been proposed and are often used for reduction of total imaging time *(63,103–105)*. For cine MRI, these methods exploit the high degree of interframe correlation that exists between time-resolved cardiac images.

In addition, it can be shown that the velocity-induced phase shift in PC techniques is mainly encoded in the central section of k-space, which makes view sharing also suitable for PC flow measurements *(77,78)*.

APPLICATIONS: FLOW QUANTIFICATION AND FLOW VISUALIZATION

Visualization and quantification of blood flow and tissue motion using PC MRI has been widely used in a number of applications. In addition to analyzing tissue motion such as left ventricular function *(24,35,43,51,54,66,68)*, time-resolved two-dimensional (2D) and 3D PC MRI have proven to be useful tools for the assessment of blood flow within the cardiovascular system *(26–30,34,50,52,55,56,57,67,70,72)*.

Fast 2D and 3D velocity-mapping techniques can be used not only to evaluate blood flow to quantify cardiovascular performance (e.g., aortic regurgitation) but also to allow the assessment of complex 3D flow patterns, which are potentially linked to structure and remodeling of surrounding tissue. Traditionally, MRI imaging of flow is accomplished using methods that resolve two spatial dimensions (2D) in individual slices. The temporal dimension can be assessed using techniques such as k-space segmentation in combination with retrospectively or prospectively gated cine imaging. Data analysis is typically based on semiautomatic segmentation of the vascular lumen of interest and calculation of time-resolved blood flow from mean flow velocities and vascular cross-sectional area. To minimize partial volume effects that may lead to flow quantification errors, vessel segmentation and determination of lumen area should be performed on magnitude images *(32,44)*.

As an example, Fig. 6 shows the results of flow profile visualization and flow quantification in the proximal ascending aorta for a through-plane flow-encoding experiment.

Applications include the assessment of left ventricular performance (e.g., cardiac output), regurgitation volumes in case of valve insufficiency, or evaluation of flow acceleration in stenotic regions (e.g., aortic valve stenosis). Figure 7 illustrates the use of PC flow analysis in a plane transecting the aortic outflow tract for a patient with aortic insufficiency. In addition to high blood flow velocities during the systolic phase, in-plane flow encoding clearly reveals a diastolic flow jet (white arrows) associated with accelerated and reverse flow through the incompletely closed valve.

Typically, multiple slices are acquired sequentially using several breath-held measurements. Disadvantages of these techniques include the inconsistent and incomplete spatial volume coverage caused by gaps between adjacent slices, imperfect slice profiles, and breath-hold misregistration. Further, it is demanding to obtain high spatial resolution in the slice direction because of the intrinsically lower SNR of 2D vs 3D spatial encoding. Alternatively, 3D spatial encoding offers the possibility of isotropic high spatial resolution and thus the ability to measure and visualize the temporal evolution of complex flow and motion patterns in a 3D volume *(27,48,60,65,68,80)*. Such methods obtain, for each pixel within a 3D volume at each measured time-point of the cardiac cycle, anatomical and three-directional velocity information. Several groups have reported advances in the application of time-resolved 3D cine PC MRI (Fig. 8), which has the advantage of imaging blood flow with complete spatial and temporal coverage of the area of interest. Recently reported applications include analysis of blood flow through artificial valves *(60)*, ventricular flow patterns *(48,57)*, blood flow characteristics in the thoracic aorta *(27,80)*, and relative pressure mapping within the cardiovascular system *(59,61,79)*.

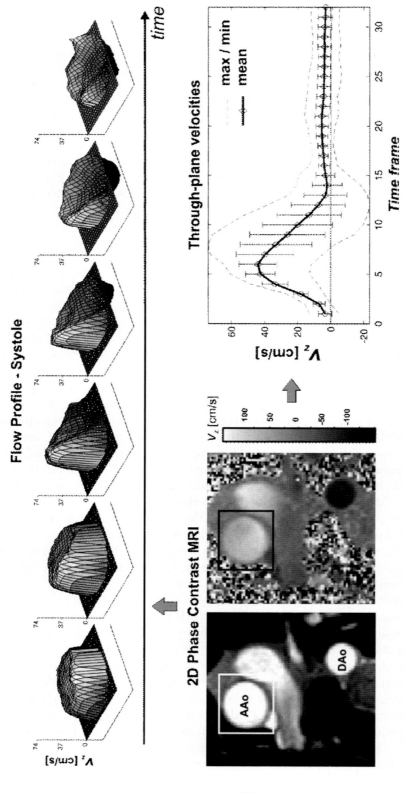

Fig. 6. Blood flow quantification in an axial slice in the proximal ascending aorta (AAo) just above the aortic valve using through-plane velocity encoding. Segmentation of vascular boundaries permits the calculation of mean, max, and min blood flow velocities (lower right), which can be used to calculate average and peak flow rates. Additional visualization of systolic through-plane flow profiles (top) provides detailed insights into the temporal evolution of the spatial distribution of blood flow velocities. The dynamic evolution of blood flow profiles extracted from ECG-synchronized phase contrast images over the entire cardiac cycle is also illustrated in supplemental Movie 2.

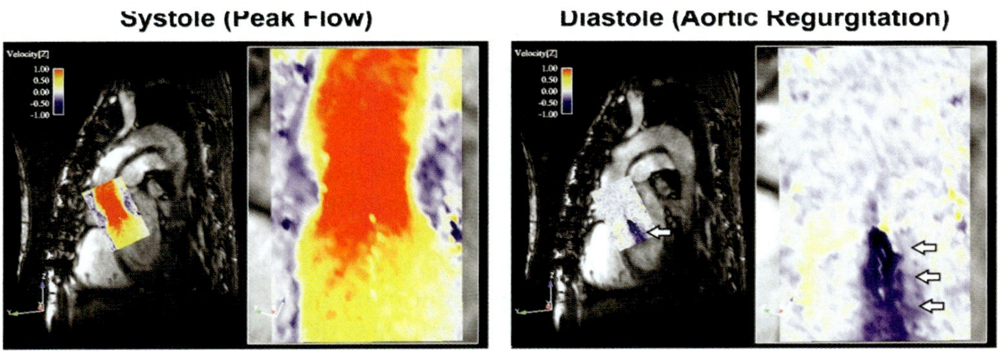

Systole (Peak Flow) **Diastole (Aortic Regurgitation)**

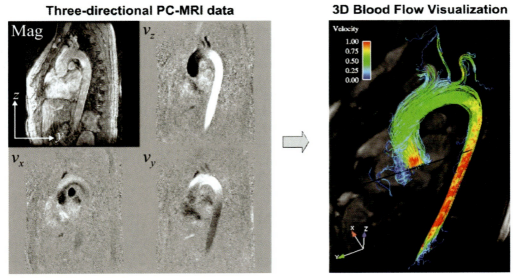

Fig. 7. Color-coded z-velocity components for a patient with aortic insufficiency overlaid onto the simultaneously acquired anatomical (magnitude) images. The systolic and diastolic time frames show in-plane blood flow velocities normal to the aortic valve. A diastolic velocity jet indicating incomplete valve closure and complex regurgitant blood flow (white arrows) is clearly visible during diastole. The temporal evolution of blood flow velocities over the entire cardiac cycle can be viewed in supplemental Movie 3.

Three-directional PC-MRI data **3D Blood Flow Visualization**

Fig. 8. (Left) Magnitude (Mag) and velocity-encoded phase difference images (v_x, v_y, and v_z) from time-resolved three-directional 3D PC MRI. The images depict a single sagittal oblique slice during systole within the acquired 3D volume. Each velocity image represents quantitative Cartesian velocity components in which the gray scale values correspond to the velocity magnitude and direction. (Right) Blood flow visualization using 3D stream lines in the thoracic aorta. The individual lines represent traces along the instantaneous velocity vector field in a systolic time frame and are color coded according to velocity magnitude in meters per second. An example for 3D visualization of the dynamics of blood flow in the thoracic aorta is also provided in supplemental Movie 4.

Because of the acquisition of at least four data sets for three-directional velocity encoding, PC MRI inherits a trade-off between spatial/temporal resolution and total scan time. For thoracic and abdominal applications, respiration control (e.g., breath holding for single-slice 2D measurements or respiratory gating for 3D methods) can therefore be necessary to avoid breathing artifacts.

SOURCES OF ERROR

PC MRI has been extensively validated in phantom and in vivo studies and has proven to be a reliable tool for the quantitative and qualitative analysis of blood flow and tissue motion *(13,22,25,29,33,39–42,52,56)*.

However, several effects can introduce imperfection in PC MRI, which causes errors in velocity measurements by affecting the velocity-induced MR signal phase. Three major sources of inaccuracy in velocity-encoded images include eddy current effects, Maxwell terms, and gradient field distortions *(30,53,64,74)*.

Field gradient switching causes a change dB/dt in magnetic flux, thereby inducing eddy currents on the conducting parts of the scanner system (coils) or in the patient, where they can cause spatially varying phase errors in the MR images. For PC MRI, the different gradient waveforms that are used for the subsequent velocity encodes lead to different eddy current-induced phase changes in the individual phase images. As a result, subtraction of phase images does not eliminate errors related to eddy currents, and additional data processing is needed to restore the original velocity-encoded signal phase.

Several correction strategies have been proposed and are typically based on the subtraction of the spatially varying eddy current-induced phases changes as estimated form static tissue. Although automatic correction algorithms have been reported, user interaction may be required to correctly identify static background signal.

In contrast, compensation for Maxwell terms (sometimes referred to as concomitant gradient terms) and for gradient field nonlinearities does not require any user interaction. Corrections can be performed during image reconstruction based on the knowledge of the gradient waveforms (Maxwell terms) and a gradient field model describing deviations between the designed and the actual velocity-encoding gradients (gradient field nonlinearities).

Additional sources of error as a result of complex flow and inadequate timing of the flow encoding include acceleration effect and spatial displacement *(58,62,76)*.

SUMMARY AND DISCUSSION

MRI provides a noninvasive method for the accurate 3D anatomic characterization of the heart and great vessels. In addition, the intrinsic sensitivity of MRI to flow and motion offers the possibility to acquire spatially registered functional information simultaneously with the morphological data within a single PC experiment.

A disadvantage of PC MRI is related to the need for multiple acquisitions for encoding a single velocity direction, resulting in long scan times. New methods based on the combination of PC MRI and fast sampling strategies such as spiral or radial imaging or other imaging strategies such as balanced steady-state free precession have been reported and are promising for further reduction in total scan time or increased spatial or temporal resolution *(37,63,71)*.

In addition, the total acquisition time or temporal and spatial resolution associated with a specific MR technique may be further improved (at the expense of SNR and artifacts) by using multicoil parallel imaging (simultaneous acquisition of spatial harmonics [SMASH], sensitivity encoding [SENSE], generalized autocalibrating partially acquisitions [GRAPPA], etc.) or partial *k*-space update methods (view sharing) *(77,78,81)*. Parallel imaging takes advantage of arrangement and spatial sensitivity of different receiver coils and has been used in numerous applications in which substantial reductions in scan time or improvements in temporal or spatial resolution could be achieved. Application of imaging acceleration to 3D MRI is particularly promising because two spatial-encoding dimensions can be optimized to accelerate data acquisition. Further promising methods for improvements in scan efficiency are based on methods that utilize symmetries in the temporal domain of the flow or motion data (temporal SENSE [TSENSE], dynamic autocalibrated parallel imaging using temporal GRAPPA [TGRAPPA], k-t broad-use linear acquisition speed-up technique [BLAST], etc).

MR velocity mapping has great potential to benefit from imaging at higher field strength because RF power deposition increase caused by SAR limitations does not pose a major problem (small flip angles). The gain in SNR associated with high field MRI can be used for improved image quality and is directly translated in reduced noise in the velocity-encoded images. Recently reported results indicate a considerable gain in SNR *(73)*, which may also be used to increase spatial or temporal resolution.

For the analysis and visualization of complex, three-directional blood flow within a 3D volume, various visualization tools, including 2D vector fields and 3D streamlines and particle traces, have been reported *(23,48,65,80)*.

To reduce the amount of information to a level at which blood flow in 3D is more easily appreciated, 3D streamlines (3D representation of the velocity vector field at a specific time), or time-resolved 3D particle traces (time-resolved path of virtual particles over the entire cardiac cycle) have been shown to produce an accurate visualization of the measured velocity field.

In addition, more advanced data quantification of directly measured (e.g., flow rates) and derived parameters (e.g., pressure difference maps, wall sheer stress, etc.) is promising for the evaluation of new clinical markers for the characterization of cardiovascular disease *(59,61,76,79)*. Noninvasive methods for estimation of pressure differences have been developed using MRI techniques. These pressure estimation techniques are based on MRI velocity data and utilize the Navier-Stokes equation, which describes the relation between the velocity field and the pressure gradient field.

APPENDIX: MAGNETIC RESONANCE SIGNAL PHASE AND VELOCITY ENCODING

The phase dependency of the MR signal to moving spins can be derived from the precession frequency of spins in local magnetic fields. The Larmor frequency of spins at the spatial location $\vec{r}$ in a static magnetic field B_0, local field inhomogeneity ΔB_0, and an added magnetic field gradient $\vec{G}$ is given by

Because flow or motion is taken into account, the spin positions are described by the time-dependent vector $\vec{r}_0(t)$. After signal reception, the acquired MR signal is demodulated with respect to the Larmor frequency $\omega_{L,0}$ in the static magnetic field B_0. This

$$\omega_L(\vec{r},t) = \gamma\, B_z(\vec{r},t) = \gamma B_0 + \gamma\Delta B_0 + \gamma\, \vec{r}(t)\vec{G}(t)$$

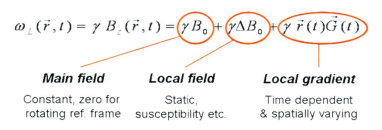

Main field   **Local field**   **Local gradient**

Constant, zero for   Static,   Time dependent
rotating ref. frame   susceptibility etc.   & spatially varying

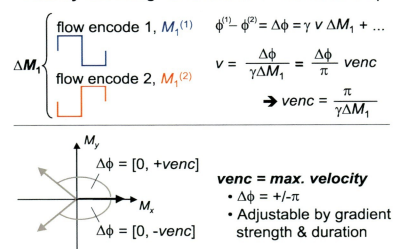

Fig. A1. Velocity encoding and definition of velocity sensitivity. Bipolar gradients with opposite polarity result in different first moments $M_1^{(1)}$ and $M_1^{(2)}$ to encode flow or motion along a single direction. Phase difference calculation eliminates the background phase and permits quantitative assessment flow or motion. Velocity aliasing occurs if the underlying motion exceeds *venc*.

corresponds to a transformation of the MR signal into a rotating reference frame such that the main field contribution to the signal frequency can be omitted for further calculation. Integration of Eq. A1 results in the phase of the precessing magnetization and thus the phase of the measured MR signal after an excitation pulse (at t_0) at TE:

$$\phi(\vec{r}, \text{TE}) \quad \phi(\vec{r}, t_0) = \int_{t_0}^{TE} \omega_L(\vec{r}, t)dt = \gamma \Delta B_0(\text{TE} \quad t_0) + \gamma \int_{t_0}^{TE} \vec{G}(t)\vec{r}(t)dt. \qquad \text{(A2)}$$

which can be expanded in the following Taylor series:

$$\phi(\vec{r}, \text{TE}) = \phi(\vec{r}, t_0) + \gamma \Delta B_0(\text{TE} \quad t_0) + \sum_{n=0}^{\infty} \phi_n(\vec{r}^{(n)}, \text{TE})$$

$$= \phi_0 + \sum_{n=0}^{\infty} \gamma \frac{\vec{r}^{(n)}}{n!} \int_{t_0}^{TE} \vec{G}(t)(t \quad t_0)^n dt, \qquad \text{(A3)}$$

with $r^{(n)}$ the nth derivative of the time-dependent spin position and ϕ_n the corresponding n^{th} order phase. Initial signal phase and field inhomogeneities result in an additional background phase ϕ_0. If the motion of the tissue under investigation does not change fast with respect to the temporal resolution of data acquisition the corresponding velocities can be approximated to be constant during the measurement of each time frame. Thus $\vec{r}_0(t)$ can be introduced as first order displacement $\vec{r}_0(t) = \vec{r}_0 + \vec{v}(t-t_0)$ with a constant velocity $\vec{v} = (v_x(\vec{r}_0), v_y(\vec{r}_0), v_z(\vec{r}_0))$. Equation A3 then simplifies to

$$\phi(\vec{r},\mathrm{TE}) = \phi_0 + \gamma\vec{r_0}\int_0^{TE}\vec{G}(t)dt + \gamma\vec{v}\int_0^{TE}\vec{G}(t)t\,dt + \dots$$

$$\underbrace{\qquad\qquad}\quad\underbrace{\qquad\qquad}\qquad\qquad\text{(A4)}$$

Gradient M_0 + M_1 + ...

moments: Static spins   Moving spins

including an unknown background phase and zeroth- and first–order components $\phi_0(\vec{r_0},\mathrm{TE})$ and $\phi_1(\vec{r_0},\mathrm{TE})$, which describe the influence of magnetic field gradients on phase components of static spins at $\vec{r_0}$ and moving spins with velocities $\vec{v}$, respectively.

The integrals describing the contribution of the magnetic field gradients are also known as n^{th}-order gradient moments M_n such that the first gradient moment M_1 determines the velocity-induced signal phase for the constant velocity approximation. As a result, appropriate control of the first gradient moment can be used to specifically encode spin flow or motion.

Velocity encoding is usually performed using bipolar gradients as depicted in Fig. A1, which, according to Eq. A4, result in zero M_0 and thus do not lead to any phase encoding of stationary spins. Moving spins, however, will experience a linear velocity-dependent phase change that is proportional to the amplitude and timing of the gradient. According to Eq. A4, velocity-induced phase shifts can be controlled by adjusting the first gradient moment M_1 by varying gradient duration T or gradient strength G and are given by (simplified gradient design without ramps)

$$\phi_1(v) = -\gamma M_1 v = \gamma G(T/2)^2 v \tag{A5}$$

However, background phase effects ϕ_0 caused by susceptibility of field inhomogeneity cannot be refocused using bipolar gradients. To filter out such phase effects, two measurements with different first moments $M_1^{(1)}$ and $M_1^{(2)}$ (e.g., inverted gradient polarities) are thus necessary to isolate the velocity-encoded phase shifts and encode the velocity v along a single direction. Subtraction of phase images from such two measurements results in phase differences $\Delta\phi$, which are directly proportional to the underlying velocities v and difference in first gradient moments $\Delta M = M_1^{(1)} - M_1^{(2)}$. Because Fourier image reconstruction resolves signal amplitudes and phases as a function of spatial locations, the encoded velocities can simply be derived from the data by dividing the pixel intensities in the calculated phase difference images by $\gamma\Delta M$.

For the gradient design in a PC MR measurement, some prior knowledge of the maximum velocities is required. For velocities larger than *venc*, the velocity-induced phase shift will exceed $\pm\pi$, and phase wrapping occurs. Velocity sensitivity ($venc = \pi/\gamma\Delta M_1$) is thus defined as the velocity that produces a phase shift $\Delta\phi$ of π radians and is determined by the difference of the first gradient moments used for velocity encoding.

REFERENCES

1. Hahn EL. Detection of sea water motion by nuclear precession. J Geophys Res 1960;65(2):776–777.
2. Morse OC, Singer JR. Blood velocity measurements in intact subjects. Science 1970;170:440–441.
3. Burt CT. NMR measurements and flow. J Nucl Med 1982;23:1044–1045.
4. Moran PR. A flow velocity zeugmatographic interlace for NMR imaging in humans. Magn Reson Imaging 1982;1:197–203.
5. Axel L. Blood flow effects in magnetic resonance imaging. AJR Am J Roentgenol 1984;143:1157–1166.

6. Bryant DJ, Payne JA, Firmin DN, Longmore DB. Measurement of flow with NMR imaging using a gradient pulse and phase difference technique. J Comput Assist Tomogr 1984;8:588–593.

7. Constantinesco A, Mallet JJ, Bonmartin A, Lallot C, Briguet A. Spatial or flow velocity phase encoding gradients in NMR imaging. Magn Reson Imaging 1984;2:335–340.

8. Van Dijk P. Direct cardiac NMR imaging of heart wall and blood flow velocity. J Comput Assist Tomogr 1984;171:429–436.

9. Feinberg DA, Crooks LE, Sheldon P, Hoenninger J 3rd, Watts J, Arakawa M. Magnetic resonance imaging the velocity vector components of fluid flow. Magn Reson Med 1985;2:555–566.

10. O'Donnell M. NMR blood flow imaging using multiecho, phase contrast sequences. Med Phys 1985;12:59–64.

11. Nayler GL, Firmin DN, Longmore DB. Blood flow imaging by cine magnetic resonance. J Comput Assist Tomogr 1986;10:715–722.

12. Axel L, Morton D. MR flow imaging by velocity-compensated/uncompensated difference images. J Comput Assist Tomogr 1987;11:31–34.

13. Firmin DN, Nayler GL, Klipstein RH, Underwood SR, Rees RS, Longmore DB. In vivo validation of MR velocity imaging. J Comput Assist Tomogr 1987;11:751–756.

14. Underwood SR, Firmin DN, Klipstein RH, Rees RS, Longmore DB. Magnetic resonance velocity mapping: clinical application of a new technique. Br Heart J 1987;57:404–412.

15. Bogren HG, Underwood SR, Firmin DN, et al. Magnetic resonance velocity mapping in aortic dissection. Br J Radiol 1988;61:456–462.

16. Walker MF, Souza SP, Dumoulin CL. Quantitative flow measurement in phase contrast MR angiography. J Comput Assist Tomogr 1988;12:304–313.

17. Firmin DN, Nayler GL, Kilner PJ, Longmore DB. The application of phase shifts in NMR for flow measurement. Magn Reson Med 1990;14:230–241.

18. Pelc NJ, Bernstein MA, Shimakawa A, Glover GH. Encoding strategies for three-direction phase-contrast MR imaging of flow. J Magn Reson Imag 1991;1:405–413.

19. Pelc NJ, Herfkens RJ, Shimakawa A, Enzmann DR. Phase contrast cine magnetic resonance imaging. Magn Reson Q 1991;7:229–254.

20. Bernstein MA, Shimakawa A, Pelc NJ. Minimizing TE in moment-nulled or flow-encoded two- and three-dimensional gradient-echo imaging. J Magn Reson Imaging 1992;2:583–588.

21. Conturo TE, Robinson BH. Analysis of encoding efficiency in MR imaging of velocity magnitude and direction. Magn Reson Med 1992;25:233–247.

22. Kraft KA, Fei DY, Fatouros PP. Quantitative phase-velocity MR imaging of in-plane laminar flow: effect of fluid velocity, vessel diameter, and slice thickness. Med Phys 1992;19:79–85.

23. Napel S, Lee DH, Frayne R, Rutt BK. Visualizing three-dimensional flow with simulated streamlines and three-dimensional phase-contrast MR imaging. J Magn Reson Imaging 1992;2:143–153.

24. Wedeen VJ. Magnetic resonance imaging of myocardial kinematics. Technique to detect, localize, and quantify the strain rates of the active human myocardium. Magn Reson Med 1992;27:52–67.

25. Frayne R, Rutt BK. Frequency response to retrospectively gated phase-contrast MR imaging: effect of interpolation. J Magn Reson Imaging 1993;3:907–917.

26. Hangiandreou NJ, Rossman PJ, Riederer SJ. Analysis of MR phase-contrast measurements of pulsatile velocity waveforms. J Magn Reson Imaging 1993;3:387–394.

27. Kilner PJ, Yang GZ, Mohiaddin RH, Firmin DN, Longmore DB. Helical and retrograde secondary flow patterns in the aortic arch studied by three-directional magnetic resonance velocity mapping. Circulation 1993;88(5 pt 1):2235–2247.

28. Mohiaddin RH, Kilner PJ, Rees S, Longmore DB. Magnetic resonance volume flow and jet velocity mapping in aortic coarctation. J Am Coll Cardiol 1993;22:1515–1521.

29. Rebergen SA, van der Wall EE, Doornbos J, de Roos A. Magnetic resonance measurement of velocity and flow: technique, validation, and cardiovascular applications. Am Heart J 1993;126:1439–1456.

30. Walker PG, Cranney GB, Scheidegger MB, Waseleski G, Pohost GM, Yoganathan AP. Semiautomated method for noise reduction and background phase error correction in MR phase velocity data. J Magn Reson Imaging 1993;3:521–530.

31. Bernstein MA, Grgic M, Brosnan TJ, Pelc NJ. Reconstructions of phase contrast, phased array multicoil data. Magn Reson Med 1994;32:330–334.

32. Hamilton CA. Correction of partial volume inaccuracies in quantitative phase contrast MR angiography. Magn Reson Imaging 1994;12:1127–1130.

33. Lauzon ML, Holdsworth DW, Frayne R, Rutt BK. Effects of physiologic waveform variability in triggered MR imaging: theoretical analysis. J Magn Reson Imaging 1994;4:853–867.

34. Mohiaddin RH, Yang GZ, Kilner PJ. Visualization of flow by vector analysis of multidirectional cine MR velocity mapping. J Comput Assist Tomogr 1994;18:383–392.
35. Pelc LR, Sayre J, Yun K, et al. Evaluation of myocardial motion tracking with cine-phase contrast magnetic resonance imaging. Invest Radiol 1994;29:1038–1042.
36. Pelc NJ, Sommer FG, Li KC, Brosnan TJ, Herfkens RJ, Enzmann DR. Quantitative magnetic resonance flow imaging. Magn Reson Q 1994;10:125–147.
37. Pike GB, Meyer CH, Brosnan TJ, Pelc NJ. Magnetic resonance velocity imaging using a fast spiral phase contrast sequence. Magn Reson Med 1994;32:476–483.
38. Dumoulin CL. Phase contrast MR angiography techniques. Magn Reson Imaging Clin North Am 1995;3:399–411.
39. Frayne R, Rutt BK. Frequency response of prospectively gated phase-contrast MR velocity measurements. J Magn Reson Imaging 1995;5:65–73.
40. Frayne R, Steinman DA, Ethier CR, Rutt BK. Accuracy of MR phase contrast velocity measurements for unsteady flow. J Magn Reson Imaging 1995;5:428–431.
41. Lingamneni A, Hardy PA, Powell KA, Pelc NJ, White RD. Validation of cine phase-contrast MR imaging for motion analysis. J Magn Reson Imaging 1995;5:331–338.
42. McCauley TR, Pena CS, Holland CK, Price TB, Gore JC. Validation of volume flow measurements with cine phase-contrast MR imaging for peripheral arterial waveforms. J Magn Reson Imaging 1995;5:663–668.
43. Pelc NJ, Drangova M, Pelc LR, et al. Tracking of cyclic motion with phase-contrast cine MR velocity data. J Magn Reson Imaging 1995;5:339–345.
44. Tang C, Blatter DD, Parker DL. Correction of partial-volume effects in phase-contrast flow measurements. J Magn Reson Imaging 1995;5:175–180.
45. Xiang QS. Temporal phase unwrapping for CINE velocity imaging. J Magn Reson Imaging 1995;5:529–534.
46. Andersen AH, Kirsch JE. Analysis of noise in phase contrast MR imaging. Med Phys 1996;23:857–869.
47. Polzin JA, Frayne R, Grist TM, Mistretta CA. Frequency response of multi-phase segmented k-space phase-contrast. Magn Reson Med 1996;35:755–762.
48. Wigstrom L, Sjoqvist L, Wranne B. Temporally resolved 3D phase-contrast imaging. Magn Reson Med 1996;36:800–803.
49. Yang GZ, Kilner PJ, Wood NB, Underwood SR, Firmin DN. Computation of flow pressure fields from magnetic resonance velocity mapping. Magn Reson Med 1996;36:520–526.
50. Bogren HG, Mohiaddin RH, Kilner PJ, Jimenez-Borreguero LJ, Yang GZ, Firmin DN. Blood flow patterns in the thoracic aorta studied with three-directional MR velocity mapping: the effects of age and coronary artery disease. J Magn Reson Imaging 1997;7:784–793.
51. Drangova M, Zhu Y, Pelc NJ. Effect of artifacts due to flowing blood on the reproducibility of phase-contrast measurements of myocardial motion. J Magn Reson Imaging 1997;7:664–668.
52. Lee VS, Spritzer CE, Carroll BA, et al. Flow quantification using fast cine phase-contrast MR imaging, conventional cine phase-contrast MR imaging, and Doppler sonography: in vitro and in vivo validation. AJR Am J Roentgenol 1997;169:1125–1131.
53. Bernstein MA, Zhou XJ, Polzin JA, et al. Concomitant gradient terms in phase contrast MR: analysis and correction. Magn Reson Med 1998;39:300–308.
54. Hennig J, Schneider B, Peschl S, Markl M, Krause T, Laubenberger J. Analysis of myocardial motion based on velocity measurements with a black blood prepared segmented gradient-echo sequence: methodology and applications to normal volunteers and patients. J Magn Reson Imaging 1998;8:868–877.
55. Mohiaddin RH, Pennell DJ. MR blood flow measurement. Clinical application in the heart and circulation. Cardiol Clin 1998;16:161–187.
56. van der Geest RJ, Niezen RA, van der Wall EE, de Roos A, Reiber JH. Automated measurement of volume flow in the ascending aorta using MR velocity maps: evaluation of inter- and intraobserver variability in healthy volunteers. J Comput Assist Tomogr 1998;22:904–911.
57. Kilner PJ, Yang GZ, Wilkes AJ, Mohiaddin RH, Firmin DN, Yacoub MH. Asymmetric redirection of flow through the heart. Nature 2000;404:759–761.
58. Thunberg P, Wigstrom L, Wranne B, Engvall J, Karlsson M. Correction for acceleration-induced displacement artifacts in phase contrast imaging. Magn Reson Med 2000;43:734–738.
59. Ebbers T, Wigstrom L, Bolger AF, Engvall J, Karlsson M. Estimation of relative cardiovascular pressures using time-resolved three-dimensional phase contrast MRI. Magn Reson Med 2001;45:872–879.

60. Kozerke S, Hasenkam JM, Pedersen EM, Boesiger P. Visualization of flow patterns distal to aortic valve prostheses in humans using a fast approach for cine 3D velocity mapping. J Magn Reson Imaging 2001;13:690–698.

61. Ebbers T, Wigstrom L, Bolger AF, Wranne B, Karlsson M. Noninvasive measurement of time-varying three-dimensional relative pressure fields within the human heart. J Biomech Eng 2002;124:288–293.

62. Thunberg P, Wigstrom L, Ebbers T, Karlsson M. Correction for displacement artifacts in 3D phase contrast imaging. J Magn Reson Imaging 2002;16:591–597.

63. Markl M, Alley MT, Pelc NJ. Balanced phase-contrast steady-state free precession (PC-SSFP): a novel technique for velocity encoding by gradient inversion. Magn Reson Med 2003;49:945–952.

64. Markl M, Bammer R, Alley MT, et al. Generalized reconstruction of phase contrast MRI: analysis and correction of the effect of gradient field distortions. Magn Reson Med 2003;50:791–801.

65. Bogren HG, Buonocore MH, Valente RJ. Four-dimensional magnetic resonance velocity mapping of blood flow patterns in the aorta in patients with atherosclerotic coronary artery disease compared to age-matched normal subjects. J Magn Reson Imaging 2004;19:417–427.

66. Jung B, Schneider B, Markl M, Saurbier B, Geibel A, Hennig J. Measurement of left ventricular velocities: phase contrast MRI velocity mapping vs tissue-Doppler-ultrasound in healthy volunteers. J Cardiovasc Magn Reson 2004;6:777–783.

67. Korperich H, Gieseke J, Barth P, et al. Flow volume and shunt quantification in pediatric congenital heart disease by real-time magnetic resonance velocity mapping: a validation study. Circulation 2004;109:1987–1993.

68. Kvitting JP, Ebbers T, Engvall J, Sutherland GR, Wranne B, Wigstrom L. Three-directional myocardial motion assessed using 3D phase contrast MRI. J Cardiovasc Magn Reson 2004;6:627–636.

69. Nasiraei-Moghaddam A, Behrens G, Fatouraee N, Agarwal R, Choi ET, Amini AA. Factors affecting the accuracy of pressure measurements in vascular stenoses from phase-contrast MRI. Magn Reson Med 2004;52:300–309.

70. Ringgaard S, Oyre SA, Pedersen EM. Arterial MR imaging phase-contrast flow measurement: improvements with varying velocity sensitivity during cardiac cycle. Radiology 2004;232:289–294.

71. Thompson RB, McVeigh ER. Flow-gated phase-contrast MRI using radial acquisitions. Magn Reson Med 2004;52:598–604.

72. van der Weide R, Viergever MA, Bakker CJ. Resolution-insensitive velocity and flow rate measurement in low-background phase-contrast MRA. Magn Reson Med 2004;51:785–793.

73. Lotz J, Doker R, Noeske R, et al. In vitro validation of phase-contrast flow measurements at 3 T in comparison to 1.5 T: precision, accuracy, and signal-to-noise ratios. J Magn Reson Imaging 2005;21:604–610.

74. Peeters JM, Bos C, Bakker CJ. Analysis and correction of gradient nonlinearity and B_0 inhomogeneity related scaling errors in two-dimensional phase contrast flow measurements. Magn Reson Med 2005;53:126–133.

75. Oshinski JN, Ku DN, Bohning DE, Pettigrew RI. Effects of acceleration on the accuracy of MR phase velocity measurements. J Magn Reson Imaging 1992;2:665–670.

76. Oshinski JN, Ku DN, Mukundan S Jr, Loth F, Pettigrew RI. Determination of wall shear stress in the aorta with the use of MR phase velocity mapping. J Magn Reson Imaging 1995;5:640–647.

77. Markl M, Hennig J. Phase contrast MRI with improved temporal resolution by view sharing: k-space related velocity mapping properties. Magn Reson Imaging 2001;19:669–676.

78. Foo TK, Bernstein MA, Aisen AM, Hernandez RJ, Collick BD, Bernstein T. Improved ejection fraction and flow velocity estimates with use of view sharing and uniform repetition time excitation with fast cardiac techniques. Radiology 1995;195:471–478.

79. Tyszka JM, Laidlaw DH, Asa JW, Silverman JM. Three-dimensional, time-resolved (4D) relative pressure mapping using magnetic resonance imaging. J Magn Reson Imaging 2000;12:321–329.

80. Markl M, Draney MT, Hope MD, et al. Time-resolved 3-dimensional velocity mapping in the thoracic aorta: visualization of 3-directional blood flow patterns in healthy volunteers and patients. J Comput Assist Tomogr 2004;28:459–468.

81. Thunberg P, Karlsson M, Wigstrom L. Accuracy and reproducibility in phase contrast imaging using SENSE. Magn Reson Med 2003;50:1061–1068.

9

Fast-Imaging Techniques

Bruno Madore

INTRODUCTION

The constant motion of the heart poses great challenges when developing cardiac imaging strategies. There is the beating motion of the heart, rich in clinically relevant information such as wall thickening and ejection fraction, and the respiration-induced motion of the heart, with little clinical importance other than the artifacts it may cause. The most common approach to handle these two types of motion consists of freezing the respiratory motion through breath holding while resolving the beating motion through electrocardiogram (ECG) gating (Chapter 2). Alternatively, one may freeze all motions at once using a suitably short scan time in real-time imaging. When breath holding is used, we need to image fast for patients to comply, and without breath holding, we need to image fast to freeze all motions involved. The need for fast imaging is ever present in cardiac imaging as speed is central to our strategies for handling motion.

Traditional Ways of Increasing Imaging Speed

Traditional ways of increasing speed have involved pulse sequence design and hardware developments. A fast pulse sequence must spend as much of the available time as possible actually acquiring data to minimize idle time. Such fast-imaging pulse sequences include, for example, echo-planar imaging (EPI) *(1,2)*, rapid acquisition with relaxation enhancement (RARE; also commercially called fast spin echo or turbo spin echo) *(3,4)*, and "steady-state free precession" (SSFP; also commercially called TrueFISP, Fiesta, or balanced FFE) *(5,6)*.

From: *Contemporary Cardiology: Cardiovascular Magnetic Resonance Imaging*
Edited by: Raymond Y. Kwong © Humana Press Inc., Totowa, NJ

On the hardware front, the importance of having good performance gradient sets can be appreciated through an analogy with auto racing. The acquisition process involves "driving" through all the needed data point locations in a space called k-space. The maximum gradient strength corresponds to the maximum speed of the car; the gradient slew rate corresponds to acceleration, braking, and steering. Accordingly, strong gradients that can be switched on and off rapidly allow fast racing through k-space and short scan times. Along the way, the transverse magnetization used to generate the acquired signal disappears because of decay, and occasional pit stops may be required to replenish it (i.e., radio-frequency [RF] excitation pulses). Although fast-imaging sequences offer efficient itineraries through k-space with only small amounts of idle time or few pit stops, it is the hardware, especially gradient sets, that determines how fast one can navigate around.

Partially Sampled Methods for Increased Speed

Running fast-imaging pulse sequences on modern magnetic resonance (MR) systems with good performance gradient sets enables fast imaging. But technology and safety impose limits on achievable hardware performance, and physics imposes limits on how efficient a pulse sequence can be. Once traditional approaches have reached their limit and further imaging speed is still required, more drastic solutions have to be considered. These solutions involve further increasing imaging speed by skipping some of the data that should normally be acquired. The skipped data can be calculated, based on the data we do acquire, using assumptions/prior knowledge. By calculating instead of acquiring parts of the data set, the corresponding k-space itinerary can be shortened, and acquisition time is reduced. This chapter is dedicated to the study of these partially sampled methods able to carry imaging speed manyfold beyond the limits technology and physics would seem, at first sight, to impose.

A large array of partially sampled methods have been developed. They propose different strategies regarding which parts of a k-space matrix can be skipped and which parts must be acquired, and on the assumptions/prior knowledge used to fill in the missing data. Many of these methods are mentioned and briefly described; three are discussed in more detail. These three approaches are parallel imaging, partial Fourier imaging, and unaliasing by Fourier encoding the overlaps in the temporal dimension (UNFOLD). We also consider hybrid approaches in which a number of individual techniques are merged for increased performance. We look at how these methods function and how they can be used in a cardiac imaging context. First, because these fast-imaging techniques work by skipping parts of k-space data sets, we start by looking in more detail at the nature of k-space and at the way it is populated with data points as part of a magnetic resonance imaging (MRI) scan.

A GUIDED TOUR INTO k-SPACE

The term k-space is an alternate name for Fourier space, and simply means the space with coordinates that are represented using the letter k, such as k_x, k_y, and k_z. This is because different k-space locations correspond to different spatial frequencies, also sometimes referred to as wave numbers; it is customary in physics to use the letter k to represent wave numbers. This tradition along with terms such as k-trajectory and k-space were extended to the MRI field by Twieg *(7)*.

Below, we focus on the nature of k-space and on the frequency-encoding and phase-encoding processes used to populate it with data during an MRI scan. We then consider the consequences of skipping parts of the k-space acquisition to increase acquisition speed.

Fourier Space, Frequency Encoding, and Spatial Resolution

Celebrated scientist and administrator Jean Baptiste Joseph Fourier (1768–1830) introduced the idea, controversial to his contemporaries, that any function can be decomposed into a sum of sine and cosine functions. In 1798, Fourier followed Napoleon's troops in their invasion of Egypt as a scientific advisor. Egypt's climate may well have been an inspiration for him as heat became a major theme of both his theoretical work and his daily life. Back in France, bundled in clothes in overheated rooms, Fourier laid down the equations for heat transfer and invented what was to become Fourier analysis to help solve these equations. The Fourier transform plays a vital role in a wide array of scientific endeavors, especially since the advent of computers, and the introduction of the fast Fourier transform (FFT) algorithm in 1965 *(8)* to greatly reduce processing time.

A Fourier transform can pull apart the various frequencies that compose any given signal. In a concert, although baritones and sopranos might combine their voices to create a sound wave that makes your eardrum vibrate, a Fourier transform of these vibrations would show how much of each tone is present, from low pitch to high pitch. In MRI, eardrums are replaced by receiver coils and pressure waves by electromagnetic waves. The contents of the imaged pixels "sing" at a precise frequency: the Larmor frequency, which is proportional to the magnetic field strength (Chapter 1).

Imagine for one short moment that we would like to make a one-dimensional (1D) image of a long and thin object, like a particularly straight and thin snake, for example. In this case, the desired image consists of a single row of pixels. By applying a magnetic field gradient along the length of the object, different pixels are made to feel slightly different fields and thus sing slightly different notes. All pixels contribute to the received signal, and an FFT of this signal shows how much of each note is present, that is, how much material is found in each pixel. This process, by which different pixels are resolved by making them sing at different frequencies, is referred to as *frequency encoding* and is used to resolve one of the dimensions involved in most two-dimensional (2D) and three-dimensional (3D) clinical MR images.

To distinguish materials in close proximity (i.e., to get good spatial resolution), one can make the corresponding tones as different as possible by applying as strong a gradient as possible and/or listening for a long time so that even small differences in tone might become noticeable through a beating phenomenon. Both of these factors, gradient strength and readout duration, are included into the calculation of k-space coordinates, and as a consequence, spatial resolution in the image is determined by how far in k-space the data collection gets (*see* Fig. 1B as compared to Fig. 1A). The direction resolved using frequency encoding is traditionally called the x-direction and is obtained by applying an FFT to the k_x direction in k-space. As explained next, a related process called phase encoding is used to resolve the second (and third) dimension in 2D (and 3D) images.

Phase Encoding and How It Can Be Understood From Old Monster Movies

To make a 2D image, pixels along two axes, x and y, must be resolved. Unlike what is done for the frequency-encoded x-direction, typically no gradient is applied along the

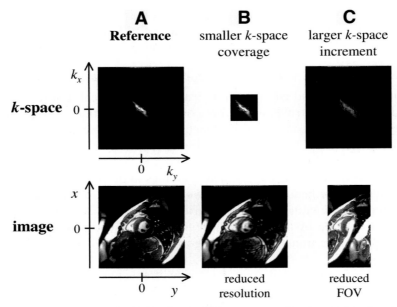

Fig. 1. (A) *k*-space data (top row) is shown along with its corresponding image data (bottom row). One goes from *k*-space data to image data by applying a type of Fourier transform called an inverse Fourier transform to all dimensions. The k_x and k_y axes become, respectively, the frequency-encoding (x) and phase-encoding (y) axes. Notice that in this particular case, the frequency-encoded x direction happens to be vertical. **(B)** As compared to the reference, one can see that reducing the covered range in *k*-space reduces spatial resolution in the corresponding image. **(C)** The *k*-space increment was increased by skipping one *k*-space line every two. In the figure, skipped lines are simply filled with zeros and appear black. The effect of increasing the distance between sampled lines is to reduce the size of the FOV. Because the object is now bigger than the FOV along y, the corresponding image is corrupted by aliasing artifacts as different parts of the anatomy overlap onto each other in the same image pixels. Unlike the phase-encoding process, the frequency-encoding process is mostly immune to aliasing problems, as explained further in the text.

y-direction while data is recorded. Accordingly, all pixels along y sing the same tone, which depends only on their x location. To understand how different y locations can be distinguished from each other, it may be useful to think of a cinematographic process called "stop motion animation."

Widely used in older movies to bring dinosaurs and monsters to life, the technique was first popularized by Willis O'Brien in his 1925 *The Lost World,* and in his 1933 *King Kong.* A scene is created one frame at a time by taking a photograph of a puppet, moving slightly the puppet, taking another photograph, moving the puppet again, and so on (Fig. 2).

When properly assembled, a large number of pictures can be played rapidly on a screen so beastly puppets appear to move around, as if alive. Although an uninformed observer looking at the shooting process might only see a team of grown-up people playing with puppets, someone acquainted with the technique would understand that a coherent scene is under construction one frame at a time.

Similarly, *k*-space matrices are built one *k*-space line at a time. Although different x locations precess at different frequencies in true time, as data are acquired, different y locations precess at different frequencies along an artificial time axis, constructed by

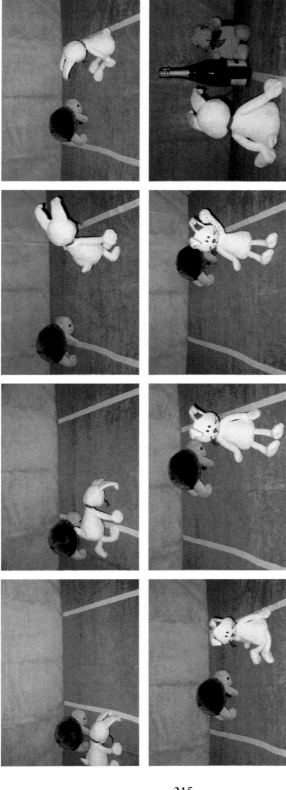

Fig. 2. In stop motion animation, a large number of photographs with puppets in different positions are assembled to create an illusion of continuous motion when played on a movie screen. An analogy to "stop motion animation" is used here to help explain how phase encoding works. For most people learning about MRI, phase encoding typically proves much more difficult to understand and to grasp than frequency encoding. In fact, the two encoding processes are essentially identical. As explained in more detail in the text, the only difference is that frequency encoding is performed in true time, and phase encoding occurs along an artificial stop-motion-animated kind of time axis assembled one shot at a time.

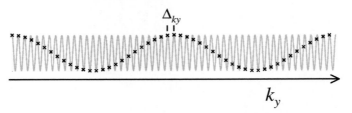

Fig. 3. Evenly spaced sampled locations, indicated with an X, clearly seem to outline a slow oscillation (two cycles from left to right), but the faster oscillation shown with a gray line also agrees with all sampled locations. Aliasing artifacts occur when material at different spatial locations, "singing" at different Larmor frequencies, appear identical to the phase-encoding process.

properly assembling a large number of different shots. In the present analogy, the application of a phase-encoding y-gradient pulse is analogous to adjusting the puppet's position, and acquiring data is analogous to taking a photograph. The process is repeated many times, varying the strength of the phase-encoding pulse from shot to shot.

Just as many snapshots of a puppet in different positions can appear like continuous motion, many readout repetitions with different amounts of phase encoding can appear like data acquired while a y-gradient is applied continuously, that is, like frequency encoding. Once all shots are properly assembled along a k_y axis, materials at different y locations appear to precess at different frequencies along this axis. An FFT along k_y, that is, across the collection of assembled shots, can resolve the signal at different y locations. Frequency encoding and phase encoding are essentially identical processes except that the former is performed in true time, and the latter in an artificial, stop-motion-animated, kind of time.

The Aliasing Problem

The analogy with stop motion animation can be taken one step further to help understand the aliasing problem that plagues the phase-encoding process. When shooting a movie scene in true time, there is no fundamental limit on how many frames per second can be recorded. The finite speed of the human eye and how much money can be spent on camera equipment may be the main factors determining frame rate. But, shooting one frame at a time along an artificial time axis, as in stop motion animation, is a painstakingly slow process. Patience and time become limiting factors, and one will certainly be inclined to keep the total number of frames to a bare minimum.

Figure 3 depicts the aliasing problem. At first sight, the points sampled every Δ_{ky} and shown with X marks in Fig. 3 clearly seem to represent a slow oscillation, with two full cycles from the leftmost to the rightmost edge of the plot. But, closer inspection reveals that, in addition to the obvious slow oscillation, every sample point also falls on top of a faster, higher-frequency oscillation, shown with a gray line in Fig. 3. There is ambiguity about the sampled signal: two different frequencies, corresponding to different y locations, appear identical at all sampled k_y locations (X marks in Fig. 3).

With Δ_{ky} representing the increment between consecutive k-space lines, any pair of points in the object separated by a distance $1/\Delta_{ky}$ along y cannot be distinguished and appear overlapped in the same image pixel, as in Fig. 1C. To avoid such aliasing artifacts, one must set the phase-encoding increment Δ_{ky} so the field-of-view (FOV) along y, $1/\Delta_{ky}$ is at least as large as the imaged object. Although a small increment along k_x (and a large FOV along x) is readily obtained because data are recorded in true time, building a large FOV along y is a painstaking task requiring a large number of individual shots.

Complex Numbers in Simple Terms

The acquired k-space signal consists of complex numbers, MR images are also made of complex numbers, and the Fourier transform is a complex number operation. Because complex numbers are ever present in MRI and because these concepts will be useful in this chapter, it would seem worthwhile at this point to take a moment to explain what is really meant by terms such as complex, real, and imaginary numbers.

Complex numbers have two distinct parts that do not readily mix: a so-called real part and a so-called imaginary part. These exotic objects were originally brought to life by mathematicians who needed ways to handle some puzzling expressions, obtained when solving polynomial equations, that featured the square root of negative numbers. Although $\sqrt{4}$ can readily be understood as either 2 or −2, a number like $\sqrt{-4}$, on the other hand, does not seem at first sight to make any sense and is called an imaginary number. Mathematicians, including the ubiquitous Karl Friedrich Gauss (1777–1855), developed tools and notations to handle complex numbers that were so convenient and successful that people from essentially all fields of engineering and physics routinely use complex numbers, even if they first have to introduce artificially the square root of a negative number somewhere just to gain access to these tools and notations. Because complex numbers are made of two separate components, they turn out to be analogous to vectors in a plane, with one component along one axis (e.g., x or the real axis) and another component along another axis (e.g., y or the imaginary axis). In science in general, whenever one has to deal with vectors in planes, it is common practice to describe these vectors using complex numbers.

In MRI, the measured signal comes from the transverse magnetization, that is, from magnetization flipped in the transverse plane by an RF pulse (Chapter 1). The transverse magnetization can be visualized as a vector in a plane perpendicular to the main B_0 field. Of course, there is nothing imaginary about transverse magnetization, but because it is a vector in a plane, complex numbers are used to represent it, as a mathematical convenience. MRI sequences are typically designed so the transverse magnetization is expected along the so-called real axis in the plane, hence the statement that the imaged object is expected to be real.

But, a number of factors may cause the orientation of the transverse magnetization to deviate from its expected orientation, such as spatial variations in the magnetic field caused by magnetic susceptibility, for example. Such variations tend to make the imaged object complex—in other words, to give it a nonzero component along the imaginary axis. It is common practice in the MRI literature, when displaying k-space or image data, to show only the magnitude of the corresponding complex numbers—in other words, their length. Their orientation, or phase, with respect to the real and imaginary axes is often not shown (notable exceptions include velocity encoding and temperature monitoring, for which useful information is encoded and displayed through the phase of the MR signal).

In the section entitled "Fourier Space, Frequency Encoding, and Spatial Resolution," it was mentioned that a Fourier transform is used to pull apart different materials singing at different frequencies. All of the oscillations in Fig. 4 have the same spatial frequency as the spacing between consecutive crests is the same in all cases. But, they

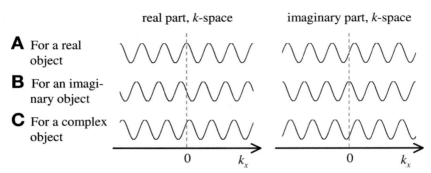

Fig. 4. Because k-space is made of complex numbers, it contains information not only about frequency, but also about phase. The three rows in the figure depict signals having the same spatial frequency but different phases. The significant difference between each signal is the location of the wave crests and valleys with respect to the $k_x = 0$ location.

have different phases because their crests and valleys do not line up along k_x (*see* dashed vertical gray lines). The Fourier transform does more than just separate tones; it also finds the "phase" of each tone. Real material would give rise to an oscillation like that in Fig. 4A, with a maximum real component and a zero imaginary component at $k_x = 0$. Figure 4B,C corresponds to songs from imaginary and complex materials, respectively.

Skipping Parts of k-Space

The fast-imaging techniques described here involve acquiring only a partial data set. As a reference, Fig. 5A depicts a fully sampled k-space matrix. Although in reality k-space matrices typically contain up to a few hundred lines, only 12 lines are actually depicted in Fig. 5 to keep the drawings visually simple. Figure 5B–I depicts a number of different ways in which data can be skipped to speed the image acquisition process. Full black lines represent acquired data; gray lines represent data that are skipped.

In Fig. 5B, the central region of k-space is sampled normally (black lines), but the outer regions are completely skipped (gray lines). As explained in the section "Fourier Space, Frequency Encoding, and Spatial Resolution," how far one reaches into k-space determines spatial resolution. Accordingly, any fast-imaging technique that speeds the acquisition by skipping the outer parts of k-space along k_y must include a strategy to somehow recover the lost spatial resolution along y. In Fig. 5C, every second line is skipped, or in other words, the k-space increment along k_y, Δ_{ky}, is doubled. As seen in Fig. 1C, doubling the k-space increment halves the FOV along y, which causes aliasing artifacts in the resulting image. Accordingly, any fast-imaging technique that functions by increasing Δ_{ky} must include a strategy to somehow recover the loss of FOV along y.

Because frequency encoding and phase encoding are essentially identical processes, as explained in the section on understanding phase encoding, it should not come as a surprise that the two can be mixed and matched in a number of hybrid ways. For example, instead of covering k-space with a series of parallel lines, one could use a series of radial lines (Fig. 5D) or a number of interleaved spirals (Fig. 5E). The regular, rigid sampling scheme depicted in Fig. 5A–C is called Cartesian after the philosopher and mathematician René Descartes (1596–1650), who introduced the idea of a gridlike coordinate system. It follows that sampling patterns not bound to a regular grid, such as those in Fig. 5D,E, can be referred to as non-Cartesian. In a way similar to Fig. 5C, the subsampled

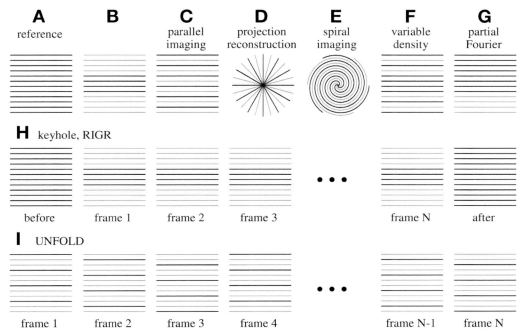

Fig. 5. The various *k*-space subsampling schemes used in partially sampled methods are depicted. The vertical direction represents k_y and the horizontal direction k_x. Although a typical *k*-space matrix contains up to a few hundred k_y lines, only 12 k_y lines are depicted in each matrix here, to keep the drawings simple.

patterns in Fig. 5D,E cover the correct area in *k*-space (i.e., full spatial resolution) but do so in an overly sparse fashion (i.e., reduced FOV). It is typical that fast-imaging techniques using a sampling strategy like that of Fig. 5C could be generalized to include non-Cartesian sampling patterns also, such as those in Fig. 5D,E.

As we have seen, common ways of reducing the amount of acquired *k*-space data include reducing how far one goes in *k*-space (Fig. 5B) or increasing the step size (Fig. 5C). But, a number of variations on these themes can also be imagined. A fairly straightforward combination of the two approaches gives a variable-density sampling scheme (Fig. 5F) by which outer regions are sampled more sparsely than the central region. Alternatively, one could sample normally on one side of *k*-space but skip most of the other side (Fig. 5G). In dynamic applications, when a time series of images is acquired, one has a new dimension available, and different sampling strategies can be chosen for different time frames (Fig. 5H,I).

Although Fig. 5 depicts a number of different ways of skipping *k*-space data to accelerate the acquisition process, the main challenge lies in recovering the missed information through calculations. In the following sections, we focus on specific methods and explain how they function, as well as how they can be used in cardiac imaging applications.

PARTIAL FOURIER IMAGING

Partial Fourier imaging is probably by far the most commonly used partially sampled fast-imaging technique. Its name simply means that the *k*-space matrix is only partially sampled. Note that the same statement could possibly be made of all the methods

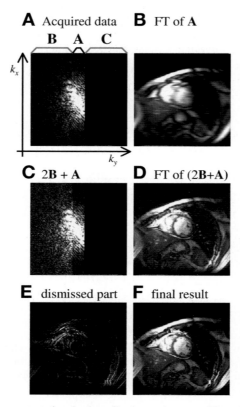

Fig. 6. A partial Fourier reconstruction is described step by step. Note that clinically the sampled region (A + B) would typically cover about 75% of the k-space matrix, unlike in the more extreme example shown here, where only 56% of the data are present. *See* text for more details.

considered here, but as partial Fourier imaging was probably the first partially sampled MR technique ever introduced, no ambiguity existed yet at the time it was named.

Partial Fourier imaging uses a sampling strategy like that depicted in Fig. 5G and seen in Fig. 6A. Note that the phase-encoding direction happens to be horizontal in Fig. 6. The missing data, on one side of k-space, can be obtained fairly directly from the acquired data on the other side whenever the imaged object is real. Although any reasonable person might be puzzled at the idea of introducing anything but real objects into a scanner, words like *real*, *imaginary*, and *complex* are to be understood in the context presented in the section entitled "Complex Numbers in Simple Terms."

Ideally, All Imaged Objects Would Be Real

If the imaged object was purely real, or in other words if the transverse magnetization always pointed exactly where it is supposed to, a partial Fourier reconstruction would be nearly trivial. The k-space matrix would have Hermitian symmetry, meaning that for every point on one side of k-space there would be a mirror point on the other side with the exact same real value and an imaginary value differing only by its sign (positive values on one side become negative on the other and vice versa). This symmetry is owing to the fact that with a real object, any deviation from realness in k-space can be caused only by the Fourier transform itself, which involves real terms containing a cosine and imaginary terms containing a sine function. Cosine functions have a so-called even symmetry because $\cos(\theta) = \cos(-\theta)$, and sine functions have an odd symmetry because $\sin(\theta) = -\sin(-\theta)$. As a result, any k-space matrix corresponding to a real object has a real component with even symmetry and an imaginary component with odd symmetry, called in short Hermitian symmetry after the French mathematician Charles Hermite (1822–1901). A complex conjugate operator, which keeps the real part untouched and flips the sign of the imaginary part, could turn each k-space point on one side of k-space into its mirror point on the other side, making the acquisition of only one half of a k-space data set necessary.

In Real Life, Imaged Objects Are Complex

In general, the imaged object cannot be considered purely real, and the k-space matrices acquired in MRI do not have Hermitian symmetry. Partial Fourier imaging feeds on the assumption that, although imaged objects are typically not real, the phenomenon responsible for making them deviate from realness has an effect that varies only slightly from one pixel to the next in an image.

Many different versions of partial Fourier imaging have been proposed (e.g., *9–13*), and one particular version, the popular and relatively simple homodyne reconstruction algorithm *(12)*, is depicted in Fig. 6. As shown in Fig. 6A, the k-space matrix can be divided into three zones: a central region **A** is fully sampled; a region **C** is entirely skipped to speed data acquisition; and a region **B**, the same size as region **C** but on the other side of the k-space matrix, is fully sampled. Using only the fully sampled region **A**, one gets a first, low-resolution image of the object (Fig. 6B). The image has low resolution because region **A** has a limited extent along k_y.

To partly compensate for the missing region **C**, one can multiply its mirror region **B** by a factor of 2 (Fig. 6C). A Fourier transform along both k_x and k_y yields an image with full spatial resolution but possibly contaminated with artifacts (Fig. 6D) as doubling region **B** does not fully compensate for the lack of region **C**. Note that the low-resolution image obtained in Fig. 6B contains information about how much, and where, the object deviates from the zero-phase result that would be expected from a real object. The phase of the low-resolution image from Fig. 6B is used to correct the phase of the data from Fig. 6D to effectively convert the imaged complex object into a real one. After the phase correction, the imaginary part of the image is expected to contain all of the artifacts caused by region **C** being absent, and none of the useful object signal (Fig. 6E). On the other hand, the real part of the phase-corrected images is expected to contain the signal for the object (Fig. 6F). The imaginary part (Fig. 6E) is simply dismissed; the real part (Fig. 6F) becomes the final result produced by the algorithm.

Clinical Use of Partial Fourier Imaging

Partial Fourier imaging relies on the assumption that the object's phase is sufficiently smooth spatially that it can be faithfully captured in a low-resolution image (e.g., Fig. 6B). In cardiac imaging, this assumption is challenged by the proximity of the air-filled lungs because of the magnetic susceptibility difference between air and water. More conservative partial Fourier settings may be appropriate for cardiac imaging compared to other applications for which no air-filled regions are found near the anatomy of interest.

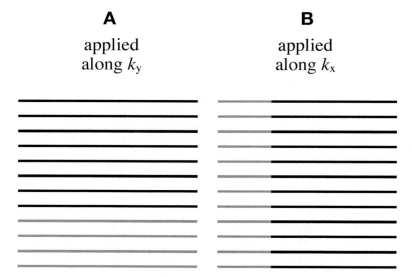

Fig. 7. Partial Fourier imaging can be applied in either the k_y direction or the k_x direction.

In general, a partial Fourier setting of about 70 or 75% could be considered typical. For example, a 75% partial Fourier setting is obtained when region **C** in Fig. 6A covers 25% of the k-space matrix, region **B** another 25%, and region **A** the remaining 50%. When using partial Fourier imaging, one should keep in mind that artifacts, if any, tend to appear in the vicinity of sharp transitions between regions of different magnetic susceptibility, such as air–water, air–fat, or water–fat transitions.

Instead of applying partial Fourier imaging along the k_y axis to diminish the number of acquired k-space lines (Fig. 7A), it can be applied along the k_x axis to reduce the length of each line (Fig. 7B). The same algorithm, depicted in Fig. 6, can be applied to either scenario. For example, when using a 75% partial Fourier algorithm along k_y, one reduces by 25% the number of k_y lines to acquire, which typically also reduces scan time by 25%. On the other hand, applying partial Fourier along k_x does not reduce the number of repetition time (TR) intervals required and has little effect on scan time. The main desired effect in this case is to reduce the amount of time required to gather a single line in k-space and thus reduce the echo time (TE).

In the presence of flow, the motion that occurs during TE may lead to blood vessels appearing displaced from their true location or to blood signal vanishing because of a loss of phase coherence called *intravoxel dephasing*. To suppress these undesirable effects, it is common practice to use partial Fourier along the k_x direction to help decrease TE as much as possible in angiography and in flow imaging applications. Note that Hermitian symmetry can be exploited only along one direction at a time; that is, partial Fourier imaging in one given direction (e.g., k_x) cannot be combined with partial Fourier imaging in any other direction.

Partial Fourier imaging is readily available on clinical scanners, although it may be referred to by a number of different names. For example, on GE systems, to enter a number of averages smaller than 1.0, which at first sight may seem a surprising concept, means using partial Fourier along the k_y direction (e.g., averaging by a factor 0.7

means using a 70% partial Fourier algorithm). Asking for the minimum TE involves using partial Fourier along the k_x direction to help bring TE to its smallest possible value; asking for the minimum full value does not use partial Fourier and leads to longer TE values.

CHANGING THE SAMPLING FROM FRAME TO FRAME WITH UNFOLD

Cardiac MRI applications often involve acquiring a time series of images to capture either the beating motion of the heart or the signal enhancement caused by a bolus of contrast agent. UNFOLD is a temporal strategy designed for dynamic applications that involves changing the set of k-space locations that are sampled from one time frame to the next, as depicted in Fig. 5I.

Forcing Aliased Signals to Behave in a Peculiar/Conspicuous Manner

To speed the image acquisition process, UNFOLD uses an FOV smaller than the imaged anatomy, causing the acquired images to be corrupted with aliasing artifacts (e.g., Fig. 1C). From time frame to time frame, the k-space sampling function is modified. As depicted in Fig. 5I, the range covered in k-space remains essentially unchanged and so does the k-space increment Δ_{ky}, but the set of locations to be sampled is shifted along the k_y axis from one time frame to the next.

Figure 8 explains the effect of such a shift. Figure 8A is a zoomed version of a portion of Fig. 3, and shows how aliasing is caused by ambiguity in the acquired data, as different frequencies appear identical at all sampled k_y locations. In Fig. 8B, the X marks representing the sampled locations are shifted along the k_y axis with respect to those in Fig. 8A (*see* dashed vertical lines). First, notice that, as in Fig. 8A and in Fig. 3, a faster oscillation can be found in Fig. 8B that agrees with all of the sampled data points (*see* gray line). The oscillation in Fig. 8B has precisely the same frequency as the one in Fig. 8A but a different phase, as can be seen from the fact that the location of the crests do not match (*see* dashed vertical lines). On the other hand, notice that the slower oscillation, the one readily picked up by a human eye when looking at the X marks in Fig. 8 and Fig. 3, is represented equally well in Fig. 8A and Fig. 8B without any phase shift (crest remains at the same location).

As the phase-encoding process attempts to distinguish different y locations by associating them with different frequencies along k_y, the fact that different frequencies appear the same at all sampled points means that different y locations can be confused and are not pulled apart by the phase-encoding process. This is the aliasing artifact problem, discussed previously and visible in Fig. 1C. The fact that the same frequencies are involved in Fig. 8A and Fig. 8B means that shifting the sampling function does not change which y locations are overlapped. As depicted in Fig. 8, the effect of a shift in the sampling function is to change the phase of aliased material (the higher frequency in Fig. 8A,B) while leaving unchanged the phase of nonaliased material (the lower frequency in Fig. 8A and Fig. 8B).

Shifting the sampling function along k_y allows the phase of the aliased signals to be controlled. By changing this shift from time frame to time frame, aliased signals can be forced to behave in a peculiar manner through time, making them conspicuous, identifiable, and thus removable *(14)*.

A Reference, zoomed version of Fig. 3

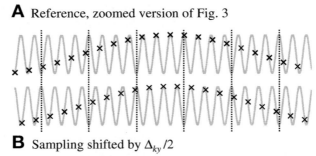

B Sampling shifted by $\Delta_{ky}/2$

Fig. 8. The X marks represent sampled k_y locations, and the spacing between consecutive marks gives Δ_{ky}, the k_y increment. In the lower row, the sampled locations are shifted by $\Delta_{ky}/2$ compared to the top row. The effect of this shift is to change the phase of the fast modulation that passes by all sampled points (gray line), as can be noticed looking at the vertical dashed lines. Any vertical dashed line passing through a crest in (**A**) passes through a valley in (**B**) and vice versa, meaning the $\Delta_{ky}/2$ shift in the sampling function modified the phase of aliased signal by 180°. *See* text for more details.

A Useful Special Case: A Phase That Evolves Linearly in Time

By shifting the sampling function from time frame to time frame, UNFOLD imposes changes on the phase of aliased signals. One particularly useful type of change involves forcing the phase of the aliased signals to change linearly (i.e., regularly) from one time frame to the next. For example, any given spoke in a bicycle wheel has an orientation, or phase, that evolves linearly in time whenever the bicycle rolls along at a constant speed. A phase that evolves linearly with time means that it always takes the same amount of time to make one full turn, or cycle. In this case, a single, precise frequency can be defined for this rotation.

As mentioned, a Fourier transform separates different frequencies. For one particular pixel in an image, by looking at how this particular pixel changes from time frame to time frame and Fourier transforming this time function, one obtains a so-called temporal frequency spectrum (Fig. 9A). By forcing the phase of aliased signals to evolve linearly in time at a certain rate, one can decide where in the temporal frequency spectrum the aliased signals should appear. A linear phase evolution is obtained by shifting the k-space sampled locations by a fixed increment from one time frame to the next, as depicted in Fig. 5I. Note that k-space lines pushed over the edge of the k-space matrix because of the shift are simply brought back to the other side of the matrix to fill in locations left vacant by the shift. In other words, the sampled region remains roughly centered around the point $k_x = 0$ and $k_y = 0$ despite the repeated shifts (Fig. 5I).

Displacing Spectra in the Temporal Frequency Domain

UNFOLD is applied along the time dimension in applications for which many different time frames are acquired. Consider a single spatial location, or pixel, in the acquired images. This pixel may feature both nonaliased and aliased signals, that is, signal that actually belongs there and signal aliased into this pixel from elsewhere. UNFOLD aims at separating such aliased and nonaliased signals, overlapped in a given pixel. Images potentially free of aliasing artifacts are obtained as UNFOLD is typically applied, in turn, to each one of the pixels in the imaged FOV.

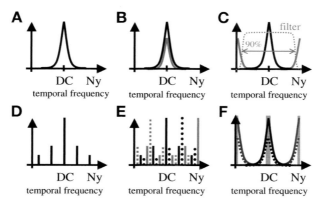

Fig. 9. UNFOLD can displace, in the temporal frequency domain, the spectra from aliased materials. Full black lines represent nonaliased signal; lines that are gray or dashed represent aliased material. Comparing (**B**) and (**C**), the action of displacing the aliased component (gray line) to the edge of the bandwidth, away from the main bulk of the nonaliased signal, allows aliased and nonaliased signals to be separated using a filter. In (**E**) and (**F**) as well, spectra were displaced to avoid, or at least reduce, the amount of overlap. The amount of overlap is reduced by UNFOLD in (**F**) as only two of the four individual spectra overlap in the regions shown shaded.

In a time series of images, a given pixel can take on different (complex) values from one time frame to the next. For example, one could plot the real part, imaginary part, magnitude, or phase of a given pixel as a function of time. The (complex) values assumed by a given pixel from frame to frame form a time function, and a so-called temporal frequency spectrum is obtained by applying a Fourier transform to this time function.

An example of a temporal frequency spectrum is depicted in Fig. 9A. The temporal frequency DC, an abbreviation borrowed from electromagnetism meaning direct current, corresponds to signal that does not change at all as a function of time. The temporal frequency Ny, for Nyquist, corresponds to the highest rate of change detectable in our time series of images, obtained when a signal completely reverses its phase from one time frame to the next (e.g., signal flip-flopping between a value +1 and −1 from one time frame to the next). The highest frequency faithfully captured by a sampling process, the Nyquist frequency, is named after the Swedish-American physicist Harry Nyquist (1889–1976), an important contributor to the field known as information theory. A temporal frequency spectrum (e.g., Fig. 9A) displays how much of each rate of change from DC (no change at all) to Nyquist (maximum rate) is present in the temporal variations undergone by a given pixel. Just like k-space values are expected to be particularly large for the low spatial frequencies near k-space center (e.g., Fig. 1, top row), temporal frequency spectra are expected to have particularly large values at low temporal frequencies, and this is why the spectrum depicted in Fig. 9A is sharply peaked around the DC (zero-frequency) point.

In Fig. 9B, two different signals are depicted: a nonaliased signal (black line) and an aliased signal (gray line). By shifting the k-space sampling function from one time frame to the next, UNFOLD forces the aliased signal to change more rapidly in time than it normally would. As a result, the aliased signal is displaced toward higher rates of change in the temporal frequency domain, potentially all the way to the Nyquist frequency (Fig. 9C). Most of this unwanted aliased signal is removed using a filter (dashed gray line in Fig. 9C). The filter removes aliased, fast-changing signal near the Nyquist frequency while preserving most of the desired, nonaliased signal near DC.

In some situations like in functional MRI, for which particular frequencies are not expected to feature any significant signal (Fig. 9D), the ability to move spectra around the temporal frequency domain can allow a large number of individual spectra, from a large number of aliased points, to be interleaved so they do not overlap. Because they are interleaved and not overlapped, the individual spectra can be readily separated from each other (Fig. 9E) *(14)*. Figure 9F shows a case where UNFOLD reduces, but does not eliminate, the amount of overlap by moving half of the individual spectra, two of four, all the way to the Nyquist frequency. Reducing the amount of overlap is useful in the context of hybrid approaches, for which a second method would be combined with UNFOLD to finish the work and resolve any remaining overlap.

An Example of How UNFOLD Works

Figure 10A shows part of a time series of *k*-space matrices acquired during a myocardial perfusion exam. Only half the lines were obtained in each matrix to reduce scan time by a factor of 2 and allow twice the normal number of slices to be acquired per R–R interval. A close inspection of Fig. 10A reveals that half of the lines appear black because they were not acquired and are simply filled with zeros. Furthermore, any line sampled in one given time frame gets skipped (i.e., appears black) in the next time frame. The odd *k*-space lines were sampled for odd time frames and the even *k*-space lines for even time frames.

Figure 10B shows the corresponding images corrupted by aliasing artifacts. Because of the changes in the sampling function from time frame to time frame (Fig. 10A), the phase of any aliased signal was forced to change by 180° from one frame to the next. In Fig. 10C, only data from coil elements placed on the chest (and not the back) were used for display purposes to better show the phase of cardiac tissues. Looking at Fig. 10C, notice that the phase of nonaliased cardiac tissues (thin black arrow) does not change appreciably from frame to frame; the phase of the aliased copy of the heart (white arrow) clearly undergoes drastic changes from frame to frame. These phase changes make aliased signals conspicuous, so they can be detected and suppressed. A filter was used to remove most of the aliased signals while preserving most of the desired nonaliased signals. The filter is multiplied with the temporal frequency spectra. Accordingly, signals at frequencies near Nyquist, where the filter is nearly zero (Fig. 9C), are very much suppressed. The suppressed frequency region has a half-width half-maximum equal to 10% of the whole bandwidth. Accordingly, 90% of the bandwidth was preserved for the nonaliased signals (Fig. 9C). Looking at the results in Fig. 10D, notice that most of the aliased material has been removed, and that contrast enhancement was captured.

PARALLEL IMAGING

Parallel imaging is a powerful approach well on its way to impact every MRI field in need of extra acquisition speed. As depicted in Fig. 11, parallel imaging relies on the fact that the imaged object can be "seen" simultaneously by a number of different coils placed at different locations around the imaged anatomy. The approach was introduced independently by a number of investigators well over a decade ago *(15–19)*, but it was only when Sodickson and Manning developed their SMASH (simultaneous acquisition

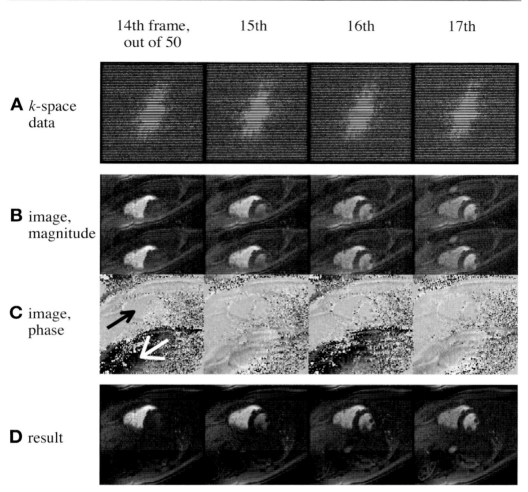

Fig. 10. (**A**) In this example, only half of the *k*-space locations are acquired, and the missing locations are simply filled with zeros. (**B**) Accordingly, the corresponding images are corrupted with aliasing artifacts. (**C**) The phase of aliased material (*see* white arrow) varies rapidly from frame to frame, unlike that of nonaliased material (*see* black arrow). (**D**) Applying a filter, as depicted in Fig. 9c, removes nearly all of the aliased material, leaving mostly intact the nonaliased signal.

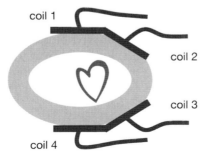

Fig. 11. Parallel imaging feeds on the fact that the object is seen simultaneously by a number of different coils. Although only 4 coil elements are depicted here, higher numbers are often used.

of spatial harmonics) algorithm and presented in vivo images *(20)* that the potential of parallel imaging became more apparent. In the years that followed, a number of different versions of parallel imaging were introduced, such as sensitivity encoding (SENSE) *(21)*, sensitivity profiles from an array of coils for encoding and reconstruction in parallel (SPACE RIP) *(22)*, generalized autocalibrating partially parallel acquisitions (GRAPPA) *(23)*, and generalized SMASH *(24)*, among others. Currently, the Cartesian version of SENSE is still probably by far the most commonly used parallel imaging method because of its relative simplicity and short image reconstruction times.

An Example of How Parallel Imaging Works

GETTING THE SENSITIVITY DATA

Parallel imaging methods require, as prior knowledge, information about the imaging coils used. In Cartesian SENSE, this prior knowledge consists of sensitivity maps showing how sensitive a given coil is to the MR signal emitted by the imaged object. Figure 12A shows sensitivity maps for four coil elements involved in acquiring the cardiac data shown in Fig. 12B,C.

Looking at Fig. 12A, notice that coil number 1 is very sensitive (high values in its sensitivity map) to tissues located near the anterior part of the thoracic cage and rather insensitive (low values) to tissues near the back. As could be expected, this is because coil number 1 was physically placed against the anterior part of the thoracic cage. On the other hand, coil number 4 was placed against back soft tissues and is sensitive mostly to tissues nearby.

Although Fig. 12A displays the strength, or magnitude, of the sensitivity, it should be mentioned that sensitivity maps are complex valued, with a phase component that is not displayed here. The most common way of generating sensitivity maps involves acquiring an extra scan, a so-called reference scan, typically right before the actual parallel imaging acquisition *(21)*. Alternately, the reference scan can be fused with the actual scan in so-called self-referenced approaches (also called self-calibrated or autocalibrated) *(23,25–27)*. Fusing reference and actual scans has the advantage of eliminating all risks that motion might occur between the two scans, unlike when a separate reference scan is performed. The maps in Fig. 12A were obtained through a self-calibrated approach described in ref. *27*.

GENERATING AN IMAGE

To speed the image acquisition, the FOV along *y* was reduced by a factor of 2, leading to the images in Fig. 12B. The corresponding *k*-space acquisition scheme is depicted in Fig. 5C. Most of the signal visible in the image from coil number 1 in Fig. 12B corresponds to tissues located near the anterior part of the thoracic cage, as could be expected from its sensitivity map in Fig. 12A. Similarly, most of the signal seen in the image from coil number 4 represents tissues in close proximity to the patient's back. As a consequence, when reconstructing the image in Fig. 12C, much weight is given to data from coil number 1 for pixels located near the patient's chest; data from coil number 4 is given much weight near the patient's back.

We now look in more detail at how Fig. 12C is generated. Imagine a small cube of back muscle tissues found at a given location (*x,y*) within the patient. Because of the aliasing problem, explained in Fig. 3 and clearly visible in Fig. 12B, the phase encoding mechanism is incapable of distinguishing signal from this parcel of tissues and

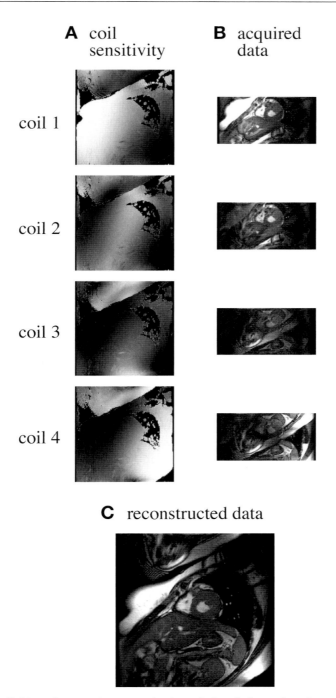

Fig. 12. (**A**) Parallel imaging requires, as prior knowledge, information about the sensitivity of the imaging coils. In this example, the sensitivity maps were obtained using a self-referenced approach *(27)*. (**B**) To speed data acquisition, only a small FOV was acquired, leading to images corrupted by aliasing artifacts. (**C**) Combining the data from all coils, along with information from the sensitivity maps, allows a mostly artifact-free image to be reconstructed. *See* text for more details.

another one aliased on top of it. With d_y the size of the reconstructed full FOV in Fig. 12, points separated by $d_y/2$ in the phase-encoding direction are overlapped in the acquired images (Fig. 12B), and tissues located at (x,y) overlap with tissues located at $(x,y + d_y/2)$.

Consider the image I_1 acquired using coil number 1. The pixel location (x,y) has a value $I_1(x,y)$ in image I_1. This value is determined in part by how much object signal $O(x,y)$ is found at (x,y), weighted by how sensitive coil number 1 happens to be at this particular location, given by $S_1(x,y)$. Another contribution to $I_1(x,y)$ comes from the aliased tissues located a distance $d_y/2$ away, $O(x,y + d_y/2)$, weighted by how sensitive coil number 1 turns out to be at this second location, $S_1(x,y + d_y/2)$. As a result of both contributions, from (x,y) and from the aliased location $(x,y + d_y/2)$, $I_1(x,y)$ is given by

$$I_1(x,y) = S_1(x,y) \times O(x,y) + S_1(x,y + d_y/2) \times O(x,y + d_y/2)$$

Similar relations are obtained for the other coils:

$$I_2(x,y) = S_2(x,y) \times O(x,y) + S_2(x,y + d_y/2) \times O(x,y + d_y/2)$$

$$I_3(x,y) = S_3(x,y) \times O(x,y) + S_3(x,y + d_y/2) \times O(x,y + d_y/2)$$

$$I_4(x,y) = S_4(x,y) \times O(x,y) + S_4(x,y + d_y/2) \times O(x,y + d_y/2)$$

In these equations, some quantities are known, and some are unknown. All of the sensitivity values S are known as prior knowledge (Fig. 12A). The values I are also known because they were acquired (Fig. 12B). The amount of object signal from different locations O constitutes the unknown quantity. Looking at these four complex equations, for a given pixel (x_0, y_0), one can see that there are two complex unknowns: $O(x_0, y_0)$ and $O(x_0, y_0 + d_y/2)$. Through algebraic manipulations of these equations, one can isolate the unknown quantities and evaluate them. Because the unknown O's always appear with a power of 1 (they never appear squared or in a square root, for example), these equations are said to be linear, and the algebraic manipulations required for their solution turn out to be equivalent to inverting a matrix having two columns and four rows and containing all of the S values from the equations. Consequently, in the literature, the reconstruction problem is typically presented in terms of a matrix inversion.

By solving these equations, one separates the object signal $O(x_0, y_0)$ from the aliased signal $O(x_0, y_0 + d_y/2)$ to resolve the aliasing problem seen in Fig. 12B. In summary, the acquired FOV is reduced to gain imaging speed, and images corrupted by aliasing artifacts are obtained (Fig. 12B). Repeating the process described above for all pixels, $O(x,y)$ is evaluated at all (x,y) locations, giving rise to a dealiased image (Fig. 12C).

Practical Differences Between Algorithms

The example in the preceding section was based on the Cartesian SENSE method. But, several other approaches have been described in the literature. One useful way to compare them is according to the type of k-space data they are meant to handle. As shown in Table 1, Cartesian SENSE *(21)* is meant to handle data sampled on a regular Cartesian grid in k-space. When the k-space lines are not evenly spaced along k_y, more general methods are required to reconstruct the data.

Methods such as GRAPPA *(23)*, SPACE RIP *(22)*, generalized SMASH *(24)*, or variable-density SENSE (vdSENSE) *(27)* can handle such variations in sampling density along the k_y direction. For other types of sampling schemes, such as radial or spiral trajectories, a more general algorithm can be used to reconstruct the data, such as general SENSE *(21)* (although GRAPPA can be extended to handle spiral sampling schemes [*28*]). Complexity and image reconstruction time tends to greatly increase the further one departs from a regular, Cartesian sampling scheme.

For example, general SENSE is expected to require much longer reconstruction times than SPACE RIP, which in turn requires much more processing than Cartesian SENSE. Typically, a given data set should be reconstructed with one of the simplest methods able to handle it. For instance, in an application for which data are sampled on a Cartesian grid, using an algorithm able to handle arbitrary sampling schemes might lead to unnecessarily long reconstruction times and extra implementation difficulties. In addition to the type of sampling scheme handled, the use of approximations may also greatly influence reconstruction time. Some methods, such as GRAPPA or vdSENSE, may feature greatly reduced reconstruction times compared to methods that solve more exact versions of the reconstruction problem, such as SPACE RIP or generalized SMASH. All of the methods mentioned here can be extended fairly directly, at least in principle, to include 3D imaging.

It would seem that a majority of the parallel imaging scans performed now use a regular, Cartesian sampling scheme and use Cartesian SENSE for image reconstruction. A notable exception involves self-calibrated scans. Such scans typically require the region near *k*-space center to be sampled more densely, as depicted in Fig. 5F. Coil sensitivity information is obtained from this central region *(23,25)*, and methods such as GRAPPA, SPACE RIP, generalized SMASH, or vdSENSE, for example, can be used to reconstruct the resulting unevenly spaced data.

Clinical Use of Parallel Imaging

The Cartesian SENSE parallel imaging method is named iPAT on Siemens scanners, ASSET on GE scanners, SENSE on Philips scanners, and SPEEDER on Toshiba scanners. Parallel imaging can be used to speed the data acquisition process in cardiac imaging. For example, it can be used to increase the number of slices acquired per R–R interval in myocardial perfusion imaging, to reduce the breath-hold duration in cine imaging of cardiac function, or to improve spatial resolution. It should be noted that different uses of the method come at different prices in terms of signal-to-noise ratio (SNR).

Using parallel imaging to reduce scan time by a factor of n comes with a price tag of at least $\sqrt{n}$ in SNR. Leaving scan time unchanged and using parallel imaging to improve spatial resolution by a factor of n reduces SNR by at least a factor of n. In dynamic imaging, improving the temporal resolution by a factor of n by reducing the acquisition time of any given frame and increasing the total number of time frames accordingly may come at arguably no cost in SNR. Although individual time frames become noisier in the process, there are more of them, and the two factors tend to offset each other (as long as images are viewed dynamically, in a movie loop, so that noise has a chance to average out in the reader's eyes).

Unlike partial Fourier imaging or UNFOLD, parallel imaging has a tendency to amplify noise. That is why the words *at least* were used in the preceding paragraph to describe SNR penalties. Although physics and noise statistics impose limits on how small the noise penalties can be, in principle at least there is no upper limit on how large a noise penalty parallel imaging can introduce. In practice, noise amplification is kept minimal through careful coil designs, conservative settings for the acceleration factor, and elaborate regularization algorithms *(29,30)*.

Note that, because of possible noise amplification, it would typically make little sense to use parallel imaging along with signal averaging. Although parallel imaging spends SNR to buy speed, signal averaging spends speed to buy SNR. Because parallel imaging sometimes overpays when buying speed (noise amplification), it would make little sense to turn around right away and spend the newly acquired speed to purchase back some (but maybe not all) of our original SNR.

Parallel imaging is already a powerful approach to speed data acquisition and is getting more powerful still as vendors are in the process of rapidly increasing the number of independent channels and receiver coils that can be used simultaneously.

OTHER METHODS AND COMBINATIONS OF METHODS

In addition to the three methods described (partial Fourier imaging, UNFOLD, and parallel imaging), several other partially sampled methods have been proposed and implemented for fast imaging. A number of these methods are briefly reviewed next.

Reduced FOV Methods

Several of the partially sampled MR methods proposed to this day involve reducing the FOV for increased acquisition speed and then suppressing the resulting artifacts caused by aliasing. We have seen two such methods, parallel imaging and UNFOLD.

An early method of this type was proposed by Hu and Parrish (31), where aliased materials are suppressed by assuming they do not change, or move, from one time frame to the next. Accordingly, all dynamic changes are assumed to originate from the nonaliased materials only. The signal from the nonchanging aliased tissues is evaluated once and can be extracted from all time frames to evaluate the nonaliased signal. The method was later improved, in terms of SNR, by Fredrickson and Pelc (32). A different approach, the multiple-region MRI method by Nagle and Levin (33), is able to exploit the fact that some objects are sparse. If areas within the object are known to be void of signal, then one can reduce the amount of acquired data and still manage to reconstruct artifact-free images.

Yet another way to avoid aliasing artifacts involves using more elaborate RF pulses to excite only part of the object in the phase-encoding direction (34,35). Because the magnetization of the aliased materials does not get flipped into the transverse plane, these materials do not have any signal with which to cause artifacts. These more elaborate 2D RF pulses, however, can be significantly longer than normal slice-selective 1D pulses, imposing constraints on how short TE and TR can be.

Other Methods

Feature-recognizing MRI (36,37) and singular-value decomposition (SVD) imaging (38,39) are partially sampled methods that feed on prior knowledge about the shape of the object imaged to speed the image acquisition process. While feature-recognizing MRI uses a library of images to figure out how the image of a knee, or a heart, is expected to look, SVD imaging uses a training scan performed with the patient *in situ*. In both cases, the acquisition process can focus on acquiring only the information that appears to be most relevant to the task at hand, leading to a reduction in the amount of data to acquire.

In dynamic imaging, when a time series of images is acquired, the keyhole (40–42) and reduced-encoding imaging with generalized-series reconstruction (RIGR) (43,44) methods

Results from UNFOLD-SENSE

A Patient 1, myocardial perfusion, acceleration 3.0, with 8 coils

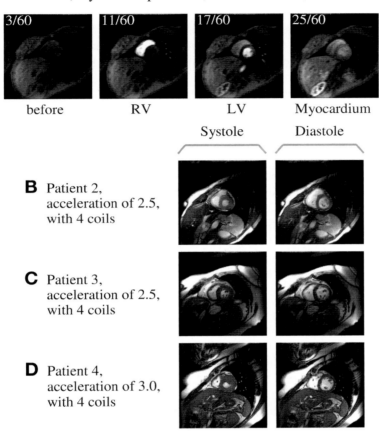

Fig. 13. Examples of results obtained using our UNFOLD-SENSE method *(27)*. The approach is self-calibrated (no separate, reference scan is required), and it includes an UNFOLD-based artifact suppression scheme. It can be used to speed image acquisition in myocardial perfusion studies and in the cine imaging of ventricular function. The number in the left upper corner of the images in (**A**) gives the frame number of 60 frames. In (**B**) through (**D**), two specific frames were selected for display from each data set, one near midsystole and one near middiastole. In (**A**), the approach was used to reduce the number of echoes per TR from four to two and to slightly increase the number of slices per R–R interval. In (**B**), the acceleration allowed temporal resolution to be improved to a value of 22 ms. In (**C**), scan time was reduced to about a 5-second breath hold per slice; in (**D**), the acceleration allowed improvements in both temporal resolution (30 ms) and scan time (about 8 seconds per slice). Without acceleration, a scan time of 12 seconds per slice and a temporal resolution around 40–50 ms could be considered typical.

can accelerate image acquisition through the sampling scheme depicted in Fig. 5H. A full *k*-space matrix is acquired before and/or after the dynamic acquisition, but during the actual dynamic scan, only a central region in *k*-space is sampled for increased speed. The missing data are filled in through models that differ in the two approaches. The keyhole model involves adding the acquired low-resolution dynamic data to high-resolution information; RIGR uses a multiplicative model in which low-resolution dynamic information gets multiplied with high-resolution information to generate images.

Combinations of Methods

The methods presented to this point could be thought of as building blocks to be assembled, mixed, and matched in a number of different ways. When different methods feed on different types of assumptions and prior knowledge, they can often be combined for added performance. For example, partial Fourier imaging is the only one of these methods feeding on Hermitian symmetries, and it has been successfully combined with essentially all of the other methods discussed here, such as with parallel imaging in ref. *45*.

In a somewhat similar fashion, because UNFOLD is a temporal strategy but many other methods function along spatial dimensions, UNFOLD has proved compatible with several different approaches. More specifically, the method seems to have found a special niche as a helper to parallel imaging, leading to hybrid methods such as temporal SENSE (TSENSE) *(26)* and UNFOLD-SENSE *(27,46)*. Examples obtained using our UNFOLD-SENSE method are shown in Fig. 13 for myocardial perfusion and cardiac cine applications.

An approach similar to UNFOLD has also been combined with a training scan strategy, leading to *k-t* broad-use linear acquisition speed–up technique (*k-t* BLAST), which in turn has been combined with parallel imaging to give *k-t* SENSE *(47)*. UNFOLD has also been combined with a 2D RF reduced-FOV approach in a temperature-monitoring application *(48)*. In a work by Mitsouras et al. *(49)*, a strategy based on training scans was combined with parallel imaging. This list is ofcourse not meant to be exhaustive.

CONCLUSION

Because of all the motion present, cardiac MRI has considerable needs in terms of imaging speed. Once traditional means of increasing speed have been exhausted, the remaining option is to acquire only partial data sets, and filling–in the missing data using prior knowledge. Many different methods, using a variety of different types of prior knowledge, have been presented in the literature. The development, and the combination, of partially sampled methods currently form a particularly active field of MR research. As a result, the available imaging speed has been rapidly increasing and can be expected to do so for some time, until fundamental SNR-related limits are reached and impede further progress.

ACKNOWLEDGMENTS

I want to thank Drs. Robert Mulkern, W. Scott Hoge, Jeffrey Duryea, and Ms. Joscelyne Bluteau for their precious help, both in proofreading the manuscript and in identifying key bibliographical references.

REFERENCES

1. Mansfield P. Multi-planar image formation using NMR spin echoes. J Phys C 1977;10:L55–L58.
2. Mansfield P, Maudsley AA. Planar spin imaging by NMR. J Magn Reson 1977;27:101–119.
3. Hennig J, Nauerth A, Friedburg H. RARE imaging: a fast imaging method for clinical MR. Magn Reson Med 1986;3:823–833.
4. Mulkern RV, Wong ST, Winalski C, Jolesz FA. Contrast manipulation and artifact assessment of 2D and 3D RARE sequences. Magn Reson Imaging 1990;8:557–566.
5. Patz S, Hawkes RC. The application of steady-state free precession to the study of very slow fluid flow. Magn Reson Med 1986;3:140–145.
6. van der Meulen P, Groen JP, Tinus AM, Bruntink G. Fast field echo imaging: an overview and contrast calculations. Magn Reson Imaging 1988;6:355–368.

7. Twieg DB. The k-trajectory formulation of the NMR imaging process with applications in analysis and synthesis of imaging methods. Med Phys 1983;10:610–621.
8. Cooley JW, Tukey JW. An algorithm for the machine calculation of complex Fourier series. Math Comput 1965;19:297–301.
9. Feinberg D, Hale J, Watts J, Kaufman L, Mark A. Halving MR imaging time by conjugation: demonstration at 3.5 kG. Radiology 1986;156:527–531.
10. Margosian P, Schmitt F, Purdy D. Faster MR imaging: imaging with half the data. Healthcare Instr 1986;1:195–197.
11. Haacke E, Lindskog E, Lin W. A fast, iterative, partial-Fourier technique capable of local phase recovery. J Magn Reson 1991;92:126–145.
12. Noll D, Nishimura D, Macovski A. Homodyne detection in magnetic resonance imaging. IEEE Trans Med Imaging 1991;10:154–163.
13. McGibney G, Smith MR, Nichols ST, Crawley A. Quantitative evaluation of several partial Fourier reconstruction algorithms used in MRI. Magn Reson Med 1993;30:51–59.
14. Madore B, Glover GH, Pelc NJ. Unaliasing by Fourier-encoding the overlaps using the temporal dimension (UNFOLD), applied to cardiac imaging and fMRI. Magn Reson Med 1999;42:813–828.
15. Hutchinson M, Raff U. Fast MRI data acquisition using multiple detectors. Magn Reson Med 1988;6:87–91.
16. Kelton JR, Magin RL, Wright SM. An algorithm for rapid image acquisition using multiple receiver coils. Paper presented at: SMRM; Amsterdam, The Netherlands; 1989.
17. Kwiat D, Einav S, Navon G. A decoupled coil detector array for fast image acquisition in magnetic resonance imaging. Med Phys 1991;18:251–265.
18. Ra JB, Rim CY. Fast imaging using subencoding data sets from multiple detectors. Magn Reson Med 1993;30:142–145.
19. Carlson JW, Minemura T. Imaging time reduction through multiple receiver coil data acquisition and image reconstruction. Magn Reson Med 1993;29:681–687.
20. Sodickson DK, Manning WJ. Simultaneous acquisition of spatial harmonics (SMASH): fast imaging with radiofrequency coil arrays. Magn Reson Med 1997;38:591–603.
21. Pruessmann KP, Weiger M, Scheidegger MB, Boesiger P. SENSE: sensitivity encoding for fast MRI. Magn Reson Med 1999;42:952–962.
22. Kyriakos WE, Panych LP, Kacher DF, et al. Sensitivity profiles from an array of coils for encoding and reconstruction in parallel (SPACE RIP). Magn Reson Med 2000;44:301–308.
23. Griswold MA, Jakob PM, Heidemann RM, et al. Generalized autocalibrating partially parallel acquisitions (GRAPPA). Magn Reson Med 2002;47:1202–1210.
24. Bydder M, Larkman DJ, Hajnal JV. Generalized SMASH imaging. Magn Reson Med 2002;47:160–170.
25. McKenzie CA, Yeh EN, Ohliger MA, Price MD, Sodickson DK. Self-calibrating parallel imaging with automatic coil sensitivity extraction. Magn Reson Med 2002;47:529–538.
26. Kellman P, Epstein FH, McVeigh ER. Adaptive sensitivity encoding incorporating temporal filtering (TSENSE). Magn Reson Med 2001;45:846–852.
27. Madore B. UNFOLD-SENSE: a parallel MRI method with self-calibration and artifact suppression. Magn Reson Med 2004;52:310–320.
28. Heidemann RM, Griswold MA, Seiberlich N, Kruger G, Kannengiesser SA, Kiefer B, Wiggins G, Wall LL, Jakob PM. Direct parallel imaging reconstructions for spiral trajectories using GRAPPA. Magn Reson Med 2006;56:317–326.
29. Lin FH, Kwong KK, Belliveau JW, Wald LL. Parallel imaging reconstruction using automatic regularization. Magn Reson Med 2004;51:559–567.
30. Hoge WS, Brooks DH, Madore B, Kyriakos WE. A tour of accelerated parallel MR imaging from a linear systems perspective. Concepts MR 2005;27A:17–37.
31. Hu X, Parrish T. Reduction of field of view for dynamic imaging. Magn Reson Med 1994;31:691–694.
32. Fredrickson JO, Pelc NJ. Temporal resolution improvement in dynamic imaging. Magn Reson Med 1996;35:621–625.
33. Nagle SK, Levin DN. Multiple region MRI. Magn Reson Med 1999;41:774–786.
34. Pauly J, Nishimura D, Macovski A. A k-space analysis of small-tip-angle excitation. J Magn Reson 1989;81:43–56.
35. Pauly J, Le Roux P, Nishimura D, Macovski A. Parameter relations for the Shinnar-Le Roux selective excitation pulse design algorithm. IEEE Trans Med Imaging 1991;10:53–65.
36. Cao Y, Levin DN. Feature-recognizing MRI. Magn Reson Med 1993;30:305–317.

37. Cao Y, Levin DN. Using prior knowledge of human anatomy to constrain MR image acquisition and reconstruction: half k-space and full k-space techniques. Magn Reson Imaging 1997;15:669–677.
38. Zientara GP, Panych LP, Jolesz FA. Dynamically adaptive MRI with encoding by singular value decomposition. Magn Reson Med 1994;32:268–274.
39. Panych LP, Oesterle C, Zientara GP, Hennig J. Implementation of a fast gradient-echo SVD encoding technique for dynamic imaging. Magn Reson Med 1996;35:554–562.
40. van Vaals JJ, Brummer ME, Dixon WT, et al. "Keyhole" method for accelerating imaging of contrast agent uptake. J Magn Reson Imaging 1993;3:671–675.
41. Jones RA, Haraldseth O, Muller TB, Rinck PA, Oksendal AN. k-Space substitution: a novel dynamic imaging technique. Magn Reson Med 1993;29:830–834.
42. Bishop JE, Santyr GE, Kelcz F, Plewes DB. Limitations of the keyhole technique for quantitative dynamic contrast-enhanced breast MRI. J Magn Reson Imaging 1997;7:716–723.
43. Liang ZP, Lauterbur PC. An efficient method for dynamic magnetic resonance imaging. IEEE Trans Med Imaging 1994;13:677–687.
44. Hanson JM, Liang ZP, Wiener EC, Lauterbur PC. Fast dynamic imaging using two reference images. Magn Reson Med 1996;36:172–175.
45. Bydder M, Robson MD. Partial fourier partially parallel imaging. Magn Reson Med 2005;53:1393–1401.
46. Madore B. Using UNFOLD to remove artifacts in parallel imaging and in partial-Fourier imaging. Magn Reson Med 2002;48:493–501.
47. Tsao J, Boesiger P, Pruessmann KP. k-t BLAST and k-t SENSE: dynamic MRI with high frame rate exploiting spatiotemporal correlations. Magn Reson Med 2003;50:1031–1042.
48. Zhao L, Madore B, Panych LP. Reduced field-of-view MRI with two-dimensional spatially-selective RF excitation and UNFOLD. Magn Reson Med 2005;53:1118–1125.
49. Mitsouras D, Hoge WS, Rybicki FJ, Kyriakos WE, Edelman A, Zientara GP. Non-Fourier-encoded parallel MRI using multiple receiver coils. Magn Reson Med 2004;52:321–328.

10 Contrast Agents for Cardiovascular MRI

Hale Ersoy, Frank Rybicki, and Martin Prince

CONTENTS

INTRODUCTION

In the last two decades, magnetic resonance imaging (MRI) has revolutionized clinical cardiovascular imaging. Its major advantages over other noninvasive diagnostic modalities are its safety, operator-independent reproducibility, and multiplanar two-dimensional (2D) and three-dimensional (3D) imaging capability with high spatial and temporal resolution. MRI does not deliver ionizing radiation and does not utilize inherently nephrotoxic iodinated contrast media. The intrinsic tissue contrast offered by MRI has been even further expanded by the introduction of paramagnetic magnetic resonance (MR) contrast agents. These agents improve the image signal-to-noise ratio (SNR) and contrast-to-noise ratio (CNR), thereby increasing the sensitivity, specificity, and accuracy of MRI.

GENERAL CONSIDERATIONS IN CONTRAST ENHANCEMENT

Contrast

MRI contrast refers to the relative difference in signal intensity (SI) between two adjacent tissues. MR pulse sequences are designed to capitalize the inherent contrast between tissues, such as differences in proton density and magnetic relaxation times of the tissues, in-flow phenomena, magnetization transfer, susceptibility, and numerous additional minor effects. Before moving to the contrast mechanisms, it is important to understand some basic concepts of signal acquisition in MRI.

From: *Contemporary Cardiology: Cardiovascular Magnetic Resonance Imaging*
Edited by: Raymond Y. Kwong © Humana Press Inc., Totowa, NJ

T_1 *and* T_2 *Relaxation Times of Tissues*

T_1 (longitudinal relaxation time) is a time constant that corresponds to the approximate time for protons to align along with the external magnetic field (B_0). Once protons align with the external magnetic field, a radio-frequency (RF) pulse is applied to obtain MR signal (referred to as echo). This MR signal is emitted for a time, referred to as T_2 (transverse relaxation time), which varies from tissue to tissue. T_1 relaxation occurs by transferring the energy to the adjacent structures (spin-lattice relaxation). Because the energy transfer is more efficient among slow-rotating molecules, the T_1 relaxation time of the water molecules bound to a macromolecule is faster compared to the free water molecules *(1–3)*. T_2 relaxation primarily occurs because of loss of phase coherence of spins (spin-spin relaxation). T_2 relaxation time is always shorter than T_1.

R_1 ($1/T_1$) is the longitudinal relaxation rate (s^{-1}), and r_1 ($mM^{-1}\ s^{-1}$) is the increase in R_1 in a given medium per unit concentration of contrast agent. R_2 ($1/T_2$) is the transverse relaxation rate (s^{-1}), and r_2 ($mM^{-1}s^{-1}$) is the increase in R_2 in a given medium per unit concentration of the contrast agent. R_2* ($1/T_2$*) is the effective transverse relaxation rate in gradient echo MR sequences.

An image emphasizing T_1 contrast (T_1 weighted) can be obtained by repeating the RF pulses at a rate (repetition time, TR) that is shorter than the T_1 relaxation time of some tissues but longer than other tissues. Protons in the tissues with shorter T_1 compared to the TR realign with the external magnetic field in between pulses, resulting in high signal. For those tissues with longer T_1 compared to the TR, the protons do not have time to realign with the external magnetic field in between the RF pulses, therefore producing low signal.

Because it is not possible to change tissue proton density, paramagnetic contrast agents are routinely used to change tissue relaxation times. Contrast agents shorten both T_1 and T_2 relaxation times of water protons in their vicinity and thus increase the strength of the magnetic field in the local environment. Increase in the local magnetic strength creates microenvironment magnetic field inhomogeneities that interact with protons undergoing Brownian motion. The effect on T_1 is more prominent, and thus clinical tissue enhancement pertains with T_1-weighted imaging. Although T_1 shortening increases the tissue SI, T_2 shortening results in signal decrease.

Paramagnetic Metals

Lanthanide metals with unpaired electrons have the potential to be paramagnetic. However, most of the metals with unpaired electrons are not suitable for clinical MRI because of the unmatched metal spin relaxation time and proton Larmor frequency. Those lanthanide metals with suitable characteristics include gadolinium (Gd^{3+}), dysprosium (Dy^{3+}), manganese (Mn^{+2}), and iron (Fe^{3+}). The number of the unpaired electrons directly correlates with the strength of the magnetic moment of the element *(4)*. Gd^{3+} has seven unpaired electrons and a long electronic relaxation time, thus a strong magnetic moment. This property of Gd^{3+} makes it an excellent paramagnetic contrast agent. Dy^{3+}, Mn^{2+}, and Fe^{3+} have five unpaired electrons. Note that hydrogen (H^+), the natural source of the MR signal, has only one (unpaired) electron. Paramagnetic contrast agents do not have protons in their structures and thus do not produce MR signal by themselves. At present, most commonly used contrast agents in routine clinical work are Gd based.

Gd-based contrast agents shorten the tissue relaxation times by transiently binding the water molecules. The water protons interacting with Gd^{3+} produce high signal on the images because of their shortened T_1 relaxation times. As these protons pass through the magnetic field gradients within their microenvironment, both T_1 and T_2 relaxations speed up roughly proportional to the Gd-based contrast agent concentration as follows:

$$1/T_1(\text{with Gd}) = 1/T_1(\text{without Gd}) + R_1 \times [\text{Gd}] \qquad (1)$$

where T_1 is the relaxation time of the tissue, R_1 and [Gd] are the relaxation rate and concentration of the Gd-based contrast agent, respectively. Therefore, the performance of paramagnetic contrast agents is highly dependent on their r_1 relaxivities. Equation 1 is maintained at the concentrations used in routine clinical imaging. However, of note, the linear relationship of Eq. 1 is not preserved at very low or very high concentrations *(5,6)*. Extremely high concentrations actually reduce the SI because the T_2 shortening effect of the contrast agent becomes prominent. This offset is more pronounced at low magnetic fields compared to high fields.

Contrast Localization

Although contrast agents increase the SI, the clinical benefit depends on the ability to localize the contrast agent within a single tissue compartment. Contrast localization can be controlled in several ways. The first is bolus timing; during the first pass, contrast agent is transiently localized to the injected vein, then pulmonary circulation, and finally the arterial system. This principle forms the basis of contrast-enhanced MR angiography (MRA). Several sophisticated bolus-timing methods have been developed into MR pulse sequences to facilitate imaging the contrast agent at the optimal moment to capture a specific vessel of interest.

The second contrast localization method is associated with the molecular size of the contrast agent. Specifically, larger molecules remain within the blood vessels (e.g., blood pool agents); smaller molecules redistribute into extracellular fluid compartments (e.g., extracellular contrast agents). At present, all Gd-based contrast agents approved by the Food and Drug Administration (FDA) in the United States are extracellular agents. For cardiac MRI, these agents are useful because they are excluded from viable myocytes but are taken up avidly in infarcted tissue, which is predominately extracellular.

The third contrast agent localization method is based on special moieties on the contrast agents that selectively bind to specific tissues. For example EP-2104R (Epix Medical, Mallinckrodt, St. Louis, MO) binds to fibrin and localizes within thrombus. Necrotic tissue-specific *bis*-gadolinium mesoporphyrin (Gadophrin-2; Schering AG, Berlin, Germany) localize within necrotic tissue to identify infarct, abscess, and necrotic tumors. Albumin-binding agents, such as MS-325 (Vasovist; Epix Medical, Mallinckrodt) remain localized within the blood pool.

The fourth localization method corresponds to the portal of entry into the body. Intravenous contrast agents must reach their target by distribution via the circulatory system. Gaseous contrast agents (e.g., helium 3 or xenon 129) enter into the lungs via inhalation. At present, cardiovascular applications do not exist because experiments using gaseous contrast agents primarily investigate pulmonary physiology. Xenon changes its resonant peak between the gaseous phase and dissolved phase, allowing the exciting potential of studying gas exchange, diffusion, and absorption into the blood. MR lymphography is performed by injecting Gd-based contrast agent into the feet and imaging after the material has tracked to the lymphatic pathways.

Contrast Agent-Related Artifacts

Understanding principles of contrast agents is important for detecting and properly interpreting artifacts. For example, an important aspect of contrast agent delivery is the dilution of the agent as it redistributes into a gradually increasing volume fraction of the body. The concentration in the injected vein is very high and decreases as the contrast reaches the central circulation because of mixing with the large volume of blood returning to the heart from the other body parts. At the site of venous injection, the concentration is so great that both T_1 and T_2 shortening effects become important. Near the site of injection (e.g., within the right axillary vein after a right antecubital vein injection), T_2 becomes shorter than the echo time, and thus the signal decays before the echo, resulting in a low SI in the vein. Thus, for venous evaluation, it is important to inject the patient on the side opposite to the region of interest (i.e., nonsymptomatic side). If this cannot be performed, then it is necessary to dilute the contrast agent (approximately 20-fold for Gd-based agents). Some contrast agents (e.g., iron oxide) have more T_2 effect. Thus, these agents can more readily cause signal drop with high concentrations in the region of interest.

Another reason for suboptimal signal on contrast-enhanced images is magnetic susceptibility. The T_2 relaxation time, or spin-spin relaxation time, is strongly affected by the tissue microenvironment. Magnetic field inhomogeneity induces faster spin dephasing and thus faster signal decay. Because this is an effect of magnetic field inhomogeneity rather than a tissue property, it is referred to as T_2*. During first-pass imaging, the Gd bolus increases the magnetic field strength within capillaries. Tissues with high capillary density develop magnetic gradients between the capillaries and the adjacent tissues, resulting in an increase in tissue T_2* and thus a signal drop on susceptibility-weighted imaging (e.g., gradient echo imaging with long echo time [TE]). Because the signal drop is proportional to capillary density, T_2* effect can be used as a perfusion imaging technique.

CLASSIFICATION OF MAGNETIC RESONANCE CONTRAST AGENTS

MR contrast agents represent a heterogeneous group of pharmacological structures. There are different classification methods, but the most commonly used is based on contrast agent biodistribution in tissues: extracellular, intracellular, tissue specific, and blood pool/intravascular contrast agents (Table 1).

EXTRACELLULAR CONTRAST AGENTS

The four most commonly used MR contrast agents approved by the U.S. FDA for intravenous use are gadopentetate dimeglumine, gadoteridol, gadodiamide, and gadoversetamide. These four Gd-based contrast agents are approved for clinical use in adults and at a single dose of 0.05–0.1 mmol/kg in the pediatric population over 2 years of age. Gadobenate dimeglumine (Gd-BOPTA) was approved by U.S. FDA for central nervous system MRI in adults.

Table 1
Biochemical Properties of Gadolinium-Based Extracellular Contrast Agents

Generic name	Other terms	Molecular structure	Concentration (mol/L)	Osmolality (mOsm/kg H_2O at 37°C)	Viscosity (mPa; 37°C)	Molecular weight	Thermodynamic stability constant	(log Keq) r_1 ($mM^{-1} s^{-1}$)	Excess chelate
Gadopentetate dimeglumine	Gd-DTPA	Linear, ionic	0.5	1690	2.9	938	22.1	4.9[a]	0.4
Gadoterate meglumine	Gd-DOTA	Macrocyclic, ionic	0.5	1350	2	25.8	4.3	0	
Gadoteridol	Gd-HP-DO3A	Macrocyclic, nonionic	0.5	630	1.3	559	23.8	5.4[b]	0.23
Gadobutrol	Gd-BT-DO3A	Macrocyclic, non-ionic	0.5/1	557/1603	4.96	605	21.8	5.6	N/A
Gadodiamide	Gd-DTPA-BMA	Linear, nonionic	0.5	789	1.4	574	16.9	5.4[b]	12
Gadoversetamide injection	Gd-DTPA-BMEA	Linear, nonionic	0.5	1110	2	1110	16.9	N/A	28.4
Gadobenate dimeglumine	Gd-BOPTA	Linear, ionic	0.5	1970	5.3	1058	22.6	9.7[a]	0
Gadoxetic acid disodium	Gd-EOB-DTPA	Linear, ionic	0.25	880	1.22	884	N/A	8.2	N/A

[a]In heparinized human plasma at 39°C.
[b]In citrated human plasma at 37°C.

241

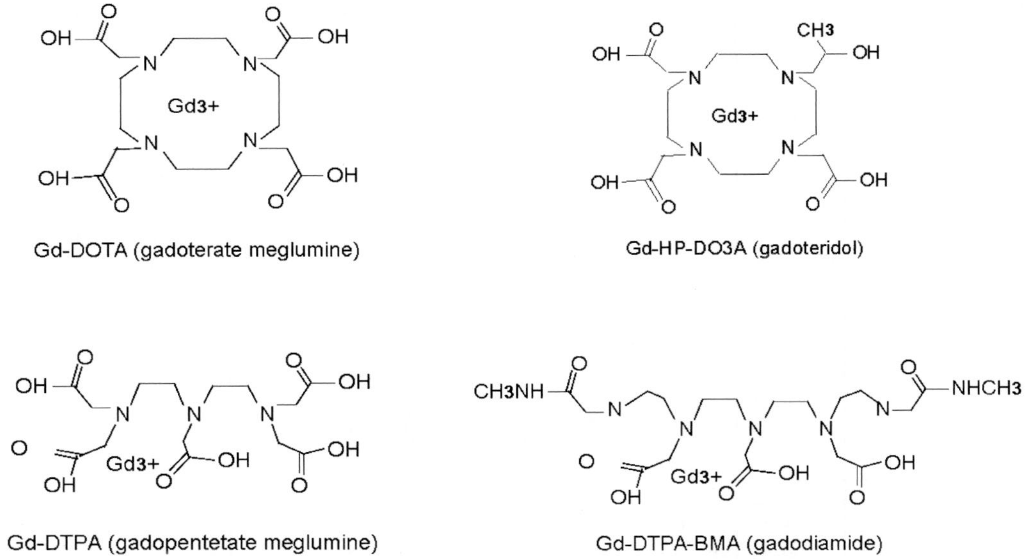

Fig. 1. The chemical structures of the most commonly used gadolinium chelates.

Biochemical Properties, Biodistribution, and Elimination of Extracellular Contrast Agents

Clinical extracellular contrast agents are Gd based. Free Gd^{3+} ions are toxic; therefore, they must be complexed with organic molecules, referred to as ligands or chelators, before intravenous administration. The ideal chelator prevents interactions between Gd^{3+} ions and endogenous tissue (including blood components), thereby allowing renal excretion of the complex without significant biotransformation. On the other hand, chelators decrease the T_1 shortening effect by keeping the Gd^{3+} ions away from the protons and alter the pharmacokinetic profile of Gd (7). The renal excretion rate of chelated Gd^{3+} ions increases enormously (approximately 500-fold) compared with the excretion rate of the free Gd^{3+} ions (8,9). Biochemical differences among Gd-based contrast agents are determined by the chemical structure of the chelators. Biochemical properties and r_1 relaxivities of the Gd-based contrast agents are summarized in Table 2 (10,11). The chelator can be linear or macrocyclic, ionic or nonionic. The chemical structures of the most commonly used Gd chelates are illustrated in Fig. 1.

After injection, water-soluble Gd chelates initially distribute into the intravascular space. With careful adjustments of the pulse sequence parameters, it is possible to capture the contrast media in the arterial, venous, and equilibrium phases. The arterial phase is defined as the time between contrast arrival in the region of interest and subsequent venous filling. The duration may change depending on the patient's cardiac output, but it is typically less than 20 seconds. The contrast agent then rapidly diffuses across the vascular membranes into the interstitial spaces. The concentration of extracellular contrast agent in the veins is not as high as in the arteries because although the extracellular agent diffuses into the interstitial space, there is excretion via glomerular filtration. The equilibrium phase occurs approximately 10 minutes after intravenous injection. In this stage, the extracellular contrast agent redistributes into interstitial spaces. Tissues with

Table 2
Classification of MR Contrast Agents With Potential for Cardiovascular Applications

Generic name	Other terms	Vendor
Extracellular agents		
Gadopentetate dimeglumine	Gd-DTPA	Magnevist (Berlex Laboratories, Wayne, NJ)
Gadoterate meglumine	Gd-DOTA	Dotarem (Guerbet Research, Aulnay Sous Bois, France)
Gadoteridol	Gd-HP-DO3A	Prohance (Bracco, Milan, Italy)
Gadobutrol	Gd-BT-DO3A	Gadovist (Schering AG, Berlin, Germany)
Gadodiamide	Gd-DTPA-BMA	Omniscan (GE Healthcare, Milwaukee, WI)
Gadoversetamide injection	Gd-DTPA-BMEA	Optimark (Mallinckrodt, St Louis, MO)
Gadobenate dimeglumine	Gd-BOPTA	Multihance (Bracco SpA, Milan, Italy)
Gadoxetic acid disodium	Gd-EOB-DTPA	Primovist (Schering AG, Berlin, Germany)
Intracellular agents		
Mangafodipir trisodium	Mn-DPDP	Teslascan (GE Healthcare, Milwaukee, WI)
EVP 1001–1		
Tissue-directed agents		
Bis-gadolinium mesoporphyrin	Bis-Gd-MP	Gadophrin-2 (Schering AG, Berlin, Germany)
Intravascular/blood pool agents		
Gadolinium based		
Gadofosveset trisodium	MS-325	Vasovist (Epix Medical, Mallinckrodt)
Gadomer-17	(Gd-DTPA)-17, SH L 643A	Gadomer-17 (Schering AG, Berlin, Germany)
Gadomeritol	P792	Vistarem (Guerbet, France)
Gadocoletic acid	B-22956	Bracco SpA, Milan, Italy
Iron oxides		
Ferumoxide	AMI-25	Feridex I.V (Berlex Laboratories, Wayne, NJ), Endorem (Guerbet, France)
Ferucarbotran	SH U 555A	Resovist (Schering AG, Berlin, Germany)
Ferucarbotran	SH U 555C	Supravist (Schering AG, Berlin, Germany)
Ferrumoxtran-10	AMI-227, Code 7227, BMS 180549	Combidex (Advanced Magnetics, Cambridge, MA), Sinerem (Guerbet, Aulneysous-Bois, France)
Ferumoxytol	Code 7228	Advanced Magnetics, Cambridge, MA
Feruglose	NC100150	PEG-Feron

leaky capillaries and large interstitial spaces enhance in this phase more than the other phases, such as inflamed tissue, scar, and malignant tumors. Brain and testicular tissue capillaries are impermeable to the contrast agents; therefore, there is no interstitial space distribution in these tissues when the blood–tissue barrier is intact.

Extracellular contrast agents are excreted via glomerular filtration without biotransformation. Therefore, the plasma half-life of the agent is mainly determined by the glomerular filtration rate, typically 90 minutes in patients with normal renal function (7).

When a Gd chelate is bound to a protein or other large molecular structure, its rate of tumbling slows, and the relaxivity increases (1,12,13). Gd-BOPTA and gadoxetic acid disodium (Gd-EOB-DTPA) are different from the other Gd-based agents because they have a noncovalent interaction with the plasma albumin; therefore, their in vivo relaxivities are higher than those of the other Gd compounds (10,14). However, the plasma protein interactions of these two Gd chelates are weak and transient (15); therefore, they do not act like blood pool agents.

Tissues may alter the kinetics by changing the distribution volume of the contrast agents. For example, in infarcted myocardium, extracellular agents can become nearly tissue specific because of the delayed diffusion from the infarct tissue. This feature forms the basis of MR viability studies, referred to as myocardial delayed-enhancement imaging. Delayed imaging at 10–20 minutes tailored to visualize only the retained contrast in the infarct tissue allows differentiation of infarcted tissue from normal myocardium (16–19).

The enhancement mechanisms of different contrast agents in myocardial tissue have been widely investigated. Lima et al. described three different contrast enhancement patterns when using extracellular contrast agents based on the SI ratio of myocardium to blood as a function of time after contrast injection. In normal myocardium, the SI ratio (myocardium/blood) is constant. In infarcted myocardium with open arteries, the ratio increases rapidly over the first 2 minutes and then reaches a plateau. In infarcted myocardium with closed arteries, the ratio increases over 10 minutes following contrast administration. These findings suggest two possible mechanisms for hyperenhancement in the infarcted tissues. The first is the impairment of contrast wash-in/wash-out kinetics; the second is the expanded extracellular space caused by the edema and loss of cellular membrane (i.e., the intracellular space becomes integrated into the extracellular space) (19).

Safety of Gd-Based Contrast Agents

SIDE EFFECTS AND ADVERSE REACTIONS

Gd-based extracellular contrast agents are considered safe, with an extremely low overall incidence of adverse events that are mostly minor (20–28). These adverse events can be classified into two groups: nonallergic reactions (i.e., headache, fatigue, arthralgia, taste perversion, flushed feeling, nausea, or vomiting) and idiosyncratic reactions resembling allergy (i.e., hives, diffuse erythema, respiratory distress, chest tightness, respiratory distress, periorbital edema). Adverse reaction incidence is higher in patients with a history of asthma or allergy, in patients who received contrast agent at a faster injection rate, and in patients with previous reactions to a Gd-based or iodinated contrast agent (28). There may be crossreactivity between different Gd chelates.

Cochran et al. published an adverse reaction rate of 0.07% with Gd-based contrast agents in 28,340 administrations with only 1 bronchospasm (0.0035%) (29). Murphy et al.

reported an overall adverse event rate of 0.17% with 2 anaphylactic reactions (0.01%) in 21,000 contrast-enhanced MR studies (30). Neindorf et al. reported severe adverse event rate of 0.0003% in an estimated total of more than 2 million applications (31). The safety profile of Gd-based contrast agents in the pediatric population under 2 years of age and pregnant women is not known. Gd-based contrast agents can cross the placenta into the fetal circulation and are excreted by fetal kidneys into the amniotic fluid; therefore, they should be avoided in pregnancy.

In general, Gd chelates are considered nonnephrotoxic in clinically recommended doses for MRI and MRA (22,32–35). The plasma elimination half-life of the Gd chelates is approximately 70–90 minutes in individuals with normal kidney function, and approximately 98% of the injected dose of the contrast agent is cleared from plasma within 24 hours. However, in patients with renal impairment, the plasma half-life of the Gd chelate is lengthened, inversely proportional to the residual glomerular function (36,37). Gd chelates can be dialyzed; thus, they are tolerated by patients undergoing either hemodialysis or continuous ambulatory peritoneal dialysis (36,38). The experience with human subjects confirms that Gd-based contrast agent excretion via liver is negligible, even among the patients with severely reduced renal function the substance will be completely excreted by the kidneys (37). Rapid elimination of the contrast agents from the body is important to minimize the time period of Gd chelate decomplexation and subsequent toxicity. In theory, the Gd chelates with high stability may be preferred in patients with renal insufficiency.

Off-label use of high-dose Gd chelates for examinations such as computed tomography and digital subtraction angiography in humans (39,40) has led the increased concerns about safety profiles of these agents. At high doses (>0.3 mmol/kg), Gd chelates are nephrotoxic in animals and may cause transient osmotic (albuminuria) and chemotoxic (renal enzyme excretion in urine) injury on kidneys (41,42). In fact, review of the experimental data on animals suggests that Gd-based contrast media may be more nephrotoxic than iodinated contrast agents at doses for equivalent X-ray attenuation. Therefore, they are not recommended for radiographic examinations, particularly in patients with renal insufficiency (43,44).

In vitro studies show that deoxygenated sickle erythrocytes align perpendicular to the magnetic field (45). In theory, increased local magnetic moments following the contrast agent administration may increase the perpendicular alignment; thus, it may induce vaso-occlusive complications. However, a later study in patients with sickle cell anemia did not reveal supporting findings (46), and so far in the literature there are no reported vaso-occlusive complications induced by contrast agent injection in patients with sickle cell anemia. Therefore, the proposed risk in the package inserts has never been a clinical concern in routine contrast-enhanced MRI or MRA applications.

NEPHROGENIC SYSTEMIC FIBROSIS (NSF)

NSF is a disorder that primarily involves the skin, but it may also affect other organs such as the lungs, liver, muscle, and the heart in patients with renal failure. Grobner was the first to suggest that MR contrast media containing Gd might trigger NSF (47). Recently, researchers have documented the presence of gadolinium in biopsy specimens of patients with NSF (48,49). The incidence of NSF among patients with GFR < 30 mL/minute is 3–5% (50–52). The majority of patients with NSF had moderate to severe renal failure and received gadodiamide, gadobenate dimeglumine followed by gadodiamide and gadopentetate dimeglumine *(47–56)*. Although editorials by Kuo *(57)* and Bongartz *(58)* mention fewer cases have been reported in the US and Europe after the administration of other linear Gd-based contrast agents (gadoversetamide, gadopentetate dimeglumine and gadobenate dimeglumine). Most patients who developed NSF had received high doses or standard doses of Gd agents several times in a short period of time. Therefore, it is important to develop MR protocols that minimize the volume of contrast for the specific clinical indication, particularly in patients with moderate to severe renal failure.

There is no definite consensus among the authors regarding the most important in vivo stability parameter, and it would be wrong to speculate that some Gd-chelates are more stable than the others by taking a single parameter into account. Other factors, including the concentration of competing ions or ligands, and the interaction time between the Gd-chelate and the competitors are important as well *(59,60)*. The association with renal failure can be explained by the fact that dissociation of Gd-chelates is more likely to occur when it remains inside the body for an extended period of time.

TOXICITY

Gd chelates cannot be differentiated based on the rate or the severity of the adverse events; however, the differences in their thermodynamic stability can have important consequences with respect to the in vivo transmetallation and in vitro interferences with laboratory assays.

Gd chelates have the theoretical possibility of substantial toxicity from release of the Gd^{3+} ions as well as the free chelator. Free Gd^{3+} ion has a biological half-life of several weeks *(61)*. Therefore, the ideal chelator must be highly selective and tightly bound to the Gd^{3+} ion to avoid release into the circulation. Once released into the body, free Gd^{3+} ions are rapidly sequestered in the bone and liver and may persist for years or even for the patient's lifetime. Potential complications are interactions with physiological systems such as the reticuloendothelial system (RES) or inhibition of the activity of some enzymes such as Ca^{2+}-activated Mg-ATPase (magnesium-adenosine triphosphatase), some dehydrogenases, and aldolase via noncompetitive inhibition of Ca^{2+} binding *(62,63)*.

The ideal chelator should have high thermodynamic stability constant. This constant reflects the in vitro energy required for breaking the structure of the chelator in which the Gd^{3+} ion is bound, as well as the selectivity of the chelator to the Gd^{3+} ions *(64)*. If the selectivity is weak, chelator may release the Gd^{3+} and bind other ions. This condition is referred to as *transmetallation*.

In addition to the thermodynamic stability constant, the possibility of transmetallation also depends on the concentration of competing ions or ligands as well as the interaction time between the Gd chelate and the competitors *(11,65)*. In vivo transmetallation may be a consequence of endogen Zn^{2+}, Cu^{2+}, and Ca^{2+} ions *(9,66–68)*. However, Fe^{3+} ions are tightly bound to the storage proteins (ferritin and hemosiderin); therefore, they are essentially unavailable for transmetallation. Among these endogenous metal ions, Zn^{2+} is considered to be the most important competitor; thus, Zn^{2+} is the most likely cause of acute or subacute toxicity in animal studies.

The findings of subchronic rodent toxicity experiments are similar to those caused by Zn deficiency *(9)*. The median lethal dose (LD_{50}) of the Gd chelates are 60- to 300-fold of the typical MR application dose of 0.1 mmol/kg (7,69). In vitro studies demonstrated that Gd^{3+} competitively inhibits Ca^{2+} ion binding to the transport sites on purified sarcoplasmic reticulum Ca-ATPase (calcium-adenosine triphosphatase) (70). This may explain the hemodynamic disturbances that were observed in animal toxicity studies.

Molecular structure of the Gd chelates plays an important role in propensity for transmetallation. The linear Gd complexes (Gd-DTPA-BMA, Gd-DTPA-BMEA, and Gd-DTPA) are more prone to transmetallation when compared to the macrocyclic Gd complexes (Gd-DOTA and Gd-HP-DO3A) (11,67,71–73). In humans, Gd-DTPA-BMA increases the urinary Zn excretion more than Gd-DTPA. On the other hand, Gd-HP-DO3A does not interfere with Zn excretion. Gd chelates may cause some decrease in the serum Zn level, although the differences among the agents are not statistically significant (65). Gd-DTPA and Gd-DTPA-BMA have a significant inhibition effect on Zn-dependent angiotensin-converting enzyme activity, whereas no significant interference is seen with Gd-DOTA and Gd-HP-DO3A. The inhibitory effect was shown to be decreased by adding Zn ions into the environment (73). In an animal study, it was shown that the Gd-DTPA-BMA left 2.5 times more Gd^{3+} in the bone when compared to Gd-HP-DO3A (74). These results reflect the different transmetallation potentials of the Gd chelates related to their chelator structures.

Adding excess of free chelator or Ca-bound chelate is a commonly used formulation method to ensure the absence of free Gd^{3+} in the solutions during their shelf lives (67,73). The commercial formulations of Gd-DTPA-BMA and Gd-DTPA-BMEA injection include the largest amount of excess free or Ca-bound chelator, probably because of their lower thermodynamic stability constants (see Table 2). In fact, the excess Ca-DTPA-BMA in the Gd-DTPA-BMA formulation significantly prevents Gd^{3+} sequestration in the body, even more than macrocyclic chelates (67).

Gd chelates may cause blood pressure disturbances, nonspecific electrocardiogram changes, prolonged PR interval, tachycardia, atrioventricular conduction defects, and atrial and ventricular arrhythmias. Muhler et al. observed a dose-dependent hemodynamic depressive effect following Gd-DTPA (linear ionic) injection via a central vein, whereas they did not observe significant cardiovascular deterioration after Gd-DTPA-BMA (linear nonionic) administration in animals (75).

Based on these observations, the ionicity of the Gd chelates has been suggested as a possible reason for hemodynamic disturbances. All Gd-based contrast agents with FDA approval carry only one Gd^{3+} atom in each molecule; this is why the molar concentration of each agent is equivalent. However, the osmolality is determined by the ionicity. The ionic complexes contain a carboxylic group and a cation, methylglucamine. This structure with osmotically active particles provides the high osmolality of the Gd-DTPA, Gd-DOTA, and Gd-BOPTA formulations.

Oksendal and Hals also observed hemodynamic adverse events with ionic chelates, especially at high doses and injection rates (7). However, a more recent animal study did not substantiate these results; Gd-DTPA (linear ionic) and Gd-DTPA-BMA (linear nonionic) Gd chelates caused hypotension, whereas Gd-DOTA (macrocyclic ionic) did not interfere with the blood pressure. Therefore, ionicity of the contrast agent does not appear to be enough to explain cardiovascular adverse events. Moreover, the hypotensive effects of the linear agents (both ionic and nonionic) were corrected by Ca infusion. Based on these findings, the authors concluded that the transmetallation of the Gd^{3+} ions with endogen Ca^{2+} ions was the possible reason for the transient drop in blood pressure following the contrast injection. They also observed an increase in blood pressure following Gd-HP-DO3A injection, probably because of its positive inotropic effect *(76)*.

CONTRAST AGENT EXTRAVASATION AND OSMOTIC TISSUE DAMAGE

The increasing number of MR applications using high-dose Gd chelate at fast injection rates, often with a power injector, has led to concerns of extravasation and associated tissue damage, such as necrosis, edema, and inflammation. The tissue damage has been more severe with contrast agents with higher osmolality *(77)*.

POTENTIAL EFFECT ON MEASURED SERUM CALCIUM AND OTHER SERUM LABORATORY VALUES

The propensity of the Gd chelates to interfere with the colorimetric serum Ca assays was reported in two in vitro studies *(64,78)*. Lin et al. demonstrated decomplexation of Gd-DTPA-BMA in the presence of *o*-cresol-phthalein complexone or methylthymol blue, reagents used for colorimetric Ca measurement, and the rate of the decomplexation increased proportional to the concentration of the Gd chelate in the serum sample, whereas no interference was seen with Gd-DTPA or Gd-DOTA. The authors concluded that the weak thermodynamic stability of the Gd-DTPA-BMA was the possible mechanism for interference. According to their theory, the colorimetric assay reagents recruit the Gd^{3+} ions from the chelator, and the free DTPA-BMA binds Ca^{2+} ions. Because the available Ca^{2+} and the free colorimetric reagent levels are low, the measured Ca level is low even though the actual serum Ca level is normal *(64)*.

The relevance of interference between Gd chelates and colorimetric serum Ca measurements in humans was demonstrated in a retrospective study by Prince et al. *(11)*. The authors reported a spurious decrease in serum Ca measurements from normal to hypocalcemia (<8.5 mg/dL) in 16%, a decrease of more than 2 mg/dL in 4%, and decreases to a level below 6 mg/dL (critical hypocalcemia) in 2.4% of MR examinations with Gd-DTPA-BMA. The decrease in Ca levels was greater in patients who received high-dose (>2 mmol/kg) of Gd-DTPA-BMA and in patients with renal insufficiency. Subsequently, in vitro experiments revealed reduced serum Ca measurements in serum samples mixed with different concentrations of Gd-DTPA-BMA and Gd-DTPA-BMEA but not with Gd-HP-DO3A, Gd-DTPA, and Gd-BOPTA. Gd-DTPA-BMA and Gd-DTPA-BMEA have lower stability constants than the others *(11,79)*.

Awareness of this effect of Gd chelates on colorimetric Ca measurements is important. If a Ca measurement obtained after contrast-enhanced MRI or MRA is thought to be in error, it is appropriate to measure the serum Ca level with another method, such as the ionized calcium assay.

Gd chelates may also interfere with the colorimetric assays for angiotensin-converting enzyme; total iron-binding capacity; and Fe, Mg, and Zn in serum samples of patients who have recently received Gd-based contrast media. Gd-DTPA-BMA and Gd-DTPA-BMEA may cause clinically significant negative interference with colorimetric assays for serum angiotensin-converting enzyme, Ca, and Zn *(80)*; significant positive interference with colorimetric measurements of Mg and total iron-binding capacity; and both positive and negative interferences with Fe assays *(20,80)*. Gd-DTPA may increase the serum ferritin level transiently and produce negative interference with colorimetric Zn assays *(80)*.

INTRACELLULAR CONTRAST AGENTS

Manganese (Mn^{2+}) is an essential trace metal of human diet and a powerful paramagnetic lanthanide metal with five unpaired electrons. Its free form is toxic if directly administered to the circulation. To minimize the potential toxicity and to increase the tolerance, Mn^{2+} must be chelated to a molecule such as mangafodipir trisodium (Mn-DPDP) or mixed with calcium ions (EVP-1001).

However, Mn-DPDP has a potential future use in cardiovascular imaging because it produces significant myocardial enhancement caused by the Mn^{2+} accumulation in the myocytes. First-pass distribution of the Mn in the myocardium is directly correlated with blood flow. Mn has dynamics similar to thallium 201 (^{201}Tl); the uptake by the injured myocytes is slower than in the normal myocytes, and the clearance from normal myocardium is slower compared to infarcted myocardium *(81)*. Thus, Mn-based contrast agents are promising for the viability studies when they are used with delayed-phase T_1-weighted MR pulse sequences *(82)*.

TISSUE-SPECIFIC CONTRAST AGENTS

Porphyrins have been known as indicators of some metabolic disorders and disease states. Their metal-chelated forms show selective retention in tumor tissue *(83,84)*. Originally, *bis*-gadolinium mesoporphyrin (*bis*-Gd-MP: Gadophrin-2) was developed for tumor-specific imaging. Studies in myocardium have drawn attention to possible future use. Specifically, metalloporphyrins have demarcated irreversibly infarcted myocardium from viable myocardium *(85–88)*. Thus, these agents also show promise in viability studies.

INTRAVASCULAR/BLOOD POOL AGENTS

At present, no intravascular/blood pool agents have FDA approval. Thus, their use in the United States is investigational. In contrast to the extracellular contrast agents, blood pool agents remain in the intravascular space (i.e., do not rapidly diffuse into interstitial space). Therefore, blood pool agents hold the promise of imaging the vascular system hours after the intravascular injection. The permeability of the capillaries to the contrast agents depends on the size, charge, and molecular shape of the agent as well as the existence or absence of ischemic injury, inflammation, or tumor *(89)*. When contrast agents gain access to the interstitial and intracellular spaces, they provide different enhancement patterns. Among the promising blood pool agents, Gd-based gadofesevet trisodium (MS-325) has been approved for clinical use in Europe. MS-325 (Vasovist; Epix Medical, Mallinckrodt) is an albumin-targeted intravascular contrast agent. Unlike conventional MRI contrast agents, this small gadolinium chelate expresses intravascular behavior by reversible albumin binding. Thus, MS-325 avoids renal clearance and moves with the blood for an extended period of time, enabling imaging up to 50 minutes after the injection *(90)*. Its serum half-life is about 2–3 hours *(91)*.

Superparamagnetic iron oxide (SPIO) particles are composed of a water-insoluble crystalline magnetic core (magnetite or maghemite) and a dextran or starch derivate coat. The particles are classified according to their mean hydrated diameter, which includes both the core and the coat. The mean hydrated diameter of SPIO particles, ultrasmall SPIO (USPIO) particles, and monocrystalline iron oxide nanoparticles

(MION) are 50–180, 20–50, and 10–20 nm, respectively. All iron oxide particles for intravenous injection first distribute into the intravascular space as blood pool agents. They are subsequently internalized and degraded by the macrophages of the RES in the liver, lymph nodes, and bones. They enter into the total body iron storage after the degradation in the RES *(92)*.

Iron oxide particles shorten T_1, T_2, and T_2^* relaxation times. However, the r_2 of the iron oxide particles are always higher than their r_1. When used for imaging, all iron oxide particles have "negative" contrast because of the dominant T_2/T_2^* shortening effect. As the concentration of the SPIO in certain location increases, the SI decreases because of the enhanced T_2 effect *(93)*. The USPIO particles and MION have a lower R_2/R_1 ratio than those of SPIO particles *(94)*, and they significantly reduce both T_1 and T_2 relaxation times. Therefore, USPIO particles are more suitable for MRA or first-pass perfusion imaging. They can act as "positive" enhancers if their T_2/T_2^* shortening effect is minimized and T_1 relaxivity is enhanced by using short TE gradient echo pulse sequences. The more the sequence is T_1 weighted, the greater the positive enhancement.

CONCLUSION

At present, Gd-based agents are widely utilized and safe for routine clinical cardiovascular MRI. Although many of these applications have become routine, they continue to expand and evolve. Moreover, there are many applications only used at the research level. These have common themes: understanding and determining enhancement mechanisms, developing new agents, and exploring molecular MRI. These ongoing refinements and developments will undoubtedly lead to more choices for patients, who will benefit from noninvasive imaging in the near future.

REFERENCES

1. Henrotte V, Laurent S, Gabelica V, Elst L, Depauw E, Muller R. Investigation of non-covalent interactions between paramagnetic complexes and human serum albumin by electrospray mass spectrometry. Rapid Commun Mass Spectrom 2004;18:1919–1924.
2. Koenig S, Brown R. Relaxation of solvent protons by paramagnetic ions and its dependence on magnetic field and chemical environment: implications for NMR imaging. Magn Reson Med 1984;1:478–495.
3. Outhred R, George E. A nuclear magnetic resonance study of hydrated systems using the frequency dependence of the relaxation processes. Biopolymers 1973;13:83–96.
4. Runge V, Clanton J, Lukehart C, Partain C, James AJ. Paramagnetic agents for contrast-enhanced NMR imaging: a review. AJR Am J Roentgenol 1983;141:1209–1215.
5. Rinck P, Muller R. Field strength and dose dependence of contrast enhancement by gadolinium-based MR contrast agents. Eur Radiol 1999;9:998–1004.
6. Runge V, Clanton J, Herzer W, et al. Intravascular contrast agents suitable for magnetic resonance imaging. Radiology 1984;153:171–176.
7. Oksendal A, Hals P. Biodistribution and toxicity of MR imaging contrast media. J Magn Reson Imaging 1993;3:157–165.
8. Chang C. Magnetic resonance imaging contrast agents. Design and physicochemical properties of gadodiamide. Invest Radiol 1993;28(suppl 1):S21–S27.
9. Cacheris W, Quay S, Rocklage S. The relationship between thermodynamics and the toxicity of gadolinium complexes. Magn Reson Imaging 1990;8:467–481.
10. de Haen C, Cabrini M, Akhnana L, Ratti D, Calabi L, Gozzini L. Gadobenate dimeglumine 0.5 M solution for injection (MultiHance) pharmaceutical formulation and physicochemical properties of a new magnetic resonance imaging contrast medium. J Comput Assist Tomogr 1999;suppl 1:S161–S168.
11. Prince M, Erel H, Lent R, et al. Gadodiamide administration causes spurious hypocalcemia. Radiology 2003;227:627–628.

12. Nicolle G, Toth E, Schmitt-Willich H, Raduchel B, Merbach A. The impact of rigidity and water exchange on the relaxivity of a dendritic MRI contrast agent. Chemistry 2002;8:1040–1048.

13. Toth EE, Vauthey S, Pubanz D, Merbach A. Water exchange and rotational dynamics of the dimeric gadolinium(III) complex [BO{Gd(DO3A)(H(2)O)}(2)]: a variable-temperature and -pressure (17)O NMR study(1). Inorg Chem 1996;35:3375–3379.

14. Huppertz A, Balzer T, Blakeborough A, et al. EES. Improved detection of focal liver lesions at MR imaging: multicenter comparison of gadoxetic acid-enhanced MR images with intraoperative findings. Radiology 2004;230:266–275.

15. Cavagna F, Maggioni F, Castelli P, et al. Gadolinium chelates with weak binding to serum proteins. A new class of high-efficiency, general purpose contrast agents for magnetic resonance imaging. Invest Radiol 1997;32:780–796.

16. Lund G, Stork A, Saeed M, et al. Acute myocardial infarction: evaluation with first-pass enhancement and delayed enhancement MR imaging compared with 201Tl SPECT imaging. Radiology 2004;232:49–57.

17. Van Hoe L, Vanderheyden M. Ischemic cardiomyopathy: value of different MRI techniques for prediction of functional recovery after revascularization. AJR Am J Roentgenol 2004;182:95–100.

18. de Roos A, van Rossum A, van der Wall E, et al. Reperfused and nonreperfused myocardial infarction: diagnostic potential of Gd-DTPA—enhanced MR imaging. Radiology 1989;172:717–720.

19. Lima J, Judd R, Bazille A, Schulman S, Atalar E, Zerhouni E. Regional heterogeneity of human myocardial infarcts demonstrated by contrast-enhanced MRI: potential mechanisms. Circulation 1995;92:1117–1125.

20. Goldstein H, Kashanian F, Blumetti R, Holyoak W, Hugo F, Blumenfield D. Safety assessment of gadopentetate dimeglumine in U.S. clinical trials. Radiology 1990;174:17–23.

21. Aslanian V, Lemaignen H, Bunouf P, Svaland M, Borseth A, Lundby B. Evaluation of the clinical safety of gadodiamide injection, a new nonionic MRI contrast medium for the central nervous system: a European perspective. Neuroradiology 1996;38:537–541.

22. Harpur E, Worah D, Hals P, Holtz E, Furuhama K, Nomura H. Preclinical safety assessment and pharmacokinetics of gadodiamide injection, a new magnetic resonance imaging contrast agent. Invest Radiol 1993;28:S28–S43.

23. Carvlin M, De Simone D, Meeks M. Phase II clinical trial of gadoteridol injection, a low-osmolal magnetic resonance imaging contrast agent. Invest Radiol 1992;27:S16–S21.

24. Grossman R, Rubin D, Hunter G, et al. Magnetic resonance imaging in patients with central nervous system pathology: a comparison of OptiMARK (Gd-DTPA-BMEA) and Magnevist (Gd-DTPA). Invest Radiol 2000;35:412–419.

25. Kirchin M, Pirovano G, Venetianer C, Spinazzi A. Safety assessment of gadobenate dimeglumine (MultiHance): extended clinical experience from phase I studies to post-marketing surveillance. J Magn Reson Imaging 2001;14:281–294.

26. Chanalet S, Masson B, Boyer L, Laffont J, Bruneton J. [Comparative studies of the tolerability of gadodiamide, dimeglumine gadopentetate and meglumine gadoterate in MRI tests of the central nervous system]. J Radiol 1995;76:417–421.

27. Staks T, Schuhmann-Giampieri G, Frenzel T, Weinmann H, Lange L, Platzek J. Pharmacokinetics, dose proportionality, and tolerability of gadobutrol after single intravenous injection in healthy volunteers. Invest Radiol 1994;29:709–715.

28. Nelson K, Gifford L, Lauber-Huber C, Gross C, Lasser T. Clinical safety of gadopentetate dimeglumine. Radiology 1995;196:439–443.

29. Cochran S, Bomyea K, Sayre J. Trends in adverse events after IV administration of contrast media. AJR Am J Roentgenol 2001;176:1385–1388.

30. Murphy K, Brunberg J, Cohan R. Adverse reactions to gadolinium contrast media: a review of 36 cases. AJR Am J Roentgenol 1996;167:847–849.

31. Niendorf H, Haustein J, Cornelius I, Alhassan A, Clauss W. Safety of gadolinium-DTPA: extended clinical experience. Magn Reson Med 1991;22:222–228.

32. Prince M, Arnoldus C, Frisoli J. Nephrotoxicity of high-dose gadolinium compared with iodinated contrast. J Magn Reson Imaging 1996;6:162–166.

33. Swan S, Lambrecht L, Townsend R, et al. Safety and pharmacokinetic profile of gadobenate dimeglumine in subjects with renal impairment. Invest Radiol 1999;34:443–448.

34. Townsend R, Cohen D, Katholi R, et al. Safety of intravenous gadolinium (Gd-BOPTA) infusion in patients with renal insufficiency. Am J Kidney Dis 2000;36:1207–1212.

35. Haustein J, Niendorf H, Krestin G, et al. Renal tolerance of gadolinium-DTPA/dimeglumine in patients with chronic renal failure. Invest Radiol 1992;27:153–156.

36. Joffe P, Thomsen H, Meusel M. Pharmacokinetics of gadodiamide injection in patients with severe renal insufficiency and patients undergoing hemodialysis or continuous ambulatory peritoneal dialysis. Acad Radiol 1998;5:491–502.

37. VanWagoner M, O'Toole M, Worah D, Leese P, Quay S. A phase I clinical trial with gadodiamide injection, a nonionic magnetic resonance imaging enhancement agent. Invest Radiol 1991;26:980–986.

38. Normann P, Joffe P, Martinsen I, Thomsen H. Quantification of gadodiamide as Gd in serum, peritoneal dialysate and faeces by inductively coupled plasma atomic emission spectroscopy and comparative analysis by high-performance liquid chromatography. J Pharm Biomed Anal 2000;22:939–947.

39. Coche E, Hammer F, Goffette P. Demonstration of pulmonary embolism with gadolinium-enhanced spiral CT. Eur Radiol 2001;11:2306–2309.

40. Spinosa D, Kaufmann J, Hartwell G. Gadolinium chelates in angiography and interventional radiology: a useful alternative to iodinated contrast media for angiography. Radiology 2002;223:319–325.

41. Thomsen H, Dorph S, Larsen S, et al. Urine profiles and kidney histology after intravenous injection of ionic and nonionic radiologic and magnetic resonance contrast media in normal rats. Acad Radiol 1994;1:128–135.

42. Leander P, Allard M, Caille J, Golman K. Early effect of gadopentetate and iodinated contrast media on rabbit kidneys. Invest Radiol 1992;27:922–926.

43. Thomsen H, Almen T, Morcos S, Contrast Media Safety Committee of the European Society of Urogenital Radiology E. Gadolinium-containing contrast media for radiographic examinations: a position paper. Eur Radiol 2002;12:2600–2605.

44. Elmstahl B, Nyman U, Leander P, Chai C, Frennby B, Almen T. Gadolinium contrast media are more nephrotoxic than a low osmolar iodine medium employing doses with equal X-ray attenuation in renal arteriography: an experimental study in pigs. Acad Radiol 2004;11:1219–1228.

45. Brody A, Sorette M, Gooding C, et al. AUR Memorial Award. Induced alignment of flowing sickle erythrocytes in a magnetic field. A preliminary report. Invest Radiol 1985;20:560–566.

46. Brody A, Embury S, Mentzer W, Winkler M, Gooding C. Preservation of sickle cell blood-flow patterns during MR imaging: an in vivo study. AJR Am J Roentgenol 1988;151:139–141.

47. Grobner T. Gadolinium–a specific trigger for the development of nephrogenic fibrosing dermopathy and nephrogenic systemic fibrosis? Nephrol Dial Transplant 2006.

48. Boyd AS, Zic JA, Abraham JL. Gadolinium deposition in nephrogenic fibrosing dermopathy. J Am Acad Dermatol 2007;56:27–30.

49. High WA, Ayers RA, Chandler J, Zito G, Cowper SE. Gadolinium is detectable within the tissue of patients with nephrogenic systemic fibrosis. J Am Acad Dermatol 2007;56:21–26.

50. Broome DR, Girguis MS, Baron PW, Cottrell AC, Kjellin I, Kirk GA. Gadodiamide-associated nephrogenic systemic fibrosis: why radiologists should be concerned. AJR Am J Roentgenol 2007;188:586–592.

51. Marckmann P, Skov L, Rossen K, et al. Nephrogenic systemic fibrosis: suspected causative role of gadodiamide used for contrast-enhanced magnetic resonance imaging. J Am Soc Nephrol 2006; 17:2359–2362.

52. Sadowski EA, Bennett LK, Chan MR, et al. Nephrogenic systemic fibrosis: risk factors and incidence estimation. Radiology 2007.

53. Khurana A, Runge VM, Narayanan M, Greene JF, Jr., Nickel AE. Nephrogenic systemic fibrosis: a review of 6 cases temporally related to gadodiamide injection (Omniscan). Invest Radiol 2007; 42:139–145.

54. Lim YL, Lee HY, Low SC, Chan LP, Goh NS, Pang SM. Possible role of gadolinium in nephrogenic systemic fibrosis: report of two cases and review of the literature. Clin Exp Dermatol 2007.

55. Marckmann P, Skov L, Rossen K, Heaf JG, Thomsen HS. Case-control study of gadodiamide-related nephrogenic systemic fibrosis. Nephrol Dial Transplant 2007.

56. Deo A, Fogel M, Cowper S. Nephrogenic Systemic Fibrosis: A population study examining the relationship of disease development to gadolinium exposure. Clin J Am Soc Nephrol 2007;2:264–267.

57. Kuo PH, Kanal E, Abu-Alfa AK, Cowper SE. Gadolinium-based MR contrast agents and nephrogenic systemic fibrosis. Radiology 2007.

58. Bongartz G. Imaging in the time of NFD/NSF: do we have to change our routines concerning renal insufficiency? Magma 2007;20:57–62.

59. Puttagunta N, Gibby W, Smith G. Human in vivo comparative study of zinc and copper transmetallation after administration of magnetic resonance imaging contrast agents. Invest Radiol. 1996; 31:739–742.

60. Prince M, Erel H, Lent R, et al. Gadodiamide administration causes spurious hypocalcemia. Radiology 2003;227:627–628.
61. Kanal E, FG S. Safety manual on magnetic resonance imaging contrast agents. Cedar Knolls, NJ: Lippincott-Raven Health Care; 1996.
62. Krasnow N. Effects of lanthanum and gadolinium ions on cardiac sarcoplasmic reticulum. Biochim Biophys Acta 1972;282:187–194.
63. Bourne G, Trifaro J. The gadolinium ion: a potent blocker of calcium channels and catecholamine release from cultured chromaffin cells. Neuroscience 1982;7:1615–1622.
64. Lin J, Idee J, Port M, et al. Interference of magnetic resonance imaging contrast agents with the serum calcium measurement technique using colorimetric reagents. J Pharm Biomed Anal 1999;21:931–943.
65. Puttagunta N, Gibby W, Smith G. Human in vivo comparative study of zinc and copper transmetallation after administration of magnetic resonance imaging contrast agents. Invest Radiol 1996;31:739–742.
66. Tweedle M, Hagan J, Kumar K, Mantha S, Chang C. Reaction of gadolinium chelates with endogenously available ions. Magn Reson Imaging 1991;9:409–415.
67. Tweedle M, Wedeking P, Kumar K. Biodistribution of radiolabeled, formulated gadopentetate, gadoteridol, gadoterate, and gadodiamide in mice and rats. Invest Radiol 1995;30:372–380.
68. Puttagunta N, Gibby W, Smith G. Human in vivo comparative study of zinc and copper transmetallation after administration of magnetic resonance imaging contrast agents. Invest Radiol 1669;31:739–742.
69. Weinmann H, Gries H, Speck U. Gd-DTPA and low osmolar Gd chelates. In: Runge V, ed. Enhanced magnetic resonance imaging. St. Louis, MO: Mosby; 1989, pp. 74–86.
70. Ogurusu T, Wakabayashi S, Shigekawa M. Functional characterization of lanthanide binding sites in the sarcoplasmic reticulum Ca(2+)–ATPase: do lanthanide ions bind to the calcium transport site? Biochemistry 1991;30:9966–9973.
71. Laurent S, Elst L, Copoix F, Muller R. Stability of MRI paramagnetic contrast media: a proton relaxometric protocol for transmetallation assessment. Invest Radiol 2001;36:115–122.
72. Puttagunta N, Gibby W, Puttagunta V. Comparative transmetallation kinetics and thermodynamic stability of gadolinium-DTPA bis-glucosamide and other magnetic resonance imaging contrast media. Invest Radiol 1996;31:619–624.
73. Corot C, Idee J, Hentsch A, et al. Structure-activity relationship of macrocyclic and linear gadolinium chelates: investigation of transmetallation effect on the zinc-dependent metallopeptidase angiotensin-converting enzyme. J Magn Reson Imaging 1998;8:695–702.
74. Gibby W, Gibby K, Gibby W. Comparison of Gd DTPA-BMA (Omniscan) vs Gd HP-DO3A (ProHance) retention in human bone tissue by inductively coupled plasma atomic emission spectroscopy. Invest Radiol 2004;39:138–142.
75. Muhler A, Saeed M, Brasch R, Higgins C. Hemodynamic effects of bolus injection of gadodiamide injection and gadopentetate dimeglumine as contrast media at MR imaging in rats. Radiology 1992;183:523–528.
76. Idee J, Berthommier C, Goulas V, et al. Haemodynamic effects of macrocyclic and linear gadolinium chelates in rats: role of calcium and transmetallation. Biometals 1998;11:113–123.
77. Runge V, Dickey K, Williams N, Peng X. Local tissue toxicity in response to extravascular extravasation of magnetic resonance contrast media. Invest Radiol 2002;37:393–398.
78. Normann P, Froysa A, Svaland M. Interference of gadodiamide injection (OMNISCAN) on the colorimetric determination of serum calcium. Scand J Clin Lab Invest 1995;55:421–426.
79. Lowe A, Balzer T, Hirt U. Interference of gadolinium-containing contrast-enhancing agents with colorimetric calcium laboratory testing. Invest Radiol 2005;40:521–525.
80. Proctor K, Rao L, Roberts W. Gadolinium magnetic resonance contrast agents produce analytic interference in multiple serum assays. Am J Clin Pathol 2004;121:282–292.
81. Bremerich J, Saeed M, Arheden H, Higgins C, Wendland M. Normal and infarcted myocardium: differentiation with cellular uptake of manganese at MR imaging in a rat model. Radiology 2000;216:524–530.
82. Brurok H, Skoglund T, Berg K, Skarra S, Karlsson J, Jynge P. Myocardial manganese elevation and proton relaxivity enhancement with manganese dipyridoxyl diphosphate. Ex vivo assessments in normally perfused and ischemic guinea pig hearts. NMR Biomed 1999;12:364–372.
83. Patronas N, Cohen J, Knop R, et al. Metalloporphyrin contrast agents for magnetic resonance imaging of human tumors in mice. Cancer Treat Rep 1986;70:391–395.
84. Saini S, Jena A, Dey J, Sharma A, Singh R. MnPcS4: a new MRI contrast enhancing agent for tumor localisation in mice. Magn Reson Imaging 1995;13:985–990.

85. Choi S, Choi S, Kim S, et al. Irreversibly damaged myocardium at MR imaging with a necrotic tissue-specific contrast agent in a cat model. Radiology 2000;215:863–868.
86. Lee S, Goo H, Park S, et al. MR imaging of reperfused myocardial infarction: comparison of necrosis-specific and intravascular contrast agents in a cat model. Radiology 2003;229:608–609.
87. Saeed M, Lund G, Wendland M, Bremerich J, Weinmann H, Higgins C. Magnetic resonance characterization of the peri-infarction zone of reperfused myocardial infarction with necrosis-specific and extracellular nonspecific contrast media. Circulation 2001;103:871–876.
88. Marchal G, Ni Y, Herijgers P, et al. Paramagnetic metalloporphyrins: infarct avid contrast agents for diagnosis of acute myocardial infarction by MRI. Eur Radiol 1996;6:2–8.
89. Bonnemain B. Superparamagnetic agents in magnetic resonance imaging: physicochemical characteristics and clinical applications. A review. J Drug Target 1998;6:167–174.
90. Grist T, Korosec F, Peters D, et al. Steady-state and dynamic MR angiography with MS-325: initial experience in humans. Radiology 1998;207:539–544.
91. Parmelee D, Walovitch R, Ouellet H, Lauffer R. Preclinical evaluation of the pharmacokinetics, biodistribution, and elimination of MS-325, a blood pool agent for magnetic resonance imaging. Invest Radiol 1997;32:741–747.
92. Wang Y, Hussain S, Krestin G. Superparamagnetic iron oxide contrast agents: physicochemical characteristics and applications in MR imaging. Eur Radiol 2001;11:2319–2331.
93. Chambon C, Clement O, Le Blanche A, Schouman-Claeys E, Frija G. Superparamagnetic iron oxides as positive MR contrast agents: in vitro and in vivo evidence. Magn Reson Imaging 1993;11:509–519.
94. Knollmann F, Bock J, Rautenberg K, Beier J, Ebert W, Felix R. Differences in predominant enhancement mechanisms of superparamagnetic iron oxide and ultrasmall superparamagnetic iron oxide for contrast-enhanced portal magnetic resonance angiography. Preliminary results of an animal study original investigation. Invest Radiol 1998;339637–339643.

11

Safety and Monitoring for Cardiac Magnetic Resonance Imaging

Saman Nazarian, Henry R. Halperin, and David A. Bluemke

CONTENTS

OVERVIEW

Because of unsurpassed soft tissue resolution, lack of ionizing radiation, and multi-planar imaging capability, magnetic resonance imaging (MRI) has become an important tool in the evaluation and treatment of cardiovascular disorders. However, an increasing proportion of patients with cardiovascular disease have higher acuity of disease and ferromagnetic implants with potential for interaction with the MRI environment. Familiarity with each device class and its potential for electromagnetic interaction is essential for radiologists and cardiologists performing MRI examinations in this population of patients.

Currently, there is a remarkable range of implanted medical devices, many of which have the potential for interaction with powerful magnetic fields imposed by the MRI scanner as well as the radio-frequency (RF) energy that is deposited in the patient. The final decision to perform MRI is frequently made by considering the potential benefit of MRI relative to the attendant risks associated with various devices. Minimization of risk may also involve considerations of alternative methods of diagnostic imaging (e.g., computed tomography or ultrasound) relative to MRI. If multiple MRI scanners are available, then MRI risk may also be lower in magnets with low field strength relative to high field units. Because of the wide range of circumstances encountered in the MRI suite, the descriptions that follow should not be construed as recommendations that are appropriate for all patients. The reader is therefore encouraged to consult Web sites of the device manufacturers, those related to listing of device safety with MRI (e.g.,

From: *Contemporary Cardiology: Cardiovascular Magnetic Resonance Imaging*
Edited by: Raymond Y. Kwong © Humana Press Inc., Totowa, NJ

www.mrisafety.com), or standard handbooks for MRI safety that provide more specific information regarding individual devices and specific device testing details.

PATIENT CONDITION AND MONITORING

As the indications for cardiovascular MRI expand, patients with higher acuity of disease and increased dependence on monitoring and intervention are referred for MRI. Patients with cardiovascular disease are often referred for imaging in the setting of brady- and tachyarrhythmias, hypotension, myocardial ischemia, or congestive heart failure. Contrast administration, prolonged supine imaging, and interaction with implantable or temporary devices may lead to changes in patient condition during the MRI examination. Appropriate monitoring with continuous electrocardiogram (ECG) telemetry, pulse oximetry, and noninvasive blood pressure measurements in addition to monitoring of patient symptoms is essential. To perform MRI safely, some devices may have to be disabled, and patient monitoring is limited. To increase safety, steps need to be taken to replace the disabled function of the device with a well-rehearsed plan for monitoring and treatment.

Potential for Interaction With Implanted Devices

Ferromagnetic materials in a magnetic field are subject to force and torque. The potential for movement of an implanted device in the MRI environment depends on the magnetic field strength, ferromagnetic properties of the material, the implant distance from the magnet bore, and the stability of the implant *(1)*.

The RF and pulsed gradient magnetic fields in the MRI environment may induce electrical currents in leads and other ferromagnetic wires within the field. Implant length (vs the RF wavelength) and conformations such as loops favor improved transition of energy to the implanted device. RF pulses may also lead to implant heating and tissue damage at the device–tissue interface.

Sophisticated electronic implants, such as those in neurostimulators, pacemakers, and implantable cardioverter defibrillators, have the potential for receiving electromagnetic interference in the MRI environment, resulting in programming changes or loss of function.

Patient Screening

Given the potential risks listed, it is essential to conduct a systematic review of the patient's condition, implanted devices, and safety for MRI. At our institution, all patients are asked to review and answer a safety questionnaire (Fig. 1). The latest data regarding the MRI safety of devices commonly used in cardiovascular patients are reviewed here.

DEVICES WITH POTENTIAL FOR INTERACTION WITH MAGNETIC RESONANCE IMAGING

ECG Leads

Metallic telemetry leads used routinely for patient monitoring can induce artifacts and may heat in the MRI environment, resulting in skin burns. Specially designed non-ferromagnetic ECG leads and filtered monitoring systems have been designed for the MRI environment (e.g., S/5 MRI Monitor, Datex-Ohmeda, Finland). Such systems also offer continuous SpO_2 monitoring, which in our experience is an invaluable tool for

**THE JOHNS HOPKINS HOSPITAL
DEPARTMENT OF RADIOLOGY AND
RADIOLOGICAL SCIENCE**

M R I   P a t i e n t   S c r e e n i n g

for addressograph plate

This section is to be filled out by the PATIENT:

The M R I room contains a very strong magnet. Before you go into the M R I room, we must know if you have any metal in your body. Please complete the following:

Pacemaker/Wires	☐ Yes ☐ No		Recent Stent Placement	☐ Yes	☐ No
Aneurysm Clips	☐ Yes ☐ No		Shunt	☐ Yes	☐ No
Surgical Clips	☐ Yes ☐ No		Ear Implant	☐ Yes	☐ No
Eye Implant	☐ Yes ☐ No		IUD	☐ Yes	☐ No
Internal Defibrillator	☐ Yes ☐ No		Blood Vessel Coil	☐ Yes	☐ No
Bullets, pellets, BBs	☐ Yes ☐ No		Heart Valve	☐ Yes	☐ No
Stimulator/Wires	☐ Yes ☐ No		Artificial Limb	☐ Yes	☐ No
Infusion Pump	☐ Yes ☐ No		Cochlear Device	☐ Yes	☐ No
Penile Prosthesis	☐ Yes ☐ No		Tracheostomy	☐ Yes	☐ No

Have you ever been a machinist, welder, or metal worker? ☐ Yes ☐ No

Have you ever had a facial injury from metal? ☐ Yes ☐ No

Have you ever had metal removed from your eye(s)? ☐ Yes ☐ No

Are you pregnant? ☐ Yes ☐ No

(Last menstrual period: _____)

Do you have any allergies?

If 'Yes', please specify: _____

Current Medications: _____

Weight: _____   Patient Signature: _____   Date: _____

This section is to be filled out by the RADIOLOGY STAFF:

Operations ☐ Yes ☐ No _____

Orbit Films ☐ Yes ☐ No   If 'Yes', cleared by radiologist?   Name: _____

Disposition of Valuables: ☐ Family Member ☐ M R I Locker #: _____ ☐ No Valuables
Patient/Family has key

Anyone attending patient in the M R I room has been cleared for M R I safety requirements. ☐ Yes ☐ No

Radiology Staff Signature/Title: _____   Date: _____

FORM #JH4-18-22001 (10-03-97)   GRAPHICS BY JHH CENTER FOR INFORMATION SERVICES   JH1008 - 642

Fig. 1. Sample patient safety questionnaire.

monitoring of the cardiac rhythm, especially when the ECG signal, despite filtering, becomes unreadable in the setting of specific MRI pulse sequences.

Sternal Wires

Sternal wires used for closure after thoracotomy procedures are typically made of stainless steel, which is minimally ferromagnetic. Animal studies have suggested the safety of MRI in this setting *(2)*. Over the course of 15 years in a large acute care hospital setting, one patient had chest discomfort that was classified as "possibly" related to sternal wires; the MRI in this case was discontinued, with resolution of symptoms and no further complications. However, sternal wires, similar to any other metallic implant, typically induce susceptibility artifacts in the immediate area and may limit imaging of the anterior right ventricle *(3)*.

Epicardial Wires

Temporary epicardial pacing wires are routinely cut short at the skin and left in place after cardiac surgery. There are reports of safe performance of MRI in patients with such retained temporary wires *(4,5)*. Permanent epicardial pacing leads and patches placed at cardiac surgery, however, have more ferromagnetic materials and are prone to heating in the MRI environment. Unlike endovascular leads, these devices are not cooled by the blood pool, and in experimental models up to 20°C of heating has been observed *(6)*. For this reason, at our institution we do not scan patients with permanent epicardial leads and patches. Temporary epicardial wires are removed prior to MRI whenever possible.

Prosthetic Valves and Annuloplasty Rings

Ex vivo studies of a variety of current prosthetic valves and annuloplasty rings, including the mechanical St. Jude, Bjork Shiley, and Carbo-Medics and bioprosthetic (with metal struts) such as the Hancock, have shown minimal torque and heating (<0.8°C) at 1.5 T and with specific absorption rates limited to 1.1 W/kg *(7–9)*. Artifact size correlated with the amount of metal in the device and was exaggerated on gradient echo pulse sequences.

Shellock also evaluated prosthetic valve and annuloplasty ring safety at 3 T, revealing minor magnetic field interactions *(10)*. Studies to determine the force required to cause partial or total detachment of a heart valve prosthesis in patients with degenerative valvular disease have found that forces significantly higher than those induced at 4.7 T would be required to pull a suture through the valve annulus tissue *(11)*.

The only prosthetic valves thought to have potential for experiencing enough force and torque to cause clinically concerning problems are the Star-Edwards pre-6000 series prostheses. Deflection measurements at 1.5 T revealed forces similar to peak forces exerted by the beating heart itself *(7)*, leading to initial recommendations to exclude patients with this device series from MRI procedures. However, later studies revealed lower peak forces exerted even on this prosthetic series *(12)*. Mechanical valves do not appear to be prone to induced lead currents *(9)*.

Although there are no reports of patient injury in the MRI environment caused by the presence of a heart valve, there are theoretical concerns about MRI at 1.5 T and higher field strengths *(12)*. One such theoretical concern is the tendency of a metallic object to develop an opposing magnetic field to that through which it moves (the Lenz effect). Such a secondary magnetic field may result in a resistive pressure to opening and closing of a disk prosthesis within the valve *(13)*. Björk-Shiley convex/concave heart valves (Shiley, Irvine, CA) are associated with an increased risk of mechanical failure because of outlet strut fracture. These valves are associated with large susceptibility artifacts under MRI, and such artifacts may increase in size in fractured valves *(14)*.

Edwards et al. evaluated multiple heart valve prostheses for MRI-related forces in static fields up to 4.7 T. Most were found to be safe based on current criteria. However, valves made of Elgiloy, a Ni-Co-Cr base paramagnetic engineering material *(15)*, such as the Carpentier Edwards Physio Ring were found to be prone to rotational forces at such high field strengths *(16)*.

Coronary Stents

In vitro studies have shown minimal heating of coronary stents in the MRI environment *(17)*. Stent dislodgement, even microdislodgement, is of theoretical concern because of the potential for dissection, embolism, and thrombosis. However, most stents are made of materials with little or no ferromagnetism, such as stainless steel, nitinol, or titanium. In vitro and in vivo studies of stent movement have shown minimal movement caused by MRI *(18,19)*. Despite manufacturer recommendations to wait 8 weeks after stent placement prior to imaging, no adverse effects have been noted because of MRI even in the acute poststent period *(20,21)*.

A study of acute MRI after deployment of drug-eluting coronary stents (Taxus, Boston Scientific, Natick, MA; Cypher, Cordis, Johnson & Johnson, New Brunswick, NJ) revealed no acute thrombosis and 9-months adverse events comparable to that expected without MRI *(22)*. In vitro testing of another drug-eluting stent (Endeavor, cobalt alloy, Medtronic Vascular, Santa Rosa, CA) has also been performed, revealing minor magnetic field interactions, heating (+0.5°C), and artifacts *(23)*. Most recently, prototype "active" stents designed to act as electric resonating circuits, thus functioning as inductively coupled transmit coils to allow high-resolution imaging of in-stent restenosis, are under development *(24)*.

Noncoronary Stents

MRI of nonferromagnetic nickel titanium aortic stents has been safely performed in patients with minimal artifact *(25)*. Ex vivo studies have revealed no deflection forces and minimal heating, limited to 1.1°C *(25)*. Despite the recommendation by some authorities to delay MRI for 6 weeks after implant in the case of ferromagnetic large-vessel stents *(26)*, safe imaging has been reported in the acute postimplant period *(27)*.

Coils

In vitro tests of nonferromagnetic platinum microcoils has revealed no coil migration and minimal susceptibility artifacts *(28)*. Three-dimensional time-of-flight MRI has been performed for follow-up of patients with Guglielmi detachable coils within a week postdeployment for treatment of intracranial aneurysms *(29)*. Substitution of digital subtraction angiography by MRI in this patient population was safe, produced minimal artifact, and helped identify thromboembolic events associated with balloon-assisted deployment *(30,31)*. Chronic studies have revealed that time-of-flight MRI is not only safe, but also may indeed be more sensitive at identifying residual flow in coiled aneurysms than traditional plain radiographs and digital subtraction angiography *(32,33)*. In a case series of diffusion and perfusion MRI in patients with ruptured and unruptured intracranial aneurysms treated by intravascular coiling, no MRI-related complications were reported, and stents and platinum coils added negligible effects on the quality of images *(34)*.

Filters

Initial testing of Greenfield filters for deflection at 1.5 T found large variations in the amount of deflection experienced by each device *(35)*. However, in vivo studies showed no evidence of migration *(35,36)*. Although the stainless steel filters such as Tulip and Bird's Nest filters cause extensive signal voids, the susceptibility artifacts associated with most filters appear to be minimal *(37)*. Imaging of the tantalum or titanium alloy filters is associated with such minimal artifact that even intraluminal tilting of the device, postfilter turbulence, and thrombi trapped within the filters can be visualized *(38–40)*. A study comparing the sensitivity of MRI vs ultrasound to assess inferior vena caval patency in the setting of Simon nitinol filters concluded that MRI is the superior modality *(41)*.

Placement of vena caval filters guided by MRI has been attempted; however, it is limited by only passive visualization of the implanted device *(42)*. Techniques to improve real-time visualization of the vessel and interventional instruments are under development *(43)*.

Septal Defect Closure Devices

An in vitro study to evaluate the safety of 12 different occluders used to treat patients with patent ductus arteriosus, atrial septal defects, and ventricular septal defects in a 1.5-T system was performed by Shellock and Morisoli. Occluders made of 304 stainless steel were ferromagnetic and displayed deflection forces of 248–299 dynes, whereas those made of MP35n were nonferromagnetic. Artifacts were variable depending on the type and amount of metal used to construct the implant. The authors recommended a waiting period of 6 weeks postimplant to allow tissue growth and a stronger implant-tissue interface prior to MRI *(44)*.

Real-time MRI guidance with the use of intravascular antenna guidewires has been used to image atrial septal defects and deploy Amplatzer Septal Occluders in swine *(45)*. CardioSEAL Septal Repair and STARFlex Septal Repair Implants have been tested for MRI compatibility at 3 T. Only minor translational attraction or torque was noted, leading the authors to conclude that MRI even at 3 T could be performed immediately postimplantation. Temperature rises were limited to 0.5°C, and artifacts were minimal *(46)*.

Vascular Access Ports and Catheters

Shellock and Shellock tested a variety of vascular access catheters made of titanium, polysulfone, barium sulfate, or silicone, such as the commonly used Vital-Port and Hickman catheters, for MRI safety. At 1.5 T, no magnetic attraction was noted, temperature changes were limited to 0.3°C, and minimal artifacts were noted *(47)*.

Guidewires, Angiography, and Electrophysiology Catheters

Guidewires are typically made from stainless steel or nitinol (nickel/titanium alloy) and are prone to heating and lead currents in the MRI environment. However, the use of guidewires with RF decoupling to reduce heating may lead to successful MRI-guided wire and catheter placement *(48)*. Angiography and electrophysiology catheters with any form of internal or external conductive wire may be prone to heating or induced lead currents and are contraindicated in the MRI environment *(1)*. However, multifunctional electrophysiology catheters that also act as long loop receivers, allowing for catheter visualization, intracardiac electrogram recording, and ablation during MRI have been developed and are currently under testing *(49)*.

Swan-Ganz and Thermodilution Catheters

Swan-Ganz and thermodilution catheters contain long wires made of paramagnetic or magnetic materials, and the tips are not fixed. Therefore, they may be prone to movement, heating *(26)*, and induction of current and are not safe in the MRI environment.

Implantable Monitors

The Reveal (Medtronic, Minneapolis, MN) implantable loop recorder is an ECG recording device that can be activated by preset heart rate limits or a patient trigger. Scanning patients with this family of implantable recorders has been performed safely *(50)*. However, the device frequently records artifacts as arrhythmia because of electromagnetic interference in the setting of MRI. Care should be taken to clear episodes recorded during MRI to prevent future misinterpretation of artifact as clinically significant arrhythmia.

Temporary Pacemakers

To our knowledge, there are no studies assessing the safety of temporary pacemakers in the MRI environment. Unlike permanent devices, temporary pacemakers typically have unfixed leads and are more prone to movement. Furthermore, the leads are longer and may be more prone to induction of lead currents. Finally, the electronic platform of external temporary pacemakers is less sophisticated and has less filtering compared to modern implantable pacemakers. Therefore, such devices are likely more susceptible to electromagnetic interference.

Permanent Pacemakers and Implantable Cardioverter Defibrillators

Because of underlying structural heart disease and accompanying conduction system disease or risk of ventricular arrhythmia, a significant proportion of patients referred for cardiac MRI have permanent pacemakers and implantable defibrillators *(51–55)*. It has been estimated that a patient with a pacemaker or implanted defibrillator has a 50–75% likelihood of having a clinically indicated MRI over the lifetime of their device *(56)*. The potential for movement of the device *(57)*, programming changes, asynchronous pacing, activation of tachyarrhythmia therapies, inhibition of demand pacing *(58)*, and induced lead currents leading to heating and cardiac stimulation *(59)* have led to concerns from device manufacturers *(60–62)* and MRI authorities *(1,63,64)* regarding the performance of MRI procedures in cardiac implantable device recipients.

However, several case series have reported the safety of MRI in the setting of pacemakers *(65–70)*. A small case series has also reported neurological MRI in the setting of selected implantable cardioverter defibrillator systems *(71)*. Overall, safety has been reported, but acute changes in battery voltage, lead thresholds *(68)*, and programming *(71)* can be seen.

At our institution, we have developed a protocol including (1) device selection based on previous in vitro and in vivo testing (6), (2) device programming to minimize inappropriate activation or inhibition of brady-/tachyarrhythmia therapies, and (3) limitation of the specific absorption rate of MRI sequences (less than 2.0 W/kg using a Signa CV/I Scanner, General Electric Healthcare Technologies, Waukesha, WI). The protocol (Fig. 2) is unique in selecting device generators previously tested under worst-case scenario (imaging over the region containing the generator, and specific absorption rate [SAR] up to 3.5 W/kg) MRI conditions (6). It also describes suggested steps to identify and exclude patients with leads that are more prone to movement and heating.

Programming steps to reduce the risk of inappropriate pacemaker inhibition or activation or inappropriate activation of tachyarrhythmia functions are summarized in Figure 2 (72). It is important to note, however, that because of poor correlation of heating at different specific absorption rates across different scanners even within those of the same manufacturer, the specific absorption rates from the authors' results should not be directly applied to other MRI systems (73).

Neurostimulation Systems

In vitro studies of a chronic deep brain stimulation system (Soletra model 7426, Medtronic) at 1.5 T have revealed temperature rises as high as 25°C depending on the type of RF coil used, positioning of the electrodes, and the specific absorption rate of sequences (64,74). Such excessive heating was thought to be avoidable by using send/receive head RF coils and limiting the SAR of sequences to 2.4 W/kg using a 1.5-T/64-mHz Vision MR imaging system (Siemens Medical Systems, Iselin, NJ) (75). Another in vitro study using a 1.5-T Sonata MRI system (Siemens Medical Systems) to scan bilateral neurostimulation systems (Soletra 7246, 7495, and 3389, Medtronic) revealed temperature rises limited to 2.1°C (76).

Note should be made that a study has revealed poor correlation of heating at different SAR across different scanners even within those of the same manufacturer, and therefore the results of the previous studies *should not be applied* to other MRI systems (73). Importantly, several reports of injury during MRI of patients with neurostimulation systems exist in the literature, and experts advise judicious use of MRI, only when clinically warranted, following the specific guidelines of the manufacturer, using send/receive head RF coils, and limiting the SAR to 0.4 W/kg (77–80). Note that limiting SAR in combination with send/receive RF coils is not currently approved for all MRI scanners in conjunction with deep brain stimulators.

Intra-Aortic Balloon Pumps

An animal study assessed the recovery of left ventricular function after myocardial infarction with and without balloon counterpulsation via MRI. During this study, the intra-aortic balloon pump was paused during the scan. Although MRI safety was not the primary outcome assessed, no untoward side effects of MRI in this setting were reported (80). More studies are needed to assess the safety of MRI in the setting of intra-aortic balloon counterpulsation prior to human studies with MRI.

Ventricular Assist Devices

Ventricular assist devices have high metal content, complicated circuitry, and in some cases magnetic field dependence for appropriate function. There is no literature regarding MRI in patients with implanted assist devices. Because of the issues listed

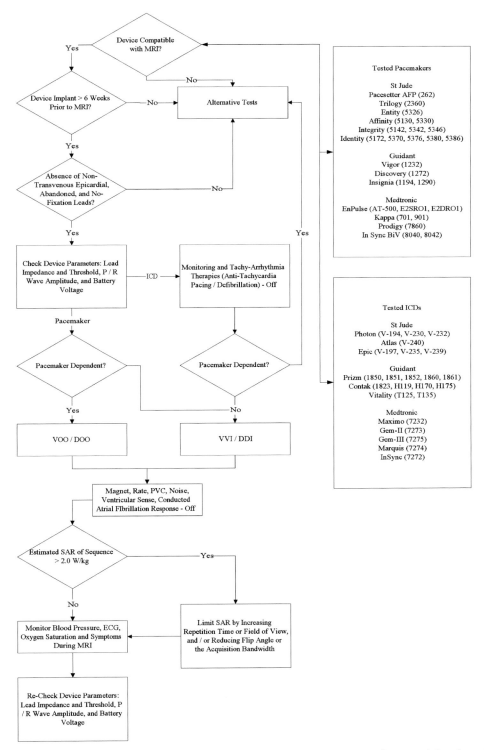

Fig. 2. Safety protocol for MRI of patients with permanent pacemakers and implantable defibrillators (From ref. *72*).

and high potential for catastrophic device failure, MRI is an absolute contraindication in patients with current ventricular assist devices.

Orthopedic Implants

Most orthopedic implants have been reported to be nonferromagnetic or weakly ferromagnetic and therefore are safe for undergoing MRI at 1.5 T *(81–86)*. The Perfix interference screw (Instrument Macar, Okemos, MI) used for anterior cruciate ligament reconstruction is the only hardware found to be highly ferromagnetic. However, the strength of the surrounding tissue provides sufficient retentive force to provide for safe imaging of patients with these implants *(87)*.

Shellock tested a variety of orthopedic implants at 3 T and found low torque measurements for most devices except for the bone fusion stimulator. However, this device is also likely safe for imaging given its typical position in the patient with respect to the static magnetic field of MRI and retentive strength of the subcutaneous and granulation tissue *(10)*.

IMAGE ARTIFACTS

The presence of ferromagnetic materials can cause variations in the surrounding magnetic field, resulting in image distortion, signal voids or bright areas, and poor fat suppression *(88)*. Susceptibility artifacts appear to be most pronounced on inversion recovery and steady-state free precession sequences.

In our experience, artifacts on inversion recovery prepared delayed cardiac MRI show high signal intensity and can mimic areas of delayed enhancement, which would otherwise indicate myocardial scar. Correlation of suspect areas on different pulse sequences can help avoid misidentification of artifact. Using imaging planes perpendicular to the plane of the device generator, shortening of the echo time, and using spin echo and fast spin echo sequences appears to reduce the qualitative extent of artifact.

SUMMARY

As indications for referral of patients for cardiovascular MRI evolve, acuity of illness and potential for interaction with implanted devices in those referred will likely increase. Although techniques for safe imaging in the setting of certain devices have been developed, the potential for catastrophic complications exists and dictates a high degree of vigilance for safe imaging. The reader is encouraged to consult Web sites that provide more specific information regarding individual devices (e.g., www.mrisafety.com) for specific device testing details.

REFERENCES

1. Prasad SK, Pennell DJ. Safety of cardiovascular magnetic resonance in patients with cardiovascular implants and devices. Heart 2004;90:1241–1244.
2. Manner I, Alanen A, Komu M, Savunen T, Kantonen I, Ekfors T. MR imaging in the presence of small circular metallic implants. Assessment of thermal injuries. Acta Radiol 1996;37:551–554.
3. Okamura Y, Yamada Y, Mochizuki Y, et al. [Evaluation of coronary artery bypass grafts with magnetic resonance imaging]. Nippon Kyobu Geka Gakkai Zasshi 1997;45:801–805.
4. Hartnell GG, Spence L, Hughes LA, Cohen MC, Saouaf R, Buff B. Safety of MR imaging in patients who have retained metallic materials after cardiac surgery. AJR Am J Roentgenol 1997;168:1157–1159.
5. Murphy KJ, Cohan RH, Ellis JH. MR imaging in patients with epicardial pacemaker wires. AJR Am J Roentgenol 1999;172:727–728.

6. Roguin A, Zviman MM, Meininger GR, et al. Modern pacemaker and implantable cardioverter/defibrillator systems can be magnetic resonance imaging safe: in vitro and in vivo assessment of safety and function at 1.5 T. Circulation 2004;110:475–482.

7. Soulen RL, Budinger TF, Higgins CB. Magnetic resonance imaging of prosthetic heart valves. Radiology 1985;154:705–707.

8. Edwards MB, Taylor KM, Shellock FG. Prosthetic heart valves: evaluation of magnetic field interactions, heating, and artifacts at 1.5 T. J Magn Reson Imaging 2000;12:363–369.

9. Shellock FG. Prosthetic heart valves and annuloplasty rings: assessment of magnetic field interactions, heating, and artifacts at 1.5 T. J Cardiovasc Magn Reson 2001;3:317–324.

10. Shellock FG. Biomedical implants and devices: assessment of magnetic field interactions with a 3.0-T MR system. J Magn Reson Imaging 2002;16:721–732.

11. Edwards MB, Draper ER, Hand JW, Taylor KM, Young IR. Mechanical testing of human cardiac tissue: some implications for MRI safety. J Cardiovasc Magn Reson 2005;7:835–840.

12. Shellock FG. Magnetic resonance safety update 2002: implants and devices. J Magn Reson Imaging 2002;16:485–496.

13. Condon B, Hadley DM. Potential MR hazard to patients with metallic heart valves: the Lenz effect. J Magn Reson Imaging 2000;12:171–176.

14. van Gorp MJ, van der Graaf Y, de Mol BA, et al. Bjork-Shiley convexoconcave valves: susceptibility artifacts at brain MR imaging and mechanical valve fractures. Radiology 2004;230:709–714.

15. Ho JC, Shellock FG. Magnetic properties of Ni-Co-Cr-base Elgiloy. J Mater Sci Mater Med 1999;10:555–560.

16. Edwards MB, Ordidge RJ, Hand JW, Taylor KM, Young IR. Assessment of magnetic field (4.7 T) induced forces on prosthetic heart valves and annuloplasty rings. J Magn Reson Imaging 2005;22:311–317.

17. Strohm O, Kivelitz D, Gross W, et al. Safety of implantable coronary stents during [1]H-magnetic resonance imaging at 1.0 and 1.5 T. J Cardiovasc Magn Reson 1999;1:239–245.

18. Scott NA, Pettigrew RI. Absence of movement of coronary stents after placement in a magnetic resonance imaging field. Am J Cardiol 1994;73:900–901.

19. Hug J, Nagel E, Bornstedt A, Schnackenburg B, Oswald H, Fleck E. Coronary arterial stents: safety and artifacts during MR imaging. Radiology 2000;216:781–787.

20. Kramer CM, Rogers WJ Jr, Pakstis DL. Absence of adverse outcomes after magnetic resonance imaging early after stent placement for acute myocardial infarction: a preliminary study. J Cardiovasc Magn Reson 2000;2:257–261.

21. Gerber TC, Fasseas P, Lennon RJ, et al. Clinical safety of magnetic resonance imaging early after coronary artery stent placement. J Am Coll Cardiol 2003;42:1295–1298.

22. Porto I, Selvanayagam J, Ashar V, Neubauer S, Banning AP. Safety of magnetic resonance imaging 1 to 3 days after bare metal and drug-eluting stent implantation. Am J Cardiol 2005;96:366–368.

23. Shellock FG, Forder JR. Drug eluting coronary stent: in vitro evaluation of magnet resonance safety at 3 T. J Cardiovasc Magn Reson 2005;7:415–419.

24. Busch M, Vollmann W, Bertsch T, et al. On the heating of inductively coupled resonators (stents) during MRI examinations. Magn Reson Med 2005;54:775–782.

25. Engellau L, Olsrud J, Brockstedt S, et al. MR evaluation ex vivo and in vivo of a covered stent-graft for abdominal aortic aneurysms: ferromagnetism, heating, artifacts, and velocity mapping. J Magn Reson Imaging 2000;12:112–121.

26. Ahmed S, Shellock FG. Magnetic resonance imaging safety: implications for cardiovascular patients. J Cardiovasc Magn Reson 2001;3:171–182.

27. Stables RH, Mohiaddin R, Panting J, Pennell DJ, Pepper J, Sigwart U. Images in cardiovascular medicine. Exclusion of an aneurysmal segment of the thoracic aorta with covered stents. Circulation 2000;101:1888–1889.

28. Marshall MW, Teitelbaum GP, Kim HS, Deveikis J. Ferromagnetism and magnetic resonance artifacts of platinum embolization microcoils. Cardiovasc Intervent Radiol 1991;14:163–166.

29. Okahara M, Kiyosue H, Hori Y, Yamashita M, Nagatomi H, Mori H. Three-dimensional time-of-flight MR angiography for evaluation of intracranial aneurysms after endosaccular packing with Guglielmi detachable coils: comparison with 3D digital subtraction angiography. Eur Radiol 2004;14: 1162–1168.

30. Soeda A, Sakai N, Sakai H, et al. Thromboembolic events associated with Guglielmi detachable coil embolization of asymptomatic cerebral aneurysms: evaluation of 66 consecutive cases with use of diffusion-weighted MR imaging. AJNR Am J Neuroradiol 2003;24:127–132.

31. Albayram S, Selcuk H, Kara B, et al. Thromboembolic events associated with balloon-assisted coil embolization: evaluation with diffusion-weighted MR imaging. AJNR Am J Neuroradiol 2004;25: 1768–1777.
32. Cottier JP, Bleuzen-Couthon A, Gallas S, et al. Follow-up of intracranial aneurysms treated with detachable coils: comparison of plain radiographs, 3D time-of-flight MRA and digital subtraction angiography. Neuroradiology 2003;45:818–824.
33. Yamada N, Hayashi K, Murao K, Higashi M, Iihara K. Time-of-flight MR angiography targeted to coiled intracranial aneurysms is more sensitive to residual flow than is digital subtraction angiography. AJNR Am J Neuroradiol 2004;25:1154–1157.
34. Cronqvist M, Wirestam R, Ramgren B, et al. Diffusion and perfusion MRI in patients with ruptured and unruptured intracranial aneurysms treated by endovascular coiling: complications, procedural results, MR findings and clinical outcome. Neuroradiology 2005;47:855–873.
35. Williamson MR, McCowan TC, Walker CW, Ferris EJ. Effect of a 1.5 T magnetic field on Greenfield filters in vitro and in dogs. Angiology 1988;39:1022–1024.
36. Liebman CE, Messersmith RN, Levin DN, Lu CT. MR imaging of inferior vena caval filters: safety and artifacts. AJR Am J Roentgenol 1988;150:1174–1176.
37. Honda M, Obuchi M, Sugimoto H. Artifacts of vena cava filters ex vivo on MR angiography. Magn Reson Med Sci 2003;2:71–77.
38. Teitelbaum GP, Ortega HV, Vinitski S, et al. Low-artifact intravascular devices: MR imaging evaluation. Radiology 1988;168:713–719.
39. Teitelbaum GP, Ortega HV, Vinitski S, et al. Optimization of gradient-echo imaging parameters for intracaval filters and trapped thromboemboli. Radiology 1990;174:1013–1019.
40. Grassi CJ, Matsumoto AH, Teitelbaum GP. Vena caval occlusion after Simon nitinol filter placement: identification with MR imaging in patients with malignancy. J Vasc Interv Radiol 1992;3:535–539.
41. Kim D, Edelman RR, Margolin CJ, et al. The Simon nitinol filter: evaluation by MR and ultrasound. Angiology 1992;43:541–548.
42. Frahm C, Gehl HB, Lorch H, et al. MR-guided placement of a temporary vena cava filter: technique and feasibility. J Magn Reson Imaging 1998;8:105–109.
43. Bucker A, Neuerburg JM, Adam GB, et al. Real-time MR guidance for inferior vena cava filter placement in an animal model. J Vasc Interv Radiol 2001;12:753–756.
44. Shellock FG, Morisoli SM. Ex vivo evaluation of ferromagnetism and artifacts of cardiac occluders exposed to a 1.5-T MR system. J Magn Reson Imaging 1994;4:213–215.
45. Rickers C, Jerosch-Herold M, Hu X, et al. Magnetic resonance image-guided transcatheter closure of atrial septal defects. Circulation 2003;107:132–138.
46. Shellock FG, Valencerina S. Septal repair implants: evaluation of magnetic resonance imaging safety at 3 T. Magn Reson Imaging 2005;23:1021–1025.
47. Shellock FG, Shellock VJ. Vascular access ports and catheters: ex vivo testing of ferromagnetism, heating, and artifacts associated with MR imaging. Magn Reson Imaging 1996;14:443–447.
48. Razavi R, Hill DL, Keevil SF, et al. Cardiac catheterisation guided by MRI in children and adults with congenital heart disease. Lancet 2003;362:1877–1882.
49. Susil RC, Yeung CJ, Halperin HR, Lardo AC, Atalar E. Multifunctional interventional devices for MRI: a combined electrophysiology/MRI catheter. Magn Reson Med 2002;47:594–600.
50. Gimbel JR, Zarghami J, Machado C, Wilkoff BL. Safe scanning, but frequent artifacts mimicking bradycardia and tachycardia during magnetic resonance imaging (MRI) in patients with an implantable loop recorder (ILR). Ann Noninvasive Electrocardiol 2005;10:404–408.
51. Brown DW, Croft JB, Giles WH, Anda RF, Mensah GA. Epidemiology of pacemaker procedures among Medicare enrollees in 1990, 1995, and 2000. Am J Cardiol 2005;95:409–411.
52. Moss AJ, Zareba W, Hall WJ, et al. Prophylactic implantation of a defibrillator in patients with myocardial infarction and reduced ejection fraction. N Engl J Med 2002;346:877–883.
53. Abraham WT, Fisher WG, Smith AL, et al. Cardiac resynchronization in chronic heart failure. N Engl J Med 2002;346:1845–1853.
54. Bristow MR, Saxon LA, Boehmer J, et al. Cardiac-resynchronization therapy with or without an implantable defibrillator in advanced chronic heart failure. N Engl J Med 2004;350: 2140–2150.
55. Bardy GH, Lee KL, Mark DB, et al. Amiodarone or an implantable cardioverter-defibrillator for congestive heart failure. N Engl J Med 2005;352:225–237.
56. Kalin R, Stanton MS. Current clinical issues for MRI scanning of pacemaker and defibrillator patients. Pacing Clin Electrophysiol 2005;28:326–328.

57. Shellock FG, Tkach JA, Ruggieri PM, Masaryk TJ. Cardiac pacemakers, ICDs, and loop recorder: evaluation of translational attraction using conventional ("long-bore") and "short-bore" 1.5- and 3.0-T MR systems. J Cardiovasc Magn Reson 2003;5:387–397.

58. Erlebacher JA, Cahill PT, Pannizzo F, Knowles RJ. Effect of magnetic resonance imaging on DDD pacemakers. Am J Cardiol 1986;57:437–440.

59. Hayes DL, Holmes DR Jr, Gray JE. Effect of 1.5 T nuclear magnetic resonance imaging scanner on implanted permanent pacemakers. J Am Coll Cardiol 1987;10:782–786.

60. Smith JM. Industry viewpoint: guidant: pacemakers, ICDs, and MRI. Pacing Clin Electrophysiol 2005;28:264.

61. Stanton MS. Industry viewpoint: Medtronic: pacemakers, ICDs, and MRI. Pacing Clin Electrophysiol 2005;28:265.

62. Levine PA. Industry viewpoint: St. Jude Medical: pacemakers, ICDs and MRI. Pacing Clin Electrophysiol 2005;28:266–267.

63. Shellock FG, Crues JV. MR procedures: biologic effects, safety, and patient care. Radiology 2004; 232:635–652.

64. Faris OP, Shein MJ. Government viewpoint: U.S. Food and Drug Administration: pacemakers, ICDs and MRI. Pacing Clin Electrophysiol 2005;28:268–269.

65. Gimbel JR, Johnson D, Levine PA, Wilkoff BL. Safe performance of magnetic resonance imaging on five patients with permanent cardiac pacemakers. Pacing Clin Electrophysiol 1996;19:913–919.

66. Sommer T, Vahlhaus C, Lauck G, et al. MR imaging and cardiac pacemakers: in-vitro evaluation and in-vivo studies in 51 patients at 0.5 T. Radiology 2000;215:869–879.

67. Vahlhaus C, Sommer T, Lewalter T, et al. Interference with cardiac pacemakers by magnetic resonance imaging: are there irreversible changes at 0.5 T? Pacing Clin Electrophysiol 2001;24:489–495.

68. Martin ET, Coman JA, Shellock FG, Pulling CC, Fair R, Jenkins K. Magnetic resonance imaging and cardiac pacemaker safety at 1.5-T. J Am Coll Cardiol 2004;43:1315–1324.

69. Del Ojo JL, Moya F, Villalba J, et al. Is magnetic resonance imaging safe in cardiac pacemaker recipients? Pacing Clin Electrophysiol 2005;28:274–278.

70. Shellock FG, Fieno DS, Thomson LJ, Talavage TM, Berman DS. Cardiac pacemaker: in vitro assessment at 1.5 T. Am Heart J 2006;151:436–443.

71. Gimbel JR, Kanal E, Schwartz KM, Wilkoff BL. Outcome of magnetic resonance imaging (MRI) in selected patients with implantable cardioverter defibrillators (ICDs). Pacing Clin Electrophysiol 2005;28:270–273.

72. Nazarian S, Roguin A, Zviman MM, Lardo AC, Dickfeld TL, Calkins H, Weiss RG, Berger RD, Bluemke DA, Halperin HR. Clinical utility and safety of a protocol for noncardiac and cardiac magnetic resonance imaging of patients with permanent pacemakers and implantable-cardioverter defibrillators at 1.5 tesla. Circulation 2006 Sep 19;114(12):1277–1284.

73. Baker KB, Tkach JA, Nyenhuis JA, et al. Evaluation of specific absorption rate as a dosimeter of MRI-related implant heating. J Magn Reson Imaging 2004;20:315–320.

74. Rezai AR, Finelli D, Nyenhuis JA, et al. Neurostimulation systems for deep brain stimulation: in vitro evaluation of magnetic resonance imaging-related heating at 1.5 T. J Magn Reson Imaging 2002;15:241–250.

75. Finelli DA, Rezai AR, Ruggieri PM, et al. MR imaging-related heating of deep brain stimulation electrodes: in vitro study. AJNR Am J Neuroradiol 2002;23:1795–1802.

76. Bhidayasiri R, Bronstein JM, Sinha S, et al. Bilateral neurostimulation systems used for deep brain stimulation: in vitro study of MRI-related heating at 1.5 T and implications for clinical imaging of the brain. Magn Reson Imaging 2005;23:549–555.

77. Rezai AR, Phillips M, Baker KB, et al. Neurostimulation system used for deep brain stimulation (DBS): MR safety issues and implications of failing to follow safety recommendations. Invest Radiol 2004;39:300–303.

78. Henderson JM, Tkach J, Phillips M, Baker K, Shellock FG, Rezai AR. Permanent neurological deficit related to magnetic resonance imaging in a patient with implanted deep brain stimulation electrodes for Parkinson's disease: case report. Neurosurgery 2005;57:E1063; discussion E1063.

79. Rezai AR, Baker KB, Tkach JA, et al. Is magnetic resonance imaging safe for patients with neurostimulation systems used for deep brain stimulation? Neurosurgery 2005;57:1056–1062; discussion 1056–1062.

80. Azevedo CF, Amado LC, Kraitchman DL, et al. The effect of intra-aortic balloon counterpulsation on left ventricular functional recovery early after acute myocardial infarction: a randomized experimental magnetic resonance imaging study. Eur Heart J 2005;26:1235–1241.

81. New PF, Rosen BR, Brady TJ, et al. Potential hazards and artifacts of ferromagnetic and nonferro-magnetic surgical and dental materials and devices in nuclear magnetic resonance imaging. Radiology 1983;147:139–148.
82. Mechlin M, Thickman D, Kressel HY, Gefter W, Joseph P. Magnetic resonance imaging of postoperative patients with metallic implants. AJR Am J Roentgenol 1984;143:1281–1284.
83. Mesgarzadeh M, Revesz G, Bonakdarpour A, Betz RR. The effect on medical metal implants by magnetic fields of magnetic resonance imaging. Skeletal Radiol 1985;14:205–206.
84. Shellock FG, Crues JV. High-field-strength MR imaging and metallic biomedical implants: an ex vivo evaluation of deflection forces. AJR Am J Roentgenol 1988;151:389–392.
85. Lyons CJ, Betz RR, Mesgarzadeh M, Revesz G, Bonakdarpour A, Clancy M. The effect of magnetic resonance imaging on metal spine implants. Spine 1989;14:670–672.
86. Shellock FG, Morisoli S, Kanal E. MR procedures and biomedical implants, materials, and devices: 1993 update. Radiology 1993;189:587–599.
87. Shellock FG, Mink JH, Curtin S, Friedman MJ. MR imaging and metallic implants for anterior cruciate ligament reconstruction: assessment of ferromagnetism and artifact. J Magn Reson Imaging 1992;2:225–228.
88. Peh WC, Chan JH. Artifacts in musculoskeletal magnetic resonance imaging: identification and correction. Skeletal Radiol 2001;30:179–191.

12

Assessment of Left Ventricular Systolic Function by MRI

Frederick H. Epstein

CONTENTS

INTRODUCTION
METHODS
CLINICAL APPLICATIONS
SUMMARY
REFERENCES

INTRODUCTION

The accurate assessment of left ventricular (LV) systolic function is clinically important in nearly all types of cardiac disease and often directly affects patient management. One example in ischemic heart disease include acute myocardial infarction (MI) for which ejection fraction and end-systolic volume are important predictors of survival *(1)* and are used to determine medical therapy. In other examples, a positive functional response to low doses of dobutamine accurately predicts recovery of function after acute MI and identifies myocardial viability in chronic MI. In the latter case, the functional response to dobutamine can be used to guide coronary revascularization therapy. In addition, the presence or absence of inducible wall motion abnormalities during stress testing indicates the presence or absence of significant coronary artery stenoses and consequently determines whether cardiac catheterization is indicated. Finally, recent research shows that the degree of LV dyssynchrony may be better than QRS morphology or width for predicting the response to cardiac resynchronization therapy in patients with heart failure.

Noninvasive imaging is the primary method for the clinical assessment of LV systolic function. Echocardiography is the most widely used modality for this application because of its efficacy, relatively low cost, portability, and widespread availability. Gated single photon emission computed tomography (SPECT) can also be used for noninvasive imaging of global and regional LV function, although it has relatively low spatial resolution. Although echocardiography and SPECT are the imaging modalities most familiar to cardiologists, magnetic resonance imaging (MRI) has in fact been shown to be the most accurate modality for the evaluation of global and regional systolic LV function in normal volunteers and patients *(2–5)*. Accordingly, the clinical use of MRI in ischemic heart disease is growing.

From: *Contemporary Cardiology: Cardiovascular Magnetic Resonance Imaging*
Edited by: Raymond Y. Kwong © Humana Press Inc., Totowa, NJ

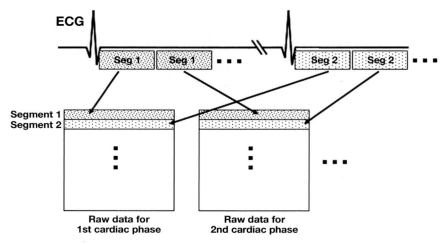

Fig. 1. Schematic diagram of ECG-gated breath-hold cine MRI. Segments of data for multiple cardiac phases are acquired over a series of heartbeats during suspended respiration. For each segment, multiple lines of the raw data matrix (*k*-space) are acquired using repetitions of either a spoiled gradient echo or steady-state free precession pulse sequence. During a single breath hold, data for all of the segments of each cardiac phase are acquired.

In this chapter, the MRI methods used to assess LV function and their application in ischemic heart disease are discussed. The section on methods covers the physics and properties of pulse sequences such as breath-hold gradient echo cine, steady-state free precession (SSFP), myocardial tagging, and real-time imaging. Applications include imaging systolic LV function in acute and chronic MI, heart failure, during dobutamine stress testing, and when assessing the synchrony of LV contraction. The chapter ends by discussing how to integrate LV function findings with other MRI data, such as delayed contrast enhancement.

METHODS

Breath-Hold Segmented k-Space Electrocardiogram-Gated Cine MRI

Multiphase, or cine, MRI commonly employs fast gradient echo imaging combined with *k*-space segmentation to acquire images during suspended respiration *(6)*. This type of breath-hold cine imaging typically has in-plane spatial resolution of around 1.5×2 mm^2, slice thickness of 5–10 mm, temporal resolution of 30–50 ms, and scan times of 8–16 seconds per slice. The acquisition of data during suspended respiration eliminates motion artifact caused by breathing. The *k*-space segmentation technique entails acquiring multiple lines of the *k*-space data, referred to as a segment of *k*-space, for each cardiac phase during each heartbeat (Fig. 1).

By acquiring a segment of *k*-space, as opposed to a single line of *k*-space, in each heartbeat, a complete image data set can be acquired in a fraction of the time required for nonsegmented techniques, enabling the acquisition of a complete set of multiphase images for a single slice within a breath hold. For example, if 96 lines of *k*-space are required per image, repetition time = 5 ms, and 8 lines of *k*-space are acquired per heartbeat, then the temporal resolution is 8 lines $\times$ 5 ms per line = 40 ms per image. The total scan time is 96 lines/8 lines per beat = 12 heartbeats.

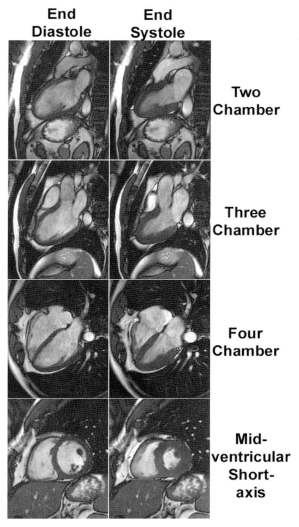

Fig. 2. Images of arbitrary scan planes can be acquired using MRI. Examples from cine data sets shown here include two-, three-, and four-chamber long-axis views as well as a short-axis view.

Multislice imaging is typically performed as a sequence of breath-hold acquisitions and can include both short-axis and long-axis views. Usually, one slice is acquired per breath hold; however, using phased-array radio-frequency (RF) receiver coils and parallel imaging methods multiple slices can be acquired per breath hold (7). Unlike echocardiography, arbitrary scan planes can be reproducibly prescribed, so that multiple short-axis planes and specific long-axis planes such as two-chamber and four-chamber views are readily acquired (Fig. 2). In general, blood appears bright, and myocardium appears gray or dark gray in these images; however, the specific appearance of blood, myocardium, and blood flow depends on whether spoiled gradient echo or SSFP is used for signal generation within the segmented k-space structure.

Spoiled Gradient Echo and Steady-State Free Precession

Prior to 1999, breath-hold cine MRI was generally performed using spoiled gradient echo imaging for signal generation (6,8). Using this method, longitudinal magnetization is converted to transverse magnetization by means of RF excitation and is subsequently sampled. Residual transverse magnetization is then spoiled prior to application of the next RF pulse by application of gradient pulses and by incrementing the phase of the RF pulse. Because residual magnetization is spoiled, signal intensity is not maximized; images are essentially proton density weighted, assuming that low flip angle excitations are used; and artifacts are minimized. Because of inflow into the imaging slice of protons that have not previously experienced RF excitation, blood typically appears bright.

Although image quality was considered quite good for spoiled gradient echo cine MRI, SSFP imaging of the heart was subsequently developed, which yields even better signal-to-noise and contrast-to-noise ratios (5,9). Using this approach, residual transverse magnetization is refocused, not spoiled, prior to the next RF pulse, signal intensity is maximized, and images are T_2/T_1 weighted. Because the T_2 of blood is quite long at approximately 200 ms, blood appears bright regardless of the degree of inflow in SSFP. Also, using an excitation flip angle of 50–70°, myocardium appears quite dark, resulting in superb myocardium–blood contrast and subsequently excellent delineation of the endocardial border. SSFP was not practical prior to around 2000 because it is prone to dark-band artifacts caused by off-resonance effects when the repetition time is longer than approximately 4–5 ms. However, because high-performance gradient systems have been available since the late 1990s, state-of-the-art 1.5-T MRI systems can now routinely achieve repetition times less than 4–5 ms and acquire artifact-free SSFP images of the heart. Example short- and long-axis images from electrocardiogram (ECG)-gated segmented acquisitions employing spoiled gradient echo and SSFP for signal generation are shown in Fig. 3.

In addition to different image contrast, SSFP and spoiled gradient echo also differ in sensitivity to turbulent flow. Specifically, because SSFP generally uses shorter echo times and is to some degree inherently motion compensated, this technique is less sensitive to dephasing-induced signal loss compared to spoiled gradient echo. This effect leads to a more uniform appearance of blood in cine images, which improves the appearance of most images. However, this effect also decreases sensitivity to turbulent flow, such as is demonstrated in Fig. 4, which shows a patient with aortic stenosis and turbulent flow in the ascending aorta.

Image Analysis

Cine images are most often subject to visual interpretation; however, they are also suitable for quantitative analysis (10). For example, indices that can be quantified from multislice short-axis cine MRI covering the LV include myocardial mass, end-diastolic volume, end-systolic volume, ejection fraction, stroke volume, wall thickness, wall thickening, and other parameters. These parameters are commonly computed following manual planimetry of the LV epicardial and endocardial borders as demonstrated in Fig. 5. The borders are typically traced at the end-diastolic and end-systolic cardiac phases for all slices. After border detection, cardiac volumes are calculated by multiplying the blood pool area (defined by the endocardial border) by the slice thickness and summing over slices. If there are gaps between the slices, then the gap can be included in an effective slice thickness (11). Myocardial mass can similarly be computed as the difference between the volumes determined by the epicardial and endocardial borders multiplied by

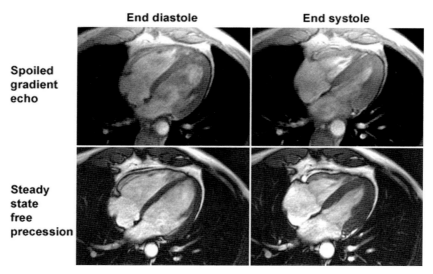

Fig. 3. Steady-state free precession (SSFP) provides greater blood–myocardium contrast compared to spoiled gradient echo. In addition, shorter repetition times are typically used for SSFP, leading to shorter scan times or improved temporal resolution.

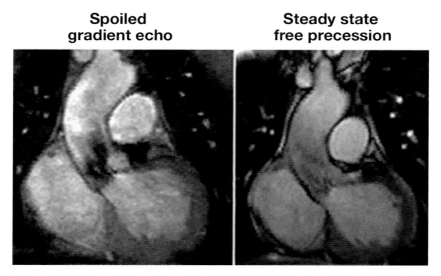

Fig. 4. Signal loss caused by turbulent flow is more pronounced using spoiled gradient echo (left) compared to SSFP (right). This may be important for the detection of valvular disease.

the specific gravity of myocardium (1.05 g/cm^3). Using these techniques, normal ranges of these parameters have been compiled for human adults *(12)* and children *(13,14)*.

The main limitation associated with quantitative analysis is the time required for manual planimetry. To address this issue, numerous automatic and semiautomatic methods for LV segmentation have been proposed. Although completely automatic segmentation remains elusive, semiautomatic approaches that rely only on manual corrections can reduce the analysis time to around 5 minutes per study *(15,16)*.

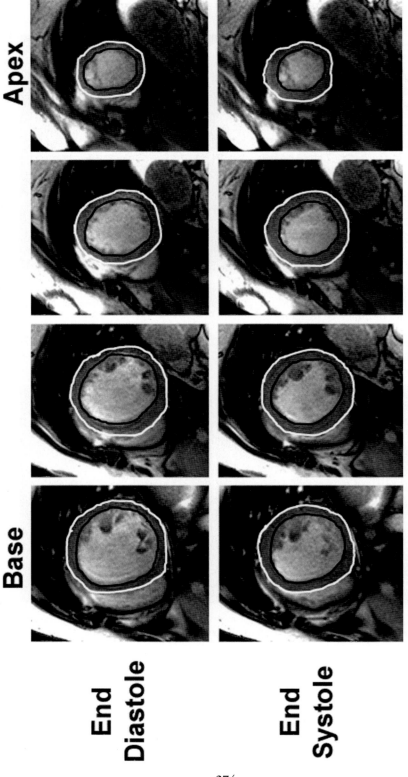

Fig. 5. LV function may be quantified by tracing the epicardial and endocardial borders on short-axis images and subsequently computing volumes, wall thickness, and wall thickening as described in the text. In this case of a patient with heart failure, eight locations were scanned for base-to-apex coverage; however, only four slices are shown.

Myocardial Tagging

In addition to cine imaging, magnetic resonance (MR) tissue-tracking methods have been developed that enable the quantitative assessment of intramyocardial contractile motion, strain, and strain rate. These techniques include myocardial tagging *(17,18)*, velocity-encoded phase contrast MRI *(19)*, harmonic phase (HARP) analysis *(20)*, and displacement encoding with stimulated echo (DENSE) *(21,22)*. Myocardial tagging is the most widely used MR tissue-tracking technique in the heart and is typically performed using breath-hold segmented *k*-space ECG-gated acquisitions *(23)*.

On detection of the ECG R-wave, which occurs before the onset of systolic contraction, RF and gradient pulses are applied that saturate the water proton magnetization in a stripe or grid pattern. Images acquired immediately after application of the tagging pulses demonstrate signal nulling in the applied stripe or grid pattern (Fig. 6, left side) because essentially no contraction has occurred between application of the tags and acquisition of the images. Because the saturated myocardial protons move coherently as the heart contracts, in subsequent cardiac phases the deformation of the stripe or grid pattern reveals intramyocardial motion (Fig. 6).

As time moves forward, the saturated protons do not retain diminished signal intensity indefinitely; rather, their magnetization recovers toward equilibrium because of T_1 relaxation. Because the T_1 of the heart at a magnetic field strength of 1.5 T is 850 ms, the tags remain adequately saturated throughout systole and into early diastole. Tag fading in late diastole because of T_1 relaxation is evident in Fig. 6. In effect, magnetically saturated protons can be tracked in a manner similar to implanted radio-opaque beads through about two-thirds of the cardiac cycle.

Like breath-hold gradient echo cine MRI, tagged cine images are generally acquired over 12–16 heartbeats during suspended respiration using a segmented *k*-space approach. Spoiled gradient echo imaging has most commonly been used for signal generation; however, studies have demonstrated better tag contrast and reduced tag fading using SSFP *(24,25)*. Also, segmented echo planar imaging has been developed for myocardial tagging during dobutamine infusion *(26)*. Example tagged long-axis images comparing LV function at rest and during dobutamine infusion (40 µg/kg/min) are shown in Fig. 7 and on the accompanying CD. Short-axis images with grid tags are often acquired, although the acquisition of two sets of short-axis images with orthogonal one-dimensional (1D) line tags, such as in Fig. 6, has also been advocated for better spatial resolution *(27)*. For more sophisticated three-dimensional (3D) analysis, tagged long-axis images can be acquired in addition to short-axis images.

Conventional strain analysis of tagged images *(28,29)* entails computer-assisted detection of the epicardial border, endocardial border, and tag lines. Border and tag detection can be performed manually or semiautomatically; however, semiautomatic techniques generally require some extent of manual correction, and either technique is usually quite time consuming.

Following border and tag detection, the computation of myocardial strain associated with tag deformation is performed automatically. Circumferential strain is the most accurately estimated element of the strain tensor from tagged images and most commonly reported component of strain. Tag detection and strain maps corresponding to the end-systolic images of Fig. 6 are shown in Fig. 8.

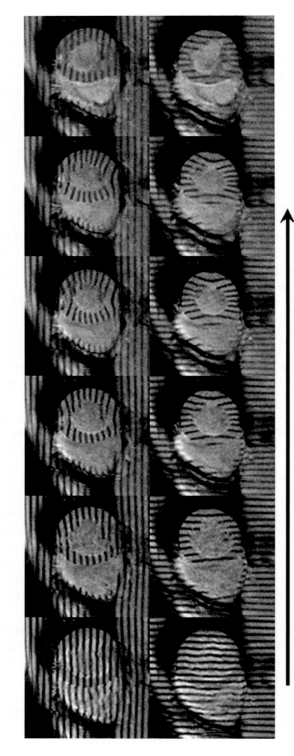

Cardiac phase

Fig. 6. Multiphase myocardial tagging of a midventricular slice using two sets of orthogonal line tags is demonstrated. The tag lines bend as the heart contracts, revealing intramyocardial motion. Tag fading over time because of T_1 relaxation is evident near the end of the cardiac cycle.

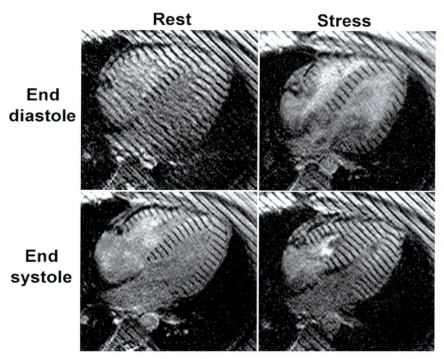

Fig. 7. Long-axis myocardial at tagging rest (left) and during high-dose dobutamine stress (right). Enhanced myocardial motion is detected at end-systole with dobutamine (bottom right) compared to rest (bottom left) (*see* movie clips in CD).

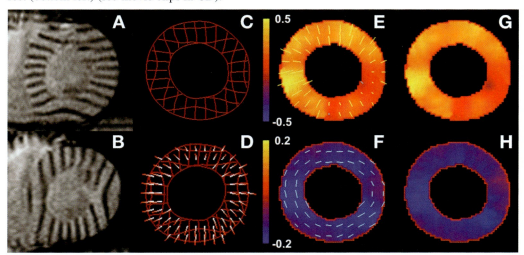

Fig. 8. Displacement and strain analysis of tagged MR images. End-systolic images with horizontal and vertical tags demonstrating systolic function are shown in (**A**) and (**B**). The results of computer-assisted tag and contour detection are shown in (**C**), and the resulting estimated 2D systolic displacement field is shown in (**D**). Myocardial strain is subsequently computed from the displacement field. The first and second principal strains, E_1 and E_2, are shown in (**E**) and (**F**), where lines indicate the direction of principal strain, and color indicates the magnitude of principal strain. In this healthy volunteer, E_1 and E_2 are oriented in approximately the radial and circumferential directions, respectively. Projecting strain into cylindrical coordinates, exact radial and circumferential strains E_{rr} and E_{cc} are shown in (**G**) and (**H**), respectively.

To overcome the time-consuming aspect of tag analysis, the HARP *(20)* and DENSE *(21,22)* techniques have been developed that do not require tag detection. Instead, the techniques encode myocardial tissue displacement into the phase of the MRI signal and then compute myocardial strain from phase-reconstructed images. These newer methods may enable the more routine clinical use of myocardial strain imaging in the future.

Real-Time Imaging

For patients who have difficulty holding their breath or when ECG gating is unreliable for either technical reasons or arrhythmias, MRI offers the ability to perform non-gated or real-time cine imaging *(30,31)*. Because real-time images are acquired without the benefit of *k*-space segmentation, image quality must be diminished in some way compared to techniques that employ *k*-space segmentation. Typically, real-time images have lower spatial and temporal resolution, and they often have more artifacts if echo planar, spiral, or undersampled radial trajectories are used. Parallel imaging techniques that use arrays of receiver coils in concert with sophisticated reconstruction algorithms to accelerate image acquisition have greatly enhanced the performance of real-time imaging *(7,32,33)*. Example real-time short-axis images with SSFP contrast, spatial resolution of 3×3 mm^2, and temporal resolution of 60 ms are shown in Fig. 9.

Although some degradation in spatial resolution, temporal resolution, and artifact are unavoidable in real-time MRI, these techniques can still be accurate for the assessment of LV systolic function. For example, Kaji et al. compared real-time spiral MRI to breath-hold segmented MRI and found that real-time imaging at rest was accurate for the measurement of LV end-diastolic volume, end-systolic volume, ejection fraction, and LV mass *(34)*. For imaging at high heart rates such as during exercise or dobutamine stress testing, although real-time MRI has not yet been directly compared to breath-hold imaging, initial results using parallel imaging appear promising. For example, echo planar images employing temporal filtering with spatial sensitivity encoding (TSENSE) parallel imaging acquired at a heart rate of 160 beats per minute immediately after vigorous exercise using an MRI-compatible ergometer are shown on the accompanying CD *(35)*.

CLINICAL APPLICATIONS

Viability in Chronic and Acute Myocardial Infarction

MRI of LV systolic function has been shown to be accurate for detecting viable myocardium in chronic ischemic heart disease. Specifically, Baer et al. and others have investigated whether the presence of contractile reserve measured by performing cine MRI at rest and during the infusion of low doses of dobutamine can predict recovery of resting function following coronary revascularization therapy. In one important study, 43 patients with documented chronic MI were studied by MRI before and 4–6 months after surgically successful coronary revascularization *(36)*. The mean LV ejection fraction was $42 \pm 10\%$ before and $51 \pm 15\%$ after revascularization. Both before and after therapy, the MRI protocol included short-axis cine imaging of the entire LV at rest and then repeated during the infusion of 10 µg/kg/min dobutamine. Cine imaging was performed either using an older nonsegmented non-breath-hold gradient echo technique or using the segmented *k*-space gradient echo technique described in this chapter. The total

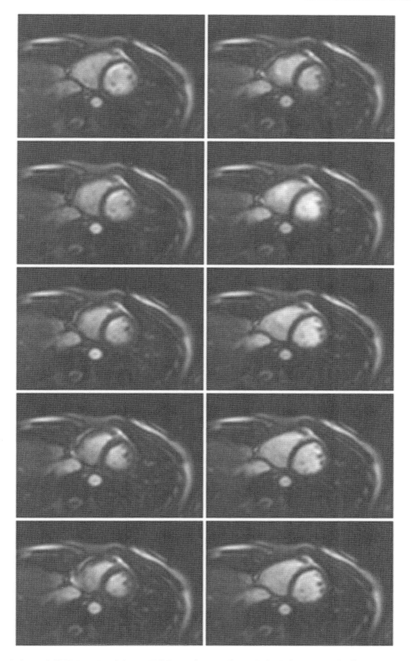

Fig. 9. Real-time SSFP MRI without ECG gating or breath holding. In this figure, time proceeds from top to bottom and then left to right. The spatial resolution is 3×3 mm^2, and the temporal resolution is 60 ms per frame (*see* movie clip in CD).

imaging time, including baseline and dobutamine imaging, was 60–80 minutes using the older technique and 20–30 minutes using the segmented sequence.

Data analysis for this study included the computation of end-diastolic wall thickness and systolic wall thickening after semiautomatic detection of the endocardial and epicardial borders. Segments were called viable if, in at least half of the segment, the end-diastolic wall thickness was 5.5 mm or greater or systolic wall thickening or dobutamine-induced systolic wall thickening was greater than 2 mm. After revascularization, resting systolic wall thickening showed that 27 of 43 patients demonstrated LV functional recovery. MRI of dobutamine-induced systolic wall thickening before therapy had a sensitivity of 89% and a specificity of 94% for detecting which patients would recover resting systolic wall thickening.

Other studies by Baer et al. comparing MRI to other modalities have shown good agreement for predicting recovery of function between MRI and positron emission tomography (37) and between MRI and transesophageal echocardiography (38). Also, a study by Dendale et al. found that the overall accuracy of older cine MRI techniques was 80% for predicting recovery of function after revascularization (39).

The transmural extent of late hyperenhancement by MRI after contrast agent infusion has been predictive of postrevascularization functional recovery independent of LV function (40). Specifically, it was shown that a greater transmural extent of hyperenhancement is related to a lower likelihood of functional recovery, and likewise, a lesser transmural extent of hyperenhancement is related to a higher likelihood of functional recovery. In particular, if the transmural extent of hyperenhancement is less than 1% or greater than 75%, then the ability to predict recovery or lack thereof, respectively, is good. However, for a transmural extent of 1–75%, the predictive value is poor.

Two studies sought to determine the concordance between low-dose dobutamine MRI and MRI of late hyperenhancement and whether low-dose dobutamine MRI of LV function could better assess recovery of function when the transmural extent of hyperenhancement is 1–75%. In the first study (41), patients were imaged only before revascularization using cine SSFP and late hyperenhancement. For those patients with an intermediate transmural extent of hyperenhancement, 61% demonstrated contractile reserve with dobutamine, whereas 39% did not, suggesting the likelihood that contractile reserve could add predictive information beyond that obtained with delayed hyperenhancement alone.

This speculation was indeed confirmed by Wellnhofer et al. who imaged patients using low-dose dobutamine and contrast enhancement before revascularization and assessed resting LV function after revascularization (42). Binary prediction of recovery was modeled by logistic regression, and different predictive models were compared by receiver operator curve–area under the curve analysis. The results showed that MRI of delayed hyperenhancement predicted the recovery or lack of recovery for 73% of segments correctly, whereas dobutamine cine MRI correctly predicted 85% of segments. Furthermore, the difference between the two techniques for predicting recovery was statistically significant, dobutamine stress magnetic resonance (DSMR) improved the performance of delayed hyperenhancement alone, and delayed hyperenhancement did not improve the performance of dobutamine cine MRI alone. It should also be noted that cine MRI in the two studies was performed with SSFP cine imaging with breath-hold durations of 7–15 heartbeats. Taken together, these studies demonstrate that dobutamine cine MRI for the assessment of global and regional LV systolic function provides an accurate assessment of myocardial viability, similar to that achieved by positron emission tomography and with better sensitivity than stress echocardiography.

Cine MRI has also shed light on LV systolic function in the setting of acute MI, for which the contractile response to dobutamine has been shown to identify stunned myocardium that, weeks later, recovers function. In one study, Geskin et al. examined 20 patients 4 ± 2 days after a first MI; the authors used breath-hold myocardial tagging applied at rest and at dobutamine doses of 5 and 10 µg/kg/minute *(43)*. Rest myocardial tagging was repeated at 8 ± 1 weeks after MI. For patients with depressed resting function and a normal peak dobutamine response of at least 5% in percentage circumferential shortening, the increase in resting percentage circumferential shortening at 8 weeks was 9 ± 9%. This increase was significantly greater than for those patients who did not demonstrate a normal initial dobutamine response, for which resting function at 8 weeks recovered only 5 ± 9%.

In a similar acute MI study, Dendale et al. investigated the sensitivity and specificity of the cine MRI dobutamine response for predicting recovery of function *(44)*. Using older non-breath-hold techniques, they reported a high sensitivity of 91% but a marginal specificity of only 69%.

Inducible Ischemia

Cine MRI of LV systolic function has also been evaluated for the detection of inducible ischemia during high-dose dobutamine stress testing. Two seminal studies of this application were published in 1999. In the first study, Nagel et al. compared DSMR to dobutamine stress echocardiography (DSE) in 208 consecutive patients with suspected coronary artery disease *(45)*. MRI was performed using segmented *k*-space gradient echo cine imaging at a field strength of 1.5 T. Imaging views included three short-axis planes and two long-axis planes, and regional wall motion was assessed using a standard 16-segment model. After acquiring baseline images, imaging was repeated at 3-minute stages with dobutamine doses of 5, 10, 20, 30, and 40 µg/kg/minute. Stress testing was stopped if heart rate reached 85% of age-predicted maximum, and atropine was added if age-predicted maximum heart rate was not reached and the stress test remained negative. DSE was performed in a similar manner and utilized second-harmonic imaging for approximately 75% of the patients. Biplane coronary angiography was performed in all patients, and significant coronary artery disease was defined as 50% or greater luminal narrowing.

Exclusion of 36 patients from the analysis was made because 18 could not be scanned by MRI for a variety of reasons and 18 had poor image quality by DSE. Coronary artery disease was diagnosed by angiography in 109 of 172 patients who successfully completed both DSE and DSMR. In these patients, the sensitivity and specificity of DSE were 74 and 70%, respectively, whereas the sensitivity and specificity of DSMR were 86 and 86%, respectively. The improvements in the sensitivity and specificity of MRI were attributed mainly to better image quality.

In the second study by Hundley et al., DSMR was performed in 153 consecutive patients who were not well suited for transthoracic echocardiography because of poor acoustic windows despite the use of second-harmonic imaging or contrast enhancement *(46)*. The MR imaging and dobutamine protocols were similar to the previous study. In the 50 patients with positive DSMR tests and subsequent coronary angiography, the sensitivity and specificity for detecting a greater than 50% luminal narrowing were 83 and 83%, respectively. For the 103 patients with negative DSMR tests, the cardiovascular occurrence-free survival rate at a mean of 228 days after DSMR was 97%.

In addition to the impressive clinical results reported in this study, the relationship between the rapid display of cine MR images and patient safety was addressed. Because the ECG cannot be monitored for ischemia in the MRI environment because of signal distortions attributed both to the magnetohydrodynamic effect and to interference from gradient pulses *(47)*, safety monitoring is accomplished in DSMR by imaging inducible wall motion abnormalities. In theory, this approach is sound because wall motion defects precede ECG changes in the ischemic cascade. In practice, this approach works best when images are rapidly reconstructed and displayed as cine loops and can be compared with other slices or dobutamine doses such as described by Hamilton et al. *(48)*.

Following up on the studies of Nagel and Hundley, Kuijpers et al. showed that visual analysis of myocardial tagging improves the ability of cine MRI to detect inducible ischemia *(49)*. Specifically, of 211 patients who underwent DSMR in this study, new wall motion abnormalities were detected in 58 patients by segmented *k*-space cine MRI and in 68 patients by myocardial tagging. Of the 68 cases detected by tagging, 65 were confirmed by angiography, demonstrating the improved sensitivity of tagging.

In addition to achieving high sensitivity and specificity, DSMR has been shown to have good prognostic utility. For example, Hundley et al. showed that the presence of inducible ischemia at DSMR when LV ejection fraction is greater than 40% identifies patients at risk for MI and cardiac death independent of conventional risk factors *(50)*. Conversely, the absence of inducible ischemia when LV ejection fraction is greater than 40% indicates a very low risk for MI and cardiac death. In addition, Kuijpers et al. showed that the presence of resting wall motion abnormalities when the stress test is negative is predictive of major adverse cardiac events, including cardiac death, MI, and clinically indicated coronary revascularization *(51)*.

Although impressive clinical results have been reported for dobutamine stress testing by MRI, it is also interesting to consider that these studies preceded or did not use some of the most recent MR methods for imaging LV function. For example, although segmented *k*-space gradient echo cine MRI was used for most studies, one might expect even better results using the newer SSFP technique. For myocardial tagging, SSFP or echo planar imaging may provide better image quality, and techniques such as HARP and DENSE could facilitate the on-line quantitation of myocardial strain. Future studies will likely determine whether these techniques further improve DSMR.

MRI of LV Synchrony

Cardiac resynchronization therapy (CRT) using biventricular pacing for patients with heart failure has recently become widespread *(52,53)*. However, although this therapy is beneficial for many patients, some do not respond, and the ability to predict response using QRS width is poor *(52)*. In this context, research has investigated echocardiography and MRI for the assessment of mechanical dyssynchrony as a better index for identifying CRT candidates. In echocardiography, spatiotemporal dyssynchrony can be assessed using tissue Doppler methods to compare the timing of mechanical function in different segments of the heart *(54)*. Some specific spatiotemporal measurements used to assess dyssynchrony include the extent of myocardium with delayed contraction and the difference in time to the onset of contraction in the lateral wall compared to the basal septum.

Studies have also begun to investigate the use of MRI to assess cardiac dyssynchrony *(55)*. For example, Wyman et al. showed, using 3D strain analysis of myocardial tagging in dogs, that markedly different mechanical activation patterns across the entire LV can be quantified when different pacing sites are employed *(56)*. Indeed, because MRI can sample a large extent of the LV compared to tissue Doppler, more comprehensive indices such as the temporal duration required for the onset of contraction to occur over 20–90% of the LV can be used.

In another MRI study using a canine model of left bundle branch block and pacing-induced heart failure, Leclercq et al. showed that both biventricular pacing and LV pacing improve LV synchrony, and interestingly, LV pacing does so without improving electrical synchrony *(57)*. Finally, although data are yet to be published regarding the ability of MRI to predict response to CRT, high temporal resolution MRI data detailing normal human spatiotemporal contraction has shown in normal volunteers that MRI detects earliest onset of contraction in the lateral wall followed by latest onset in the septum *(58)*. Also, the time for onset to occur over 20–90% of the LV is 35 ± 9 ms, whereas the time of peak contraction over 20–90% of the LV is 121 ± 22 ms. In summary, largely because of the greater spatial coverage of MRI and the ability also to perform delayed contrast-enhanced MRI of scar, these studies suggest that MRI may play a role in evaluating CRT candidates in the future.

MRI of LV Systolic Function in the Context of an Integrated Cardiovascular Magnetic Resonance Exam

Although MRI of LV systolic function is a powerful modality in its own right, this technique is typically not used alone. Rather, MRI of LV systolic function is often used in the context of an integrated cardiac MRI exam when MR methods for imaging myocardial anatomy, perfusion, perfusion reserve, and infarction can all be readily employed *(59–61)*. For example, if a resting wall motion defect is seen in a region of delayed contrast enhancement, then it is caused by a MI. However, if delayed hyperenhancement is not seen, then the resting wall motion defect may represent ischemic, stunned, or hibernating myocardium. In this case, additional wall motion imaging during dobutamine infusion may aid in the differential diagnosis. In another example, if only a small transmural extent of delayed hyperenhancement is seen and the clinical question concerns viability, then wall motion imaging during dobutamine infusion can be employed.

SUMMARY

MR is the most accurate modality for imaging LV systolic function and myocardial mass. The SSFP technique provides high spatial resolution, excellent image contrast, and short acquisition times. When breath holding or ECG gating fail, real-time MRI can be used with only minor degradation in image quality. Because MRI can be performed in arbitrary planes such as true short- and long-axis views, the assessment of LV function is very reproducible and can be accurately quantified. In addition to standard cine MRI, techniques such as myocardial tagging for quantifying intramyocardial strain exist that may improve accuracy in detecting wall motion abnormalities and may enable new applications such as quantifying mechanical dyssynchrony of the heart. Furthermore, all of these techniques may be used during pharmacological stress to detect critical coronary stenoses or viable myocardium. In summary, MR of LV systolic function can answer many clinical questions and is often most useful when used in conjunction with other MR techniques for imaging myocardial structure, perfusion, and infarction.

ACKNOWLEDGMENTS

I would like to acknowledge the important contributions of Christopher Kramer and David Isbell regarding the role of CMR in clinical cardiology, John Christopher for help acquiring images, and Moriel Vandsburger for assistance in preparing figures.

REFERENCES

1. White HD, Norris RM, Brown MA, et al. Left ventricular end-systolic volume as the major determinant of survival after recovery from myocardial infarction. Circulation 1987;76:44–51.
2. Pattynama PM, Lamb HJ, van der Velde EA, Van der Wall EE, De Roos A. Left ventricular measurements with cine and spin-echo MR imaging: a study of reproducibility with variance component analysis. Radiology 1993;187:261–268.
3. Cranney GB, Lotan CS, Dean L, et al. Left ventricular volume measurement using cardiac axis nuclear magnetic resonance imaging. Validation by calibrated ventricular angiography. Circulation 1990;82: 154–163.
4. Ichikawa Y, Sakuma H, Kitagawa K, et al. Evaluation of left ventricular volumes and ejection fraction using fast steady-state cine MR imaging: comparison with left ventricular angiography. J Cardiovasc Magn Reson 2003;5:333–342.
5. Carr JC, Simonetti O, Bundy J, Li D, Pereles S, Finn JP. Cine MR angiography of the heart with segmented true fast imaging with steady-state precession. Radiology 2001;219:828–834.
6. Atkinson DJ, Edelman RR. Cineangiography of the heart in a single breath hold with a segmented turboFLASH sequence. Radiology 1991;178:357–360.
7. Pruessmann KP, Weiger M, Boesiger P. Sensitivity encoded cardiac MRI. J Cardiovasc Magn Reson 2001;3:1–9.
8. Foo TK, Bernstein MA, Aisen AM, Hernandez RJ, Collick BD, Bernstein T. Improved ejection fraction and flow velocity estimates with use of view sharing and uniform repetition time excitation with fast cardiac techniques. Radiology 1995;195:471–478.
9. Heid O. True FISP cardiac fluoroscopy. Seventh Annual Meeting of the ISMRM 1997;320–320.
10. Moon JC, Lorenz CH, Francis JM, Smith GC, Pennell DJ. Breath-hold FLASH and FISP cardiovascular MR imaging: left ventricular volume differences and reproducibility. Radiology 2002;223:789–797.
11. Cottin Y, Touzery C, Guy F, et al. MR imaging of the heart in patients after myocardial infarction: effect of increasing intersection gap on measurements of left ventricular volume, ejection fraction, wall thickness. Radiology 1999;213:513–520.
12. Lorenz CH, Walker ES, Morgan VL, Klein SS, Graham TP Jr. Normal human right and left ventricular mass, systolic function, gender differences by cine magnetic resonance imaging. J Cardiovasc Magn Reson 1999;1:7–21.
13. Lorenz CH. The range of normal values of cardiovascular structures in infants, children, adolescents measured by magnetic resonance imaging. Pediatr Cardiol 2000;21:37–46.
14. Alfakih K, Plein S, Thiele H, Jones T, Ridgway JP, Sivananthan MU. Normal human left and right ventricular dimensions for MRI as assessed by turbo gradient echo and steady-state free precession imaging sequences. J Magn Reson Imaging 2003;17:323–329.
15. Young AA, Cowan BR, Thrupp SF, Hedley WJ, Dell'Italia LJ. Left ventricular mass and volume: fast calculation with guide-point modeling on MR images. Radiology 2000;216:597–602.
16. van der Geest RJ, Lelieveldt BP, Reiber JH. Quantification of global and regional ventricular function in cardiac magnetic resonance imaging. Topics Magn Reson Imaging 2000;11:348–358.
17. Zerhouni EA, Parish DM, Rogers WJ, Yang A, Shapiro EP. Tagging with MR imaging—a method for noninvasive assessment of myocardial motion. Radiology 1988;169:59–63.
18. Axel L, Dougherty L. Imaging of motion with spatial modulation of magnetization. Radiology 1989;171:841–845.
19. Pelc LR, Sayre J, Yun K, et al. Evaluation of myocardial motion tracking with cine-phase contrast magnetic resonance imaging. Invest Radiol 1994;29:1038–1042.
20. Osman NF, Kerwin WS, McVeigh ER, Prince JL. Cardiac motion tracking using CINE harmonic phase (HARP) magnetic resonance imaging. Magn Reson Med 1999;42:1048–1060.
21. Aletras AH, Ding S, Balaban RS, Wen H. DENSE: displacement encoding with stimulated echoes in cardiac functional MRI. J Magn Reson 1999;137:247–252.
22. Kim D, Gilson WD, Kramer CM, Epstein FH. Myocardial tissue tracking with two-dimensional cine displacement-encoded MR imaging: development and initial evaluation. Radiology 2004;230:862–871.
23. McVeigh ER, Atalar E. Cardiac tagging with breath-hold cine MRI. Magn Reson Med 1992;28:318–327.
24. Zwanenburg JJ, Kuijer JP, Marcus JT, Heethaar RM. Steady-state free precession with myocardial tagging: CSPAMM in a single breathhold. Magn Reson Med 2003;49:722–730.
25. Herzka DA, Guttman MA, McVeigh ER. Myocardial tagging with SSFP. Magn Reson Med 2003;49:329–340.

26. Kim D, Bove CM, Kramer CM, Epstein FH. Importance of *k*-space trajectory in echo-planar myocardial tagging at rest and during dobutamine stress. Magn Reson Med 2003;50:813–820.

27. McVeigh ER. MRI of myocardial function: motion tracking techniques. Magn Reson Imaging 1996;14:137–150.

28. Young AA, Imai H, Chang CN, Axel L. Two-dimensional left ventricular deformation during systole using magnetic resonance imaging with spatial modulation of magnetization [erratum appears in Circulation 1994;90:1584]. Circulation 1994;89:740–752.

29. Guttman MA, Prince JL, McVeigh ER. Tag and contour detection in tagged MR images of the left ventricle. IEEE Trans Med Imaging 1994;13:74–88.

30. Hardy CJ, Darrow RD, Nieters EJ, et al. Real-time acquisition, display, interactive graphic control of NMR cardiac profiles and images. Magn Reson Med 1993;29:667–673.

31. Kerr AB, Pauly JM, Hu BS, et al. Real-time interactive MRI on a conventional scanner [erratum appears in Magn Reson Med 1998;40:952–955]. Magn Reson Med 1997;38:355–367.

32. Jakob PM, Griswold MA, Edelman RR, Manning WJ, Sodickson DK. Accelerated cardiac imaging using the SMASH technique. J Cardiovasc Magn Reson 1999;1:153–157.

33. Guttman MA, Kellman P, Dick AJ, Lederman RJ, McVeigh ER. Real-time accelerated interactive MRI with adaptive TSENSE and UNFOLD. Magn Reson Med 2003;50:315–321.

34. Kaji S, Yang PC, Kerr AB, et al. Rapid evaluation of left ventricular volume and mass without breath-holding using real-time interactive cardiac magnetic resonance imaging system. J Am Coll Cardiol 2001;38:527–533.

35. Kellman P, Epstein FH, McVeigh ER. Adaptive sensitivity encoding incorporating temporal filtering (TSENSE). Magn Reson Med 2001;45:846–852.

36. Baer FM, Theissen P, Schneider CA, et al. Dobutamine magnetic resonance imaging predicts contractile recovery of chronically dysfunctional myocardium after successful revascularization. J Am Coll Cardiol 1998;31:1040–1048.

37. Baer FM, Voth E, Schneider CA, Theissen P, Schicha H, Sechtem U. Comparison of low-dose dobutamine-gradient-echo magnetic resonance imaging and positron emission tomography with [18F] fluorodeoxyglucose in patients with chronic coronary artery disease. A functional and morphological approach to the detection of residual myocardial viability. Circulation 1995;91:1006–1015.

38. Baer FM, Theissen P, Crnac J, et al. Head to head comparison of dobutamine-transoesophageal echocardiography and dobutamine–magnetic resonance imaging for the prediction of left ventricular functional recovery in patients with chronic coronary artery disease. Eur Heart J 2000;21:981–991.

39. Dendale P, Franken PR, Holman E, Avenarius J, Van der Wall EE, De Roos A. Validation of low-dose dobutamine magnetic resonance imaging for assessment of myocardial viability after infarction by serial imaging. Am J Cardiol 1998;82:375–377.

40. Kim RJ, Wu E, Rafael A, et al. The use of contrast-enhanced magnetic resonance imaging to identify reversible myocardial dysfunction. N Engl J M 2000;343:1445–1453.

41. Kaandorp TA, Bax JJ, Schuijf JD, et al. Head-to-head comparison between contrast-enhanced magnetic resonance imaging and dobutamine magnetic resonance imaging in men with ischemic cardiomyopathy. Am J Cardiol 2004;93:1461–1464.

42. Wellnhofer E, Olariu A, Klein C, et al. Magnetic resonance low-dose dobutamine test is superior to SCAR quantification for the prediction of functional recovery. Circulation 2004;109:2172–2174.

43. Geskin G, Kramer CM, Rogers WJ, et al. Quantitative assessment of myocardial viability after infarction by dobutamine magnetic resonance tagging. Circulation 1998;98:217–223.

44. Dendale PA, Franken PR, Waldman GJ, et al. Low-dosage dobutamine magnetic resonance imaging as an alternative to echocardiography in the detection of viable myocardium after acute infarction. Am Heart J 1995;130:134–140.

45. Nagel E, Lehmkuhl HB, Bocksch W, et al. Noninvasive diagnosis of ischemia-induced wall motion abnormalities with the use of high-dose dobutamine stress MRI: comparison with dobutamine stress echocardiography. Circulation 1999;99:763–770.

46. Hundley WG, Hamilton CA, Thomas MS, et al. Utility of fast cine magnetic resonance imaging and display for the detection of myocardial ischemia in patients not well suited for second harmonic stress echocardiography. Circulation 1999;100:1697–1702.

47. Fischer SE, Wickline SA, Lorenz CH. Novel real-time R-wave detection algorithm based on the vectorcardiogram for accurate gated magnetic resonance acquisitions. Magn Reson Med 1999;42:361–370.

48. Hamilton CA, Link KM, Salido TB, Epstein FH, Hundley WG. Is imaging at intermediate doses necessary during dobutamine stress magnetic resonance imaging? J Cardiovasc Magn Reson 2001; 3:297–302.

49. Kuijpers D, Ho KY, van Dijkman PR, Vliegenthart R, Oudkerk M. Dobutamine cardiovascular magnetic resonance for the detection of myocardial ischemia with the use of myocardial tagging. Circulation 2003;107:1592–1597.

50. Hundley WG, Morgan TM, Neagle CM, Hamilton CA, Rerkpattanapipat P, Link KM. Magnetic resonance imaging determination of cardiac prognosis. Circulation 2002;106:2328–2333.

51. Kuijpers D, van Dijkman PR, Janssen CH, Vliegenthart R, Zijlstra F, Oudkerk M. Dobutamine stress MRI. Part II. Risk stratification with dobutamine cardiovascular magnetic resonance in patients suspected of myocardial ischemia. Eur Radiol 2004;14:2046–2052.

52. Abraham WT, Fisher WG, Smith AL, et al. Cardiac resynchronization in chronic heart failure. N Engl J Med 2002;346:1845–1853.

53. Bradley DJ, Bradley EA, Baughman KL, et al. Cardiac resynchronization and death from progressive heart failure: a meta-analysis of randomized controlled trials. JAMA 2003;289:730–740.

54. Sogaard P, Egeblad H, Kim WY, et al. Tissue Doppler imaging predicts improved systolic performance and reversed left ventricular remodeling during long-term cardiac resynchronization therapy. J Am Coll Cardiol 2002;40:723–730.

55. McVeigh ER, Prinzen FW, Wyman BT, Tsitlik JE, Halperin HR, Hunter WC. Imaging asynchronous mechanical activation of the paced heart with tagged MRI. Magn Reson Med 1998;39:507–513.

56. Wyman BT, Hunter WC, Prinzen FW, McVeigh ER. Mapping propagation of mechanical activation in the paced heart with MRI tagging. Am J Physiol 1999;276:H881–H891.

57. Leclercq C, Faris O, Tunin R, et al. Systolic improvement and mechanical resynchronization does not require electrical synchrony in the dilated failing heart with left bundle-branch block. Circulation 2002;106:1760–1763.

58. Zwanenburg JJ, Gotte MJ, Kuijer JP, Heethaar RM, van Rossum AC, Marcus JT. Timing of cardiac contraction in humans mapped by high-temporal-resolution MRI tagging: early onset and late peak of shortening in lateral wall. Am J Physiol Heart Circ Physiol 2004;286:H1872–H1880.

59. Sensky PR, Jivan A, Hudson NM, et al. Coronary artery disease: combined stress MR imaging protocol-one-stop evaluation of myocardial perfusion and function. Radiology 2000;215:608–614.

60. Plein S, Ridgway JP, Jones TR, Bloomer TN, Sivananthan MU. Coronary artery disease: assessment with a comprehensive MR imaging protocol—initial results. Radiology 2002;225:300–307.

61. Kwong RY, Schussheim AE, Rekhraj S, et al. Detecting acute coronary syndrome in the emergency department with cardiac magnetic resonance imaging. Circulation 2003;107:531–537.

13 Acute Myocardial Infarction and Postinfarct Remodeling

David C. Isbell and Christopher M. Kramer

CONTENTS

ACUTE MYOCARDIAL INFARCTION

Magnetic Resonance Assessment of Left Ventricular Size and Function Postinfarction

In the wake of an acute myocardial infarction (AMI), accurate assessment of the left ventricle (LV) is of paramount importance as functional impairment or chamber dilatation predicts increased mortality *(1–3)*. In a study of 866 postinfarct patients, a resting LV ejection fraction (EF) less than 0.40 predicted higher 1-year mortality than did an LVEF greater than 0.40 *(1)*. Others have demonstrated that, following reperfusion therapy, the relationship between resting LVEF and all-cause mortality persists *(4)*. Although LVEF is a powerful predictor of postinfarct survival, end-systolic volume (ESV) is superior as a prognostic parameter. This was demonstrated by White et al., who enrolled 605 patients following AMI and followed them for an average of 78 months. Ultimately, ESV was the best predictor of survival, and neither the LVEF nor end-diastolic volume (EDV) added prognostic value.

Radionuclide imaging and transthoracic echocardiography are widely available and well-validated noninvasive techniques employed for measuring LVEF and cardiac volumes. Although studies have generally demonstrated good correlation between these modalities, both inter- and intraobserver agreement is suboptimal, and most studies have only assessed patients with normal LV dimensions and function *(5)*. Moreover, in patients following AMI, distortion of LV chamber size and geometry can exacerbate measurement error.

In contrast, cardiovascular magnetic resonance (CMR) generates a complete three-dimensional (3D) data set from apex to base with high temporal and spatial resolution (Fig. 1). Measurements made with these data set do not require geometric assumptions

From: *Contemporary Cardiology: Cardiovascular Magnetic Resonance Imaging*
Edited by: Raymond Y. Kwong © Humana Press Inc., Totowa, NJ

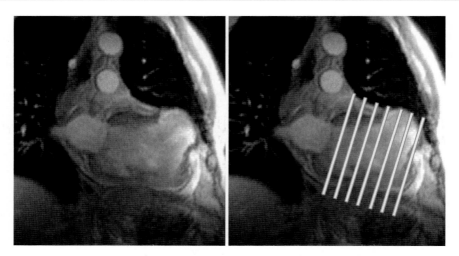

Fig. 1. End-systolic gradient echo cine MR in a two-chamber orientation from a patient 7 years following a large anterior MI (left panel) who presented with congestive heart failure. Geometric distortion is profound as this patient has a large pseudoaneurysm (2- to 3-mm thick with base wider than the neck) in the anterior wall and evidence of global remodeling. With CMR, a 3D data set is acquired in short axis (right panel), allowing for accurate measure of ventricular dimensions and function.

and are therefore less prone to error in ventricles deformed by infarction. Furthermore, the large field of view and excellent contrast generated between the myocardium and blood pool facilitate accurate assessment of chamber dimensions and both regional and global function *(6)*. Consequently, CMR is increasingly employed for prognostication and to guide therapeutic management in patients postinfarct.

Contrast-Enhanced CMR

Histopathologic studies of AMI have consistently revealed the complex, heterogeneous, and dynamic character of infarct zones *(7)*. This heterogeneity appears to be a consequence of many factors, including the presence and opening of collaterals during and after injury, magnitude of the ischemic insult, and impact of therapeutic interventions *(8)*. Furthermore, it has been demonstrated that infarcts evolve over time, generally passing through an early, necrotic phase followed by both a fibrotic and remodeling phase that is dominated by the laying down of new collagen and infarct involution *(9,10)*. In fact, infarct scar remains biologically active long after ischemic injury, populated by cells involved in collagen turnover and scar tissue contraction, and may therefore never truly reach a "stable" configuration *(7)*.

In the acute phase, at the very core of infarcts and typically within the subendocardium, there is often microvascular obstruction (MO). MO may result from embolization and platelet activation, although the exact mechanisms are unclear *(11)*. These areas are generally devoid of blood flow and have also been described as "no-reflow zones" with the extent of no reflow related to total infarct size *(12)*. Surrounding areas of no reflow are often comprised of myocytes subjected to significant, but varying, degrees of ischemic injury. Many undergo necrosis with loss of membrane integrity and depletion of cellular energy stores *(13)*. In this acute phase, tissue edema, hemorrhage, and inflammation can increase infarct volume by as much as 25% *(8)*. Beyond these necrotic regions, dysfunctional, nonnecrotic tissue coexists that has the potential for functional recovery *(14)*.

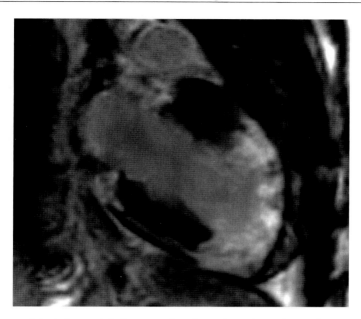

Fig. 2. LGE image of the left ventricle in a two-chamber orientation using a phase-sensitive inversion recovery technique. This image was acquired from a patient following a large anterior MI who was found to have total occlusion of the LAD artery at cardiac catheterization. The image demonstrates extensive transmural hyperenhancement extending from the mid anterior wall to the LV apex and distal one-third of the inferior wall, a pattern consistent with infarction in the territory supplied by the LAD artery. On the basis of this image, no recovery of resting function could be anticipated in the infarcted segments following revascularization.

Thus, a region of systolic dysfunction following myocardial infarction (MI) will generally consist of a combination of reversibly injured (stunned) and irreversibly injured (infarcted) myocardium, with the severity of dysfunction a poor marker for the transmural extent of necrosis *(5)*. With the development of late gadolinium-enhanced CMR, these tissue states can be distinguished within the same segment of myocardium.

Late gadolinium enhancement (LGE) refers to regions of scar, necrosis, or inflammation discriminated from normal tissue by prolonged retention of a gadolinium-based contrast agent. Since the mid-1980s, investigators have appreciated T_1 shortening (increased enhancement) in regions of infarction following gadolinium administration *(16–18)*. However, these early imaging techniques were limited by long acquisition times, artifacts, and insufficient contrast between normal and abnormal regions. With faster imaging sequences using *k*-space segmentation, LGE can be performed in a single breath hold with collection of data during the diastolic phase of the cardiac cycle when there is less cardiac motion. Implementation of an inversion recovery pulse sequence with inversion time set to null normal myocardium increases the signal difference between normal and infarcted segments by 500–1000%, allowing enhanced detection and delineation of small subendocardial infarcts *(19)*.

Kim et al. demonstrated that the spatial extent of hyperenhancement seen on CMR closely mirrored the distribution of myocyte necrosis in the early period following infarction and that of collagenous scar seen at 8 weeks ($R = 0.97$, $p < 0.001$) *(20)*; in regions of the heart subjected to reversible injury, the retention of contrast did *not* occur *(21)* (Fig. 2). LGE accurately delineates infarction as defined by the histology at various time-points following injury *(22)*.

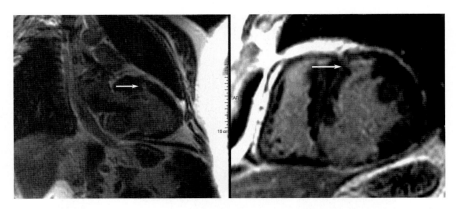

Fig. 3. A patient with known coronary disease and basal inferior aneurysm with recent percutaneous intervention of the proximal LAD artery. The intervention was complicated by a small enzyme leak. LGE images using a gradient echo inversion recovery technique in a two-chamber (left panel) and short-axis (right panel) orientation are shown. In addition to the infarct and large aneurysm of the basal inferior wall, a small region of hyperenhancement is seen in the midanterior wall (arrows) consistent with microinfarction related to recent percutaneous intervention in the LAD territory.

When compared to other noninvasive techniques, LGE is more reliable in detecting infarct scar. In a study of 91 patients with suspected or known coronary artery disease, Wagner et al. performed both LGE and single photon emission computed tomography (SPECT) imaging to evaluate the location, extent, and size of infarction *(23)*. Although SPECT correctly identified all patients with transmural or near-transmural scar seen on LGE, SPECT failed to correctly identify nearly half of those with subendocardial infarction. Klein et al. compared LGE to positron emission tomography in 31 patients with ischemic heart failure *(24)*. Infarct mass correlated well between the two modalities ($r = 0.81$, $p < 0.0001$), but LGE more frequently identified scar than positron emission tomography, again reflecting the superior spatial resolution of CMR.

Transmural extent of infarct scar, as determined on LGE is a powerful predictor of functional recovery following acute infarction. Choi et al. performed contrast-enhanced CMR on 24 MI patients within 7 days of successful revascularization. Scans were repeated at 8–12 weeks to assess functional recovery *(25)*. There was an inverse relationship between transmural extent of infarction and segmental recovery of function ($p = 0.001$). Moreover, the best predictor of improved wall thickening and global function was the extent of dysfunctional myocardium that was either without LGE or had LGE that comprised less than 25% of wall thickness.

Investigators have exploited the enhanced sensitivity of CMR to study small infarctions after both percutaneous intervention *(26,27)* and coronary artery bypass surgery *(28)*. Ricciardi et al. utilized LGE to evaluate the mechanism of creatine kinase-MB fraction (CK-MB) release after successful percutaneous coronary intervention *(27)*. Fourteen patients without evidence of prior MI were imaged following elective percutaneous intervention. Nine experienced elevation of cardiac enzymes following the procedure; 5 did not. In all patients with an enzyme leak (median CK-MB was 21 ng/mL), a discrete area of LGE was seen in the target vessel zone. This LGE persisted in all but one of the patients at follow-up scan 3–12 months later; LGE was not detected in any control patient (Fig. 3).

Evidence suggests LGE may be a valuable tool for predicting major adverse cardiac events (MACE). In a study by Kwong et al, 195 patients were evaluated for LGE in a variety of clinical circumstances, including 29% with known CAD *(29)*. After 16 months

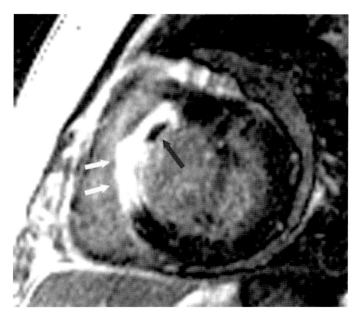

Fig. 4. LGE image of the LV in short axis using a gradient echo inversion recovery technique. Transmural LGE can be seen in the anteroseptal wall (white arrows) with small region of MO at the core of the infarct zone (black arrow). MO is associated with larger infarcts, greater remodeling, and an increase in adverse clinical outcomes.

of follow-up, LGE was found to be the strongest predictor of MACE (HR 8.29, $p <$ 0.0001). Adjusted to segmental wall motion abnormality or LVEF, LGE maintained a strong association with MACE.

Investigators have also established the clinical importance of MO, regions typically at the core of infarcts that are sometimes referred to as no-reflow zones (Fig. 4). In a study of 17 patients on day 4 post-MI with contrast-enhanced CMR, Rogers et al. demonstrated that regions with MO were nonviable as no recovery of function was noted at 7 weeks post-MI in these territories *(30)*.

At an average of 10 days after infarction, Wu et al. performed CMR on 44 patients with MO defined as hypoenhancement at 1–2 minutes after contrast injection *(31)*. Even after infarct size was controlled for, the presence of MO remained a prognostic marker of postinfarction complications ($\chi^2 = 5.17$, $p < 0.05$) and LV remodeling ($p < 0.05$).

Hombach et al. studied 110 postinfarct patients with MO defined as persistent hypoenhancement on delayed contrast imaging *(32)*. At an average of 6 days following infarct, 46% of the patients imaged had MO; none were found to have MO on follow-up. Patients with cardiac death had a lower LVEF (41.5 ± 8.3 vs $58.1 \pm 10.0\%$), larger infarcts (15.7 ± 10.1 vs $11.7 \pm 7.2\%$), and a greater extent of MO (3.6 ± 3.2 vs $1.2 \pm 2.2\%$) than survivors. Furthermore, MO was a better predictor of MACE than infarct size.

LEFT VENTRICULAR REMODELING

LV remodeling refers to maladaptive alterations in ventricular geometry and function that develop in response to myocardial injury. Remodeling is characterized by a complex series of histopathologic changes in both injured and uninjured segments that is set in motion after an ischemic insult. Early after infarction, expansion of the scar can occur with thinning of the affected region and an increase in scar surface area *(33)*. The extent of this infarct expansion is dependent on a number of factors, including infarct size, location, preload, and afterload *(34)*. As a consequence of this expansion and chamber enlargement, LV wall tension increases, which in turn results in both a mechanical and energetic disadvantage *(35)*. Further alterations in LV geometry are the result of lengthening of the noninfarcted regions in response to the increased stress *(36–38)*. From a clinical perspective, the remodeling process is maladaptive and results in higher patient mortality compared to that of postinfarct patients with preserved LV geometry following ischemic injury *(3,39)*.

Although both left ventriculography *(40)* and echocardiography *(41)* are widely used to evaluate LV size and function postinfarction, assessment of a remodeled ventricle can pose a significant challenge to these modalities. In contrast, CMR is ideally suited for the task because an enlarged, deformed ventricle influences CMR measurements to a lesser extent *(42)*. With its high spatial resolution, reproducibility, and 3D data set that requires the operator to make no geometric assumptions, CMR has evolved into the reference standard for measuring mass, chamber volumes, and EF *(42,43)*. The precision and reproducibility afforded by CMR has fueled its wide acceptance as the gold standard for the assessment of LV remodeling and led to its increased utilization for both clinical and research purposes. Already, CMR has played an important role in both understanding the natural history of LV remodeling and investigation of both pharmacological and nonpharmacological interventions employed to attenuate the remodeling process.

MR Evaluation of Ventricular Geometry and Function

LV remodeling has been investigated extensively with CMR in animal models both large *(37)* and small *(44,45)*. In a large animal model of MI induced by coronary ligation, short-axis MR images were used to follow LV mass, EDVs, and ESVs in the first 6 months after infarct *(37)*. A stepwise increase in LV mass and volumes was observed, with volumes increasing disproportionately to mass over the 6-months period. Infarct wall thickness decreased over the same period; there was no change observed in noninfarcted regions. However, there was an increase in segment length over the 6 months, suggesting that the hypertrophy in noninfarcted segments was of the eccentric type *(46)*. Additional studies showed that cellular hypertrophy in these adjacent regions was eccentric, with an increase in cell length *(47)*.

Ross et al. assessed remodeling in a mouse model of reperfused injury of the left anterior descending (LAD) artery *(45)*. On day 1 following injury, the LVEF declined by more than half and remained depressed throughout the study. By 4 weeks, a threefold increase in end systolic volume index (ESVI) and fourfold increase in end diastolic volume index (EDVI) were observed. Moreover, transmural LV wall thickening analysis demonstrated reduced contractile function in remote septal regions. Similar natural history studies of both LV and right ventricular remodeling have been published in rat models of infarction *(48,49)*.

CMR has also been employed to evaluate postinfarct LV remodeling in human subjects. Matheijessen et al. demonstrated that measurement of LV volume and mass could be performed with a high degree of precision using manual contouring methods following infarction. In their study of 7 patients, intra- and interobserver variability were in the 2–5% range for both myocardial mass and chamber volumes *(50)*. Konermann et al. employed cine CMR to study changes in LV geometry for the first 6 months following infarction in 61 patients *(51)*. Cine CMR was performed at 1, 6, and 26 weeks after the ischemic insult. LVEDV increased from 74 ± 23 to 85 ± 28 mL/m^2, LVESVI from 40 ± 19 to 51 ± 29 mL/m^2, and myocardial mass from 246 ± 66 to 276 ± 80 g over the course of the study, with the greatest increase in volumes among the subgroup of patients with anterior MI. Both size and location of infarction were found to be the best predictors of remodeling.

In 26 human subjects with anterior MI and LVEF below 50%, CMR was used to evaluate LV geometry on day 5 and week 8 after reperfusion therapy *(52)*. Although LV mass decreased during the 8-weeks follow-up, falling from 109 ± 19 to 102 ± 18 g/m^2, LVEDVI increased (83 ± 24 to 96 ± 27 m/L/m^2), and ESV failed to change significantly over the study period (52 ± 20 to 54 ± 24 mL/m^2). LVEF did improve, from $39 \pm 12\%$ to $45 \pm 14\%$, despite an increase in LVEDVI. By multivariate analysis, the only predictor of increased LVEDVI was peak creatine kinase, a surrogate marker of infarct size.

In 51 patients postinfarction, Schroeder et al. performed serial long-axis cine CMR at week 1, 13, 26, and 52 *(53)*. Early increases in LV mass were attributed to edema in the infarcted myocardium, with late increases the consequence of hypertrophy of noninfarcted segments. Interestingly, LV mass increased to a greater extent in patients who received thrombolysis compared to those who underwent percutaneous transluminal angioplasty.

A number of MR methods have been employed to study regional LV function during postinfarct remodeling. These include cine CMR, 3D wall-thickening analysis, and MR tagging. In an ovine model of remodeling, Kramer et al. used MR tagging to assess regional function at baseline and 1, 8, and 24 weeks following experimentally induced infarction *(37)*. A difference was appreciated in circumferential and longitudinal shortening between adjacent and remote noninfarcted regions during the course of the study. Although these differences were seen early as 1 week after infarct, there was partial improvement in adjacent regions during infarct healing. A similar animal model was used to demonstrate that adjacent or border zone fibers were stretched during isovolumic systole, and that this contributed to reduced fiber shortening during ejection *(54)*.

In a study of 25 patients 3 weeks after anterior MI, Holman et al. performed cine MR and analyzed functional data with a 3D wall-thickening approach. Thickening was reduced compared to normal controls in territories perfused by the LAD and left circumflex arteries. The quantity of dysfunctional myocardium correlated well with an enzymatic measure of infarct size *(55)*. A separate study of 28 patients on day 5 ± 2 after first reperfused anterior MI used MR tagging to demonstrate dysfunction within remote noninfarcted regions *(56)*. Dysfunction was observed in the apex, anterior wall, and septum relative to a normal database as well as mild dysfunction in remote noninfarcted regions. When this same group was reevaluated at 8 weeks, improvement in regional function was observed in both infarcted and noninfarcted segments *(52)*. The dysfunction seen in remote regions on day 5 resolved by week 8 and EF increased from $39 \pm 12\%$ to $45 \pm 14\%$. These improvements occurred despite an increase in LVEDVI during the same period. As in the ovine model, regional improvements in function following infarction were uncoupled from changes in LV volume.

MR Spectroscopic Evaluation of Energetics During LV Remodeling

MR spectroscopy (MRS) has been utilized to study metabolic derangements during the remodeling process. In a canine study of LV remodeling following direct current shock, Zhang and McDonald performed spatially localized ^{31}P spectroscopy to assess changes over a 12-months period. Energetics in these 11 animals with myocardial injury were compared to those seen in 8 normal animals. In the infarcted group, the phosphocreatine/adenosine triphosphate ratio (PCr/ATP) was reduced in both the subepicardium and subendocardium, evidence of an abnormal transmural distribution of high-energy phosphates in remodeled ventricles. In the same animal model, pacing reduced the endocardial/epicardial blood flow ratio. This was associated with a fall in PCr/ATP and increase in inorganic phosphate/phosphocreatine (Pi/PCr) in the subendocardium, suggesting that blood flow redistribution could lead to the alterations observed in high-energy phosphate levels in remodeled hearts. This work also suggested that the extent of remodeling correlated with the PCr/ATP ratio in the subendocardium (57).

In the perfused remodeled rat myocardium, Friedrich et al. utilized ^{31}P MRS to demonstrate changes in high-energy phosphates (58). In remodeled animals, the amount of PCr per unit mass in remodeled, noninfarcted segments was decreased compared to that seen in normal animals, and this decrease was proportional to infarct size. Interestingly, there was no difference in PCr/mass between adjacent and remote noninfarcted regions.

Zhang et al. studied a porcine model of postinfarct LV remodeling (59). In their group of 18 animals, 6 developed overt heart failure following infarction; 12 developed asymptomatic dysfunction. The PCr/ATP ratio in remodeled, noninfarcted segments was decreased to a greater extent in animals with clinical congestive heart failure compared to those with asymptomatic LV dysfunction. Hence, the extent of bioenergetic derangements reflected the severity of LV dysfunction in the remodeled ventricle, which in turn reflected the extent of the initial injury.

MRS has also been employed to study the impact on cellular energetics of both well-established and novel therapies for remodeling. Hugel et al. studied rats following coronary ligation that were treated with either angiotensin-converting enzyme (ACE) inhibitor or placebo (60). At 8 weeks, spectrophotometry, high-performance liquid chromatography, and ^{31}P MRS was performed on the isolated, intact myocardium. ACE inhibitor therapy reduced postinfarct LV remodeling as expected, but attenuation of remodeling paralleled beneficial changes in high-energy phosphate metabolism, suggesting an additional mechanism responsible for ACE benefit post-MI. Nicorandil demonstrated similar benefits on cardiac energy utilization in a swine model of remodeling (60). The majority of studies to date employing MRS have been limited to animals.

Gadolinium-Enhanced CMR and Remodeling

Gadolinium chelates, extracellular/interstitial contrast agents have proven to be a valuable tool for studying the natural history of remodeling postinfarction. The two most useful techniques for this purpose are first-pass perfusion and delayed hyperenhancement. First-pass perfusion imaging, in addition to identifying regions of ischemia, has the ability to delineate no-reflow zones. LGE occurs within infarcts because of the increased extracellular matrix in these regions and delayed washout of contrast as a consequence of reduced capillary density (62). LGE accurately defines the spatial extent of myocyte necrosis in the acute setting and collagenous scar at later time-points (20).

In animal models, incorporation of LGE has enabled investigators to simultaneously chronicle changes in both infarct scar and LV function and geometry following injury.

3 Days   8 Weeks

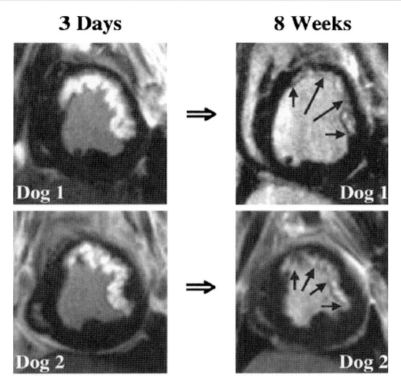

Fig. 5. Short-axis LGE images from two dogs following MI. At 3 days (left panels), large, nearly transmural infarcts are appreciated in the anterolateral wall of both animals. Infarct thinning and involution can be seen after 8 weeks (right panels). (From ref. *62* with permission.)

Fieno et al. imaged 10 dogs following MI at day 3, 10, and 28 using both stacked 5-mm short-axis cines and a T_1-weighted inversion recovery turboflash pulse sequence postcontrast *(63)*. Animals were divided into three groups: transient LAD occlusion for 45 minutes, transient LAD occlusion for 90 minutes, and permanent LAD occlusion. Although infarct mass decreased over the course of the study in all animals, resorption occurred more rapidly in reperfused animals and was consistently associated with thinning of the myocardial wall (Fig. 5). Mean radial infarct thickness also decreased progressively and at final study averaged only $38 \pm 6\%$ of values observed at 3 days. In noninfarcted segments, mass increased over the study period in both the 90-minutes occlusion group and complete occlusion group with a time-course that differed from that of infarct resorption.

Using contrast-enhanced CMR, Judd et al. found that regions of myocardial hypoenhancement correlated with zones of MO as determined by microsphere measures of blood flow *(64)*. With respect to remodeling, Gerber et al. demonstrated the importance of MO in 17 dogs following 90-minutes occlusion of the LAD *(64a)*. Gadolinium-enhanced first-pass perfusion CMR was performed 4–6 and 48 hours (8 animals) and 10 days (9 animals) after reperfusion. Multivariate analysis found that the extent of MO predicted the increase in LV volumes post-MI better than overall infarct size, and a strong inverse relationship existed between magnitude of first principal strain ($r = -0.80$, $p < 0.001$) and relative extent of MO within infarcted myocardium.

The relationship between infarct remodeling and global changes in the LV has also been investigated. In 110 patients post-AMI, Hombach et al. found that absolute infarct size, as defined by extent of LGE, decreased from $11.4 \pm 7.2\%$ to $7.8 \pm 5.3\%$ (a decline of 32%) from day 6 to month 9 post-MI (32). Similar changes in infarct size were observed in another study of 20 AMI patients (65). At follow-up, the region defined as infarct by LGE correlated well with the LVEF ($r = 0.86$, $p < 0.001$). However, infarct size decreased from $16 \pm 12\%$ to $11 \pm 9\%$ ($p < 0.003$) over the course of the study.

Choi et al. confirmed this phenomenon in his study of 25 patients on week 1 and 8 following reperfused MI (66). Between studies, the contrast defect area fell from 1729 ± 970 to 1270 ± 706 mm^2 ($p < 0.001$). The transmural extent of infarction also declined over this period (71 ± 22 to $63 \pm 24\%$, $p < 0.001$), and involution was observed to a greater degree among patients with MO. However, myocardial segments with both LGE and MO failed to demonstrate functional improvement over the study period; partial recovery of function was seen in LGE segments devoid of MO.

Changes in infarct size as determined by LGE may be a relatively early phenomenon. In a study looking at infarct size at an average of 11 days compared to 6 months following acute reperfused MI, no difference in size was observed using LGE (20.8 and 21.9%; $p = not$ significant) (67). Although apoptosis and cellular loss likely play a role in infarct involution (12), early interstitial edema and inflammation within the infarct zone (not surrounding viable regions) augment the interstitial compartment of the necrotic tissue (68) and increase the volume of the infarct zone. Although LGE accurately depicts this expanded infarct region, the ultimate extent of the collagenous scar is less as edema and inflammation subsides. This phenomenon of *infarct evolution* (as defined by the area of LGE) has important implications for the use of LGE in clinical trials in which infarct size is used as a therapeutic end point.

Therapy in LV Remodeling

ANIMAL STUDIES

Unrivaled in its reproducibility, CMR is ideal for the study of therapeutic interventions for LV remodeling. Utilizing CMR to assess LV volumes, mass, and function, a variety of animal models have been employed to explore pharmacological therapy designed to attenuate this maladaptive process. One of the first studies using CMR evaluated the effects of the ACE inhibitor cilazapril in a rat model of remodeling (69). Cilazapril preserved wall thickness and limited the increase in chamber surface area compared to that observed in untreated controls. Similar results were observed with ACE inhibition in an ovine model of remodeling. Therapy during the first 2 months following infarction limited the increase in LVEDV. Furthermore, ACE inhibitor-treated animals had preserved function in noninfarcted segments (70).

A canine model of injury induced by direct current has also been used extensively to assess pharamacological therapy for remodeling with CMR. In one example, dogs were subjected to direct current injury and then administered nitrates (71). Nitrate therapy attenuated the increase in LV mass and LVEDV compared to animals in the control group. In the same model, McDonald et al. investigated the effects of four pharmacological interventions on postinfarct remodeling (72). Although high-dose ACE inhibition attenuated remodeling, low-dose ACE, α_1-receptor blockade, and angiotensin II type 1 receptor inhibition failed to limit the remodeling process.

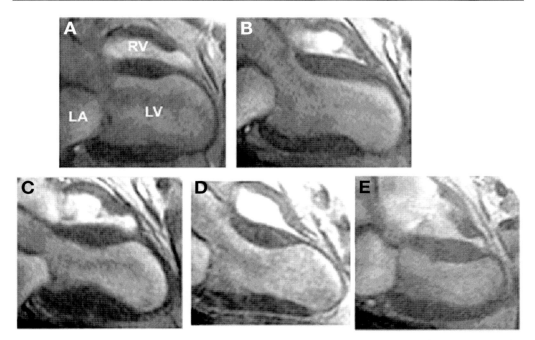

Fig. 6. End-systolic four-chamber, long-axis gradient echo cine at 8 weeks postinfarction in an ovine model of LV remodeling after coronary ligation-induced anteroapical MI. Shown are examples of five medically treated groups: control (no therapy) (**A**), angiotensin type 1 receptor (AT_1) antagonism (**B**), standard dose angiotensin-converting enzyme (ACE) inhibition (**C**), high-dose ACE inhibition (**D**), and combination therapy with AT_1 antagonism and standard dose ACE inhibition (**E**). Note that there is visually less infarct expansion with combination therapy.

This group went on to study the relative importance of bradykinin in ACE inhibitor-mediated attenuation of remodeling *(73)*. At 24 hours after myocardial injury, dogs were assigned to one of three groups: control, 10 mg ramipril twice daily, and 10 mg ramipril twice daily plus subcutaneous infusion of HOE 40, a bradykinin-2 receptor antagonist. Bradykinin antagonism counteracted the reduction in LV mass observed with ACE inhibition alone and confirmed the importance of this compound in facilitating some of the benefits of ACE inhibition.

The relative importance of β-blockade in both acute and chronic remodeling has also been investigated in animal models using CMR-based methods. In one study, infarcted dogs were assigned to 3 months of therapy with captopril, metoprolol, or control several months after myocardial injury *(74)*. Both therapies resulted in reductions in LV mass and EDV compared to untreated animals. In an ovine model of anteroapical infarction, Kramer et al. demonstrated that the combination of β-blockade and ACE inhibition resulted in an increase in LVEF over an 8-weeks period compared to ACE inhibition alone *(75)*. The same model was used to demonstrate that the combination of ACE and angiotensin II type 1 receptor antagonism was superior to ACE alone in attenuating remodeling *(76)* (Fig. 6).

Many studies have employed complex, genetically engineered animal models with the aim of developing novel pharmacological strategies to attenuate remodeling *(77,78)*. One promising target that is under exploration with MR is the angiotensin II type 2 receptor. Yang et al. found that overexpression of this receptor in the infarcted mouse heart resulted in improved EF and smaller ESVs and EDVs compared to wild-type controls over a 28-days period following MI *(79)*.

The mechanisms underlying the benefits of angiotensin II type 2 receptor (AT2R) overexpression are also under elucidation. Although administration of the nitric oxide synthase inhibitor N(G)-nitro-l-arginine methyl ester attenuates the beneficial effects of AT2R overexpression *(80)*, simultaneous knockout of the bradykinin 2 receptor does not alter its antiremodeling effects *(81)*.

Another promising target currently under study is inducible nitric oxide synthase (iNOS). In an iNOS knockout (KO) mouse, Gilson et al. studied 12 wild-type and 12 iNOS KO mice after reperfused anterior infarction. Using short-axis cine and MR tagging sequences, they found that circumferential strain in border zone regions improved in KO animals compared to wild type, and the improvement persisted through day 28. The circumferential extent of wall thinning was also reduced in KO animals *(82)*. As novel targets and pharmacotherapies emerge, MR-based animal models will continue to play a central role in the study interventions designed to allay remodeling.

HUMAN STUDIES

Because of its precision, low interobserver variability, and relatively small cohorts required to demonstrate significance, CMR is employed with increasing frequency in clinical studies of LV remodeling as a means of objectively quantifying end points. In one early example, Schulman et al. enrolled 43 patients with AMI and randomly assigned them to the ACE inhibitor enalapril IV followed by 1 month of oral ACE therapy or placebo within 24 hours of presentation *(83)*. At 1 month, 23 patients underwent MR evaluation of the infarct to assess expansion. The infarct expansion index was defined as the ratio of the infarct to noninfarct endocardial segment length. Treated patients had a reduced infarct segment length and lower infarct expansion index compared to controls, and this difference was most evident in patients with anterior infarction.

CMR was used to evaluate 35 patients with LVEF of more than 40% after infarction at 1 week and 3 months postinjury. Although ACE inhibitor therapy in this subgroup of AMI patients failed to alter measures of function and volume compared to placebo, LV mass was reduced compared to controls at 3 months. In contrast, patients with AMI and EF below 40% had improved function despite a decrease in both mass-to-volume ratio and wall thickness-to-volume ratio in noninfarcted segments *(84)*.

In one recent study, CMR was used to study cardiac remodeling after intracoronary progenitor cell treatment *(85)*. Following reperfused AMI, 28 patients received circulating blood (CPC) or bone marrow-derived (BMC) progenitor cells by catheter into the infarct territory 4.7 ± 1.7 days after the initial event. Serial, contrast-enhanced CMR was performed initially and at 4 months after injection. A significant increase in LVEF was observed over the study period ($44 \pm 10\%$ to $49 \pm 10\%$; $p = 0.003$) with a decrease in LVESV (69 ± 26 to 60 ± 28 mL; $p = 0.003$). Infarct size, measured by LGE, also decreased over the study period and correlated with global LVEF improvement (46 ± 32 to 37 ± 28 mL; $p < 0.05$). Although tantalizing, the results of the recent study have to be interpreted cautiously as no control group was employed, and the natural history of a reperfused infarct is scar involution and functional improvement over time *(62,64–66)*.

Wollert et al. subsequently studied intracoronary autologous bone marrow transfer with a control arm *(86)*. Mean time from precutaneous coronary intervention (PCI) to baseline CMR was 3–5 days, with implantation of bone marrow cells at day 4–8. Follow-up CMR was then performed at 6 months. No difference was observed between groups with respect to LVEDV index, LVESV index, LV mass index, and delayed contrast enhancement (infarct size) from baseline to 6 months. A small, but appreciable, improvement was observed in resting LVEF in the treated arm.

The importance of infarct artery patency has also been documented with serial CMR. At 10 ± 4 days after a first anterior wall MI with an occluded LAD and akineses, 16 patients were evaluated in a serial fashion (87). One group had opening of the infarct artery at 2 weeks; the other had it on a delayed basis. CMR was then performed at 3 months and 12 months. With delayed reperfusion, LVEF, infarct zone wall motion, and LV volumes did not improve during the study; early reperfusion (2 weeks) led to improvements in LVEF, ESV, and regional function.

Baks et al. assessed the impact of primary angioplasty on remodeling in AMI (88). Twenty-two patients underwent cine CMR, first-pass perfusion, and LGE imaging 5 days after successful placement of a drug-eluting stent in the infarct-related coronary artery. At 5 months, EF increased from 48 ± 11 to 55 ± 9% ($p < 0.01$), with changes in both EF and ESV most dependent on size of LGE regions ($R^2 = 0.65$; $p > 0.001$ and $R^2 = 0.78$; $p < 0.001$, respectively). Long-term effects of primary angioplasty have also been evaluated.

In a study of patients investigated initially at a median of 11 days and again at 6 months after PCI, Peterson et al. found that regional wall motion improved significantly in LGE zones (percentage wall thickening 21.9 and 37.9%, $p < 0.05$) in contrast to remote normal myocardium (46.4 and 38.4%; p = not significant) (67). Although interesting from a natural history perspective, it is difficult to interpret either of these studies as demonstrating the remodeling benefits of reperfusion therapy in the absence of a control arm.

Nonpharmacological therapies have also been assessed postinfarction. In a study of 25 patients with post-MI LV dysfunction, Dubach et al. randomized one group to 2 months of physical rehabilitation and the other to control (89). Despite improvements in exercise capacity, no changes in LV volumes, mass, or EF were noted between the groups, in contrast to prior studies suggesting deleterious effects of exercise training on LV remodeling (90). At 1 year, the improvement in exercise capacity was sustained, and no adverse changes in LV geometry or function were noted (91).

CONCLUSIONS

CMR is well suited for studying patients with AMI. Not only can this technique reliably follow changes in LV size, shape, and function following MI, but also it has the ability to accurately discriminate regions of infarction from noninfarcted tissue. Increasingly, investigators are employing CMR in both animal and clinical studies to study the effects of pharmacological and other interventions on AMI and the remodeling process. With its inherent precision and accuracy, CMR enables these studies to be performed using fewer subjects, thereby increasing cost-effectiveness.

REFERENCES

1. Risk stratification and survival after myocardial infarction. N Engl J Med. 1983;309:331–336.
2. Mock MB, Ringqvist I, Fisher LD, et al. Survival of medically treated patients in the coronary artery surgery study (CASS) registry. Circulation 1982;66:562–568.

3. White HD, Norris RM, Brown MA, Brandt PW, Whitlock RM, Wild CJ. Left ventricular end-systolic volume as the major determinant of survival after recovery from myocardial infarction. Circulation 1987;76:44–51.

4. Zaret BL, Wackers FJ, Terrin ML, et al. Value of radionuclide rest and exercise left ventricular ejection fraction in assessing survival of patients after thrombolytic therapy for acute myocardial infarction: results of Thrombolysis in Myocardial Infarction (TIMI) phase II study. The TIMI Study Group. J Am Coll Cardiol 1995;26:73–79.

5. van der Wall EE, Bax JJ. Different imaging approaches in the assessment of left ventricular dysfunction: all things equal? Eur Heart J 2000;21:1295–1297.

6. Isbell DC, Kramer CM. Cardiovascular magnetic resonance: structure, function, perfusion, and viability. J Nucl Cardiol 2005;12:324–336.

7. Sun Y, Kiani MF, Postlethwaite AE, Weber KT. Infarct scar as living tissue. Basic Res Cardiol 2002; 97:343–347.

8. Reimer KA, Jennings RB. The changing anatomic reference base of evolving myocardial infarction. Underestimation of myocardial collateral blood flow and overestimation of experimental anatomic infarct size due to tissue edema, hemorrhage and acute inflammation. Circulation 1979; 60:866–876.

9. Fishbein MC, Maclean D, Maroko PR. The histopathologic evolution of myocardial infarction. Chest 1978;73:843–849.

10. Jugdutt BI, Amy RW. Healing after myocardial infarction in the dog: changes in infarct hydroxyproline and topography. J Am Coll Cardiol 1986;7:91–102.

11. Reffelmann T, Kloner RA. Microvascular alterations after temporary coronary artery occlusion: the no-reflow phenomenon. J Cardiovasc Pharmacol Ther 2004;9:163–172.

12. Kramer CM. The prognostic significance of microvascular obstruction after myocardial infarction as defined by cardiovascular magnetic resonance. Eur Heart J 2005;26:532–533.

13. Kloner RA, Ganote CE, Jennings RB. The "no-reflow" phenomenon after temporary coronary occlusion in the dog. J Clin Invest 1974;54:1496–1508.

14. Rahimtoola SH. The hibernating myocardium. Am Heart J 1989;117:211–221.

15. Lieberman AN, Weiss JL, Jugdutt BI, et al. Two-dimensional echocardiography and infarct size: relationship of regional wall motion and thickening to the extent of myocardial infarction in the dog. Circulation 1981;63:739–746.

16. Rehr RB, Peshock RM, Malloy CR, et al. Improved in vivo magnetic resonance imaging of acute myocardial infarction after intravenous paramagnetic contrast agent administration. Am J Cardiol 1986;57:864–868.

17. Peshock RM, Malloy CR, Buja LM, Nunnally RL, Parkey RW, Willerson JT. Magnetic resonance imaging of acute myocardial infarction: gadolinium diethylenetriamine pentaacetic acid as a marker of reperfusion. Circulation 1986;74:1434–1440.

18. de Roos A, Doornbos J, van der Wall EE, Van Voorthuisen AE. MR imaging of acute myocardial infarction: value of Gd-DTPA. AJR Am J Roentgenol 1988;150:531–534.

19. Thomson LE, Kim RJ, Judd RM. Magnetic resonance imaging for the assessment of myocardial viability. J Magn Reson Imaging 2004;19:771–788.

20. Kim RJ, Fieno DS, Parrish TB, et al. Relationship of MRI delayed contrast enhancement to irreversible injury, infarct age, and contractile function. Circulation 1999;100:1992–2002.

21. Rehwald WG, Fieno DS, Chen EL, Kim RJ, Judd RM. Myocardial magnetic resonance imaging contrast agent concentrations after reversible and irreversible ischemic injury. Circulation 2002; 105:224–229.

22. Fieno DS, Kim RJ, Chen EL, Lomasney JW, Klocke FJ, Judd RM. Contrast-enhanced magnetic resonance imaging of myocardium at risk: distinction between reversible and irreversible injury throughout infarct healing. J Am Coll Cardiol 2000;36:1985–1991.

23. Wagner A, Mahrholdt H, Holly TA, et al. Contrast-enhanced MRI and routine single photon emission computed tomography (SPECT) perfusion imaging for detection of subendocardial myocardial infarcts: an imaging study. Lancet 2003;361:374–379.

24. Klein C, Nekolla SG, Bengel FM, et al. Assessment of myocardial viability with contrast-enhanced magnetic resonance imaging: comparison with positron emission tomography. Circulation 2002; 105:162–167.

25. Choi KM, Kim RJ, Gubernikoff G, Vargas JD, Parker M, Judd RM. Transmural extent of acute myocardial infarction predicts long-term improvement in contractile function. Circulation 2001; 104:1101–1107.

26. Choi JW, Gibson CM, Murphy SA, Davidson CJ, Kim RJ, Ricciardi MJ. Myonecrosis following stent placement: association between impaired TIMI myocardial perfusion grade and MRI visualization of microinfarction. Catheter Cardiovasc Interv 2004;61:472–476.

27. Ricciardi MJ, Wu E, Davidson CJ, et al. Visualization of discrete microinfarction after percutaneous coronary intervention associated with mild creatine kinase-MB elevation. Circulation 2001;103: 2780–2783.
28. Steuer J, Bjerner T, Duvernoy O, et al. Visualisation and quantification of peri-operative myocardial infarction after coronary artery bypass surgery with contrast-enhanced magnetic resonance imaging. Eur Heart J 2004;25:1293–1299.
29. Kwong RY, Chan AK, Brown KA, et al. Impact of unrecognized scar detected by cardiac magnetic resonance imaging on event-free survival in patients presenting with signs or symptoms of coronary artery disease. *Circulation* 2006;113:2733–2743.
30. Rogers WJ Jr, Kramer CM, Geskin G, et al. Early contrast-enhanced MRI predicts late functional recovery after reperfused myocardial infarction. Circulation 1999;99:744–750.
31. Wu KC, Zerhouni EA, Judd RM, et al. Prognostic significance of microvascular obstruction by magnetic resonance imaging in patients with acute myocardial infarction. Circulation 1998;97:765–772.
32. Hombach V, Grebe O, Merkle N, et al. Sequelae of acute myocardial infarction regarding cardiac structure and function and their prognostic significance as assessed by magnetic resonance imaging. Eur Heart J 2005;26:549–557.
33. Schuster EH, Bulkley BH. Expansion of transmural myocardial infarction: a pathophysiologic factor in cardiac rupture. Circulation 1979;60:1532–1538.
34. Jugdutt BI, Warnica JW. Intravenous nitroglycerin therapy to limit myocardial infarct size, expansion, and complications. Effect of timing, dosage, and infarct location. Circulation 1988;78:906–919.
35. Pfeffer JM, Pfeffer MA, Fletcher PJ, Braunwald E. Progressive ventricular remodeling in rat with myocardial infarction. Am J Physiol 1991;260:H1406–H1414.
36. Olivetti G, Capasso JM, Meggs LG, Sonnenblick EH, Anversa P. Cellular basis of chronic ventricular remodeling after myocardial infarction in rats. Circ Res 1991;68:856–869.
37. Kramer CM, Lima JA, Reichek N, et al. Regional differences in function within noninfarcted myocardium during left ventricular remodeling. Circulation 1993;88:1279–1288.
38. Mitchell GF, Lamas GA, Vaughan DE, Pfeffer MA. Left ventricular remodeling in the year after first anterior myocardial infarction: a quantitative analysis of contractile segment lengths and ventricular shape. J Am Coll Cardiol 1992;19:1136–1144.
39. Hammermeister KE, DeRouen TA, Dodge HT. Variables predictive of survival in patients with coronary disease. Selection by univariate and multivariate analyses from the clinical, electrocardiographic, exercise, arteriographic, and quantitative angiographic evaluations. Circulation 1979;59:421–430.
40. McKay RG, Pfeffer MA, Pasternak RC, et al. Left ventricular remodeling after myocardial infarction: a corollary to infarct expansion. Circulation 1986;74:693–702.
41. Picard MH, Wilkins GT, Ray PA, Weyman AE. Natural history of left ventricular size and function after acute myocardial infarction. Assessment and prediction by echocardiographic endocardial surface mapping. Circulation 1990;82:484–494.
42. Bellenger NG, Burgess MI, Ray SG, et al. Comparison of left ventricular ejection fraction and volumes in heart failure by echocardiography, radionuclide ventriculography and cardiovascular magnetic resonance; are they interchangeable? Eur Heart J 2000;21:1387–1396.
43. Bellenger NG, Davies LC, Francis JM, Coats AJ, Pennell DJ. Reduction in sample size for studies of remodeling in heart failure by the use of cardiovascular magnetic resonance. J Cardiovasc Magn Reson 2000;2:271–278.
44. Franco F, Thomas GD, Giroir B, et al. Magnetic resonance imaging and invasive evaluation of development of heart failure in transgenic mice with myocardial expression of tumor necrosis factor-α. Circulation 1999;99:448–454.
45. Ross AJ, Yang Z, Berr SS, et al. Serial MRI evaluation of cardiac structure and function in mice after reperfused myocardial infarction. Magn Reson Med 2002;47:1158–1168.
46. Grossman W, Jones D, McLaurin LP. Wall stress and patterns of hypertrophy in the human left ventricle. J Clin Invest 1975;56:56–64.
47. Kramer CM, Rogers WJ, Park CS, et al. Regional myocyte hypertrophy parallels regional myocardial dysfunction during post-infarct remodeling. J Mol Cell Cardiol 1998;30:1773–1778.
48. Nahrendorf M, Hu K, Fraccarollo D, et al. Time course of right ventricular remodeling in rats with experimental myocardial infarction. Am J Physiol Heart Circ Physiol 2003;284:H241–H248.
49. Jones JR, Mata JF, Yang Z, French BA, Oshinski JN. Left ventricular remodeling subsequent to reperfused myocardial infarction: evaluation of a rat model using cardiac magnetic resonance imaging. J Cardiovasc Magn Reson 2002;4:317–326.
50. Matheijssen NA, Baur LH, Reiber JH, et al. Assessment of left ventricular volume and mass by cine magnetic resonance imaging in patients with anterior myocardial infarction intra-observer and inter-observer variability on contour detection. Int J Card Imaging 1996;12:11–19.

51. Konermann M, Sanner BM, Horstmann E, et al. Changes of the left ventricle after myocardial infarction—estimation with cine magnetic resonance imaging during the first 6 months. Clin Cardiol 1997; 20:201–212.

52. Kramer CM, Rogers WJ, Theobald TM, Power TP, Geskin G, Reichek N. Dissociation between changes in intramyocardial function and left ventricular volumes in the eight weeks after first anterior myocardial infarction. J Am Coll Cardiol 1997;30:1625–1632.

53. Schroeder AP, Houlind K, Pedersen EM, Nielsen TT, Egeblad H. Serial magnetic resonance imaging of global and regional left ventricular remodeling during 1 year after acute myocardial infarction. Cardiology 2001;96:106–114.

54. Moulton MJ, Downing SW, Creswell LL, et al. Mechanical dysfunction in the border zone of an ovine model of left ventricular aneurysm. Ann Thorac Surg 1995;60:986-997.

55. Holman ER, Buller VG, de Roos A, et al. Detection and quantification of dysfunctional myocardium by magnetic resonance imaging. A new three-dimensional method for quantitative wall-thickening analysis. Circulation 1997;95:924–931.

56. Kramer CM, Rogers WJ, Theobald TM, Power TP, Petruolo S, Reichek N. Remote noninfarcted region dysfunction soon after first anterior myocardial infarction. A magnetic resonance tagging study. Circulation 1996;94:660–666.

57. Zhang J, McDonald KM. Bioenergetic consequences of left ventricular remodeling. Circulation 1995;92:1011–1019.

58. Friedrich J, Apstein CS, Ingwall JS. ^{31}P nuclear magnetic resonance spectroscopic imaging of regions of remodeled myocardium in the infarcted rat heart. Circulation 1995;92:3527–3538.

59. Zhang J, Wilke N, Wang Y, et al. Functional and bioenergetic consequences of postinfarction left ventricular remodeling in a new porcine model. MRI and ^{31}P-MRS study. Circulation 1996;94:1089–1100.

60. Hugel S, Horn M, Remkes H, Dienesch C, Neubauer S. Preservation of cardiac function and energy reserve by the angiotensin-converting enzyme inhibitor quinapril during postmyocardial infarction remodeling in the rat. J Cardiovasc Magn Reson 2001;3:215–225.

61. Murakami Y, Wu X, Zhang J, Ochiai K, Bache RJ, Shimada T. Nicorandil improves myocardial high-energy phosphates in postinfarction porcine hearts. Clin Exp Pharmacol Physiol 2002;29:639–645.

62. Wu KC, Lima JA. Noninvasive imaging of myocardial viability: current techniques and future developments. Circ Res 2003;93:1146–1158.

63. Fieno DS, Hillenbrand HB, Rehwald WG, et al. Infarct resorption, compensatory hypertrophy, and differing patterns of ventricular remodeling following myocardial infarctions of varying size. J Am Coll Cardiol 2004;43:2124–2131.

64. Judd RM, Lugo-Olivieri CH, Arai M, et al. Physiological basis of myocardial contrast enhancement in fast magnetic resonance images of 2-days-old reperfused canine infarcts. Circulation 1995;92:1902–1910.

64a. Gerber BL, Rochitte CE, Melin JA, et al. Microvascular obstruction and left ventricular remodeling early after acute myocardial infarction. *Circulation* 2000;101:2734–2741.

65. Ingkanisorn WP, Rhoads KL, Aletras AH, Kellman P, Arai AE. Gadolinium delayed enhancement cardiovascular magnetic resonance correlates with clinical measures of myocardial infarction. J Am Coll Cardiol 2004;43:2253–2259.

66. Choi CJ, Haji-Momenian S, Dimaria JM, et al. Infarct involution and improved function during healing of acute myocardial infarction: the role of microvascular obstruction. J Cardiovasc Magn Reson 2004; 6:917–925.

67. Petersen SE, Voigtlander T, Kreitner KF, et al. Late improvement of regional wall motion after the subacute phase of myocardial infarction treated by acute PTCA in a 6-months follow-up. J Cardiovasc Magn Reson 2003;5:487–495.

68. Steenbergen C, Hill ML, Jennings RB. Volume regulation and plasma membrane injury in aerobic, anaerobic, and ischemic myocardium in vitro. Effects of osmotic cell swelling on plasma membrane integrity. Circ Res 1985;57:864–875.

69. Saeed M, Wendland MF, Seelos K, Masui T, Derugin N, Higgins CB. Effect of cilazapril on regional left ventricular wall thickness and chamber dimension following acute myocardial infarction: in vivo assessment using MRI. Am Heart J 1992;123:1472–1480.

70. Kramer CM, Ferrari VA, Rogers WJ, et al. Angiotensin-converting enzyme inhibition limits dysfunction in adjacent noninfarcted regions during left ventricular remodeling. J Am Coll Cardiol 1996;27:211–217.

71. McDonald KM, Francis GS, Matthews J, Hunter D, Cohn JN. Long-term oral nitrate therapy prevents chronic ventricular remodeling in the dog. J Am Coll Cardiol 1993;21:514–522.

72. McDonald KM, Garr M, Carlyle PF, et al. Relative effects of α_1-adrenoceptor blockade, converting enzyme inhibitor therapy, and angiotensin II subtype 1 receptor blockade on ventricular remodeling in the dog. Circulation 1994;90:3034–3046.

73. McDonald KM, Mock J, D'Aloia A, et al. Bradykinin antagonism inhibits the antigrowth effect of converting enzyme inhibition in the dog myocardium after discrete transmural myocardial necrosis. Circulation 1995;91:2043–2048.

74. McDonald KM, Rector T, Carlyle PF, Francis GS, Cohn JN. Angiotensin-converting enzyme inhibition and β-adrenoceptor blockade regress established ventricular remodeling in a canine model of discrete myocardial damage. J Am Coll Cardiol 1994;24:1762–1768.

75. Kramer CM, Nicol PD, Rogers WJ, Seibel PS, Park CS, Reichek N. β-Blockade improves adjacent regional sympathetic innervation during postinfarction remodeling. Am J Physiol 1999;277:H1429–H1434.

76. Mankad S, d'Amato TA, Reichek N, et al. Combined angiotensin II receptor antagonism and angiotensin-converting enzyme inhibition further attenuates postinfarction left ventricular remodeling. Circulation 2001;103:2845–2850.

77. Ramani R, Mathier M, Wang P, et al. Inhibition of tumor necrosis factor receptor-1-mediated pathways has beneficial effects in a murine model of postischemic remodeling. Am J Physiol Heart Circ Physiol 2004;287:H1369–H1377.

78. Askari AT, Brennan ML, Zhou X, et al. Myeloperoxidase and plasminogen activator inhibitor 1 play a central role in ventricular remodeling after myocardial infarction. J Exp Med 2003;197:615–624.

79. Yang Z, Bove CM, French BA, et al. Angiotensin II type 2 receptor overexpression preserves left ventricular function after myocardial infarction. Circulation 2002;106:106–111.

80. Bove CM, Yang Z, Gilson WD, et al. Nitric oxide mediates benefits of angiotensin II type 2 receptor overexpression during post-infarct remodeling. Hypertension 2004;43:680–685.

81. Isbell DC, Voros S, Yang Z. Bradykinin does not mediate the anti-remodeling effects of angiotensin II type 2 receptor overexpression following myocardial infarction [abstract]. J Cardiovasc Magn Reson 2005;7:27–28.

82. Gilson WD, Epstein FH, Roy RJ, Yang Z, French BA. Cine MRI and myocardial tagging reveal improved border zone function and reduced wall thinning in postinfarction iNOS knockout mice [abstract]. Circulation 2004;110:686.

83. Schulman SP, Weiss JL, Becker LC, et al. Effect of early enalapril therapy on left ventricular function and structure in acute myocardial infarction. Am J Cardiol 1995;76:764–770.

84. Foster RE, Johnson DB, Barilla F, et al. Changes in left ventricular mass and volumes in patients receiving angiotensin-converting enzyme inhibitor therapy for left ventricular dysfunction after Q-wave myocardial infarction. Am Heart J 1998;136:269–275.

85. Britten MB, Abolmaali ND, Assmus B, et al. Infarct remodeling after intracoronary progenitor cell treatment in patients with acute myocardial infarction (TOPCARE-AMI): mechanistic insights from serial contrast-enhanced magnetic resonance imaging. Circulation 2003;108:2212–2218.

86. Wollert KC, Meyer GP, Lotz J, et al. Intracoronary autologous bone-marrow cell transfer after myocardial infarction: the BOOST randomised controlled clinical trial. Lancet 2004;364:141–148.

87. Pfisterer ME, Buser P, Osswald S, Weiss P, Bremerich J, Burkart F. Time dependence of left ventricular recovery after delayed recanalization of an occluded infarct-related coronary artery: findings of a pilot study. J Am Coll Cardiol 1998;32:97–102.

88. Baks T, van Geuns RJ, Biagini E, et al. Recovery of left ventricular function after primary angioplasty for acute myocardial infarction. Eur Heart J 2005;26:1070–1077.

89. Dubach P, Myers J, Dziekan G, et al. Effect of exercise training on myocardial remodeling in patients with reduced left ventricular function after myocardial infarction: application of magnetic resonance imaging. Circulation 1997;95:2060–2067.

90. Jugdutt BI, Michorowski BL, Kappagoda CT. Exercise training after anterior Q wave myocardial infarction: importance of regional left ventricular function and topography. J Am Coll Cardiol 1988;12:362–372.

91. Myers J, Goebbels U, Dzeikan G, et al. Exercise training and myocardial remodeling in patients with reduced ventricular function: 1-year follow-up with magnetic resonance imaging. Am Heart J 2000;139:252–261.

14 Stress Cine MRI

Eike Nagel

CONTENTS

INTRODUCTION

Cardiovascular magnetic resonance (CMR) imaging is increasingly used to detect the presence of coronary artery disease (CAD) and to assess its hemodynamic significance *(1)*. The development of rapid gradient systems and consequently very short measurement times allows us to perform high-resolution cine imaging of the heart at rest and under stress conditions up to heart rates of 200 beats per minute. The standard sequence used today for visualization of cardiac wall motion (steady-state free precession) provides an excellent endocardial border definition independent of limiting acquisition windows because of the high blood-myocardium contrast without the need for application of contrast agents *(2)*. This endocardial border definition is highly superior to state-of-the-art echocardiographic image quality.

The limited space within the scanner necessitates the application of pharmacological stress agents (usually dobutamine) for the detection of inducible wall motion abnormalities.

STRESS AGENTS

Pharmacological stress is a well-documented alternative stress method to ergometry and is superior in patients who are not able to exert themselves adequately.

Even though vasodilator (adenosine/dipyridamole) stress has been suggested for the induction of ischemic wall motion abnormalities and considered interchangeable to

From: *Contemporary Cardiology: Cardiovascular Magnetic Resonance Imaging*
Edited by: Raymond Y. Kwong © Humana Press Inc., Totowa, NJ

dobutamine stress, a significantly lower diagnostic accuracy for the detection of epicardial coronary stenoses both with magnetic resonance (MR) and echocardiography has been reported for vasodilator vs dobutamine stress wall motion imaging *(3)*.

DOBUTAMINE STRESS MAGNETIC RESONANCE PROTOCOL

The pharmacological stress protocol for magnetic resonance imaging (MRI) follows the standard high-dose dobutamine/atropine regimen as used in stress echocardiography. After acquisition of cine scans in the diagnostic standard views (apical, mid- and basal short-axis view; four-chamber, two-chamber, and three-chamber view) at rest, dobutamine is infused intravenously at 3-minute intervals at doses of 10, 20, 30, and 40 µg/kg/minute, and imaging is repeated in all standard views at each level. If target heart rate, which is age-predicted submaximal heart rate ([220 – Age] × 0.85), is not reached at the maximal dobutamine dose, a maximal dose of 2 mg atropine is applied in 0.25-mg fractions. Termination criteria are identical to those of dobutamine stress echocardiography *(4)*.

Safety and Flexibility of Dobutamine Stress Magnetic Resonance

Of patients, 4–6% are unable to lie in the scanner because of claustrophobia. In addition, MRI is contraindicated in patients with noncompatible biometallic implants and pacemakers or implanted defibrillators (implantable cardioverter defibrillators, ICDs). Coronary stents, sternal wires after thoracic surgery, and the majority of prosthetic valve types do not represent a contraindication for cardiac MRI and do not interfere with image quality.

Wahl et al. *(5)* reported data from a 5-years experience in performing high-dose dobutamine stress magnetic resonance (DSMR) in 1000 consecutive patients and showed a safety profile almost identical to dobutamine stress echocardiography: only 1 patient suffered sustained ventricular tachycardia with successful defibrillation, and no cases of death or myocardial infarction occurred. The patients included into this study had an intermediate pretest likelihood, and over half had ischemia induced at the time of stress CMR, thereby closely reflecting the clinical practice. In addition, DSMR resulted in a high number of diagnostic examinations (89.5%) in patients without contraindications to MRI.

Monitoring

Heart rate and rhythm need to be monitored throughout the dobutamine stress infusion. ST segment changes are nondiagnostic in the magnetic field because of the magneto-hydrodynamic effect, however, because wall motion abnormalities precede ST segment changes and the former can readily be detected with MRI, monitoring is effective without a diagnostic electrocardiogram (ECG) *(4)*.

Blood pressure monitoring can easily be done with a conventional monitoring system outside the scanner room with an extension line placed through a waveguide in the radio-frequency cage, or special CMR-compatible equipment may be used that already exists at many MR sites.

In general, monitoring during a MR examination requires the same precautions and emergency equipment as any other stress test. A physician appropriately trained in basic and advanced cardiac life support must be present throughout the stress examination and during the recovery phase. In addition, precautions for rapid patient removal must be taken. The staff should regularly practice the maneuver for rapid patient evacuation, and two staff members should be able to start resuscitation outside the scanner room in less than 30 seconds.

Imaging Technique

MR cine imaging is usually performed with the patient in the supine position using a 1.5-T magnet. Multiple-element phased-array coils for signal detection allow application of parallel imaging techniques. Preferably, cardiac synchronization should be performed with a multichannel ECG (vector-ECG). Routinely, a steady-state free precession sequence in combination with parallel image acquisition and retrospective ECG gating are used for MR cine imaging, resulting in the acquisition of more than 25 phases/cardiac cycle during an end-expiratory breath hold of 4–6 seconds up to heart rates of 190–200 beats per minute. The in-plane spatial resolution of MR cine scans usually lies in the range of 1.6×1.6 mm (slice thickness of 8 mm).

Image Display

During the pharmacological stress procedure, the examiner continuously evaluates the MR cine images in an "automatic view" window as displayed on the console of the scanner. The reconstruction speed of the phase images has become very fast and allows on-line visual assessment of wall motion with the cine loops displayed less than 1 second after data acquisition. Alternatively, with a workstation next to the scanner console, the cine loops can be automatically transferred and displayed in a synchronized quadscreen.

DIAGNOSTIC CRITERIA

Visual assessment is usually applied to grade wall motion because quantification has not be shown superior to visual assessment. Always, all segments need to be assessed. For image interpretation, multiple synchronized cine loop display is recommended to view one or more imaging planes at each dose level simultaneously. The ventricle is analyzed for 17 segments per stress level according to the standards suggested by the American Society of Echocardiography *(6)*. Image quality is graded as good, acceptable, or bad, and the number of diagnostic segments is reported. Segmental wall motion is classified as normokinetic, hypokinetic, akinetic, or dyskinetic and assigned 1–4 points. The sum of points is divided by the number of analyzed segments and yields a wall motion score. Normal contraction results in a wall motion score of 1; a higher score is indicative of wall motion abnormalities. During dobutamine stress with increasing doses, a lack of increase in the wall motion or systolic wall thickening or a reduction of the wall motion or thickening are both regarded as pathological findings (Fig. 1).

DIAGNOSTIC PERFORMANCE

In single-center trials DSMR has been shown to be superior to dobutamine stress echocardiography for the detection of inducible wall motion abnormalities in patients with suspected CAD *(7)*, patients with wall motion abnormalities at rest *(8)*, and patients not well suited for second-harmonic echocardiography *(9)* (Table 1).

In a head-to-head comparison of dobutamine stress echocardiography and high-dose dobutamine/atropine stress MR (DSMR), with X-ray coronary angiography as the standard of reference in a larger patient cohort *(7)*, we found a high accuracy of

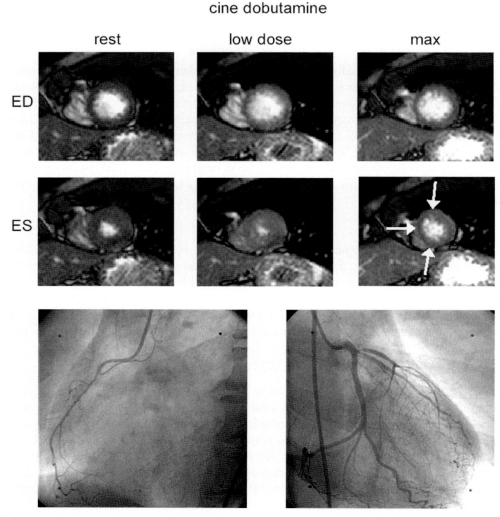

Fig. 1. DSMR cine images (four-chamber view) of a patient with suspected CAD complaining about typical anginal pain.

Normal regional wall motion at rest and with 20 (µg/kg/minute dobutamine. At maximum stress, an inducible wall motion abnormally was detected in the apical, septal, and apical anterior segments (white arrows).

X-ray coronary angiography.

Single-vessel disease of the left anterior descending artery with high-grade proximal stenosis and septal branch collaterals.

(Reprinted with permission from ref. *3*).

DSMR for the detection of inducible wall motion abnormalities related to the presence of epicardial coronary stenosis in patients with suspected CAD. Diagnostic accuracy was 86% (sensitivity 86%; specificity 86%), which was superior to dobutamine stress echocardiography (76% accuracy). In patients with limited echocardiographic image quality, Hundley et al. reported a similar diagnostic performance of DSMR (accuracy 83%; sensitivity 83%; specificity 83%). The superiority of DSMR

Table 1
Diagnostic Accuracy of Dobutamine Stress Magnetic Resonance Imaging in Detecting Angiographically Proven Coronary Artery Disease

Author	Year	Population	Significant CAD	Total no. of patients	Dobutamine dosage, μg/kg/minute	Sensitivity, %	Specificity, %	PPV, %	NPV, %	Overall accuracy, %
(10)	1992	Exercise chest pain, abnormal exercise ECG	<50%	25	20	91	—	—	—	—
(11)	1994	Angiographically proven CAD	≥70%	26	20	85	—	—	—	—
(12)	1994	Suspected CAD	≥50%	39	20	91	80	—	—	90
(7)	1999	Suspected CAD	≥50%	172	40	86	86	91	78	86
(9)	1999	Suspected CAD	<50%	41	40	83	83	—	—	83
(3)	2004	Known and suspected CAD	<50%	79	40	89	80	91	77	86
(8)	2004	Resting WMA, postrevascularization	≥50%	160	40	89	84	94	73	88

PPV, positive predictive value; NPV, negative predictive value; WMA, wall motion abnormality.

has been attributed primarily to the consistently high endocardial border definition inherent to the MR cine sequences *(3)*, which is independent of limited acquisition windows, thereby allowing for the detection of subtle wall motion abnormalities. Thus, the gain in diagnostic accuracy is particularly high in those patients with inadequate acoustic windows or limited echocardiographic image quality despite the use of second-harmonic imaging.

FUNCTIONAL ASSESSMENT OF VIABLE MYOCARDIUM

In addition to the assessment of ischemia, DSMR offers the possibility to detect viable myocardium after myocardial infarction. This information can be extracted from every dobutamine stress test and is based on the contractile response to low-dose dobutamine stimulation. Low-dose dobutamine stimulates recruitment of hibernating myocardium at a dose of 10–20 µg/kg/minute. Thus, in areas with viable myocardium, a "biphasic response" is observed with a wall motion abnormality at rest, improvement at low-dose dobutamine, and deterioration at high-dose dobutamine. When low-dose dobutamine stimulation was compared with scar imaging, it was found that low-dose dobutamine is superior to scar imaging in predicting recovery of function after revascularization *(4)*. This observation was most pronounced in segments with nontransmural scar.

As an explanation, it was suggested that even though scar imaging depicts the area of myocardial fibrosis, it does not assess the functional state of the surrounding (potentially viable) myocardium, and thus its capability for the prediction of functional recovery of nontransmurally scarred myocardium is limited.

PROGNOSTIC VALUE OF DOBUTAMINE STRESS MAGNETIC RESONANCE

Only data from single-center studies are available on the prognostic information provided by high-dose DSMR: in a retrospective study, Hundley et al. *(5)* reported the usefulness of DSMR for determination of patient prognosis and found that the presence of inducible wall motion abnormalities during DSMR identifies those patients at risk of myocardial infarction and cardiac death independent of the presence of traditional risk factors for CAD. A low cardiac event rate was demonstrated in case of a negative DSMR testing (2% over 2 years for patients with left ventricular ejection fraction >40% and 0% over 2 years for patients with left ventricular ejection fraction ≥60%).

Similarly, the value of DSMR for the assessment of preoperative cardiac risk in patients undergoing noncardiac surgery has been examined *(6)*. In the subgroup of patients with intermediate clinical predictors of future cardiac events, a positive DSMR test proved to be an independent factor for predicting myocardial infarction, cardiac death, or congestive heart failure during or after the surgery.

OUTLOOK

Tagged MRI (i.e., image acquisition with a grid deforming with myocardial contraction) can be used to quantify wall motion in systole and diastole and to detect the early occurrence of ischemic responses *(7)*. Visual analysis of tagged images has led to a higher diagnostic accuracy for the tagged vs the conventional cine approach *(7)*.

New real-time analysis tools for tagged MR images may facilitate direct visualization of regional myocardial strain (e.g., fast harmonic phase imaging [FastHARP]) *(9)*; these imaging techniques are currently reviewed in clinical trials.

CONCLUSIONS

DSMR can be regarded as the imaging method of choice in patients with moderate or worse echocardiographic image quality. It provides prognostically relevant information and can be used for preoperative assessment of patients scheduled for noncardiac surgery.

In addition, functional assessment of viable myocardium with low-dose DSMR is superior to myocardial scar imaging if scar transmurality is less than 75%. This information is readily at hand in all patients with resting wall motion abnormalities referred for ischemia testing with DSMR.

REFERENCES

1. Pennell DJ, Sechtem UP, Higgins CB, et al. Clinical indications for cardiovascular magnetic resonance (CMR): Consensus Panel report. Eur Heart J 2004;25:1940–1965.
2. Thiele H, Nagel E, Paetsch I, et al. Functional cardiac MR imaging with steady-state free precession (SSFP) significantly improves endocardial border delineation without contrast agents. J Magn Reson Imaging 2001;14:362–367.
3. Paetsch I, Jahnke C, Wahl A, et al. Comparison of dobutamine stress magnetic resonance, adenosine stress magnetic resonance, and adenosine stress magnetic resonance perfusion. Circulation 2004; 110:835–842.
4. Nagel E, Lorenz C, Baer F, et al. Stress cardiovascular magnetic resonance: consensus panel report. J Cardiovasc Magn Reson 2001;3:267–281.
5. Wahl A, Paetsch I, Gollesch A, et al. Safety and feasibility of high-dose dobutamine-atropine stress cardiovascular magnetic resonance for diagnosis of myocardial ischaemia: experience in 1000 consecutive cases. Eur Heart J 2004;25:1230–1236.
6. Cerqueira MD, Weissman NJ, Dilsizian V, et al. American Heart Association Writing Group on Myocardial Segmentation and Registration for Cardiac Imaging. Standardized myocardial segmentation and nomenclature for tomographic imaging of the heart: a statement for healthcare professionals from the Cardiac Imaging Committee of the Council on Clinical Cardiology of the American Heart Association. Circulation. 2002 Jan 29;105 (4):533–542.
7. Nagel E, Lehmkuhl HB, Bocksch W, et al. Noninvasive diagnosis of ischemia-induced wall motion abnormalities with the use of high-dose dobutamine stress MRI: comparison with dobutamine stress echocardiography. Circulation 1999;99:763–770.
8. Wahl A, Paetsch I, Roethemeyer S, Klein C, Fleck E, Nagel E. High-dose dobutamine-atropine stress cardiovascular MR imaging after coronary revascularization in patients with wall motion abnormalities at rest. Radiology 2004;233:210–216.
9. Hundley WG, Hamilton CA, Thomas MS, et al. Utility of fast cine magnetic resonance imaging and display for the detection of myocardial ischemia in patients not well suited for second harmonic stress echocardiography. Circulation 1999;100:1697–1702.
10. Pennell DJ, Underwood SR, Manzara CC, et al. Magnetic resonance imaging during dobutamine stress in coronary artery disease. Am J Cardiol. 1992 Jul 1;70 (1):34–40.
11. Baer FM, Voth E, Theissen P, Schicha H, Sechtem U. Gradient-echo magnetic resonance imaging during incremental dobutamine infusion for the localization of coronary artery stenoses. Eur Heart J. 1994 Feb;15 (2):218–225.
12. van Rugge FP, van der Wall EE, Spanjersberg SJ, et al. Magnetic resonance imaging during dobutamine stress for detection and localization of coronary artery disease. Quantitative wall motion analysis using a modification of the centerline method. Circulation. 1994 Jul;90 (1):127–138.
13. Nagel E, Lehmkuhl HB, Klein C, et al. Influence of image quality on the diagnostic accuracy of dobutamine stress magnetic resonance imaging in comparison with dobutamine stress echocardiography for the noninvasive detection of myocardial ischemia.

14. Wellnhofer E, Olariu A, Klein C, et al. Magnetic resonance low-dose dobutamine test is superior to scar quantification for the prediction of functional recovery. Circulation 2004;109:2172–2174.
15. Hundley WG, Morgan TM, Neagle CM, Hamilton CA, Rerkpattanapipat P, Link KM. Magnetic resonance imaging determination of cardiac prognosis. Circulation 2002;106:2328–2333.
16. Rerkpattanapipat P, Morgan TM, Neagle CM, Link KM, Hamilton CA, Hundley WG. Assessment of preoperative cardiac risk with magnetic resonance imaging. Am J Cardiol 2002;90:416–419.
17. Paetsch I, Foll D, Kaluza A, et al. Magnetic resonance stress tagging in ischemic heart disease. Am J Physiol Heart Circ Physiol. 2005 Jun;288 (6):H2708–H2714.
18. Kuijpers D, Ho KY, van Dijkman PR, Vliegenthart R, Oudkerk M. Dobutamine cardiovascular magnetic resonance for the detection of myocardial ischemia with the use of myocardial tagging. Circulation 2003;107:1592–1597.
19. Kraitchman DL, Sampath S, Castillo E, et al. Quantitative ischemia detection during cardiac magnetic resonance stress testing by use of FastHARP. Circulation 2003;107:2025–2030.

15 Myocardial Perfusion Using First-Pass Gadolinium-Enhanced Cardiac Magnetic Resonance

Andrew E. Arai and Li-Yueh Hsu

Although cardiovascular magnetic resonance (CMR) can image myocardial perfusion with many methods, first-pass perfusion studies using gadolinium contrast have the highest signal-to-noise ratio and most extensive published experience. This chapter focuses primarily on the basic principles and clinical applications of first-pass myocardial perfusion studies.

BASIC PRINCIPLES OF CONTRAST-ENHANCED FIRST-PASS PERFUSION IMAGING

The fundamental principle of first-pass perfusion imaging is relatively simple. Multiple imaging planes through the heart are taken every heartbeat or every other heartbeat. These images are used to track an intravenous bolus of contrast dynamically as it courses through the cardiac chambers and into the myocardium. A heavily T_1-weighted image acquisition protocol is selected to make the images sensitive to the effects of the gadolinium-based contrast agents. Because the gadolinium primarily shortens T_1 relaxation, the heart appears dark until contrast is delivered via blood flow or perfusion (Fig. 1). Thus, when the contrast arrives in the right ventricle,

From: *Contemporary Cardiology: Cardiovascular Magnetic Resonance Imaging*
Edited by: Raymond Y. Kwong © Humana Press Inc., Totowa, NJ

A Normal perfusion (*see* figure A, movie 1, in CD)

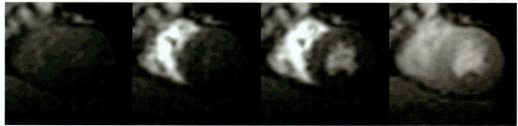

B Severe subendocardial perfusion defect (*see* figure B, movie 2, in CD)

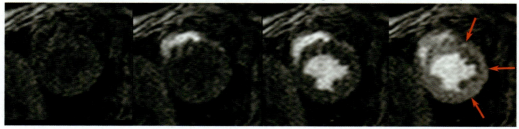

C Severe transmural perfusion defect

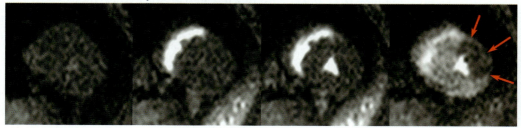

Fig. 1. Appearance of a first-pass perfusion study as a function of time.

this chamber brightens, but the remainder of the heart stays dark. Several heartbeats later, the contrast traverses the pulmonary circulation and reenters the left atrium and left ventricle (LV). A few heartbeats later, contrast is ejected into the aorta and courses through the coronary arteries. Thus, the myocardium starts to brighten about two heartbeats after the LV cavity and enhances at a slower rate. In a normal heart, signal enhancement should be relatively uniform throughout the myocardium and should have intermediate gray signal intensity.

Analysis of myocardial perfusion can be done at different levels, including qualitative, semiquantitative, and fully quantitative analysis. Most investigators have relied on qualitative visual interpretation of clinical studies because the dynamic acquired images contain all of the first-pass perfusion information. However, basic science studies provide a framework that can help physicians understand the relationships between image intensity and myocardial perfusion.

Because the signal intensity in perfusion images is related to the contrast concentration, many investigators measure signal intensity in regions of the heart as a function of time (Fig. 2). In such plots, the temporal characteristics of signal intensity in the right ventricle,

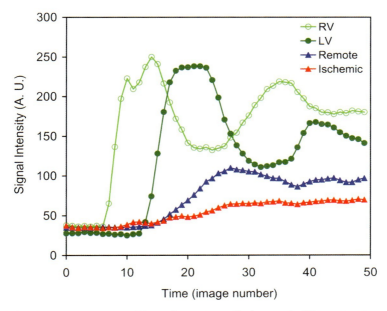

Fig. 2. Time intensity curves measured from first-pass perfusion study. The open green circles were measured in the right ventricular cavity. The dark green circles were measured in the left ventricular cavity. The blue triangles were measured in a sector representing normal vasodilated myocardium. The red triangles came from a region of the myocardium with severely reduced perfusion.

the LV, and the myocardium are well delineated. These time signal intensity plots follow the same temporal relationships as the qualitative description of the images in Fig. 1. Both semiquantitative and fully quantitative measurements can be derived from the time signal intensity curves of these plots. Some of these semiquantitative measures are strongly related to perfusion; others are significantly affected by factors other than perfusion. Even when interpreting images qualitatively, it is important to know which characteristics of perfusion images correlate most closely with perfusion.

Semiquantitative analysis provides an indirect assessment of myocardial perfusion. The simplest semiquantitative measure of perfusion is *contrast enhancement*, which represents how much the image brightens. This can be determined by measuring signal intensity of the myocardium prior to contrast arrival and at the time of peak myocardial enhancement (Fig. 3). Contrast enhancement is related to the amount of contrast that accumulates in the myocardium but ignores temporal considerations such as the rate of contrast delivery. Measuring the rate of enhancement or *upslope* of signal intensity is one important step more closely related to perfusion because this parameter incorporates information about the rate of contrast delivery. By normalizing to the rate of enhancement in the LV cavity or aorta, upslope analysis can account for variable delivery of contrast to the heart related to cardiac output and dispersion in the heart and pulmonary vasculature.

The myocardial *upslope integral* is another semiquantitative approach that can be measured on time signal intensity curves, and it correlates well with microsphere measures of perfusion *(1,2)*. The upslope integral or the area under the initial upslope of myocardial time intensity curves incorporates information about the rate of enhancement and the amount of enhancement. Compared with the upslope, the main advantage of the upslope integral is lower measurement noise. By performing the analysis at rest and

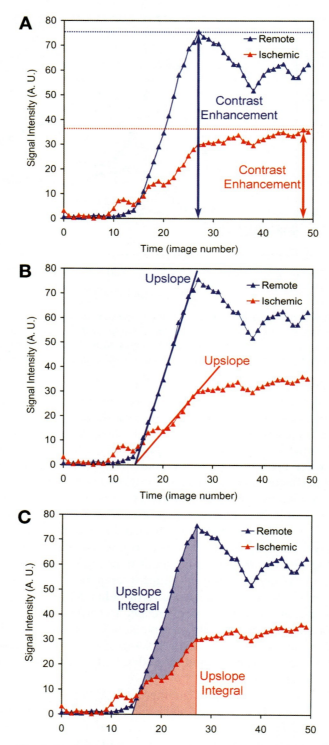

Fig. 3. Methods for semiquantitative analysis of perfusion.

stress, one can report a myocardial perfusion reserve index (MPR_i). The term *index* is generally associated with semiquantitative analysis because these measurements do not carry perfusion units and are not linearly related to myocardial perfusion. Despite these limitations, the MPR_i measurement of the perfusion upslope has been used successfully in many studies *(3–5)*.

Fully quantitative analysis of myocardial perfusion in units of milliliters per minute per gram can be obtained with deconvolution methods *(6)* and compartmental analysis *(7)*. Such studies provide insight into contrast dynamics by using simple tracer kinetic models from a system approach to derive myocardial perfusion measurements. In a population study, quantitative CMR measurement of perfusion by deconvolution inversely correlated with Framingham risk scores *(8)*. It is also encouraging that fully quantitative perfusion correlated with microspheres over a wide range of myocardial blood flow and had good limits of agreement in Bland Altman analysis *(9)*. However, all of the semiquantitative perfusion indices underestimated vasodilated blood flow. The contrast enhancement ratio was the worst of the three semiquantitative indices. Furthermore, these images have the resolution to analyze perfusion in subgram regions of interest *(9,10)*.

Compartmental analysis can also provide CMR estimates of myocardial perfusion in units of milliliters per minute per gram of tissue. Quantitative perfusion by this type of analysis has been shown to correlate inversely with the degree of stenosis in patients *(11)*. However, in a comparison with positron emission tomography (PET), perfusion measurements from compartmental analysis underestimated myocardial perfusion reserve.

It is important to recognize that there are many factors, including contrast dose, image acquisition parameters, and analysis methods, that may affect any type of quantitative perfusion measurements. Other aspects of quantitative perfusion modeling such as collateral-dependent myocardium can also be assessed by first-pass contrast CMR studies. Experimental results indicate that collateral-dependent myocardium is often characterized by a delay in the arrival of the contrast and reduced overall perfusion *(12)*.

From a practical perspective, visual interpretation of perfusion images is most likely to be used clinically because semiquantitative and fully quantitative approaches are still time consuming. The next section of this chapter reviews how well various groups have detected significant coronary artery disease in comparison to reference standards.

DETECTION OF CORONARY ARTERY DISEASE

The CMR first-pass perfusion methods translate reasonably well into clinical practice. However, there remains uncertainty about the best techniques to use when diagnosing coronary artery disease. Despite this uncertainty, it is possible to directly visualize perfusion abnormalities and resolve the transmural extent of perfusion defects qualitatively (Figs. 1, 4, and 5). Such anecdotes support the efficacy of the methods and hint to their clinical utility. Many publications validate the use of first-pass perfusion CMR methods for detecting coronary artery disease in patients.

Table 1 summarizes all CMR first-pass perfusion studies that reported sensitivity and specificity for detection of coronary artery disease in a sample size of at least 25 subjects (PubMed search April 2006). These 20 clinical studies describe experience with adenosine or dipyridamole stress CMR in 1392 patients. It is important to note that many smaller studies have been published that could not be included in this chapter

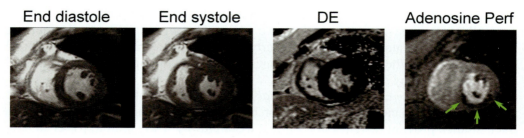

Fig. 4. Stress perfusion study in a patient with severe coronary artery disease but no myocardial infarction (*see* figure 4 movies A and C in CD).

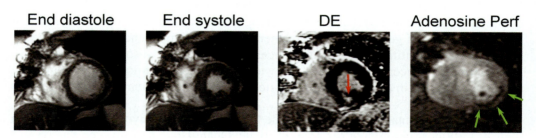

Fig. 5. Stress perfusion study in a patient with prior myocardial infarction but also with peri-infarct ischemia (*see* figure 5 movies A and C in CD).

because of space limitations. A few trends that warrant further discussion are evident from these studies.

The overall sensitivity for detecting coronary artery disease is approximately 83% (Table 1). However, only one study using the newer hybrid echo-planar imaging (EPI) methods reported less than 80% sensitivity. Overall specificity is about 82%, but 3 of the 11 studies using hybrid EPI methods had less than 80% specificity. Nonetheless, the overall sensitivity and specificity are clinically relevant.

Some variability originates from the comparisons and reference standards used for a given study. For example, in the study by Schwitter et al. *(13)*, the sensitivity and specificity of adenosine perfusion CMR was 91 and 94%, respectively, when PET perfusion was the reference standard but 87 and 85%, respectively, when quantitative coronary angiography was the reference standard. The majority of studies used visual assessment of the invasive coronary angiogram as the reference standard. It is well accepted that visual assessment frequently results in some overestimation of stenosis severity. Thus, the reference standards used and the thresholds selected influence the sensitivity and specificity.

Ishida et al. *(14)* compared dipyridamole stress CMR perfusion with single photon emission computed tomography (SPECT) imaging for detecting a 70% stenosis on coronary angiography. CMR had higher sensitivity and specificity than SPECT. In receiver operator curve analysis, CMR outperformed SPECT over a wide range of diagnostic thresholds. They also documented cases in which triple-vessel disease was misdiagnosed by SPECT but was evident as a diffuse subendocardial perfusion defect by CMR. Schwitter et al. *(13)* found that dipyridamole CMR perfusion had similar diagnostic performance as a PET perfusion study in careful receiver operator curve analysis when both tests were compared with quantitative coronary angiography.

Table 1
Sensitivity and Specificity of Vasodilator Stress Perfusion Studies for Detecting Coronary Artery Disease

Year	Reference	n	Stress	Dose (Gd)	Technique	Comparisons	Analysis	Sensitivity (%)	Specificity (%)
2006	16	92	Adenosine	0.065	Hybrid EPI	Cath <70%	Qualitative	89	87
2006	15	135	Adenosine	0.1	Hybrid EPI	Prognosis	Qualitative	100	93
2005	37	33	Dipyridamole	0.05	Hybrid EPI	Cath <75%	Qualitative	84	87
2005	38	40	Dipyridamole	0.03	GRE	Cath <70%	Qualitative	81	68
2005	39	92	Adenosine	0.05	GRE	Cath <70%	SLP	88	82
2004	40	102	Dipyridamole	0.1	Hybrid EPI	Cath <50%	Qualitative	93	85
2004	41	49	Adenosine	0.05, 0.1, 0.15	Hybrid EPI	Cath <75%	Qualitative	79	75
2004	42	79	Adenosine	0.05	Hybrid EPI	QCA <50%	Qualitative	91	62
2004	43	99	Adenosine	0.05, 0.1, 0.15	Hybrid EPI	QCA <70%	Qualitative	93	75
2004	44	32	Adenosine	0.05	GRE	Cath <70%	SLP	75	80
						SPECT		97	91
2004	17	72	Adenosine	0.05	GRE	Cath <70%	Qualitative	88	83
2004	45	35	Adenosine	0.05	GRE	Cath <50%	SLP	74	71
2003	5	84	Adenosine	0.025	Hybrid EPI	Cath <75%	SLP	88	90
2003	14	104	Dipyridamole	0.075	Hybrid EPI	Cath <70%	Qualitative	84	82
2003	46	184	Dipyridamole	0.04	GRE	QCA <70%	SLP	57	52
						SPECT		78	82
2003	47	27	Dipyridamole	0.1	GRE	Cath 75–90%	Qualitative	55	77
						Cath <90%		77	81
2002	48	25	Adenosine	0.05	Hybrid EPI	QCA <75%	SLP	69	89
2001	13	48	Dipyridamole	0.1	Hybrid EPI	QCA <50%	SLP	87	85
						PET		91	94
2001	36	26	Adenosine	0.05	SE-EPI	Cath <50%	SLP, CE, TPK	79, 72, 60	77
							Qualitative	83, 83, 43	83
2000	3	34	Dipyridamole	NA	NA	Cath <75%	SLP	90	83

Cath, coronary angiography; QCA, quantitative coronary angiography; SPECT, single photon emission computed tomography; PET, positron emission tomography; EPI, echo-planar imaging; GRE, gradient-recalled echo; SLP, signal intensity upslope; CE, contrast enhancement; TPK, time to peak contrast enhancement; NA, information not available.

Ingkanisorn et al. *(15)* used adenosine stress CMR perfusion to assess patients who presented to an emergency department with chest pain but had acute myocardial infarction excluded by serial electrocardiogram (ECG) and cardiac biomarkers. No patients with a negative adenosine CMR developed adverse cardiovascular end points during approximately 1-year follow-up (100% sensitivity); a large percentage of subjects with a positive adenosine CMR had a new diagnosis or complication of coronary disease confirmed during follow-up (specificity 91%).

Klem et al. *(16)* developed a practical and rapid qualitative approach to detecting coronary artery disease that relies on a combination of delayed enhancement, stress perfusion, and rest perfusion imaging. In patients presenting to the emergency department with chest pain but no prior history of myocardial infarction, a simple three-step algorithm provided high diagnostic accuracy and could be performed in a few minutes. By avoiding any quantitative analysis, this approach is clinically feasible and efficient. In step 1, evidence of any myocardial infarction using delayed enhancement imaging in such a patient is highly specific for coronary artery disease and further workup or hospitalization appears warranted. In step 2, if stress perfusion imaging is normal, then the patient does not need further testing for coronary artery disease. In step 3, rest perfusion images help decide if the stress perfusion defects are real. In their algorithm, a real stress perfusion defect is present only if a similiar artifact or possible perfusion defect is not also present on rest perfusion images.

One advantage of CMR is the complementary nature of cine, perfusion, viability, and coronary imaging. In general, many studies have shown substantial benefit to combined analysis of all available CMR data rather than relying on a single component. This was nicely documented by Plein et al. *(17)* in a study of patients with known or suspected acute coronary syndrome. In that study, adenosine perfusion had the highest diagnostic accuracy of any single component of the CMR examination. However, a combined interpretation of perfusion, coronary magnetic resonance angiography, delayed enhancement, and cine MRI had higher diagnostic accuracy than any individual component. Importantly, the authors ignored or discounted poor-quality images and relied only on those methods that provided highest diagnostic confidence.

ASSESSING THE RESPONSE TO MYOCARDIAL REVASCULARIZATION

CMR is capable of detecting improvement in myocardial perfusion before and after revascularization (Table 2) *(4,18–20)*. For example, Lauerma et al. *(18)* studied 10 patients with single-vessel coronary artery disease located in the proximal left anterior descending coronary artery before and after percutaneous intervention. They found that myocardial time intensity curves differentiated ischemic myocardium from normal myocardium on the initial study, and that these abnormalities generally improved with revascularization.

In 35 patients undergoing percutaneous intervention for known severe coronary stenosis, the MPR_i prior to intervention was lower than for a group of normal control subjects *(4)*. After percutaneous intervention, MPR_i improved in all subjects and normalized in all but 4 patients. Intriguingly, all 4 subjects that received percutaneous intervention but failed to improve stress perfusion into the normal range had angioplasty without a stent.

Taylor et al. *(21)* found that there was a delay in the arrival of contrast in the myocardium distal to a successful percutaneous intervention, which they interpreted

Table 2

MRI Perfusion Studies for Assessing the Response of Myocardial Revascularization

Year	Reference	Subjects	n	Stress	Rest	Primary finding
2006	21	PCI	15	No	Yes	PCI resulted in a delay of regional contrast arrival and a reduction in SLP; regional systolic thickening was not different
2004	49	Laser or thoracic sympathectomy	20 (15 CMR)	Yes	Yes	Laser had greater clinical benefit than thoracic sympathectomy early after surgery, but no perfusion differences were found
2004	24	Infarcted (pre- and postrevascularization)	18	No	Yes	Perfusion CMR had a poor predictive value for functional recovery
2002	20	PCI	6	Yes	Yes	Perfusion reserve of remote and ischemic myocardium was different before PCI; perfusion reserve improved in ischemic sectors after PCI; PCI reduced the number of ischemic segments
2002	50	Laser	15	No	Yes	Laser did not improve SPECT perfusions; however, CMR perfusion showed a smaller underperfused area during follow-up and improved regional function
2000	19	CABG (pre and post)	10	Yes	No	Viable myocardium assessment was more accurate in cine, perfusion, and delay-enhanced CMR than PET
2000	22	Revascularization (pre and post)	12	No	Yes	Perfusion did not predict viability as well as delayed enhancement imaging
2000	4	CAD (pre and postintervention)	35	Yes	Yes	Perfusion reserve was abnormally low distal to a significant stenosis and improved with revascularization
1997	18	CAD (pre and postrevascularization)	11	Yes	Yes	Stress perfusions were abnormal before treatment and improved after revascularization; SPECT and CMR defect size agreed well

Abbreviations are the same as in Table 1 unless otherwise stated. PCI, percutaneous coronary intervention; laser, laser revascularization; CAD, coronary artery disease; CABG, coronary artery bypass graft.

321

as evidence of a postprocedure abnormality in blood flow regulation. Whether this intriguing finding is a result of plaque rupture or other mechanisms warrants further investigation.

Regarding predicting myocardial viability, Sandstede et al. *(22)* found that cine magnetic resonance imaging (MRI) and delayed enhancement imaging were more useful in predicting recovery of regional myocardial function after revascularization compared with rest perfusion imaging. The high predictive value of delayed enhancement *(23)* relegates the main benefit of perfusion imaging to further defining the pathophysiology of segments with intermediate degrees of delayed enhancement or in special circumstances where the presence of myocardial ischemia is in question despite the presence of some degree of coronary stenosis. Van Hoe et al. *(24)* came to similar conclusions.

Although the number of CMR studies evaluating perfusion before and after myocardial revascularization remains fairly limited, a few trends are evident. The first-pass perfusion studies are capable of detecting significant stenosis. Most perfusion parameters improve or normalize after the procedure. Based on this limited information, delayed enhancement appears to be a better measure of viability than resting first-pass perfusion imaging.

SOME TECHNICAL CONSIDERATIONS REGARDING CARDIAC MAGNETIC RESONANCE PERFUSION IMAGING

The choice of contrast dose varies substantially from study to study (Table 1). Although 10 studies used a gadolinium dose of 0.05 mmol/kg, 6 studies used double that dose (0.1 mmol/kg), and few studies used three times (0.15 mmol/kg) as much contrast. Choice of contrast dose is not simple. There is an important interplay between the dose of contrast, the image acquisition parameters, and even the analysis of the images. In general, it is desirable for signal intensity to remain proportional to contrast concentration over the range of values encountered. This is most likely to occur at low doses of contrast (approximately 0.05 mmol/kg). If the analysis is not dependent on the LV cavity signal, then it might be advantageous to use higher doses to get more contrast enhancement within the myocardium. Newer methods use a combination of either two different boluses of contrast *(9,25,26)* or two imaging parameters *(27)* to get accurate measurements in both the LV cavity and the myocardium.

The choice of image acquisition sequence is also quite variable. The simplest image acquisition method relies on a gradient echo (GRE) image readout as used in 5 of the 20 studies listed in Table 1. The biggest advantage of this method is lower likelihood of image artifacts. It comes at the cost of being slower and having lower image signal-to-noise ratio compared with the other methods. The hybrid EPI methods typically acquire 4 or 6 lines of raw data for each radio-frequency excitation *(10)*. This accelerates how fast a perfusion image can be acquired by a factor of about 2.5 compared with the simpler GRE readouts. Thus, the user can get about 2.5 times as many slices of the heart per heartbeat with a hybrid EPI acquisition compared with a GRE readout. Newer studies may use a steady-state free precession acquisition (various trade names FISP [fast imaging with steady-state precession], fast imaging employing steady state acquisition (FIESTA), balanced turbo filled echo (TFE)) *(28)*.

As of the time this chapter was written, no publications reported sensitivity and specificity in more than 25 patients with a steady-state free precession acquisition perfusion method. Theoretically, steady-state free precession methods are as fast as hybrid EPI methods and have better signal-to-noise ratio than either competing method. The extent to which steady-state free precession techniques get used will be determined by the amount of artifact on the images and diagnostic accuracy of studies using this method.

USE OF FIRST-PASS PERFUSION IN ACUTE MYOCARDIAL INFARCTION

CMR perfusion studies have been used in the setting of acute myocardial infarction and also after stabilization after myocardial infarction. In general, a rest perfusion study can be used to detect microvascular obstruction assuming that the coronary artery was successfully reperfused. Wu et al. *(29)* noted that patients with microvascular obstruction after acute myocardial infarction had worse prognosis than those patients without microvascular obstruction.

FIRST-PASS PERFUSION IN MISCELLANEOUS CONDITIONS

First-pass perfusion imaging has many applications beyond traditional stress testing to detect coronary artery disease. Table 3 lists a number of studies that have used these CMR perfusion methods to address disease states or conditions that did not easily fit in the prior portions of this chapter.

First-pass perfusion imaging has helped resolve a long-standing question about the pathophysiology of hibernating myocardium in patients. Basic science studies have indicated prolonged moderate reductions of myocardial perfusion cause downregulation of myocardial function *(30)* and metabolism *(31,32)*. Clinically, it has been uncertain whether the regional myocardial dysfunction is a result of repetitive myocardial stunning or whether a state of myocardial hibernation exists.

Selvanayagam et al. *(33)* used quantitative analysis to measure rest myocardial perfusion before and after angioplasty in 27 carefully selected patients with severe coronary artery disease and a regional wall motion abnormality that was not explainable by myocardial infarction. Based on successful recovery of function after revascularization, these segments meet clinical criteria to qualify as hibernating myocardium. Their quantitative perfusion analysis indicated that subendocardial perfusion was lower in hibernating myocardium compared to normal tissue.

The response to dipyridamole in "normal myocardium" varies with the age and health of the subject. There is a significant stepwise trend toward reduced myocardial perfusion in regions served by coronary arteries of patients with the following characteristics: (1) in patients with no abnormality detected in the coronary arteries by invasive coronary angiography; (2) in segments downstream from angiographically normal arteries in patients with coronary artery disease elsewhere; (3) in segments with less than a 40% stenosis; (4) in segments with 40–70% stenosis; and (5) with lowest perfusion in segments distal to a 70% stenosis *(34)*.

Wang et al. *(8)* measured adenosine stress myocardial blood flow in 222 asymptomatic participants of the Multi-Ethnic Study of Atherosclerosis (MESA), an epidemiological study funded by the National Heart, Lung, and Blood Institute. Men had lower rest and hyperemic myocardial blood flow than women. Age, hypertension, and dyslipidemia were all associated with lower myocardial perfusion reserve. There was also an inverse correlation between peak myocardial blood flow and the 10-years risk of coronary

Table 3

MRI Perfusion Studies in Miscellaneous Conditions

Year	Reference	Subjects	n	Stress	Rest	Primary finding
2006	51	Normal	18	Yes	Yes	CMR perfusion reserve was lower than PET (compartmental analysis); CMR rest perfusion was higher than PET, but stress was comparable; correlation of CMR and PET was good
2006	26	Normal	10	Yes	Yes	SLP and CE underestimated perfusion reserve compared to quantitative perfusion
2006	8	Asymptomatic	222	Yes	Yes	Stress perfusion and perfusion reserve correlated inversely with 10-years Framingham risk scores
2006	34	CAD	37	Yes	Yes	Perfusion was lower in patients with increasing evidence of CAD
2005	33	PCI	27	No	Yes	Rest perfusion was abnormal distal severe coronary stenoses consistent with one leading theory about hibernating myocardium
2005	52	Heart transplant	15	No	Yes	Perfusion was different for transplant recipients with normal cath and with transplant arteriopathy
2005	53	Inferior attenuation on SPECT	30	Yes	Yes	CMR perfusion abnormalities were detected in 23% of patients with inferior attenuation on SPECT
2005	54	DCM	7	Yes	Yes	Perfusion was not different at rest but was abnormal during stress comparing DCM patients and normal subjects
2005	55	CAD, valvular, and myocarditis	13	No	Yes	12 array coil improved SNR, SLP, CE, and INT perfusion parameters
2005	56	Systemic sclerosis	18	Yes	Yes	SLP increased after nifedipine treatment
2005	57	AMI and myocarditis	55 (31, 24)	No	Yes	96% of myocarditis patients had normal rest perfusion; 100% AMI patients had a segmental distribution of subendocardial defects
2004	58	AMI	60	No	Yes	Perfusion images detected MO in 38% of patients; these patients had larger MI at delay enhancement than patients without MO

324

Year	Ref	Condition	N			Findings
2004	59	AMI	20, 10	No	Yes	A contrast delay longer than 2 seconds and transmural infarction were independent predictors of impaired LV systolic thickening at 3 months
2004	60	HCM, DCM, CAD, and abnormal ECG but normal Cath	12 (5, 2, 4, 1)	Yes	Yes	Stress perfusion increased in patients with normal cath or after PCI but not in patients with CAD; stress perfusion increased in HCM but not in DCM patients
2004	61	Congenital and pediatric	17	Some	Yes	Good agreement in perfusion and cine CMR with cath and SPECT.
2003	62	AMI	27	No	Yes	Perfusion parameters (INT, SLP, CE) correlated with myocardial wall thickening and degree of coronary artery stenosis
2003	63	Tx-CHD	27	Yes	Yes	Tx-CHD had educed myocardial perfusion reserve and transmural perfusion gradient
2002	64	Syndrome X	20	Yes	Yes	Stress SLP increased in normal subjects and in patient subepi segments but not in patient subendo segments
2002	35	Diabetes	19 (9 AN+, 10 AN–)	Yes	Yes	Perfusion was similar in normal, AN+, and AN– groups at rest but was lower in AN+ patients than in AN– or normal groups; perfusion reserve correlated with blood pressure during stress
2001	65	CAD, microvascular dysfunction, and DCM	14 (9, 3, 2)	Some (3)	Yes	Good intraobserver and interobserver agreement in quantitative perfusion measurements.

Abbreviations are the same as in Table 1 unless otherwise stated. DCM. dilated cardiomyopathy; HCM. hypertrophic cardiomyopathy; ECG, electrocardiograms; Tx-CHD, transplant arteriopathy; AMI, acute myocardial infarction; AN, autonomic neuropathy; MO, microvascular obstruction; INT, signal intensity upslope integral.

heart disease estimated by the Framingham model. Thus, at least at a population level, vasodilator stress perfusion appears capable of detecting preclinical levels of abnormal vasodilator reserve associated with traditional risk factors for coronary artery disease.

Taskiran et al. *(35)* measured myocardial perfusion at rest and during stress in subjects with diabetes. Diabetic patients with dysautonomia averaged about 35% lower stress perfusion than normal volunteers. Diabetic patients without evidence of dysautonomia averaged about 90% of that seen in normal subjects. This study further supports the concept that CMR can detect subtle differences in myocardial perfusion. Thus, first-pass perfusion is a powerful tool that can provide insights into the regulation of myocardial perfusion.

Panting et al. *(64)* studied patients with microvascular coronary regulation abnormalities caused by syndrome X. In general, this type of patient is ideally suited for CMR perfusion studies because this technique has adequate resolution to resolve subendocardial perfusion from subepicardial perfusion. Thus, CMR can detect uniformity or diffusely abnormal subendocardial perfusion that might be missed on a lower resolution test like SPECT. Diffuse subendocardial perfusion abnormalities are also a hallmark of the relatively uncommon but important "balanced" three-vessel disease *(14)*.

Although Table 3 cannot comprehensively survey the literature, it is clear that various investigators have found value in CMR perfusion imaging in a wide range of clinical situations, including transplant arteriopathy, congenital heart disease, and certain types of cardiomyopathy. Thus, one can expect an expanding role of CMR perfusion in understanding a wide range of disease.

ACKNOWLEDGMENTS

This work was supported by the Intramural Research Program of the National Heart, Lung, and Blood Institute.

REFERENCES

1. Klocke FJ, Simonetti OP, Judd RM, et al. Limits of detection of regional differences in vasodilated flow in viable myocardium by first-pass magnetic resonance perfusion imaging. Circulation 2001; 104:2412–2416.
2. Lee DC, Simonetti OP, Harris KR, et al. Magnetic resonance vs radionuclide pharmacological stress perfusion imaging for flow-limiting stenoses of varying severity. Circulation 2004;110:58–65.
3. Al-Saadi N, Nagel E, Gross M, et al. Noninvasive detection of myocardial ischemia from perfusion reserve based on cardiovascular magnetic resonance. Circulation 2000;101:1379–1383.
4. Al-Saadi N, Nagel E, Gross M, et al. Improvement of myocardial perfusion reserve early after coronary intervention: assessment with cardiac magnetic resonance imaging. J Am Coll Cardiol 2000;36: 1557–1564.
5. Nagel E, Klein C, Paetsch I, et al. Magnetic resonance perfusion measurements for the noninvasive detection of coronary artery disease. Circulation 2003;108:432–437.
6. Jerosch-Herold M, Wilke N, Stillman AE. Magnetic resonance quantification of the myocardial perfusion reserve with a Fermi function model for constrained deconvolution. Med Phys 1998;25: 73–84.
7. Larsson HB, Fritz-Hansen T, Rostrup E, et al. Myocardial perfusion modeling using MRI. Magn Reson Med 1996;35:716–726.
8. Wang L, Jerosch-Herold M, Jacobs DR Jr, et al. Coronary risk factors and myocardial perfusion in asymptomatic adults: the Multi-Ethnic Study of Atherosclerosis (MESA). J Am Coll Cardiol 2006;47:565–572.
9. Christian TF, Rettmann DW, Aletras AH, et al. Absolute myocardial perfusion in canines measured by using dual-bolus first-pass MR imaging. Radiology 2004;232:677–684.
10. Epstein FH, London JF, Peters DC, et al. Multislice first-pass cardiac perfusion MRI: validation in a model of myocardial infarction. Magn Reson Med 2002;47:482–491.

11. Cullen JH, Horsfield MA, Reek CR, et al. A myocardial perfusion reserve index in humans using first-pass contrast-enhanced magnetic resonance imaging. J Am Coll Cardiol 1999;33: 1386–1394.

12. Jerosch-Herold M, Hu X, Murthy NS, et al. Time delay for arrival of MR contrast agent in collateral-dependent myocardium. IEEE Trans Med Imaging 2004;23:881–890.

13. Schwitter J, Nanz D, Kneifel S, et al. Assessment of myocardial perfusion in coronary artery disease by magnetic resonance: a comparison with positron emission tomography and coronary angiography. Circulation 2001;103:2230–2235.

14. Ishida N, Sakuma H, Motoyasu M, et al. Noninfarcted myocardium: correlation between dynamic first-pass contrast-enhanced myocardial MR imaging and quantitative coronary angiography. Radiology 2003;229:209–216.

15. Ingkanisorn WP, Kwong RY, Bohme NS, et al. Prognosis of negative adenosine stress magnetic resonance in patients presenting to an emergency department with chest pain. J Am Coll Cardiol 2006;47:1427–1432.

16. Klem I, Heitner JF, Shah DJ, et al. Improved detection of coronary artery disease by stress perfusion cardiovascular magnetic resonance with the use of delayed enhancement infarction imaging. J Am Coll Cardiol 2006;47:1630–1638.

17. Plein S, Greenwood JP, Ridgway JP, et al. Assessment of non-ST-segment elevation acute coronary syndromes with cardiac magnetic resonance imaging. J Am Coll Cardiol 2004;44:2173–2181.

18. Lauerma K, Virtanen KS, Sipila LM, et al. Multislice MRI in assessment of myocardial perfusion in patients with single-vessel proximal left anterior descending coronary artery disease before and after revascularization. Circulation 1997;96:2859–2867.

19. Lauerma K, Niemi P, Hanninen H, et al. Multimodality MR imaging assessment of myocardial viability: combination of first-pass and late contrast enhancement to wall motion dynamics and comparison with FDG PET-initial experience. Radiology 2000;217:729–736.

20. Sensky PR, Samani NJ, Horsfield MA, et al. Restoration of myocardial blood flow following percutaneous coronary balloon dilatation and stent implantation: assessment with qualitative and quantitative contrast-enhanced magnetic resonance imaging. Clin Radiol 2002;57:593–599.

21. Taylor AJ, Al-Saadi N, Abdel-Aty H, et al. Elective percutaneous coronary intervention immediately impairs resting microvascular perfusion assessed by cardiac magnetic resonance imaging. Am Heart J 2006;151:891 e891–e897.

22. Sandstede JJ, Lipke C, Beer M, et al. Analysis of first-pass and delayed contrast-enhancement patterns of dysfunctional myocardium on MR imaging: use in the prediction of myocardial viability. AJR Am J Roentgenol 2000;174:1737–1740.

23. Kim RJ, Wu E, Rafael A, et al. The use of contrast-enhanced magnetic resonance imaging to identify reversible myocardial dysfunction. N Engl J Med 2000;343:1445–1453.

24. Van Hoe L, Vanderheyden M. Ischemic cardiomyopathy: value of different MRI techniques for prediction of functional recovery after revascularization. AJR Am J Roentgenol 2004;182:95–100.

25. Kostler H, Ritter C, Lipp M, et al. Prebolus quantitative MR heart perfusion imaging. Magn Reson Med 2004;52:296–299.

26. Hsu LY, Rhoads KL, Holly JE, et al. Quantitative myocardial perfusion analysis with a dual-bolus contrast-enhanced first-pass MRI technique in humans. J Magn Reson Imaging 2006;23:315–322.

27. Gatehouse PD, Elkington AG, Ablitt NA, et al. Accurate assessment of the arterial input function during high-dose myocardial perfusion cardiovascular magnetic resonance. J Magn Reson Imaging 2004;20:39–45.

28. Fenchel M, Helber U, Kramer U, et al. Detection of regional myocardial perfusion deficit using rest and stress perfusion MRI: a feasibility study. AJR Am J Roentgenol 2005;185:627–635.

29. Wu KC, Zerhouni EA, Judd RM, et al. Prognostic significance of microvascular obstruction by magnetic resonance imaging in patients with acute myocardial infarction. Circulation 1998;97: 765–772.

30. Vatner SF. Correlation between acute reductions in myocardial blood flow and function in conscious dogs. Circ Res 1980;47:201–207.

31. Gallagher KP, Matsuzaki M, Koziol JA, et al. Regional myocardial perfusion and wall thickening during ischemia in conscious dogs. Am J Physiol 1984;247(5, pt 2):H727–H738.

32. Arai AE, Pantely GA, Anselone CG, et al. Active downregulation of myocardial energy requirements during prolonged moderate ischemia in swine. Circ Res 1991;69:1458–1469.

33. Selvanayagam JB, Jerosch-Herold M, Porto I, et al. Resting myocardial blood flow is impaired in hibernating myocardium: a magnetic resonance study of quantitative perfusion assessment. Circulation 2005;112:3289–3296.

34. Rodrigues de Avila LF, Fernandes JL, Rochitte CE, et al. Perfusion impairment in patients with normal-appearing coronary arteries: identification with contrast-enhanced MR imaging. Radiology 2006;238:464–472.
35. Taskiran M, Fritz-Hansen T, Rasmussen V, et al. Decreased myocardial perfusion reserve in diabetic autonomic neuropathy. Diabetes 2002;51:3306–3310.
36. Panting JR, Gatehouse PD, Yang GZ, et al. Echo-planar magnetic resonance myocardial perfusion imaging: parametric map analysis and comparison with thallium SPECT. J Magn Reson Imaging 2001;13:192–200.
37. Okuda S, Tanimoto A, Satoh T, et al. Evaluation of ischemic heart disease on a 1.5 T scanner: combined first-pass perfusion and viability study. Radiat Med 2005;23:230–235.
38. Sakuma H, Suzawa N, Ichikawa Y, et al. Diagnostic accuracy of stress first-pass contrast-enhanced myocardial perfusion MRI compared with stress myocardial perfusion scintigraphy. AJR Am J Roentgenol 2005;185:95–102.
39. Plein S, Radjenovic A, Ridgway JP, et al. Coronary artery disease: myocardial perfusion MR imaging with sensitivity encoding vs conventional angiography. Radiology 2005;235:423–430.
40. Takase B, Nagata M, Kihara T, et al. Whole-heart dipyridamole stress first-pass myocardial perfusion MRI for the detection of coronary artery disease. Jpn Heart J 2004;45:475–486.
41. Paetsch I, Foll D, Langreck H, et al. Myocardial perfusion imaging using OMNISCAN: a dose finding study for visual assessment of stress-induced regional perfusion abnormalities. J Cardiovasc Magn Reson 2004;6:803–809.
42. Paetsch I, Jahnke C, Wahl A, et al. Comparison of dobutamine stress magnetic resonance, adenosine stress magnetic resonance, and adenosine stress magnetic resonance perfusion. Circulation 2004;110: 835–842.
43. Wolff SD, Schwitter J, Coulden R, et al. Myocardial first-pass perfusion magnetic resonance imaging: a multicenter dose-ranging study. Circulation 2004;110:732–737.
44. Thiele H, Plein S, Breeuwer M, et al. Color-encoded semiautomatic analysis of multi-slice first-pass magnetic resonance perfusion: comparison to tetrofosmin single photon emission computed tomography perfusion and X-ray angiography. Int J Cardiovasc Imaging 2004;20:371–384; discussion 385–377.
45. Bunce NH, Reyes E, Keegan J, et al. Combined coronary and perfusion cardiovascular magnetic resonance for the assessment of coronary artery stenosis. J Cardiovasc Magn Reson 2004;6:527–539.
46. Doyle M, Fuisz A, Kortright E, et al. The impact of myocardial flow reserve on the detection of coronary artery disease by perfusion imaging methods: an NHLBI WISE study. J Cardiovasc Magn Reson 2003;5:475–485.
47. Kinoshita M, Nomura M, Harada M, et al. Myocardial perfusion magnetic resonance imaging for diagnosing coronary arterial stenosis. Jpn Heart J 2003;44:323–334.
48. Ibrahim T, Nekolla SG, Schreiber K, et al. Assessment of coronary flow reserve: comparison between contrast-enhanced magnetic resonance imaging and positron emission tomography. J Am Coll Cardiol 2002;39:864–870.
49. Galinanes M, Loubani M, Sensky PR, et al. Efficacy of transmyocardial laser revascularization and thoracic sympathectomy for the treatment of refractory angina. Ann Thorac Surg 2004;78:122–128.
50. Laham RJ, Simons M, Pearlman JD, et al. Magnetic resonance imaging demonstrates improved regional systolic wall motion and thickening and myocardial perfusion of myocardial territories treated by laser myocardial revascularization. J Am Coll Cardiol 2002;39:1–8.
51. Parkka JP, Niemi P, Saraste A, et al. Comparison of MRI and positron emission tomography for measuring myocardial perfusion reserve in healthy humans. Magn Reson Med 2006;55:772–779.
52. Muehling OM, Panse P, Jerosch-Herold M, et al. Cardiac magnetic resonance perfusion imaging identifies transplant arteriopathy by a reduced endomyocardial resting perfusion. J Heart Lung Transplant 2005;24:1122–1123.
53. McCrohon JA, Lyne JC, Rahman SL, et al. Adjunctive role of cardiovascular magnetic resonance in the assessment of patients with inferior attenuation on myocardial perfusion SPECT. J Cardiovasc Magn Reson 2005;7:377–382.
54. Watzinger N, Lund GK, Saeed M, et al. Myocardial blood flow in patients with dilated cardiomyopathy: quantitative assessment with velocity-encoded cine magnetic resonance imaging of the coronary sinus. J Magn Reson Imaging 2005;21:347–353.
55. Hoffmann MH, Schmid FT, Jeltsch M, et al. Multislice MR first-pass myocardial perfusion imaging: impact of the receiver coil array. J Magn Reson Imaging 2005;21:310–316.

56. Vignaux O, Allanore Y, Meune C, et al. Evaluation of the effect of nifedipine upon myocardial perfusion and contractility using cardiac magnetic resonance imaging and tissue Doppler echocardiography in systemic sclerosis. Ann Rheum Dis 2005;64:1268–1273.
57. Laissy JP, Hyafil F, Feldman LJ, et al. Differentiating acute myocardial infarction from myocarditis: diagnostic value of early- and delayed-perfusion cardiac MR imaging. Radiology 2005;237:75–82.
58. Lund GK, Stork A, Saeed M, et al. Acute myocardial infarction: evaluation with first-pass enhancement and delayed enhancement MR imaging compared with 201Tl SPECT imaging. Radiology 2004;232: 49–57.
59. Taylor AJ, Al Saadi N, Abdel-Aty H, et al. Detection of acutely impaired microvascular reperfusion after infarct angioplasty with magnetic resonance imaging. Circulation 2004;109:2080–2085.
60. Nakajima T, Oriuchi N, Tsushima Y, et al. Noninvasive determination of regional myocardial perfusion with first-pass magnetic resonance (MR) imaging. Acad Radiol 2004;11:802–808.
61. Prakash A, Powell AJ, Krishnamurthy R, et al. Magnetic resonance imaging evaluation of myocardial perfusion and viability in congenital and acquired pediatric heart disease. Am J Cardiol 2004;93: 657–661.
62. Miller S, Helber U, Brechtel K, et al. MR imaging at rest early after myocardial infarction: detection of preserved function in regions with evidence for ischemic injury and non-transmural myocardial infarction. Eur Radiol 2003;13:498–506.
63. Muehling OM, Wilke N, Panse P, et al. Reduced myocardial perfusion reserve and transmural perfusion gradient in heart transplant arteriopathy assessed by magnetic resonance imaging. J Am Coll Cardiol 2003;42:1054–1060.
64. Panting JR, Gatehouse PD, Yang GZ, et al. Abnormal subendocardial perfusion in cardiac syndrome X detected by cardiovascular magnetic resonance imaging. N Engl J Med 2002;346:1948–1953.
65. Muhling OM, Dickson ME, Zenovich A, et al. Quantitative magnetic resonance first-pass perfusion analysis: inter- and intraobserver agreement. J Cardiovasc Magn Reson 2001;3:247–256.

16 Coronary Magnetic Resonance Angiography

Hajime Sakuma

CONTENTS

INTRODUCTION

Coronary artery disease is one of the leading causes of morbidity and mortality in many industrialized countries *(1)*. Catheter X-ray coronary angiography has been used as the gold standard for identifying significant luminal narrowing of the coronary arteries. However, X-ray coronary angiography entails small but definable risks *(2)*, and a considerable number of patients undergoing elective X-ray coronary angiography are found to have no significant coronary arterial disease *(3)*. Consequently, there is a strong need for a noninvasive test that can reliably delineate narrowing of the coronary arteries.

Considerable progress has been made in the field of noninvasive imaging of the coronary arteries by using magnetic resonance (MR) angiography and computed tomography (CT). Contrast-enhanced multislice spiral CT has rapidly emerged as a noninvasive method that can provide visualization of the coronary arteries and detection of the luminal narrowing. In particular, the new-generation 64-slice CT scanners are significantly improved in terms of gantry speed, spatial resolution, and temporal resolution *(4,5)*. Mollet et al. *(5)* reported that significant coronary arterial stenoses were detected using a 64-slice CT scanner with a sensitivity of 99% and a specificity of 95% compared with catheter X-ray coronary angiography.

However, multislice CT has several disadvantages of requiring rapid injection of iodinated contrast medium and of exposing the patients to ionizing radiation. Estimated effective radiation dose of 64-slice CT coronary angiography was 13–15 mSv for men and 18–21 mSv for women *(4,5)*, substantially higher than a typical radiation dose for diagnostic X-ray coronary angiography.

From: *Contemporary Cardiology: Cardiovascular Magnetic Resonance Imaging*
Edited by: Raymond Y. Kwong © Humana Press Inc., Totowa, NJ

From a patient's point of view, coronary MR angiography is more preferable to coronary CT angiography for the detection of coronary artery disease because it does not expose the patient to radiation or necessitate a rapid injection of iodinated contrast material. In addition, coronary arterial lumen can be readily visualized by coronary MR angiography in patients with heavy calcification of the atherosclerotic coronary plaques.

Despite these potential advantages of coronary MR angiography, noninvasive MR imaging of the coronary artery is technically demanding because of small size and tortuous course of the coronary arteries and their complex motion caused by cardiac contraction and respiration. Sufficient contrast between coronary arterial lumen and the surrounding tissue is crucial for the visualization of the coronary artery. In addition, high spatial resolution and volume coverage of the coronary artery trees are required, and time available for MR image data acquisition is limited to overcome complex motion of the coronary artery.

In this chapter, the techniques currently used for coronary MR angiography and new methods to improve visualization of the coronary artery are briefly reviewed. Then, the current roles of coronary MR angiography for the evaluation of coronary artery disease and other abnormalities, such as anomalous coronary artery and Kawasaki disease, are explained.

TECHNIQUES OF CORONARY MAGNETIC RESONANCE ANGIOGRAPHY

Two-Dimensional and Three-Dimensional Acquisitions

Assessment of coronary artery disease with coronary MR angiography was initiated in the early 1990s by using breath-hold two-dimensional (2D) segmented k-space gradient echo techniques *(6–8)*. The breath-hold 2D approach was relatively easy to implement and had some success in the visualization of the proximal coronary arteries. However, breath-hold 2D coronary MR angiography has several limitations, including slice misregistration because of inconsistent diaphragm positions between breath-hold scans, patient fatigue from multiple repeated breath holdings, suboptimal signal-to-noise ratio caused by 2D acquisition of thin-slice and high operator dependency to successfully image tortuous coronary arteries with 2D imaging slices.

To overcome these limitations of breath-hold 2D methods, three-dimensional (3D) gradient echo coronary MR angiography sequences were developed by employing either a breath-hold method or a respiratory-gated method. The advantages of 3D coronary MR angiography are improved signal-to-noise ratio, volumetric coverage of the coronary arteries, and no misregistration between slices within each 3D volume acquisition. These features of 3D coronary MR angiography permit 3D postprocessing of the coronary artery tree. Volume coverage, acquisition speed, and arterial contrast of 3D coronary MR angiography have substantially improved with use of steady-state free precession sequences and parallel imaging techniques, allowing for the acquisition of high-quality 3D MR angiograms encompassing all coronary arteries within a reasonably short imaging time.

The most fundamental weakness of 3D coronary MR angiography compared with recent 64-slice CT scanners is slow acquisition speed of 3D volume data. For example, imaging of 3D data with $300 \times 300 \times 100$ mm volume coverage and $0.6 \times 0.6 \times 0.6$ mm acquisition resolution necessitates more than 20,000 phase-encoding steps when a parallel imaging factor of 2 and a half-scan are employed, which corresponds to approximately

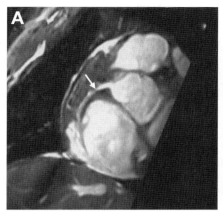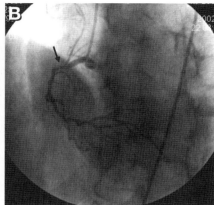

Fig. 1. Breath-hold 3D coronary MR angiography acquired with a steady state free precession sequence (FIESTA) in a patient with stenosis in the right coronary artery. **(A)** Oblique multi-planar reformatted image demonstrates significant luminal narrowing (arrow) in the proximal right coronary artery. **(B)** Conventional X-ray coronary angiography from left anterior oblique view confirms significant stenosis in the right coronary artery.

1 minutes of non-ECG (electrocardiographic)-gated imaging time with a repetition time of 3 ms. In contrast, acquisition of the same 3D volume can be completed in approximately 1s using a non-ECG-gated acquisition of a 64-slice CT scanner.

Because of slow-speed constraints of MR, acquisition of 3D coronary MR angiography remains highly challenging. Several competing requirements, including good suppression of respiratory motion, high temporal resolution in the cardiac cycle, high spatial resolution, large 3D volume coverage, and good arterial contrast to noise, need to be simultaneously satisfied.

Suppression of Respiratory Motion

BREATH-HOLD 3D CORONARY MR ANGIOGRAPHY

To overcome limitations of 2D coronary MR angiography such as slice misregistration between breath-hold scans and suboptimal signal-to-noise ratio, 3D breath-hold coronary MR angiography sequences were developed *(9–12)*. Wielopolski et al. *(11)* proposed a breath-hold 3D coronary MR angiography with volume-targeted imaging (volume coronary angiography with targeted volumes). Each coronary arterial segment was imaged with 24-mm thick double-oblique 3D volume by using a single end-expiratory breath hold. All major coronary arteries were covered in fewer than 13 breath holds.

The diagnostic accuracy of the volume coronary angiography with targeted volumes approach was evaluated in 38 patients by van Geuns et al. *(12)*. They found that 69% of segments were assessable with this approach, and the sensitivity and specificity of 3D breath-hold MR coronary angiography for the detection of more than 50% of luminal stenoses were 92 and 68%, respectively.

Breath-hold 3D coronary MR angiography has advantages in terms of time efficiency compared with free-breathing 3D coronary MA angiography *(13)* (Fig. 1). Another benefit of breath-hold 3D coronary MR angiography is that this method can utilize first-pass contrast enhancement of the coronary arterial blood following an intravenous injection of extracellular MR contrast medium such as gadolinium chelated with diethylenetriaminepentaacetic acid (Gd-DTPA) *(14–17)*.

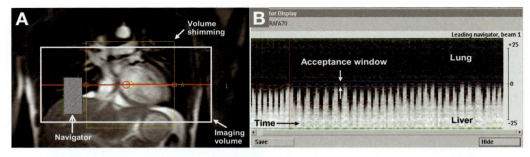

Fig. 2. Respiratory gated acquisition with a prospective real-time navigator echo method. **(A)** A selective 2D radiofrequency excitation pulse to excite a column of tissue perpendicular to the right lung-diaphragm interface. **(B)** If position of the lung-diaphragm interface is within a previously defined acceptance window at the end-expiratory level, image data are accepted and stored for image reconstruction.

Regenfus et al. obtained breath-hold 3D coronary MR angiography in 50 patients with suspected coronary artery disease by injecting extracellular MR contrast medium at a flow rate of 1 mL/second immediately prior to breath-hold 3D acquisitions *(17)*. The sensitivity and specificity were 94 and 57%, respectively, for detecting patients having significant coronary artery disease with contrast-enhanced breath-hold 3D coronary MR angiography.

Breath-hold 3D coronary MR angiography has several limitations. Short imaging time of breath-hold 3D acquisition is achieved at the expense of spatial resolution and 3D volume coverage. In addition, many patients with heart disease or pulmonary disease cannot hold their breath for a long time. Another important limitation of breath-hold MR acquisition is that breath holding does not eliminate motion of the diaphragm. A continued drift of the diaphragm position was observed during breath holding that can cause significant blurring on breath-hold 3D coronary MR angiography *(18)*.

FREE-BREATHING 3D CORONARY MR ANGIOGRAPHY

Free-breathing, respiratory-gated 3D coronary MR angiography is currently the most commonly used MR approach for the assessment of coronary arteries in patients with heart disease. Respiratory bellows belts were initially used to obtain free-breathing coronary MR angiography *(18,19)*. Oshinski et al. reported that free-breathing 2D coronary MR angiography with a respiratory belt provides improved resolution, aligned sections of coronary arteries, and improved patient tolerance *(19)*. However, respiratory motion artifacts and blurring were inevitable with the respiratory bellows belt because it cannot detect drift of the diaphragm position. Free-breathing coronary MR angiography has been substantially improved with respiratory navigators, which measure the position of the right lung–diaphragm interface using MR signal.

The initial implementations of free-breathing 3D coronary MR angiography were based on retrospective navigator gating *(20–23)*. With retrospective navigator echo sequences, image data were oversampled by acquiring each phase-encoding step data several times regardless of respiratory motion. During reconstruction, only image data acquired within a respiratory gating window were used for generating coronary MR angiography.

Retrospective navigator gating has been replaced by a prospective real-time navigator gating method *(24–27)* (Fig. 2). Current free-breathing 3D coronary MR angiography sequences utilize a selective 2D radio-frequency excitation pulse to excite a column of tissue perpendicular to the right lung–diaphragm interface. In each cardiac cycle, both navigator echo data for respiratory gating and image data were acquired. If position of the lung–diaphragm interface is within a previously defined acceptance window (typically ± 2.5 mm) at the end-expiratory level, image data are accepted and stored for image reconstruction. Otherwise, image data are rejected, and acquisition is repeated in the next cardiac cycle.

Coronary MRA data acquisition is continued until all necessary data in k-space are collected. In addition to respiratory gating, navigator echo data are used for adaptive real-time motion correction of 3D imaging volume *(24–28)*. If the lung–diaphragm interface is within an acceptance window, the superior-to-inferior position of 3D acquisition volume is corrected on a real-time basis utilizing the positional offset information of the lung-diaphragm interface measured by navigator echo.

There are several advantages in free-breathing 3D coronary MR angiography with prospective navigator gating. Because there is no constraint of imaging time caused by breath holding, 3D coronary MR images can be acquired with improved spatial resolution, larger 3D volume overage of the coronary artery tree, and improved signal-to-noise ratio. In addition, the data acquisition window in the cardiac cycle can be shortened to reduce motion blurring of the coronary artery caused by cardiac contraction.

The major disadvantage of free-breathing 3D coronary MR angiography is a long scan time, which typically ranges from several to 15 minutes. Another limitation is that acquisition of free-breathing 3D coronary MR angiography often fails in patients with an irregular breathing pattern and those showing a drift of diaphragm position over time. It is also important to remember that prospective navigator gating sequences do not directly measure respiratory motion of the coronary artery but alternatively determine the superior-inferior position of the lung–diaphragm interface. Motion of the coronary artery in the superior-to-inferior direction is less than that of the right diaphragm, and a fixed correction factor of 0.6 has been frequently used for the adaptive real-time motion correction with free-breathing 3D coronary MR angiography sequences *(24,29)*.

3D radial coronary MR angiography with self-navigated image reconstruction has been developed as a new approach for free-breathing coronary MR angiography. This self-navigation approach extracts the motional information directly from image data of the heart instead of measuring the position of the lung–diaphragm interface by navigator echo *(30)*.

Suppression of Cardiac Motion

X-ray coronary angiography can provide high-resolution images of the coronary artery in real time without using cardiac gating or respiratory gating because acquisition time per image frame is short enough (<20 ms) to eliminate motion blurring of the coronary artery. ECG gating is required in coronary MR angiography because MR imaging time is too long to freeze the motion of the coronary artery by cardiac contraction and diastolic relaxation. In most initial studies of coronary MR angiography, image data were acquired during middiastolic phase using a fixed delayed time after ECG R wave trigger. However, the optimal delay time and width of acquisition window in the cardiac cycle to minimize coronary arterial motion are different from patient to patient.

Stuber et al. proposed the following equation to calculate the delay after R wave trigger to start data acquisition: $T_d = ((t_{RR} - 350) \times 0.3) + 350$, where t_{RR} refers to the time between two consecutive ECG R waves (24). This equation is based on a principle in cardiac physiology that the systolic duration in the cardiac cycle remains relatively constant, and the diastolic duration is reduced as the heart rate increases. This standardized approach using this equation allows for an automated calculation of the acquisition delayed time in the cardiac cycle. However, the rest period of the coronary artery in the cardiac cycle is substantially different in each patient, which may cause inconsistent image quality of coronary MR angiography with the standardized ECG trigger delay calculated from heart rate (31). The use of a subject-specific data acquisition window in the cardiac cycle is recommended to improve quality of coronary MR angiography and is especially critical for the visualization of the right coronary artery (32) because the right coronary artery moves more than twice as much as the left coronary arteries.

There are several approaches to determine a subject-specific acquisition window in the cardiac cycle. Wang et al. proposed an ECG-triggered M-mode navigator echo technique to monitor cardiac motion and identify the period of minimal cardiac motion in the cardiac cycle (31). A subject-specific data acquisition window in the cardiac cycle can be optimized by acquiring high temporal resolution cine MR images (33). A trigger delay time and an interval of minimal motion of the coronary artery are visually determined on cine MR images for the subsequent coronary MR angiography acquisition. The subject-specific acquisition window is useful not only to reduce motion blurring of the coronary artery but also to shorten scan time in patients with low heart rate because the diastolic rest period of the coronary artery is considerably extended in patients with lower heart rates.

Contrast of the Coronary Artery

The contrast between luminal blood and surrounding tissue needs to be maximized for better delineation of the coronary artery on MR angiography. With "bright blood" coronary MR angiography, the pulse sequences are designed to enhance the signal from coronary arterial blood and to suppress the signal from the surrounding structures, such as pericardial fat and myocardium (7).

Suppression of fat signal can be achieved by applying a fat saturation pulse that selectively saturates the longitudinal magnetization of fat spins prior to image acquisition. Another approach to suppress fat signal is use of a spectral-selective radio-frequency pulse that selectively excites water spins. Currently, fat saturation pulses are more widely used because short repetition time, which is critical to obtain good coronary MR angiographic images with steady-state free precession sequences, is more easily achieved.

Suppression of myocardial signal is important for the visualization of distal coronary arteries and branch arteries. A T_2-weighted magnetization preparation pulse is used to suppress myocardial signal (25). Another advantage of T_2 preparation pulse is a suppression of venous blood signal in the epicardial veins. T_2 relaxation time of deoxygenated venous blood is substantially shorter than that of oxygenated arterial blood, resulting in the reduction of venous blood signal with T_2 preparation pulse.

On 2D gradient echo coronary MR angiography, high luminal blood signal is primarily generated by the inflow effect of unsaturated blood spins flowing into a thin 2D imaging slice. An introduction of 3D gradient echo coronary MR angiography eliminates many of the drawbacks of 2D coronary MR angiography. The 3D gradient echo approach has one significant downside: reduced inflow effect. Blood spins in thick 3D volume are progressively saturated by repeated radio-frequency excitations, and the arterial blood signal intensity on 3D gradient echo coronary MR angiography is substantially attenuated

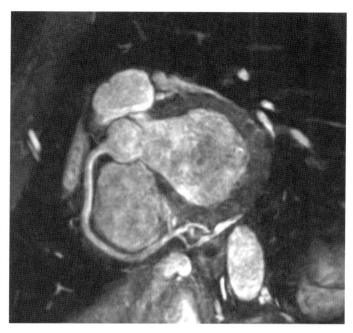

Fig. 3. Free-breathing 3D coronary MR angiography of the right coronary artery acquired with a steady state free precession sequence (balanced TFE) with fat saturation and T2 preparation and a double oblique targeted volume approach. Respiratory gating was performed with a prospective real-time navigator echo technique. Three-point planning was used to define double oblique 3D slices parallel to the right coronary artery. No stenosis in the coronary artery is demonstrated in this case.

when 3D imaging volume is large. Therefore, 3D gradient echo coronary MR angiography needs to be acquired with relatively thin 3D volume (2–3 cm total thickness) targeting to one of the major coronary arteries *(26,27)*.

3D coronary MR angiography sequences with steady-state free precession acquisition (true fast imaging in steady-state precession; balanced turbo field echo; fast imaging employing steady-state acquisition) have become available with an introduction of high-performance gradients and radio-frequency systems. Because the steady-state free precession sequence is sensitive to magnetic field inhomogeneities, short repetition time, and volume shimming capability to achieve a homogeneous magnetic field in the imaging volume are important to obtain good coronary MR angiograms. With steady-state free precession sequences, the blood signal intensity on 3D coronary MR angiography is considerably higher than that of a 3D gradient echo sequence *(34,35)* (Fig. 3). The signal intensity on steady-state free precession sequence is primarily determined by the T_2/T_1 ratio, and a high T_2/T_1 ratio of the blood acts as an intrinsic contrast medium. As a result, 3D coronary MR angiography with steady-state free precession acquisition is not dependent on inflow effect, and excellent 3D coronary MR angiograms with high blood signal can be obtained using thick 3D volume coverage.

Image quality of 3D steady-state coronary MR angiography is further improved with an optimization of *k*-space sampling strategy. Reduced motion artifacts and superior vessel sharpness were observed with the 3D steady-state coronary MR angiographic sequence with radial *k*-space sampling when compared with those by Cartesian 3D steady-state coronary MR angiography and 3D gradient echo coronary MR angiography *(36)*.

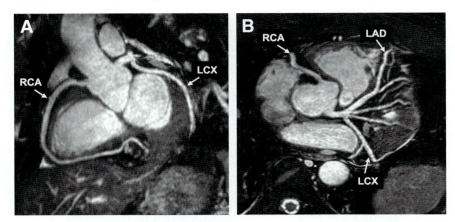

Fig. 4. Free breathing, navigator echo gated whole heart coronary MR angiography acquired with a steady state free precession sequence (balanced TFE) with fat saturation and T2 preparation in a subject with normal coronary artery. **(A)** Left anterior oblique whole heart coronary MR angiogram reformatted with curved multiplanar reformatting clearly depicts the right coronary artery (RCA) and left circumflex (LCX) arteries. **(B)** Oblique axial whole heart coronary MR angiogram reformatted with curved multiplanar reformatting visualizes the left main coronary artery, left anterior descending (LAD) artery, proximal RCA and LCX arteries. (From Sakuma H et al, Radiology. 2005;237:316)

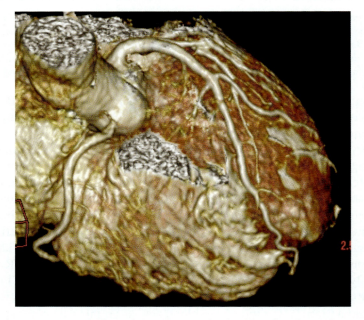

Fig. 5. Whole heart coronary MR angiography acquired with a free breathing steady state free precession sequence in a subject with normal coronary artery. Volume rendering image of whole heart coronary MR angiography is useful for three dimensional anatomical recognition of the right coronary artery, left anterior descending artery and its branches.

Whole heart coronary MR angiography using free-breathing 3D steady-state free precession has been introduced as a method that can provide visualization of all three major coronary arteries with a single 3D acquisition *(37)* (Fig. 4). Steady-state free precession sequences permit acquisition of thick 3D axial volume that encompasses the entire heart without losing arterial contrast. By using this whole heart

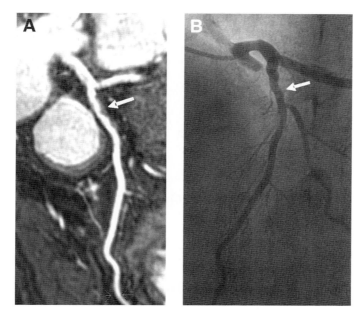

Fig. 6. Whole heart coronary MR angiography acquired with a free breathing, steady state free precession sequence in a patient with suspected coronary artery disease. (**A**) Curved multiplanar reformatted image of whole heart coronary MR angiography clearly reveals proximal and distal segments of the left anterior descending artery. Although no significant luminal narrowing is observed, MR image reveals the presence of atherosclerotic plaque in the coronary arterial wall (arrow). (**B**) X-ray coronary angiography in the same subject.

approach, one can visualize all three major coronary arteries with a reduced total examination time in comparison with targeted double-oblique 3D gradient echo MR angiography (Fig. 5). In addition, planning of whole heart coronary MR angiography is simple, eliminating the time-consuming three-point planning that was required for the targeted double-oblique approach.

Although 3D coronary MR angiography using targeted double-oblique acquisitions demonstrated relatively good accuracy for identifying stenoses in the proximal and middle coronary arterial segments, coverage of the distal segments was often limited. For example, the proportion of assessable segments was 68% for the middle left circumflex artery *(27)*. With the whole heart approach, long segments of all major coronary arteries can be imaged (Fig. 6). The proportion of distal segments exhibiting good or excellent image quality was over 90% for all major coronary arteries in our study using the whole heart approach *(38)*.

Administration of T_1 shortening MR contrast medium is useful to improve blood contrast on 3D gradient echo coronary MR angiography. In the presence of T_1 shortening MR contrast medium, magnetization of blood spins rapidly recovers after radio-frequency pulse, preventing saturation of the blood signal. With sufficient blood concentration of MR contrast medium, the blood signal intensity is primarily determined by T_1 relaxation time of the blood instead of inflow effect, and one can utilize high radio-frequency flip angle to maximize the blood signal.

In addition, contrast enhancement allows for acquiring 3D gradient echo coronary MR angiograms with large 3D volume coverage. Conventional extracellular contrast

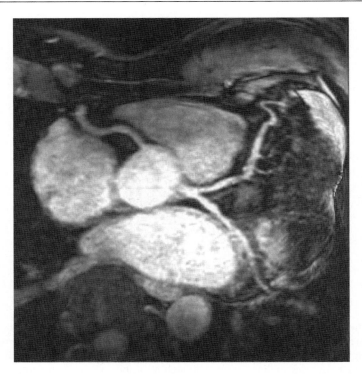

Fig. 7. 3.0 tesla whole heart coronary MR angiography acquired with a free breathing 3D segmented k-space gradient echo sequence with fat saturation and T2 preparation. At higher field strength, the signal to noise ratio of coronary MR angiography is improved (Courtesy of Matthias Stuber, Johns Hopkins University, Baltimore, USA).

media, however, exhibit nonspecific distribution in the extracellular space and rapidly extravasate from intravascular space to the interstitial space after intravenous administration. Sufficient T_1 shortening of the blood is only maintained during the first pass following venous administration (14,15). In contrast, intravascular MR contrast media remain in the blood pool longer than the extravascular contrast media. These intravascular contrast media, either iron particles (39,40) or gadolinium molecules with (41,42) and without albumin binding (43), are distributed in the blood pool and exhibited greater T_1 shortening effects in comparison with conventional extracellular contrast media.

Several investigators have demonstrated that administration of intravascular agent is highly useful in improving arterial contrast on 3D gradient echo coronary MR angiography (39–43). Further study is required to determine whether 3D gradient echo coronary MR angiography with intravascular contrast medium can provide significantly better visualization of the coronary artery and improved diagnostic accuracy in comparison with 3D steady-state coronary MR angiography without contrast.

Recent Improvements in Acquisition Speed and Resolution

Imaging speed is important not only for breath-hold 3D coronary MR angiography but also for free-breathing 3D coronary MR angiography as reduced scan time leads to improved study success rate and higher patient throughput. Parallel imaging techniques such as sensitivity encoding (SENSE) enable substantial scan time reduction in cardiac

MR imaging *(44)* and are now widely used to reduce scan time of 3D coronary MR angiography.

The major drawback of using fast-imaging techniques such as parallel imaging and half-scan is loss of signal-to-noise ratio. Therefore, it is important to have an appropriate balance between speed and image quality when determining imaging parameters of coronary MR angiography. Multichannel coils and a high-field MR system are two approaches that can provide substantial improvement in the signal-to-noise ratio of coronary MR angiography.

In a study by Reeder et al., 32-channel cardiac coils demonstrated significantly improved signal-to-noise ratio and geometry factor, which permits use of a parallel imaging acceleration factor of up to 4 *(45)*. There is increasing interest in high-field coronary MR angiography because signal-to-noise ratio increases approximately linearly with field strength, and substantial improvement in signal-to-noise ratio is expected with a magnetic field strength of 3.0 *T*. This gain in signal-to-noise ratio enables the acquisition of images with higher spatial resolution or reduced imaging time, both of which are especially important in coronary MR angiography (Fig. 7).

Stuber et al. demonstrated the feasibility of human coronary MR angiography using a 3.0*T* MR imager *(46)*. Excellent 3D coronary MR angiograms with submillimeter spatial resolution were demonstrated at 3.0 *T*. There are several potential impediments to high-field cardiac imaging, which include high radio-frequency power deposition quadratrically increased with field strength, susceptibility-related local magnetic field variations, increased sensitivity to motion artifacts, and impaired ECG R-wave triggering because of augmented magnetohydrodynamic effects. Because of these limitations, at this point coronary MR angiography at 3.0 *T* does not result in significantly improved image quality and diagnostic accuracy compared with that at 1.5 *T (47)*. With further advances in hardware and pulse sequence optimizations for high-field cardiac MRI, a 3.0-*T* MR imager might become a platform of choice for high-resolution coronary MR angiography.

CLINICAL APPLICATIONS OF CORONARY MAGNETIC RESONANCE ANGIOGRAPHY

Anomalous Coronary Arteries

Anomalous origin of the coronary artery is a relatively uncommon but important cause of chest pain and sudden cardiac death. The incidence of anomalous coronary arteries in subjects without known congenital heart disease was reported to be 0.3–0.9% *(48,49)*. Among various types of anomalous coronary arteries, the coronary arteries that pass between the aorta and pulmonary artery have a potential to impair myocardial perfusion and can cause sudden death. The diagnostic method of choice for detecting coronary artery anomalies has been catheter X-ray coronary angiography. However, X-ray coronary angiography provides only a 2D view of a vessel's complex 3D path and is associated with several limitations, including invasiveness and radiation exposure. Coronary MR angiography has been shown to have high sensitivity and specificity for detecting anomalous coronary arteries and for delineating proximal courses of the vessels *(50–52)* (Fig. 8).

A study demonstrated that anomalous coronary arteries can be accurately assessed by contrast-enhanced multislice CT as well *(53)*. However, coronary MR angiography

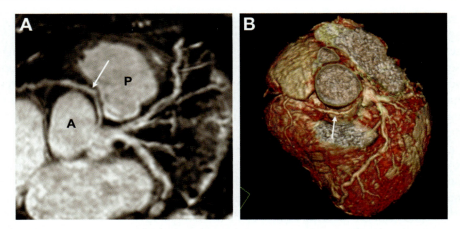

Fig. 8. Whole heart coronary MR angiography in a patient with anomalous right coronary artery. Curved multiplanar reformatted MR angiographic image (**A**) and volume rendering image (**B**) demonstrate that the anomalous right coronary artery arises from the left sinus of Valsalva. The proximal course of the right coronary artery with anomalous origin (arrow) is located between the aortic root (A) and right ventricular outflow tract to proximal pulmonary artery (P).

seems to be preferable to CT because many patients with suspected anomalous coronary arteries are younger, and MR angiography can provide equivalent diagnostic information for the detection of anomalous coronary arteries and for the identification of their proximal courses without exposing the patients to radiation.

Kawasaki Disease

Kawasaki disease is an acute febrile illness with mucosal inflammation, skin rash, and cervical lymphadenopathy in young children *(54)* and produces coronary artery aneurysms in up to 25% of untreated cases. Size of coronary artery aneurysm often changes over time and is correlated with the risk of coronary thrombosis and development of coronary artery stenoses.

Thus, serial assessment of aneurysmal size is important in risk stratification and therapeutic management. Serial evaluation with X-ray angiography in children carries risks associated with invasive catheterization and exposure to ionizing radiation. Transthoracic echocardiography is widely used and is often sufficient for the assessment of coronary artery aneurysm in young children. As children grow, however, visualization and characterization of the coronary artery become more difficult. Coronary MR angiography provides noninvasive detection and size measurement of coronary artery aneurysms in patients with Kawasaki disease and can be used as an alternative imaging method when image quality of transthoracic echocardiography is insufficient *(55)*. Another study demonstrated that MR coronary angiography and X-ray coronary angiography show excellent agreement in the diagnosis of coronary artery aneurysm, and the maximal diameter and length of the aneurysm by MR angiography and X-ray coronary angiography were similar *(56)*.

Coronary Artery Disease

As explained, coronary MR angiography has been useful in delineating proximal courses of anomalous coronary arteries and in evaluating coronary artery aneurysms in

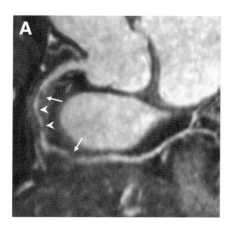
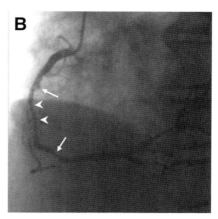

Fig. 9. Whole heart coronary MR angiography acquired with a a free breathing, steady state free precession sequence in a patient with stenoses in the right coronary artery. **(A)** Left anterior oblique whole heart coronary MR angiogram reformatted with curved multiplanar reformatting delineates significant luminal narrowing (arrows) in the proximal and mid part of the right coronary artery, and diffuse atherosclerotic plaque (arrowheads). **(B)** Conventional X-ray coronary angiography demonstrates significant luminal stenoses in the proximal and mid part of the right coronary artery (arrows). (from Sakuma H et al, Radiology. 2005;237:316)

Table 1
Detection of Significant Coronary Arterial Stenoses With Coronary MR Angiography
in Representative Previous Studies

Investigator	Reference	Method	Sensitivity (%)	Specificity (%)
Manning WJ	NEJM 1993;328:828[7]	2D breath-hold	90	92
Duerinckx AJ	Radiology 1994;193:731[57]	↑	63	82
Van Geuns RJ	Radiology 2000;217:270[12]	3D breath-hold	68	97
Regenfus M	JACC 2000;36:44[17]	↑	94	57
Woodard PK	AJR 1998;170:883[23]	3D navigator, retrospective	73	N/A
Sandstede JJ	AJR 1999;172:135[58]	↑	81	89
Sardanelli F	Radiology 2000;214:808[59]	↑	82	89
Kim WY	NEJM 2001;345:1863[27]	3D navigator, prospective	93	42
Bogaert J	Radiology 2003;226:770[60]	↑	50	90
Kefer J	JACC 2005;46:92[61]	↑	75	77

patients with Kawasaki disease. However, detection of coronary arterial stenoses with coronary MR angiography is much more challenging because sufficient spatial resolution is required to correctly identify luminal narrowing of the coronary artery.

Table 1 summarizes the sensitivity and specificity of coronary MR angiography for the detection of coronary arterial stenoses in representative previous studies *(7,12,17, 23,27,57–61)*. The sensitivity (50–94%) and specificity (42–97%) of coronary MR angiography for predicting coronary artery stenoses on X-ray coronary angiography were considerably variable in these studies. Although coronary MR angiography sequences have undergone considerable technical improvements, the diagnostic accuracy of coronary MR angiography did not exhibit significant improvement over time. Large interstudy variability may be explained by the difference in MR angiography sequences, variation in patient populations and prevalence of coronary artery disease, and different inclusion and exclusion criteria regarding which coronary arterial segments are to be assessed.

Kim et al. reported the results of an international multicenter study that evaluated the accuracy of free-breathing, navigator-gated 3D gradient echo coronary MR angiography compared with X-ray coronary angiography *(27)*. In this study, 109 patients with suspected coronary artery disease were evaluated before elective X-ray coronary angiography, and 84% (636/759) of the proximal and middle coronary artery segments were interpretable on MR angiography. In these 636 segments, 83% (78/94) of significant lesions were detected by coronary MR angiography. The sensitivity and specificity of coronary MR angiography for identifying a patient as having significant coronary artery disease were 93 and 42%, respectively. In the subgroup of patients with the left main coronary artery disease or three-vessel disease, however, coronary MR angiography demonstrated sensitivity of 100% and specificity of 85%, indicating the value of free-breathing 3D coronary MRA for excluding severe coronary artery disease.

An introduction of steady-state free precession sequences has considerably improved contrast of 3D coronary MR angiography because steady-state sequences can provide inherently high blood signal intensity without using MR contrast medium. Jahnke et al. compared the diagnostic performances of breath-hold 3D steady-state coronary MR angiography and free-breathing steady-state coronary MR angiography by using the same steady-state free precession sequence, double-oblique targeted volume acquisition, and identical spatial resolution in 40 patients *(62)*. They found that more coronary artery segments were assessable with free-breathing coronary MR angiography (79%) than with breath-hold coronary MR angiography (45%). In addition, free-breathing coronary MR angiography was superior to breath-hold coronary MR angiography in terms of both image quality and diagnostic accuracy, with overall sensitivity and specificity of 72 and 92%, respectively, by free-breathing approach and 63 and 82%, respectively, by breath-hold approach.

Free-breathing coronary MR angiography with axial 3D slices covering the whole heart has become feasible by utilizing navigator-gated 3D steady-state free precession sequence. Whole heart coronary MR angiography can provide visualization of the entire coronary artery trees in a single 3D acquisition *(37,38,63,64)*. Our initial study demonstrated that acquisition of whole heart coronary MR angiography was successful in 34 (87.2%) of 39 patients, with the averaged acquisition duration of 13.8 ± 3.8 minutes *(38)*. In addition, long segments of all major coronary arteries, including the distal segments, can be imaged. The sensitivity, specificity, positive predictive value, and negative predictive value of whole heart coronary MR angiography in 20 patients for detecting patients having at least one coronary arterial stenosis were 83.3, 75.0, 83.3, and 75.0%, respectively, in our initial study (Fig. 9).

To further improve detection of coronary artery disease, we performed whole heart coronary MR angiography in 131 patients by using an optimized acquisition window. In contrast to our previous study, a patient-specific acquisition window was set either during systole or during diastole, depending on the phase of minimal motion of the right coronary artery on cine MR images. Coronary MR angiograms were acquired

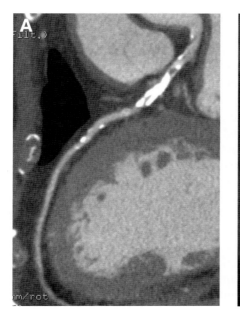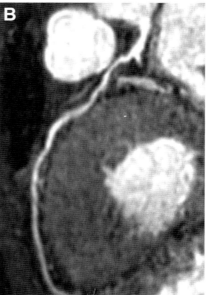

Fig. 10. Coronary CT angiography (64-slice VCT) and whole heart coronary MR angiography in a 71 year-old man with anterior chest pain on effort. **(A)** Curved multiplanar reformatted image of 64-slice contrast enhanced CT angiography demonstrates severely calcified plaque in the proximal left anterior descending artery. Luminal narrowing of the coronary artery cannot be assessed in this segment due to heavy coronary calcification. **(B)** Curved multiplanar reformatted image of non-contrast enhanced whole heart coronary MR angiography can clearly identify luminal narrowing in the proximal left anterior descending artery.

during diastole in 83 patients (delay after R-wave trigger 627 ± 64 ms) and during systole in 48 patients (delay after R-wave trigger 259 ± 39 ms). The study success rate of whole heart coronary MR angiography (86%) was not improved by using an optimized patient-specific acquisition window during either systole or diastole. However, the sensitivity, specificity, positive predictive value, and negative predictive value of whole heart coronary MR angiography for detecting patients having significant stenosis were 82, 90, 88, and 86%, respectively *(64)*, higher than the results in our previous study using subject-specific acquisition windows exclusively in the diastolic phase. These studies indicate that whole heart coronary MR angiography is useful in ruling out significant coronary artery disease in patients with suspected coronary artery disease.

Coronary MR Angiography vs Coronary CT Angiography

Free-breathing 3D steady-state coronary MR angiography has similar diagnostic accuracy when compared with 16-slice multislice CT. Kefer et al. compared the diagnostic accuracy of free-breathing 3D coronary MR angiography using a steady-state free precession sequence and double-oblique targeted volume approach with the accuracy of 16-slice multislice CT in 42 patients *(61)*. By using quantitative coronary angiography as a gold standard, the sensitivity and specificity of coronary MR angiography for the detection of luminal narrowing were 75 and 77%, respectively. These MR results were similar to the sensitivity (82%, p = not significant) and specificity (79%, p = not significant) of 16-slice multislice CT.

Newer 64-slice CT imagers have a shorter rotation time and offer shorter scan time, higher spatial resolution (0.4 mm), and higher temporal resolution (165 ms) compared with previous-generation CT scanners *(5)*. In recently published studies, 64-slice CT demonstrated sensitivity of 95–100%, specificity of 90–92%, positive predictive value of 93–97%, and negative predictive value of 93–100% in detecting patients having significant coronary artery stenoses *(4,5)*. Although there is no published study at this point that directly compared the diagnostic performances of 64-slice CT and coronary MR angiography, overall image quality and diagnostic accuracy of 64-slice coronary CT angiography seem to be superior to those of coronary MR angiography.

Despite the excellent diagnostic accuracy, coronary CT angiography has several nonnegligible limitations. Although coronary CT angiography is definitively less invasive compared with catheter X-ray angiography, estimated radiation dose during CT coronary angiography is higher than that of X-ray coronary angiography, and the rapid injection of iodinated contrast medium may cause adverse effects and complications. Coronary MR angiography and multislice coronary CT angiography are complementary to one another rather than competitive with one another, and coronary MR angiography seems to be useful in the following circumstances: (1) coronary artery anomalies, (2) coronary artery aneurysm in patients with Kawasaki disease, (3) coronary arterial stenoses in patients with renal failure, (4) coronary arterial stenoses in patients with heavy calcification, and (5) screening coronary artery disease in healthy subjects and those with low likelihood of coronary artery disease.

Coronary MR angiography can successfully delineate anomalous coronary arteries and coronary artery aneurysms in Kawasaki disease without exposing the patients to radiation. Non-contrast-enhanced coronary MR angiography is well suited for assessing coronary artery disease in patients with renal failure. Coronary MR angiography is also useful in the visualization of the coronary arterial lumen in patients with heavy coronary calcification (Fig. 10). In addition, coronary MR angiography might be of great value in screening coronary artery disease in asymptomatic healthy subjects and those with low likelihood of coronary artery disease because MR does not expose the subjects to ionizing radiation, which is associated with certain risk of radiation induced cancer. Further study is required to determine the effectiveness of coronary MR angiography in screening coronary artery disease in subjects with low prevalence of the disease.

REFERENCES

1. American Heart Association. 2004 heart disease and stroke statistical update. Dallas, TX: American Heart Association; 2003.
2. Scanlon PJ, Faxon DP, Audet AM, et al. ACC/AHA guidelines for coronary angiography. A report of the American College of Cardiology/American Heart Association Task Force on Practice Guidelines (Committee on Coronary Angiography). Developed in collaboration with the Society for Cardiac Angiography and Interventions. J Am Coll Cardiol 1999;33:1756–1824.
3. Budoff MJ, Georgiou D, Brody A, et al. Ultrafast computed tomography as a diagnostic modality in the detection of coronary artery disease: a multicenter study. Circulation 1996;93:898–904.
4. Raff GL, Gallagher MJ, O'Neill WW, Goldstein JA. Diagnostic accuracy of noninvasive coronary angiography using 64-slice spiral computed tomography. J Am Coll Cardiol 2005;46:552–557.
5. Mollet NR, Cademartiri F, van Mieghem CA, et al. High-resolution spiral computed tomography coronary angiography in patients referred for diagnostic conventional coronary angiography. Circulation 2005;112:2318–2323.
6. Edelman RR, Manning WJ, Pearlman J, Li W. Human coronary arteries: projection angiograms reconstructed from breath-hold two-dimensional MR images. Radiology 1993;187:719–722.

7. Manning WJ, Li W, Edelman RR. A preliminary report comparing magnetic resonance coronary angiography with conventional angiography. N Engl J Med 1993;328:828–832.

8. Sakuma H, Caputo GR, Steffens JC, et al. Breath-hold MR cine angiography of coronary arteries in healthy volunteers: value of multiangle oblique imaging planes. Am J Roentgenol 1994;163:533–537.

9. Wielopolski PA, Manning WJ, Edelman RR. Single breath-hold volumetric imaging of the heart using magnetization-prepared three-dimensional segmented echo planar imaging. J Magn Reson Imaging 1995;5:403–409.

10. Bornert P, Jensen D. Coronary artery imaging at 0.5 T using segmented 3D echo planar imaging. Magn Reson Med 1995;34:779–785.

11. Wielopolski PA, van Geuns RJ, de Feyter PJ, Oudkerk M. Breath-hold coronary MR angiography with volume-targeted imaging. Radiology 1998;209:209–129.

12. Van Geuns RJ, Wielopolski PA, de Bruin HG, et al. MR coronary angiography with breath-hold targeted volumes: preliminary clinical results. Radiology 2000;217:270–227.

13. Foo TK, Ho VB, Saranathan M, et al. Feasibility of integrating high-spatial-resolution 3D breath-hold coronary MR angiography with myocardial perfusion and viability examinations. Radiology 2005;235:1025–1030.

14. Goldfarb JW, Edelman RR. Coronary arteries: breath-hold, adolinium-enhanced, three-dimensional MR angiography. Radiology 1998;206:830–834.

15. Kessler W, Laub G, Achenbach S, Ropers D, Moshage W, Daniel WG. Coronary arteries: MR angiography with fast contrast-enhanced three-dimensional breath-hold imaging—initial experience. Radiology 1999;210:566–572.

16. Li D, Carr JC, Shea SM, et al. Coronary arteries: magnetization-prepared contrast-enhanced three-dimensional volume-targeted breath-hold MR angiography. Radiology 2001;219:270–277.

17. Regenfus M, Ropers D, Achenbach S, Kessler W, Laub G, Daniel WG, Moshage W. Noninvasive detection of coronary artery stenosis using contrast-enhanced three-dimensional breath-hold magnetic resonance coronary angiography. J Am Coll Cardiol 2000;36:44–50.

18. Holland AE, Goldfarb JW, Edelman RR. Diaphragmatic and cardiac motion during suspended breathing: preliminary experience and implications for breath-hold MR imaging. Radiology 1998;209: 483–489.

19. Oshinski JN, Hofland L, Mukundan S Jr, Dixon WT, Parks WJ, Pettigrew RI. Two-dimensional coronary MR angiography without breath holding. Radiology 1996;201:737–743.

20. McConnell MV, Khasgiwala VC, Savord BJ, et al. Comparison of respiratory suppression methods and navigator locations for MR coronary angiography. Am J Roentgenol 1997;168:1369–1375.

21. Li D, Kaushikkar S, Haacke EM, et al. Coronary arteries: three-dimensional MR imaging with retrospective respiratory gating. Radiology 1996;201:857–863.

22. Post JC, van Rossum AC, Hofman MB, Valk J, Visser CA. Three-dimensional respiratory-gated MR angiography of coronary arteries: comparison with conventional coronary angiography. Am J Roentgenol 1996;166:1399–1404.

23. Woodard PK, Li D, Haacke EM, et al. Detection of coronary stenoses on source and projection images using three-dimensional MR angiography with retrospective respiratory gating: preliminary experience. Am J Roentgenol 1998;170:883–888.

24. Stuber M, Botnar RM, Danias PG, Kissinger KV, Manning WJ. Submillimeter three-dimensional coronary MR angiography with real-time navigator correction: comparison of navigator locations. Radiology 1999;212:579–587.

25. Botnar RM, Stuber M, Danias PG, Kissinger KV, Manning WJ. Improved coronary artery definition with T_2-weighted, free-breathing, three-dimensional coronary MRA. Circulation 1999;99:3139–3148.

26. Stuber M, Botnar RM, Danias PG, et al. Double-oblique free-breathing high resolution three-dimensional coronary magnetic resonance angiography. J Am Coll Cardiol 1999;34:524–531.

27. Kim WY, Danias PG, Stuber M, et al. Coronary magnetic resonance angiography for the detection of coronary stenoses. N Engl J Med 2001;345:1863–1869.

28. Nagel E, Bornstedt A, Schnackenburg B, Hug J, Oswald H, Fleck E. Optimization of real-time adaptive navigator correction for 3D magnetic resonance coronary angiography. Magn Reson Med 1999;42:408–411.

29. Wang Y, Riederer SJ, Ehman RL. Respiratory motion of the heart: kinematics and the implications for the spatial resolution in coronary imaging. Magn Reson Med 1995;33:713–719.

30. Stehning C, Bornert P, Nehrke K, Eggers H, Stuber M. Free-breathing whole-heart coronary MRA with 3D radial SSFP and self-navigated image reconstruction. Magn Reson Med 2005;54:476–480.

31. Wang Y, Vidan E, Bergman GW. Cardiac motion of coronary arteries: variability in the rest period and implications for coronary MR angiography. Radiology 1999;213:751–758.

32. Kim WY, Stuber M, Kissinger KV, Andersen NT, Manning WJ, Botnar RM. Impact of bulk cardiac motion on right coronary MR angiography and vessel wall imaging. J Magn Reson Imaging 2001;14: 383–390.

33. Plein S, Jones TR, Ridgway JP, Sivananthan MU. Three-dimensional coronary MR angiography performed with subject-specific cardiac acquisition windows and motion-adapted respiratory gating. Am J Roentgenol 2003;180:505–512.

34. Carr JC, Simonetti O, Bundy J, Li D, Pereles S, Finn JP. Cine MR angiography of the heart with segmented true fast imaging with steady-state precession. Radiology 2001;219:828–834.

35. McCarthy RM, Shea SM, Deshpande VS, et al. Coronary MR angiography: true FISP imaging improved by prolonging breath holds with preoxygenation in healthy volunteers. Radiology 2003;227:283–288.

36. Spuentrup E, Katoh M, Buecker A, et al. Free-breathing 3D steady-state free precession coronary MR angiography with radial k-space sampling: comparison with Cartesian k-space sampling and Cartesian gradient-echo coronary MR angiography—pilot study. Radiology 2004;231:581–586.

37. Weber OM, Martin AJ, Higgins CB. Whole-heart steady-state free precession coronary artery magnetic resonance angiography. Magn Reson Med 2003;50:1223–1228.

38. Sakuma H, Ichikawa Y, Suzawa N, et al. Assessment of coronary arteries with total study time of less than 30 minutes by using whole-heart coronary MR angiography. Radiology 2005;237:316–321.

39. Reimer P, Bremer C, Allkemper T, et al. Myocardial perfusion and MR angiography of chest with SH U 555 C: results of placebo-controlled clinical phase i study. Radiology 2004;231:474–481.

40. Klein C, Schalla S, Schnackenburg B, et al. Improvement of image quality of non-invasive coronary artery imaging with magnetic resonance by the use of the intravascular contrast agent Clariscan (NC100150 injection) in patients with coronary artery disease. J Magn Reson Imaging 2003;17:656–662.

41. Stuber M, Botnar RM, Danias PG, et al. Contrast agent-enhanced, free-breathing, three-dimensional coronary magnetic resonance angiography. J Magn Reson Imaging 1999;10:790–799.

42. Paetsch I, Huber ME, Bornstedt A, et al. Improved three-dimensional free-breathing coronary magnetic resonance angiography using gadocoletic acid (B-22956) for intravascular contrast enhancement. J Magn Reson Imaging 2004;20:288–293.

43. Herborn CU, Barkhausen J, Paetsch I, et al. Coronary arteries: contrast-enhanced MR imaging with SH L 643A—experience in 12 volunteers. Radiology 2003;229:217–223.

44. Pruessmann KP, Weiger M, Scheidegger MB, Boesiger P. SENSE: sensitivity encoding for fast MRI. Magn Reson Med 1999;42:952–962.

45. Reeder SB, Wintersperger BJ, Dietrich O, et al. Practical approaches to the evaluation of signal-to-noise ratio performance with parallel imaging: application with cardiac imaging and a 32-channel cardiac coil. Magn Reson Med 2005;54:748–754.

46. Stuber M, Botnar RM, Fischer SE, et al. Preliminary report on in vivo coronary MRA at 3 T in humans. Magn Reson Med 2002;48:425–429.

47. Sommer T, Hackenbroch M, Hofer U, et al. Coronary MR angiography at 3.0 T vs that at 1.5 T: initial results in patients suspected of having coronary artery disease. Radiology 2005;234:718–725.

48. Donaldson RM, Raphael MJ, Yacoub MH, Ross DN. Hemodynamically significant anomalies of the coronary arteries: surgical aspects. Thorac Cardiovasc Surg 1982;30:7–13.

49. Click RL, Holmes DR Jr, Vlietstra RE, Kosinski AS, Kronmal RA. Anomalous coronary arteries: location, degree of atherosclerosis and effect on survival: a report from the Coronary Artery Surgery Study. J Am Coll Cardiol 1989;13:531–537.

50. McConnell MV, Ganz P, Selwyn AP, Edelman RR, Manning WJ. Identification of anomalous coronary arteries and their anatomic course by magnetic resonance coronary angiography. Circulation 1995;92:3158–3162.

51. Taylor AM, Thorne SA, Rubens MB, et al. Coronary artery imaging in grown up congenital heart disease: complementary role of magnetic resonance and X-ray coronary angiography. Circulation 2000;101:1670–1678.

52. Bunce NH, Lorenz CH, Keegan J, et al. Coronary artery anomalies: assessment with free-breathing three-dimensional coronary MR angiography. Radiology 2003;227:201–208.

53. Datta J, White CS, Gilkeson RC, et al. Anomalous coronary arteries in adults: depiction at multi-detector row CT angiography. Radiology 2005;235:812–818.

54. Kato H, Sugimura T, Akagi T, et al. Long-term consequences of Kawasaki disease. A 10- to 21-years follow-up study of 594 patients. Circulation 1996;94:1379–1385.
55. Greil GF, Stuber M, Botnar RM, et al. Coronary magnetic resonance angiography in adolescents and young adults with Kawasaki disease. Circulation 2002;105:908–911.
56. Mavrogeni S, Papadopoulos G, Douskou M, et al. Magnetic resonance angiography is equivalent to X-ray coronary angiography for the evaluation of coronary arteries in Kawasaki disease. J Am Coll Cardiol 2004;43:649–652.
57. Duerinckx AJ, Urman MK. Two-dimensional coronary MR angiography: analysis of initial clinical results. Radiology 1994;193:731–738.
58. Sandstede JJ, Pabst T, Beer M, et al. Three-dimensional MR coronary angiography using the navigator technique compared with conventional coronary angiography. Am J Roentgenol 1999;172:135–139.
59. Sardanelli F, Molinari G, Zandrino F, Balbi M. Three-dimensional, navigator-echo MR coronary angiography in detecting stenoses of the major epicardial vessels, with conventional coronary angiography as the standard of reference. Radiology 2000;214:808–814.
60. Bogaert J, Kuzo R, Dymarkowski S, Beckers R, Piessens J, Rademakers FE. Coronary artery imaging with real-time navigator three-dimensional turbo-field-echo MR coronary angiography: initial experience. Radiology 2003;226:707–716.
61. Kefer J, Coche E, Legros G, et al. Head-to-head comparison of three-dimensional navigator-gated magnetic resonance imaging and 16-slice computed tomography to detect coronary artery stenosis in patients. J Am Coll Cardiol 2005;46:92–100.
62. Jahnke C, Paetsch I, Schnackenburg B, et al. Coronary MR angiography with steady-state free precession: individually adapted breath-hold technique vs free-breathing technique. Radiology 2004;232:669–676.
63. Jahnke C, Paetsch I, Nehrke K, et al. Rapid and complete coronary arterial tree visualization with magnetic resonance imaging: feasibility and diagnostic performance. Eur Heart J 2005;26: 2313–2319.
64. Sakuma H, Ichikawa Y, Chino S, Hirano T, Makino K, Takeda K. Detection of coronary artery stenosis with whole heart coronary magnetic resonance angiography. J Am Coll Cardiol., 2006;48:1946–1950.

17 Myocardial Infarction and Viability With an Emphasis on Imaging Delayed Enhancement

Andrew E. Arai

CONTENTS

Cardiovascular magnetic resonance (CMR) is well suited to assessing patients with myocardial infarction. In a relatively short examination, CMR can assess myocardial anatomy, left ventricular function, perfusion, and viability—all with excellent image quality. Furthermore, the imaging planes can be programmed to provide identical views of the heart for each type of image. This facilitates intermodality comparisons.

From: *Contemporary Cardiology: Cardiovascular Magnetic Resonance Imaging*
Edited by: Raymond Y. Kwong © Humana Press Inc., Totowa, NJ

The purpose of this chapter is to review the CMR methods for assessing myocardial infarction and viability. The validations of gadolinium delayed-enhancement images form the primary emphasis of the chapter. These validations have been performed in both animal and clinical studies. Beyond the validation of delayed-enhancement imaging, it is important to recognize that there are many other CMR methods that can complement existing techniques. Thus, the field remains in a state of progressive development that is likely to continue to refine the utility of this already powerful technique.

THE PATHOPHYSIOLOGICAL BASIS OF MYOCARDIAL INFARCTION

Although the pathophysiological basis of myocardial infarction is too extensive to review in the current chapter, it is worth focusing attention on several specific and clinically relevant details. Important aspects of the pathophysiology of myocardial infarction can be imaged by CMR. Specifically, this section of the chapter discusses the theory behind the wavefront injury that results in subendocardial or transmural forms of myocardial infarction. It is also important to understand the concept of the area at risk. Finally, this section defines and differentiates reversible and irreversible forms of ischemic myocardial injury.

The high resolution of CMR infarct imaging methods brought the concept of the transmural extent of infarction from theory established by experimental studies to clinical reality. As illustrated in Fig. 1, the duration of myocardial ischemia is a major determinant of the transmural extent of infarction *(1–3)*. In a canine model, a coronary occlusion less than 20 minutes in duration will cause a regional wall motion abnormality but no permanent injury and no myocardial infarction. Myocardial infarction develops first in the subendocardium because this layer of the myocardium is metabolically most vulnerable and has the highest oxygen requirements. As a function of duration of occlusion, the transmural extent of infarction becomes progressively more extensive. After about 3–6 hours, the transmural extent of reperfused infarcts approaches that expected for nonreperfused infarcts.

Other factors can modulate the transmural extent of infarction and overall infarct size. Factors that result in high myocardial oxygen demand such as hypertension, tachycardia, or high circulating catecholamine levels will make a large or transmural infarct faster than illustrated in this diagram. Situations that compromise oxygen delivery to the heart such as anemia, hypoxia, or carbon monoxide exposure will also tend to accelerate the development of infarctions. Collateral blood flow, which is commonly present in dogs and variably present in humans, can reduce the extent of infarction. Short bouts of myocardial ischemia can also reduce infarct size *(4)*—a phenomenon known as *ischemic preconditioning (5)*.

Therapies can alter the relationship between duration of occlusion and size of infarction. Adequate reperfusion by percutaneous intervention or thrombolytic therapy can reduce infarct size. Certain medications, such as β-blockers will reduce infarct size for a given duration of occlusion. In animal studies, approximately 10 classes of medications reduce infarct size, although few have had clinical impact *(6)*. One major difference between the animal studies and their counterpart human clinical trials is the outcome measure.

In animal studies, infarct reduction is generally measured as a fraction of the area at risk. The area at risk is the myocardium that was hypoperfused during the coronary occlusion. Although several clinical trials have used sestamibi injections in the emergency

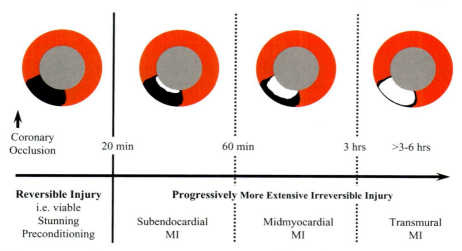

Fig. 1. The duration of ischemia is a major determinant of infarct size and the transmural extent of infarction.

department to assess the area at risk *(7)*, there are feasibility issues with this approach. Safe handling of radioactive tracers in the emergency department 24 hours/day 7 days a week taxes even the most experienced centers. Thus, there is a general need to assess not only the amount of infarcted myocardium but also the size of the area at risk. The area at risk can be imaged with T_2-weighted imaging *(8)* and is discussed in this chapter.

Despite evidence that there is some low level of myocardial regeneration after myocardial infarction *(9)*, the overall postinfarct healing process is characterized by a period of *replacement fibrosis*, by which cardiomyocytes in the infarct are replaced by a collagen scar that leaves behind a wall that is not as thick as normal myocardium. Thus, infarcted myocardium is replaced by a scar that lacks normal contractile proteins or structure. This scar impairs local myocardial contraction and diastolic properties. Importantly, the fibrotic scar of myocardial infarction can be detected with gadolinium contrast agents.

MYOCARDIAL VIABILITY: MORE THAN SIMPLY THE INVERSE OF MYOCARDIAL INFARCTION

There are two pathophysiological processes that result in reversible myocardial dysfunction. *Stunned myocardium* is a postischemic regional contractile abnormality that may persist for hours or days after an ischemic episode. The pathophysiology of stunned myocardium has been reviewed extensively *(3,10)*. As summarized in Table 1, stunned myocardium, in its simplest form, is dysfunctional myocardium that persists despite restoration of normal myocardial perfusion.

Hibernating myocardium is dysfunctional myocardium that is caused by a persistent intermediate reduction of blood flow at rest that is sufficient to cause a contractile abnormality but not severe enough to cause infarction *(11)*. This mechanism has been characterized in animal studies but is less well understood clinically because of the complexity of the pathophysiology and the high likelihood of overlap with myocardial stunning. Because resting blood flow is reduced, this condition generally requires a

Table 1
Comparison of Conditions That Can Cause Regional Myocardial Dysfunction

Infarcted myocardium
Perfusion	Normal or reduced depending on adequacy of reperfusion and presence of microvascular obstruction
Function	Reduced
Metabolism	Reduced (low FDG uptake)
Histology	Replacement fibrosis
Delayed enhancement	Subendocardial delayed enhancement that may extend to the epicardial surface; usually within a coronary distribution unless there are multiple infarcts or the patient has had bypass surgery

Stunned myocardium
Perfusion	Normal by definition
Function	Reduced but reversible with restoration of perfusion (hours to weeks)
Metabolism	Not reduced (high FDG uptake)
Histology	Normal
Delayed enhancement	Negative (unless there is a combination of stunned myocardium and infarcted myocardium)

Hibernating myocardium
Perfusion	Reduced by definition
Function	Reduced but reversible with restoration of perfusion (may take months to recover)
Metabolism	Not reduced (high FDG uptake, perfusion-metabolism mismatch)
Histology	May be normal but may also show dedifferentiation of cardiomyocytes, including loss or disarray of contractile elements within the cell
Delayed enhancement	Negative (unless there is a combination of hibernating myocardium and infarcted myocardium)

Postinfarct remodeling
Perfusion	Normal
Function	Reduced
Metabolism	Probably normal
Histology	Hypertrophy, dilatation, adverse fiber orientation
Delayed enhancement	Negative (dysfunctional myocardium remote from a large infarct appears viable)

Nonischemic cardiomyopathies
Perfusion	Normal or reduced depending on adequacy of reperfusion and presence of microvascular obstruction
Function	Reduced
Metabolism	Reduced (low FDG uptake)
Histology	Replacement fibrosis
Delayed enhancement	Variable; best recognized as midwall, epicardial, diffuse, or patchy; delayed enhancement may be absent

severe coronary stenosis. Any brief but significant increase in myocardial oxygen demand can worsen the oxygen demand/supply ratio and thus superimpose stunning on top of the hibernating process.

As a result, clinically, we generally lump stunned and hibernating myocardium into a single category of *dysfunctional but viable myocardium*. The key clinical evidence of

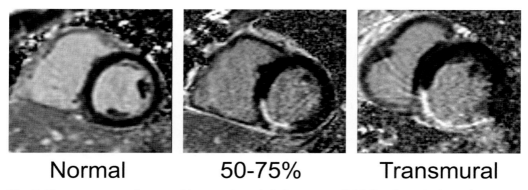

Normal   50-75%   Transmural

Fig. 2. The appearance of a normal heart and two inferior myocardial infarctions. An inversion recovery delayed-enhancement image acquisition program with phase-sensitive detection was used to acquire these images. The inversion time (a timing option) was adjusted to null the normal myocardium. Thus, normal myocardium appears uniformly dark in these midventricular short-axis images. Areas of infarction typically appear many times brighter than the dark normal myocardium and in excellent-quality studies will be brighter than the blood cavity.

viable myocardium is the recovery of function after revascularization in a setting compatible with stunned or hibernating myocardium. Positron emission tomographic (PET) studies characterize dysfunctional but viable myocardium as a region of flow/metabolism mismatch. Dysfunctional but viable myocardium on a CMR study does not exhibit significant amounts of delayed enhancement.

APPEARANCE OF MYOCARDIAL INFARCTION ON DELAYED ENHANCEMENT IMAGES

With current inversion recovery delayed-enhancement techniques, myocardial infarction should appear bright against a uniformly dark background of normal myocardium (Figs. 2 and 3). The signal intensity of blood tends to vary depending on the dose and time after contrast administration. The signal intensity of blood will tend to be relatively bright after high doses and when imaging is performed early after contrast administration. Ideally, one should acquire infarct images at a time when enough contrast has cleared out of the blood that the signal intensity of blood is an intermediate gray.

OTHER ASPECTS OF MYOCARDIAL INFARCTION THAT CAN BE IMAGED WITH CARDIAC MAGNETIC RESONANCE

Microvascular obstruction (Fig. 4) occurs commonly after acute myocardial infarction and represents a residual myocardial perfusion abnormality despite a patent infarct-related epicardial coronary artery. Microvascular obstruction is also known as the *no-reflow phenomenon.* Microvascular obstruction may occur because of one or more of the following mechanisms: (1) ischemic damage of microvessels; (2) severe tissue swelling that prevents perfusion at the tissue level; (3) thrombotic or white blood cell plugging in small blood vessels; and (4) atheroemboli. Microvascular obstruction is associated with more prolonged ischemia and more severe myocardial injury *(12).* Importantly, postinfarct microvascular obstruction appears to have adverse prognostic

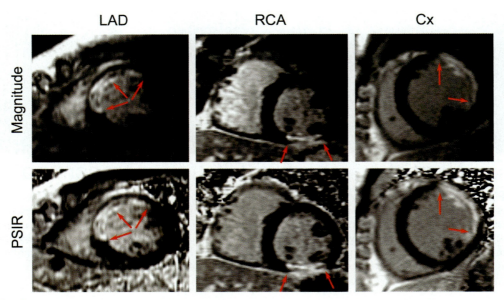

Fig. 3. Appearance of myocardial infarctions in different coronary distributions. The red arrows point to the regions of myocardial infarction. Studies of three different image qualities are included. The left anterior descending (LAD) infarct images are only fair quality because the distinction between blood and infarct is marginal. The right coronary artery (RCA) infarct images are good quality, as evidenced by better distinction between blood and the infarct. The circumflex (Cx) infarct is excellent quality, as indicated by a smooth (not grainy) appearance, good uniform myocardial null, and infarct significantly brighter than both normal myocardium and the blood. Images in the upper row were reconstructed with conventional magnitude image reconstruction methods. The bottom row images were reconstructed with phase-sensitive inversion recovery (PSIR) methods. PSIR methods significantly improve the quality of images at low signal-to-noise ratio and reduce some types of artifacts.

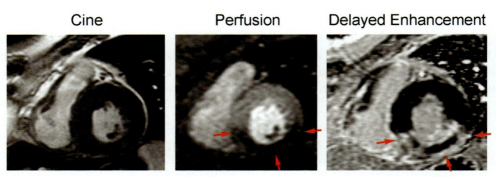

Fig. 4. Appearance of microvascular obstruction on delayed-enhancement images. On an end-systolic cine magnetic resonance image, the signal intensity of this acute inferior myocardial infarction is similar to normal myocardium. On the first-pass perfusion images, there is a severe perfusion defect (white arrows) that represents microvascular obstruction because the right coronary artery was successfully recanalized by an acute percutaneous intervention. The microvascular obstruction is severe enough that the core of the infarct did not significantly enhance even 15 minutes after the contrast injection. Note, however, that the edges of the infarct enhance substantially. This is a nice example of the delayed-enhancement phenomenon because the edges of the infarct were either dark or isointense with normal myocardium during the first-pass study but eventually become quite bright. The delayed-enhancement study also shows that the inferior right ventricular wall is infarcted.

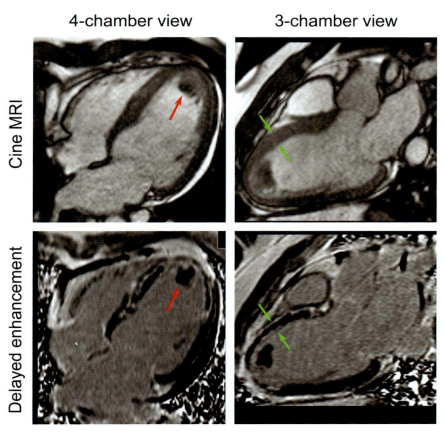

Fig. 5. Appearance of left ventricular thrombus associated with an acute anterior and apical myocardial infarction. On the steady-state free precession cine MRI image at end diastole, the apical thrombus has similar signal intensity to the myocardium but is darker than the blood. On the delayed-enhancement images, the majority of the thrombus (black arrow) does not enhance and thus appears dark. As characteristic of thrombus associated with myocardial infarction, the endocardial surface exhibits delayed enhancement consistent with myocardial infarction. The signal intensity in the myocardium is complicated by the presence of microvascular obstruction. The white arrows point to a region of the anterior septum where the blood in the left ventricular cavity is not as bright as the subendocardial rim of infarcted myocardium. The mid-left ventricular wall is dark, but the epicardial surface exhibits delayed enhancement. This case illustrates some of the subtleties in differentiating laminar thrombus from subendocardial microvascular obstruction.

significance and portends more severe long-term compromise of regional myocardial function *(13)*.

Delayed enhancement imaging is also useful in detecting and characterizing intracardiac thrombus (Fig. 5) *(14)*. Although current-generation extracellular gadolinium-based contrast agents are clearly useful in characterizing intracardiac thrombus, there is potential for molecular-targeted contrast agents that might be much more specific for thrombus *(15–19)*. Detection of intracardiac or intravascular thrombus is just one application in a growing field of molecular-specific MRI contrast agents.

In large myocardial infarctions, even myocardium remote from the infarct can undergo adverse left ventricular remodeling *(20)*. Postinfarction remodeling is caused by a complex set of interacting factors that include (1) infarct expansion; (2) neurohormonal activation; (3) myocardial hypertrophy; (4) myocardial fibrosis; (5) apoptosis; and (6) global ventricular dilatation (21). CMR is well suited to studying volumetric and mass changes associated with myocardial remodeling. Adverse left ventricular remodeling is most commonly encountered after large anterior myocardial infarctions. Because remodeling affects myocardium remote from the ischemic zone, the underlying pathophysiology appears distinct from that of stunned and hibernating myocardium.

Clinically, left ventricular remodeling is typified by a patient who survives a large anterior myocardial infarction and leaves the hospital with no definite signs of heart failure. Perhaps 6 months or a year later the patient presents with heart failure and a severely dilated left ventricle. Remodeling causes abnormal contraction in segments remote from the original infarct despite no new infarct or severe stenoses in the other coronary arteries. A large end-systolic volume has poor long-term prognosis (22).

One must also consider that left ventricular dysfunction caused by noncoronary-related etiologies is relatively common. Thus, the differential diagnosis of left ventricular dysfunction must consider this possibility, particularly when the extent of dysfunction exceeds that expected for the amount of infarcted myocardium. As summarized in the following sections, several diseases that cause nonischemic cardiomyopathies result in patterns of delayed enhancement that are atypical for myocardial infarction.

VALIDATION OF INFARCT SIZE DETERMINATION IN ANIMALS

The first descriptions of gadolinium delayed enhancement were published in the mid 1980s (23–26). High quality of validation studies using these new methods (27,28) led to a renewed appreciation of the power of extracellular gadolinium-based contrast agents for delineating regions of myocardial infarction. Improvements in the image acquisition methods used to obtain delayed enhancement images (29) enhanced the feasibility of using this method for diagnostic purposes. This section highlights studies that have validated various aspects of delayed enhancement images regarding imaging myocardial infarction.

Although early studies showed that the region of delayed enhancement correlated with myocardial infarction, there were many unanswered questions regarding which conditions led to delayed enhancement. Kim et al. validated delayed enhancement infarct size against histopathology in a landmark study published in 1999 (27). The quality of their ex vivo CMR images displayed next to histopathological specimens provided convincing evidence that delayed enhancement with gadolinium-based contrast corresponded to myocardial infarction down to a millimeter-by-millimeter basis. There were close correlations between infarct size by CMR and histopathology on day 1, day 3, and weeks 8 postinfarct. Furthermore, stunned myocardium induced by brief coronary occlusion of a noninfarct-related coronary artery did not exhibit delayed enhancement. This work was extended by the same group in 24 canine infarcts studied 4 hours, 1 day, 3 days, 10 days, 4 weeks, and 8 weeks after infarction (30). The later work used fluorescent beads to measure the area at risk and clearly demonstrated that ischemic but viable myocardium did not enhance with gadolinium. That study also documented that two different extracellular gadolinium-based contrast agents enhanced the hearts in similar patterns with no significant bias in measurement of infarct size. An example of CMR correlation with histopathologic confirmation of infarct size is shown in Fig. 6.

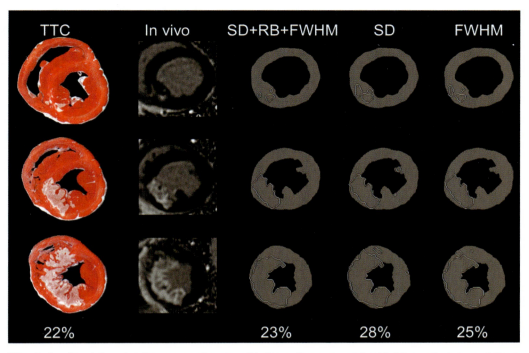

Fig. 6. In vivo delayed-enhancement images of infarct size compared with histopathology and three quantitative analysis methods. On the triphenoltetrazolium (TTC)-stained myocardium, viable tissue appears dark, and areas of myocardial infarction are white. The commonly used 2 standard deviation (SD) threshold overestimates infarct size. The full-width half-maximum (FWHM) method is more accurate but still overestimates infarct size. A more sophisticated computer program that involves stepwise incorporation of SD, regional-based feature analysis (RB), and FWHM provided the most precise approach in measuring infarct size *(31)*. (Image courtesy of L. Hsu from the National Heart, Lung, and Blood Institute.)

PATHOPHYSIOLOGICAL BASIS OF CONTRAST DISTRIBUTION IN MYOCARDIAL INFARCTION

The pathophysiological basis of delayed enhancement imaging helps one understand why myocardial infarctions usually appear bright on delayed-enhancement images. The first-generation gadolinium-based contrast agents approved by the Food and Drug Administration are in a class described as extracellular contrast agents. When injected intravenously, these agents are delivered to tissues in the body proportionally to perfusion. These gadolinium-based contrast agents rapidly diffuse into the extracellular space but, because of chemical charge and molecular size, cannot cross intact cell membranes. In other words, these agents cannot normally enter the intracellular space.

The kinetics of contrast enhancement in normal and infarcted myocardium have been well characterized *(32,33)*. After a bolus injection of gadolinium, perfusion significantly modulates arrival and clearance of contrast in normal and infarcted myocardium *(33)*. Ex vivo experiments indicated that delayed enhancement is not caused by gadolinium binding to the infarcted myocardium *(34)*.

Although normal myocardium enhances to some degree with these contrast agents, infarcted myocardium accumulates much more contrast than normal myocardium.

This is sometimes described as *hyperenhancement*, but for the purposes of this chapter the term *delayed enhancement* is preferred. This term originated from early studies that showed low signal intensity in the infarct shortly after injection. Several minutes later, however, the infarcted myocardium enhanced more than normal myocardium.

Pharmacology experiments using slow continuous infusions of gadolinium have determined that the gadolinium contrast agents distribute into the myocardium proportionately to the partition coefficient of gadolinium *(35)*. The slow infusion minimizes the influence of perfusion on gadolinium concentration within the myocardium. Although theoretically superior to bolus injections of gadolinium, these hour-long continuous infusions are not practical in patients.

High-resolution electron probe X-ray microanalysis documented that gadolinium accumulates in the myocardium with similar spatial distribution as sodium ion *(36)*. Myocardial gadolinium concentration is inversely related to potassium concentration. In normal myocardium, cell membranes pump sodium out of the cell and maintain high potassium concentration within the cell. In acutely infarcted myocardium, loss of cell membrane integrity allows sodium and gadolinium into the intracellular space. In chronic infarcts, the gadolinium also tracks with sodium *(36)*. In chronic infarcts, which have large areas of collagen scar and relatively limited intracellular space, the high gadolinium concentration represents the abnormally large extracellular space. Thus, the myocardial distribution of gadolinium provides information about the integrity cell membranes and therefore viability.

Ex vivo, high-resolution, spectrally sensitive radionuclide imaging allowed comparison of the myocardial distribution of two nuclear viability agents (^{99}Tc sestamibi and ^{18}F-FDG [^{18}F-fluorodeoxyglucose]) with ^{111}In-DTPA (diethyltriaminepentaacetic acid) in pathological specimens of myocardial infarction *(37)*. The ^{111}In-DTPA helped localize the relative distribution of DTPA in normal myocardium and regions of myocardial infarction. Gd-DTPA is a commonly used abbreviation for one of the extracellular contrast agents (generic name gadopentetate dimeglumine; chemical compound gadolinium-diethylenetriaminepentaacetic acid) approved by the Food and Drug Administration. Thus, the ^{111}In-DTPA activity in the necrotic central zone indicates there are high concentrations of DTPA, a finding consistent with gadolinium-DTPA enhancement of infarction. Both ^{99}Tc sestamibi and ^{18}F-FDG had very low activity in the collagen scar. The border zone had low perfusion based on low sestamibi activity but metabolic mismatch as evidenced by high FDG activity. In this partly viable, partly fibrosed border zone, activities from ^{111}In-DTPA correlated best with the changes in fibrosis density. This study supports the conclusion that gadolinium-DTPA distributes in the extracellular space, and this space represents a large percentage of fibrotic myocardium relative to normal myocardium.

Overall, current-generation extracellular gadolinium-based contrast agents differentiate myocardial infarction from normal myocardium based on the relative volume of distribution of contrast. In viable myocardium, intact cell membranes effectively exclude the extracellular gadolinium contrast agents from the intracellular space. Thus, gadolinium concentration tracks sodium and is inversely related to tissue potassium distribution. In acute myocardial infarction, the necrotic or dying cardiomyocytes lose cell membrane integrity, and extracellular gadolinium contrast agents can enter cells. This results in higher contrast concentrations in the area of acute myocardial infarction and consequently bright signal intensity in the infarct.

Chronic myocardial infarction also enhances, but for slightly different reasons. Fibrous scar or collagen scar is a relatively acellular tissue with a small intracellular volume found mainly in fibroblasts and other scattered cells. Because the intracellular space of collagen scar is relatively small compared to the extracellular space, this tissue enhances substantially more than normal myocardium. Thus, both acute and chronic myocardial infarctions typically appear bright on delayed enhancement images.

VALIDATION OF DELAYED-ENHANCEMENT IMAGING IN PATIENTS

The clinical validation of delayed-enhancement imaging has been comprehensive and of sufficient quality that the method is accepted as a reference standard assessment of viability (Table 2). In patients with left ventricular dysfunction associated with severe ischemic heart disease, predicting the recovery of function after revascularization is one of the better experimental designs for validating whether a clinical test is capable of assessing myocardial viability.

Kim et al. found that the transmural extent of infarction was inversely proportional to the probability of regional recovery of function after revascularization (38). This study provided the first clinical evidence that delayed-enhancement imaging was able to assess viability with recovery of function after revascularization as the reference standard. This study also provided pathophysiological insight into the role of subendocardial and transmural myocardial infarction. Kim et al. (38) found that the transmural extent of myocardial scarring predicted the probability of recovery of function. Selvanayagam et al. (39) nicely confirmed these findings in an independent study in which all patients were revascularized with coronary bypass surgery.

Recovery of function is a clinical method that has been accepted for judging whether a test can image myocardial viability. However, this method does not directly correspond to myocardial viability. There are many factors that modulate whether dysfunctional but viable myocardium will recover function after revascularization. Regional contractile function in the heart is dependent on afterload or, more precisely, wall stress. Wall stress σ is defined as left ventricular pressure P multiplied by ventricular radius R divided by wall thickness h:

$$\sigma = P \times R/h \tag{1}$$

Thus, wall thickening is affected by pressure in the left ventricular cavity, radius of the segment of the heart, and wall thickness. As wall stress increases, systolic wall thickening decreases. Theoretically, if the transmural extent of infarction is 50%, there may be too little viable myocardium to improve regional contractile function. Despite the fact that half the wall is viable, the wall stress on that segment could be twice as high as for a segment that is completely viable.

Other factors can also modulate the ability of a given segment of the heart to recover function after revascularization. When there are a large number of segments of the heart that are ischemic but viable, successful revascularization may be associated with an overall decrease in left ventricular size, leading to improved radius in the heart overall, lower afterload, and therefore improved regional function. Thus, the total number of viable but dysfunctional segments needs to be considered. Neighboring segments will also modulate the probability of regional recovery of function (50). A viable segment surrounded by transmurally infarcted segments may experience less change in local radius or may be tethered in a way that it cannot recover function as well as a segment surrounded by normal myocardium.

Table 2
Validation of Delayed-Enhancement CMR for Chronic Myocardial Infarction and Viability

Year	Reference	n	Acute vs chronic	Major findings
2005	40	48	Chronic	MI size and characteristics predict inducibility of ventricular tachycardia better than LVEF
2004	39	52	Chronic	Transmural extent of delayed enhancement correlated inversely with the likelihood of recovery of function after CABG; new CABG-related delayed enhancement predicted lack of improvement
2004	41	29	Chronic	Dobutamine CMR was slightly better than delayed enhancement for predicting recovery of regional function after revascularization
2004	42	60	Chronic	Contractile reserve varies inversely with the extent of scar; contractile reserve can be impaired with minimal delayed enhancement; conversely, thickening sometimes occurs despite extensive scar
2003	43	19	Chronic	Thick (>4.5 mm) and metabolically viable segments (>50% FDG uptake) showed functional recovery 85% of the time; thin, metabolically nonviable segments improved function 13% of the time
2003	44	26	Chronic	FDG-PET uptake was inversely correlated with the transmural extent of delayed enhancement; optimal viability threshold was 37% transmural of delayed enhancement (with PET as the reference)
2003	45	91	Chronic	In the animal validation, sensitivity for subendocardial MI was 92% CMR vs 28% SPECT; in patients with subendocardial MI by CMR, SPECT had 53% sensitivity
2002	46	15	Chronic	The unipolar voltage recorded during electro mechanical mapping varied inversely with the amount of delayed enhancement: 11.6 mV none; 6.8 mV subendocardial; and 4.6 mV transmural voltage than normal (11.6 ± 4.5 mV) segments
2002	47	20	Chronic	The reproducibility of determining infarct size was very good in a study design in which a gadolinium contrast was injected once, and two separate CMR scans were performed within about 30 minutes
2002	48	31	Chronic	CMR had 86% sensitivity and 94% specificity for detecting segmental flow/metabolism defects (PET reference standard), but 55% of subendocardial MI by delayed enhancement were normal by PET
2001	49	82	Chronic	CMR had 91% sensitivity for MI and 100% specificity; the presence and location of subendocardial and transmural MI in each coronary distribution was depicted
2000	28	50	Chronic	The likelihood of improvement in regional contractility after revascularization decreased progressively as the transmural extent of delayed enhancement before revascularization increased
	Total	523	Chronic	

CABG, coronary artery bypass graft; LVEF, left ventricular ejection fraction; MI, myocardial infarction.

Keeping in mind that factors other than viability may influence the recovery of function, there is some evidence that dobutamine CMR may predict regional recovery of function better than the transmural extent of infarction *(51,52)*. Such data can be interpreted two ways. If the primary clinical goal is predicting changes in regional function, then a physiological test that directly assesses regional function under dobutamine stimulation may be more optimal. However, there may be additional considerations, such as ischemia and arrhythmias, that are modulated by reperfusion but may not be manifest in regional assessments of function. Thus, there is likely to be a strong role for delayed enhancement imaging in the future.

Validation of delayed enhancement infarct images in humans has also relied on correlations with nuclear imaging. There was a good correlation between the amount of viable or nonviable myocardium assessed by single photon emission computed tomographic (SPECT) imaging within reasonable limits of agreement *(53,54)*. One should note that SPECT may miss smaller infarcts that are easily detected by CMR *(45)*. This has been attributed to the lower resolution of SPECT cameras and the blurring of images that occurs because of respiratory motion (or cardiorespiratory motion if the acquisitions are not cardiac gated). Despite the fact that small subendocardial infarcts can be missed on SPECT scans, the prevalence of this problem in a typical group of patients may be relatively small *(54)*.

Delayed-enhancement imaging of infarct size has also been validated against PET imaging. Klein et al. *(55)* found good correlation in infarct size between the two methods with good limits of agreement in Bland-Altman analysis. However, they noted that a large percentage of segments that showed only subendocardial infarcts on the delayed-enhancement scans were read as normal on the PET scan. Kuhl et al. *(44)* also found good correlations between PET and delayed-enhancement imaging. This work found that a threshold of less than 37% transmural extent of infarction on delayed enhancement best predicted viability as determined by the PET scan.

In the setting of acute myocardial infarction, delayed-enhancement imaging has been validated in over 300 patients (Table 3). The amount of myocardium exhibiting delayed enhancement correlates against serum biomarkers and predicts regional recovery of function *(56–58)*. The method seems to work well 1 week and even 2 days after myocardial infarction.

From the studies mentioned, it is reasonable to conclude that delayed-enhancement imaging is an excellent clinical tool for assessing myocardial infarction and viability. The method has sufficient resolution to determine the transmural extent of infarction. Delayed-enhancement imaging of myocardial infarction can predict recovery of function after revascularization. It correlates against SPECT imaging but has significant advantages in resolution for detecting small subendocardial infarctions. The amount of delayed enhancement correlates against biomarkers associated with acute myocardial infarction (at least in reperfused infarcts). Delayed-enhancement CMR is capable of determining myocardial viability in the setting of chronic coronary artery disease and within the first few days after acute myocardial infarction.

OTHER CONDITIONS THAT CAN CAUSE MYOCARDIAL DELAYED ENHANCEMENT

Understanding the pathophysiology of why extracellular gadolinium contrast agents enhance acute and chronic infarction should make it intuitively clear why other diseases that cause myocardial fibrosis and scarring should also enhance the myocardium *(69)*.

Table 3
Validation Studies of Delayed-Enhancement CMR for Acute Myocardial Infarction

Year	Reference	n	Acute vs. chronic	Major findings
2006	59	27	Acute Chronic	Delayed enhancement could predict dysfunctional segments distal to chronic total occlusions that improved after revascularization
2005	60	22	Acute chronic	Delayed enhancement predicted recovery of function after acute MI better than perfusion imaging
2005	61	33	Acute	The extent of MI was reasonably stable from 7 to 42 minutes postcontrast and correlated well with SPECT infarct size
2004	62	33 20	Acute chronic	In patients 2 days after acute PCI, MI size correlated with peak troponin; acute MI size predicted chronic LVEF and regional function; infarct size decreased from 16% of the LV to 11% of the LV
2004	63	60	Acute	SPECT and CMR infarct size correlated, but SPECT had 80% sensitivity, and CMR had 100% sensitivity; SPECT missed 6 of 30 inferior MIs
2003	57	30	Acute chronic	In patients 1 week after acute MI, there was an inverse relationship between the transmural extent of infarction and likelihood of regional recovery of function
2002	64	20	Acute chronic	In patients 4 days after acute MI, delayed enhancement predicted recovery of regional function better than perfusion images that significantly underestimated the amount of irreversible injury
2001	65	24	Acute chronic	Within 7 days of acute MI, MI size correlated with peak CKMB; there is an inverse relationship between the transmural extent of MI and likelihood of regional recovery of function
2001	66	14 6	Acute chronic	Microinfarcts were detected in patients that had PCI-related elevations in CKMB; two patterns of MI were observed: (1) small side branch occlusion and (2) distal embolization
2006	67	16 21	Acute chronic	MI size by computed tomography and CMR correlated well ($r = 0.89$), although the 2 SD limits of agreement were about 35 g; Interobserver agreement and intrastudy agreement was good
2005	68	50 24	Acute chronic	All patients with a troponin elevation (average 3.7°μg/L) associated with PCI exhibited new abnormal delayed enhancement; troponin level correlated with MI size
	Total	329	Acute	

CKMB, creatine kinase MB fraction; LVEF, left ventricular ejection fraction; MI, myocardial infarction; PCI, percutaneous coronary intervention.

There are many specific conditions that cause delayed enhancement, including myocarditis, sarcoidosis, hypertrophic cardiomyopathy, Fabrys disease, and some nonischemic cardiomyopathies. Discrimination of these nonspecific causes of delayed enhancement from myocardial infarction associated with coronary artery disease is based on the vulnerability of the subendocardium to ischemia.

As described in the pathophysiology of myocardial infarction, human infarcts typically start in the endocardium and progress toward the epicardial surface and follow the distribution of the affected coronary arteries. Other causes of delayed enhancement can often be recognized because of atypical patterns *(70)*. Refer to Chapter 19 for examples of these other diseases.

ASSESSING MYOCARDIAL INFARCTION WITH T_2-WEIGHTED IMAGING AND NEW CONTRAST AGENTS

The current power of CMR lies in the combined examination of global and regional function, myocardial perfusion, viability, and even the coronary arteries. However, there are other CMR methods that may prove valuable in the future.

T_2-weighted CMR provides images that can assess edema associated with acute myocardial infarction *(71)*. Unless otherwise indicated, CMR images rely on detecting signals from protons. The majority of protons in the body are in either water or fat. The signal intensity on T_2-weighted images is heavily influenced by the physical mobility of water protons. Edema can be detected in the myocardium after acute myocardial infarction. Because this edema resolves over approximately 1–2 months following the myocardial infarction, T_2-weighted imaging can differentiate acute from chronic infarction *(71)*. Ex vivo images suggested the edema primarily represents the area at risk during the infarction *(72)*.

Aletras et al. demonstrated that the T_2 abnormality corresponds to the area at risk *(8)*. In that study, the size of the abnormality on T_2-weighted images was compared with microsphere determinations of the area at risk. High-resolution systolic strain images also confirmed a partial recovery of function consistent with a subendocardial infarction. The ability to differentiate acute from chronic myocardial infarction is unique to CMR.

Assuming that T_2-weighted images with comparable quality to the canine images can be acquired, then it should be possible to image a patient 2 or 3 days after an acute myocardial infarction and determine how much myocardium was ischemic (i.e., measure the area at risk). Combined with high-resolution delayed-enhancement images, CMR could measure the area at risk, the amount of necrosis, and the amount of myocardial salvage. Such a measurement would be of significant value in testing therapies that alter infarct size.

Manganese can also image the area at risk associated with acute myocardial infarction. Natanzon et al. *(73)* verified that manganese chloride accumulates in normal myocardium, but regions of myocardial infarction have much lower uptake. Thus, a myocardial infarction looks dark on manganese-enhanced image, and normal myocardium is brighter.

There are other contrast agents that may be useful in imaging myocardial infarction in the future. There is a class of magnetic resonance imaging (MRI) contrast agents that has been classified as *infarct avid*. These agents accumulate in regions of myocardial infarction and can be imaged with T_1-weighted sequences *(74)*. Some of the infarct

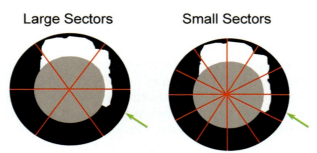

Fig. 7. Reporting the transmural extent of infarction. The *transmural extent of infarction* is defined as the percentage of each sector that exhibits delayed enhancement. Large sectors result in more variable transmural extent within a sector compared with small sectors. The transmural extent of infarction sometimes varies in the circumferential direction with a sector (arrows), a problem more likely to occur with large sectors.

avid agents are porphyrin based, but some are not. At least one of the porphyrin-based agents accurately measures the infarct size in a canine model *(75)*.

ANALYSIS AND REPORTING OF VIABILITY

The transmural extent of infarction is either visually estimated or measured in small sectors of the heart as the thickness of myocardium infarcted divided by the thickness of myocardium (reported as a percentage). This measurement is relatively straightforward for small sectors of the heart as used by Kim et al. in the landmark clinical study that defined this analysis scheme *(38)*. However, the analysis becomes more difficult when summarizing the heart in larger sectors, as recommended by the American Heart Association *(76)*, because infarcted myocardium may straddle segments or may not be evident in the full circumferential extent of a segment. Large sectors increase the likelihood that the infarct will have a complicated shape within a sector *(7)*.

The optimal threshold for classifying myocardium as normal or infarcted appears to be a signal intensity threshold about halfway between normal remote myocardium and the brightest infarcted pixels *(31,77,78)*. Thresholds based on the standard deviation of signal intensity of normal myocardium were less reliable than a full-width half-maximum threshold *(77)*. Hsu et al. *(31)* found that computer algorithms that incorporate expert knowledge can objectively analyze infarct regions with user-independent selected thresholds (Fig. 6). Incorporating advanced image-processing techniques that use feature analysis helps eliminate false-positive bright regions. Other analysis steps can identify islands of microvascular obstruction within the otherwise bright infarct as a portion of the infarct. Both studies found excellent correlations between histopathology and in vivo delayed-enhancement images of infarction *(31,79)*.

Ibrahim et al. *(53)* compared infarct size determined by SPECT in 33 patients early after acute myocardial infarction and compared CMR-determined infarct size using a wide range of signal intensity thresholds. They found that myocardium twice as bright as normal myocardium correlated most closely with infarct size determined by SPECT. Considering that their infarcts were approximately five times brighter than normal myocardium, this threshold agrees reasonably well with the animal validation studies.

Table 4
Advantages and Disadvantages of Using MRI to Assess Myocardial Infarction

Advantages	*Disadvantages*
High resolution (approximately 1 mm)	Image quality may be suboptimal if the patient has arrhythmias
Relatively simple imaging protocol	Best imaging done during breath holds; respiratory artifacts can degrade images
Gadolinium agents well tolerated	Claustrophobia prevents some subjects from completing the study
Can assess viability without stress	Dobutamine stress may predict recovery of function better than transmural extent of infarction
Comprehensive exam of function, perfusion, and viability is practical	Many obese patients cannot fit into many scanners used for cardiac imaging makers
Excellent sensitivity	Contraindications currently include pace makers and defibrillators
Excellent specificity (after excluding atypical)	Expensive technology
No ionizing radiation	

ADVANTAGES AND DISADVANTAGES OF MAGNETIC RESONANCE IMAGING IN ASSESSING MYOCARDIAL INFARCTION

Compared with conventional cardiac diagnostic tests, there are advantages and disadvantages in using MRI to assess myocardial infarction (Table 4). Overall, CMR evaluation of patients with myocardial infarction is a powerful clinical tool when performed by experienced clinicians.

TECHNICAL AND PROCEDURAL CONSIDERATIONS OF DELAYED-ENHANCEMENT IMAGING

All physicians using delayed-enhancement imaging should understand some basic aspects of the image acquisition and physics. Such information can help solve problems that arise during imaging or analysis.

The inversion recovery delayed-enhancement methods introduced by Simonetti et al. *(29)* represent a substantial improvement over prior T_1-weighted sequences. Thus, for the purposes of this chapter, the inversion recovery method is considered the conventional methodology. One must keep in mind that there are many variants of inversion recovery acquisitions. The phase-sensitive detection introduced by Kellman et al. *(80)* provides some simplicity in understanding the relationship between image acquisition parameters and signal intensity. Thus, this method is used to describe the physics of delayed-enhancement imaging.

Concept 1: T_1 *Weighting and Nulling Normal Myocardium*

Delayed-enhancement imaging of myocardial infarction depends on making the image sensitive to T_1 relaxation. To understand T_1 weighting, one must first realize that the main magnetic field B_0 of the MRI scanner is strong enough to align protons along the axis of the magnet. Outside the magnet, protons in the body are randomly oriented. Inside the magnet, protons align with the main magnetic field B_0 like the pointer of a compass. As illustrated in Fig. 4 of Chapter 1, initially more protons are aligned parallel to the magnet than antiparallel. This results in a net vector of magnetization that can be imaged.

We can use a radio-frequency pulse B_1 called the *inversion pulse* to transiently redirect the protons so that more protons are pointed antiparallel to the main magnetic field B_0 than parallel. A radio-frequency pulse is essentially a short burst of radio waves. Radio-frequency pulses are a form of electromagnetic radiation. When transmitted through the body coil in the scanner, a radio-frequency pulse can reorient the protons in the body.

After the inversion pulse, it should be intuitively sensible that nature will tend to realign the protons with the main magnetic field B_0. The T_1 relaxation rate describes the temporal characteristics of this realignment process. As a nuclear process, this realignment turns out to follow an exponential time course. One can think of T_1 as a rate constant analogous to radiation decay half-life.

As illustrated by the curve in Fig. 8a, the T_1 relaxation rate can be used to predict the signal intensity of MRI before and after an inversion pulse. In Fig. 8a, the y-axis represents magnetization but in simplistic terms can be considered the net signal that results from a given image acquisition program. If an image was acquired before the inversion pulse, then 100% signal intensity could be acquired. Immediately following the inversion pulse, the net magnetization points in the opposite direction, so the signal intensity would be –100% (assuming phase-sensitive detection was used that can differentiate a positive from a negative signal). The inversion pulse only lasts approximately 5 ms. After the inversion pulse, the protons start realigning with the main magnetic field. Thus, if an image is acquired at a short delay (inversion time) after the inversion pulse, then the number of protons aligned antiparallel with the main magnetic field (negative signal) will still outnumber the protons aligned parallel to the main magnetic field (positive signal). Thus, the net magnetization or net signal after a short inversion time still adds to a signal that is negative. With longer inversion times, the magnetization progressively grows less negative. The blue curve in Fig. 8a shows how the signal intensity of normal myocardium changes as a function of the inversion time.

Nulling normal myocardium occurs when an image is acquired at an inversion time when approximately half the protons are aligned with the main magnetic field B_0 and half the protons are aligned antiparallel to B_0. At this particular inversion time, the normal myocardium will appear uniformly dark because the signal from protons in each orientation cancels each other. In Fig. 8a, the inversion time to null normal myocardium is 275 ms, and the blue curve has a signal intensity close to zero (i.e., appears "nulled").

If an image is acquired at an even longer inversion time, then the number of protons aligned with the main magnetic field B_0 will exceed the number of protons aligned antiparallel to the magnet. The net magnetization or signal intensity will be slightly positive. Approximately 99% of the protons will be realigned with the main magnetic field B_0 at inversion times more than five times the T_1 of normal myocardium. After such a long delay, the normal myocardium will be uniformly at the maximal signal intensity achievable for a given image acquisition sequence, and the effects of the inversion pulse are no longer evident.

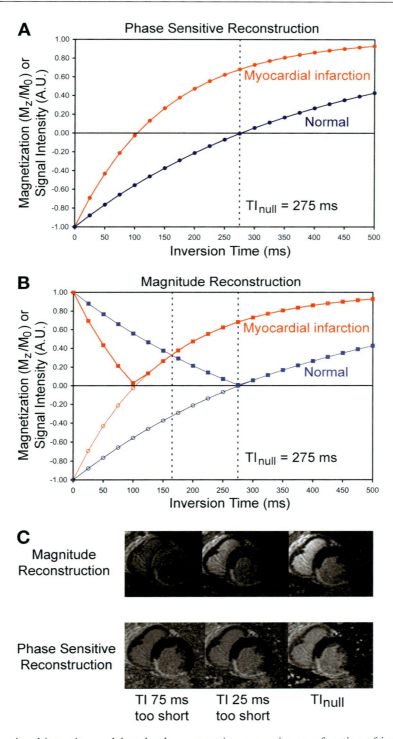

Fig. 8. How signal intensity on delayed-enhancement images varies as a function of inversion time for images reconstructed with phase-sensitive methods and conventional magnitude methods. Normal myocardium is illustrated in blue; myocardial infarction is represented in the red. See text for explanation.

Concept 2: The T_1 of the Infarct Is Shorter Than the T_1 of Normal Myocardium

Delayed-enhancement images of myocardial infarction are usually acquired at the inversion time that optimally nulls normal myocardium. There are three important reasons why the inversion time should be adjusted to null normal myocardium. As described, the normal myocardium appears uniformly dark. Because more gadolinium accumulates in the myocardial infarction than in normal myocardium, the T_1 of the infarcted myocardium is shorter than the T_1 of normal myocardium.

A shorter T_1 can be considered analogous to a short half-life. In other words, the protons in the infarct (short T_1) realign with the main magnetic field B_0 more quickly than the protons in normal myocardium (longer T_1). The faster recovery of magnetization is illustrated in Fig. 8a by the red curve. At all inversion times, the signal intensity is greater for the infarct than for normal myocardium because of the shorter T_1 (assuming phase-sensitive detection). Thus, the infarct will go through a null at a shorter inversion time. If an image is acquired at an inversion time that nulls normal myocardium, then the infarct has a bright signal intensity that contrasts well with a dark background of normal myocardium. This is the first important reason for nulling normal myocardium.

The second reason it is important to null normal myocardium is that the difference in signal intensity is close to the maximal achievable difference at this inversion time. A third reason for nulling normal myocardium also eliminates effects of surface coil intensity variations, at least for normal myocardium.

Concept 3: The Signal Intensity Can Be Misleading on Delayed-Enhancement Images When Conventional Magnitude Reconstruction Methods Are Used

Conventional MRIs use magnitude reconstruction. This means that the signal intensity on a magnitude image (Fig. 8b) is essentially the absolute value of the phase-sensitive signal intensity plotted in Fig. 8a. Most magnetic resonance scanners do not produce images with negative values. As a result, the signal intensity measured off conventional delayed-enhancement images will all be positive values. Figure 8b uses square symbols to plot the absolute values of the phase-sensitive curves, which are plotted with open circles.

There are three clinically relevant consequences related to the use of magnitude images that significantly affect the delayed-enhancement technique. First, the signal intensity on magnitude images is not simply related to gadolinium concentration. Second, it is critical to select the correct inversion time to null normal myocardium. This is because the signal intensity of the infarct on a magnitude image can be brighter, darker, or the same as normal myocardium depending on what inversion time is selected. In Fig. 8b, the signal intensity of normal myocardium is the same as the infarct at an inversion time around 165 ms. At inversion times less than 165 ms, the normal myocardium is higher than the infarct. There is even an inversion time when the infarcted myocardium appears nulled on magnitude images. Figure 8c shows that incorrect selection of the inversion time markedly affects the appearance of the heart on magnitude images, and phase-sensitive images reconstructed from the same data set are all high quality. Third, infarct size will vary if one selects the wrong inversion time. Fortunately, there are methods that can be used to help estimate the correct inversion time (81).

On the other hand, there are many advantages to using the phase-sensitive inversion recovery methods for delayed-enhancement imaging *(82,83)*. The phase-sensitive inversion recovery method has also been validated against histopathological infarct size in a canine model *(31)* and in patients *(78)*. There are also new methods that can improve the contrast between the infarct and the blood in the left ventricular cavity *(83)*. Finally, most implementations of phase-sensitive inversion recovery imaging provide both magnitude and phase-sensitive images, so one can get both types of images with a single acquisition.

CONCLUSIONS

Delayed-enhancement imaging has emerged as a reference standard method for imaging myocardial viability. There are a number of developments in the field that will nicely complement the gadolinium-based methods and further extend the utility of CMR in evaluating myocardial infarction and viability.

ACKNOWLEDGMENT

This work was supported by the Intramural Research Program of the National Heart, Lung, and Blood Institute.

REFERENCES

1. Reimer KA, Lowe JE, Rasmussen MM, Jennings RB. The wavefront phenomenon of ischemic cell death. 1. Myocardial infarct size vs duration of coronary occlusion in dogs. Circulation 1977;56:786–794.
2. Reimer KA, Jennings RB. The "wavefront phenomenon" of myocardial ischemic cell death. II. Transmural progression of necrosis within the framework of ischemic bed size (myocardium at risk) and collateral flow. Lab Invest 1979;40:633–644.
3. Kloner RA, Jennings RB. Consequences of brief ischemia: stunning, preconditioning, and their clinical implications: part 1. Circulation 2001;104:2981–2989.
4. Reimer KA, Murry CE, Yamasawa I, Hill ML, Jennings RB. Four brief periods of myocardial ischemia cause no cumulative ATP loss or necrosis. Am J Physiol 1986;251:H1306–H1315.
5. Yellon DM, Downey JM. Preconditioning the myocardium: from cellular physiology to clinical cardiology. Physiol Rev 2003;83:1113–1151.
6. Bolli R, Becker L, Gross G, Mentzer R Jr, Balshaw D, Lathrop DA. Myocardial protection at a crossroads: the need for translation into clinical therapy. Circ Res 2004;95:125–134.
7. Christian TF, Clements IP, Gibbons RJ. Noninvasive identification of myocardium at risk in patients with acute myocardial infarction and nondiagnostic electrocardiograms with technetium-99m-Sestamibi. Circulation 1991;83:1615–1620.
8. Aletras AH, Tilak GS, Natanzon A, et al. Retrospective determination of the area at risk for reperfused acute myocardial infarction with T_2-weighted cardiac magnetic resonance imaging: histopathological and displacement encoding with stimulated echoes (DENSE) functional validations. Circulation 2006;113:1865–1870.
9. Anversa P, Kajstura J, Leri A, Bolli R. Life and death of cardiac stem cells: a paradigm shift in cardiac biology. Circulation 2006;113:1451–1463.
10. Kloner RA, Jennings RB. Consequences of brief ischemia: stunning, preconditioning, and their clinical implications: part 2. Circulation 2001;104:3158–3167.
11. Braunwald E, Rutherford JD. Reversible ischemic left ventricular dysfunction: evidence for the "hibernating myocardium." J Am Coll Cardiol 1986;8:1467–1470.
12. Tarantini G, Cacciavillani L, Corbetti F, et al. Duration of ischemia is a major determinant of transmurality and severe microvascular obstruction after primary angioplasty: a study performed with contrast-enhanced magnetic resonance. J Am Coll Cardiol 2005;46:1229–1235.
13. Wu KC, Zerhouni EA, Judd RM, et al. Prognostic significance of microvascular obstruction by magnetic resonance imaging in patients with acute myocardial infarction. Circulation 1998;97:765–772.

14. Mollet NR, Dymarkowski S, Volders W, et al. Visualization of ventricular thrombi with contrast-enhanced magnetic resonance imaging in patients with ischemic heart disease. Circulation 2002;106:2873–2876.

15. Flacke S, Fischer S, Scott MJ, et al. Novel MRI contrast agent for molecular imaging of fibrin: implications for detecting vulnerable plaques. Circulation 2001;104:1280–1285.

16. Botnar RM, Perez AS, Witte S, et al. In vivo molecular imaging of acute and subacute thrombosis using a fibrin-binding magnetic resonance imaging contrast agent. Circulation 2004;109: 2023–2029.

17. Botnar RM, Buecker A, Wiethoff AJ, et al. In vivo magnetic resonance imaging of coronary thrombosis using a fibrin-binding molecular magnetic resonance contrast agent. Circulation 2004;110:1463–1466.

18. Spuentrup E, Buecker A, Katoh M, et al. Molecular magnetic resonance imaging of coronary thrombosis and pulmonary emboli with a novel fibrin-targeted contrast agent. Circulation 2005;111:1377–1382.

19. Sirol M, Fuster V, Badimon JJ, et al. Chronic thrombus detection with in vivo magnetic resonance imaging and a fibrin-targeted contrast agent. Circulation 2005;112:1594–1600.

20. Pfeffer MA. Left ventricular remodeling after acute myocardial infarction. Annu Rev Med 1995;46: 455–466.

21. Yousef ZR, Redwood SR, Marber MS. Postinfarction left ventricular remodeling: a pathophysiological and therapeutic review. Cardiovasc Drugs Ther 2000;14:243–252.

22. White HD, Norris RM, Brown MA, Brandt PW, Whitlock RM, Wild CJ. Left ventricular end-systolic volume as the major determinant of survival after recovery from myocardial infarction. Circulation 1987;76:44–51.

23. Wesbey GE, Higgins CB, McNamara MT, et al. Effect of gadolinium-DTPA on the magnetic relaxation times of normal and infarcted myocardium. Radiology 1984;153:165–169.

24. McNamara MT, Tscholakoff D, Revel D, et al. Differentiation of reversible and irreversible myocardial injury by MR imaging with and without gadolinium-DTPA. Radiology 1986;158:765–769.

25. Peshock RM, Malloy CR, Buja LM, Nunnally RL, Parkey RW, Willerson JT. Magnetic resonance imaging of acute myocardial infarction: gadolinium diethylenetriamine pentaacetic acid as a marker of reperfusion. Circulation 1986;74:1434–1440.

26. Rehr RB, Peshock RM, Malloy CR, et al. Improved in vivo magnetic resonance imaging of acute myocardial infarction after intravenous paramagnetic contrast agent administration. Am J Cardiol 1986;57:864–868.

27. Kim RJ, Fieno DS, Parrish TB, et al. Relationship of MRI delayed contrast enhancement to irreversible injury, infarct age, and contractile function. Circulation 1999;100:1992–2002.

28. Kim RJ, Wu E, Rafael A, et al. The use of contrast-enhanced magnetic resonance imaging to identify reversible myocardial dysfunction. N Engl J Med 2000;343:1445–1453.

29. Simonetti OP, Kim RJ, Fieno DS, et al. An improved MR imaging technique for the visualization of myocardial infarction. Radiology 2001;218:215–223.

30. Fieno DS, Kim RJ, Chen EL, Lomasney JW, Klocke FJ, Judd RM. Contrast-enhanced magnetic resonance imaging of myocardium at risk: distinction between reversible and irreversible injury throughout infarct healing. J Am Coll Cardiol 2000;36:1985–1991.

31. Hsu LY, Natanzon A, Kellman P, Hirsch GA, Aletras AH, Arai AE. Quantitative myocardial infarction on delayed enhancement MRI. Part I: animal validation of an automated feature analysis and combined thresholding infarct sizing algorithm. J Magn Reson Imaging 2006;23:298–308.

32. Judd RM, Lugo-Olivieri CH, Arai M, et al. Physiological basis of myocardial contrast enhancement in fast magnetic resonance images of 2-d-old reperfused canine infarcts. Circulation 1995;92:1902–1910.

33. Kim RJ, Chen EL, Lima JA, Judd RM. Myocardial Gd-DTPA kinetics determine MRI contrast enhancement and reflect the extent and severity of myocardial injury after acute reperfused infarction. Circulation 1996;94:3318–3326.

34. Decking UK, Pai VM, Wen H, Balaban RS. Does binding of Gd-DTPA to myocardial tissue contribute to late enhancement in a model of acute myocardial infarction? Magn Reson Med 2003;49:168–171.

35. Thornhill RE, Prato FS, Wisenberg G. The assessment of myocardial viability: a review of current diagnostic imaging approaches. J Cardiovasc Magn Reson 2002;4:381–410.

36. Rehwald WG, Fieno DS, Chen EL, Kim RJ, Judd RM. Myocardial magnetic resonance imaging contrast agent concentrations after reversible and irreversible ischemic injury. Circulation 2002;105:224–229.

37. Maskali F, Poussier S, Marie PY, et al. High-resolution simultaneous imaging of SPECT, PET, and MRI tracers on histologic sections of myocardial infarction. J Nucl Cardiol 2005;12:229–230.

38. Kim RJ, Wu E, Rafael A, et al. The use of contrast-enhanced magnetic resonance imaging to identify reversible myocardial dysfunction. N Engl J Med 2000;343:1445–1453.

39. Selvanayagam JB, Kardos A, Francis JM, et al. Value of delayed-enhancement cardiovascular magnetic resonance imaging in predicting myocardial viability after surgical revascularization. Circulation 2004;110:1535–1541.

40. Bello D, Fieno DS, Kim RJ, et al. Infarct morphology identifies patients with substrate for sustained ventricular tachycardia. J Am Coll Cardiol 2005;45:1104–1108.

41. Wellnhofer E, Olariu A, Klein C, et al. Magnetic resonance low-dose dobutamine test is superior to SCAR quantification for the prediction of functional recovery. Circulation 2004;109:2172–2174.

42. Nelson C, McCrohon J, Khafagi F, Rose S, Leano R, Marwick TH. Impact of scar thickness on the assessment of viability using dobutamine echocardiography and thallium single-photon emission computed tomography: a comparison with contrast-enhanced magnetic resonance imaging. J Am Coll Cardiol 2004;43:1248–1256.

43. Knuesel PR, Nanz D, Wyss C, et al. Characterization of dysfunctional myocardium by positron emission tomography and magnetic resonance: relation to functional outcome after revascularization. Circulation 2003;108:1095–1100.

44. Kuhl HP, Beek AM, van der Weerdt AP, et al. Myocardial viability in chronic ischemic heart disease: comparison of contrast-enhanced magnetic resonance imaging with (18)F-fluorodeoxyglucose positron emission tomography. J Am Coll Cardiol 2003;41:1341–1348.

45. Wagner A, Mahrholdt H, Holly TA, et al. Contrast-enhanced MRI and routine single photon emission computed tomography (SPECT) perfusion imaging for detection of subendocardial myocardial infarcts: an imaging study. Lancet 2003;361:374–379.

46. Perin EC, Silva GV, Sarmento-Leite R, et al. Assessing myocardial viability and infarct transmurality with left ventricular electromechanical mapping in patients with stable coronary artery disease: validation by delayed-enhancement magnetic resonance imaging. Circulation 2002;106:957–961.

47. Mahrholdt H, Wagner A, Holly TA, et al. Reproducibility of chronic infarct size measurement by contrast-enhanced magnetic resonance imaging. Circulation 2002;106:2322–2327.

48. Klein C, Nekolla SG, Bengel FM, et al. Assessment of myocardial viability with contrast-enhanced magnetic resonance imaging: comparison with positron emission tomography. Circulation 2002;105:162–167.

49. Wu E, Judd RM, Vargas JD, Klocke FJ, Bonow RO, Kim RJ. Visualisation of presence, location, and transmural extent of healed Q-wave and non-Q-wave myocardial infarction. Lancet 2001;357:21–28.

50. Ugander M, Cain PA, Perron A, Hedstrom E, Arheden H. Infarct transmurality and adjacent segmental function as determinants of wall thickening in revascularized chronic ischemic heart disease. Clin Physiol Funct Imaging 2005;25:209–214.

51. Wellnhofer E, Olariu A, Klein C, et al. Magnetic resonance low-dose dobutamine test is superior to SCAR quantification for the prediction of functional recovery. Circulation 2004;109:2172–2174.

52. Geskin G, Kramer CM, Rogers WJ, et al. Quantitative assessment of myocardial viability after infarction by dobutamine magnetic resonance tagging. Circulation 1998;98:217–223.

53. Ibrahim T, Nekolla SG, Hornke M, et al. Quantitative measurement of infarct size by contrast-enhanced magnetic resonance imaging early after acute myocardial infarction: comparison with single-photon emission tomography using Tc99m-sestamibi. J Am Coll Cardiol 2005;45:544–552.

54. Slomka PJ, Fieno D, Thomson L, et al. Automatic detection and size quantification of infarcts by myocardial perfusion SPECT: clinical validation by delayed-enhancement MRI. J Nucl Med 2005;46:728–735.

55. Klein C, Nekolla SG, Bengel FM, et al. Assessment of myocardial viability with contrast-enhanced magnetic resonance imaging: comparison with positron emission tomography. Circulation 2002;105:162–167.

56. Choi KM, Kim RJ, Gubernikoff G, Vargas JD, Parker M, Judd RM. Transmural extent of acute myocardial infarction predicts long-term improvement in contractile function. Circulation 2001;104:1101–1107.

57. Beek AM, Kuhl HP, Bondarenko O, et al. Delayed contrast-enhanced magnetic resonance imaging for the prediction of regional functional improvement after acute myocardial infarction. J Am Coll Cardiol 2003;42:895–901.

58. Ingkanisorn WP, Rhoads KL, Aletras AH, Kellman P, Arai AE. Gadolinium delayed enhancement cardiovascular magnetic resonance correlates with clinical measures of myocardial infarction. J Am Coll Cardiol 2004;43:2253–2259.

59. Baks T, van Geuns RJ, Duncker DJ, et al. Prediction of left ventricular function after drug-eluting stent implantation for chronic total coronary occlusions. J Am Coll Cardiol 2006;47:721–725.

60. Baks T, van Geuns RJ, Biagini E, et al. Recovery of left ventricular function after primary angioplasty for acute myocardial infarction. Eur Heart J 2005;26:1070–1077.
61. Ibrahim T, Nekolla SG, Hornke M, et al. Quantitative measurement of infarct size by contrast-enhanced magnetic resonance imaging early after acute myocardial infarction: comparison with single-photon emission tomography using Tc99m-sestamibi. J Am Coll Cardiol 2005;45:544–552.
62. Ingkanisorn WP, Rhoads KL, Aletras AH, Kellman P, Arai AE. Gadolinium delayed enhancement cardiovascular magnetic resonance correlates with clinical measures of myocardial infarction. J Am Coll Cardiol 2004;43:2253–2259.
63. Lund GK, Stork A, Saeed M, et al. Acute myocardial infarction: evaluation with first-pass enhancement and delayed enhancement MR imaging compared with 201T_1 SPECT imaging. Radiology 2004;232: 49–57.
64. Gerber BL, Garot J, Bluemke DA, Wu KC, Lima JA. Accuracy of contrast-enhanced magnetic resonance imaging in predicting improvement of regional myocardial function in patients after acute myocardial infarction. Circulation 2002;106:1083–1089.
65. Choi KM, Kim RJ, Gubernikoff G, Vargas JD, Parker M, Judd RM. Transmural extent of acute myocardial infarction predicts long-term improvement in contractile function. Circulation 2001;104: 1101–1107.
66. Ricciardi MJ, Wu E, Davidson CJ, et al. Visualization of discrete microinfarction after percutaneous coronary intervention associated with mild creatine kinase-MB elevation. Circulation 2001;103: 2780–2783.
67. Gerber BL, Belge B, Legros GJ, et al. Characterization of acute and chronic myocardial infarcts by multidetector computed tomography: comparison with contrast-enhanced magnetic resonance. Circulation 2006;113:823–833.
68. Selvanayagam JB, Porto I, Channon K, et al. Troponin elevation after percutaneous coronary intervention directly represents the extent of irreversible myocardial injury: insights from cardiovascular magnetic resonance imaging. Circulation 2005;111:1027–1032.
69. Hunold P, Schlosser T, Vogt FM, et al. Myocardial late enhancement in contrast-enhanced cardiac MRI: distinction between infarction scar and non-infarction-related disease. AJR Am J Roentgenol 2005;184:1420–1426.
70. Mahrholdt H, Wagner A, Judd RM, Sechtem U, Kim RJ. Delayed enhancement cardiovascular magnetic resonance assessment of non-ischaemic cardiomyopathies. Eur Heart J 2005;26:1461–1474.
71. Abdel-Aty H, Zagrosek A, Schulz-Menger J, et al. Delayed enhancement and T_2-weighted cardiovascular magnetic resonance imaging differentiate acute from chronic myocardial infarction. Circulation 2004;109:2411–2416.
72. Garcia-Dorado D, Oliveras J, Gili J, et al. Analysis of myocardial oedema by magnetic resonance imaging early after coronary artery occlusion with or without reperfusion. Cardiovasc Res 1993;27: 1462–1469.
73. Natanzon A, Aletras AH, Hsu LY, Arai AE. Determining canine myocardial area at risk with manganese-enhanced MR imaging. Radiology 2005;236:859–866.
74. Ni Y, Bormans G, Chen F, Verbruggen A, Marchal G. Necrosis avid contrast agents: functional similarity vs structural diversity. Invest Radiol 2005;40:526–535.
75. Pislaru SV, Ni Y, Pislaru C, et al. Noninvasive measurements of infarct size after thrombolysis with a necrosis-avid MRI contrast agent. Circulation 1999;99:690–696.
76. Cerqueira MD, Weissman NJ, Dilsizian V, et al. Standardized myocardial segmentation and nomenclature for tomographic imaging of the heart: a statement for healthcare professionals from the Cardiac Imaging Committee of the Council on Clinical Cardiology of the American Heart Association. Circulation 2002;105:539–542.
77. Amado LC, Gerber BL, Gupta SN, et al. Accurate and objective infarct sizing by contrast-enhanced magnetic resonance imaging in a canine myocardial infarction model. J Am Coll Cardiol 2004;44:2383–2389.
78. Hsu LY, Ingkanisorn WP, Kellman P, Aletras AH, Arai AE. Quantitative myocardial infarction on delayed enhancement MRI. Part II: clinical application of an automated feature analysis and combined thresholding infarct sizing algorithm. J Magn Reson Imaging 2006;23:309–314.
79. Amado LC, Gerber BL, Gupta SN, et al. Accurate and objective infarct sizing by contrast-enhanced magnetic resonance imaging in a canine myocardial infarction model. J Am Coll Cardiol 2004;44:2383–2389.

80. Kellman P, Arai AE, McVeigh ER, Aletras AH. Phase-sensitive inversion recovery for detecting myocardial infarction using gadolinium-delayed hyperenhancement. Magn Reson Med 2002;47: 372–383.
81. Gupta A, Lee VS, Chung YC, Babb JS, Simonetti OP. Myocardial infarction: optimization of inversion times at delayed contrast-enhanced MR imaging. Radiology 2004;233:921–926.
82. Kellman P, Dyke CK, Aletras AH, McVeigh ER, Arai AE. Artifact suppression in imaging of myocardial infarction using B_1-weighted phased-array combined phase-sensitive inversion recovery dagger. Magn Reson Med 2004;51:408–412.
83. Kellman P, Chung YC, Simonetti OP, McVeigh ER, Arai AE. Multi-contrast delayed enhancement provides improved contrast between myocardial infarction and blood pool. J Magn Reson Imaging 2005;22:605–613.

18 Nuclear Cardiology and CMR for the Assessment of Coronary Artery Disease

Timothy F. Christian

CONTENTS

The purpose of this chapter is not to produce a list of comparative studies between nuclear-based techniques and the cardiac magnetic resonance (MR) exam. These will change with time. It is rather to look at the two modalities in terms of physical principles and methods to determine where they differ, their degree of difference, where they are similar, and how they may be correlative. Nuclear imaging has had a long life within cardiology, and there is much magnetic resonance imaging (MRI) has to learn from it. It is a waste of resources to repeat the mistakes of the past. Consequently, practitioners of cardiovascular magnetic resonance imaging should have a foundation of the nuclear imaging past and present. The two modalities will certainly compete for the molecular imaging of the future.

LEFT VENTRICULAR FUNCTION

Radionuclide Ventriculography

Nuclear imaging pioneered the initial noninvasive measurement of ventricular function with radionuclide angiography. There are still advantages of this technique that should be considered. Determination of left ventricular ejection fraction (LVEF) is strictly count based, and gamma cameras excel at counting. Radionuclide ventriculography (RVG) acquires images of radioactively labeled red blood cells (RBC) by use of technetium 99m and tin; the latter is used as a reducing agent to allow entry of the Tc 99m into the RBC. Imaging the RBC volume is performed in a manner similar to MR imaging. The cardiac cycle is divided into 16 or 32 phases *(1)* with

From: *Contemporary Cardiology: Cardiovascular Magnetic Resonance Imaging*
Edited by: Raymond Y. Kwong © Humana Press Inc., Totowa, NJ

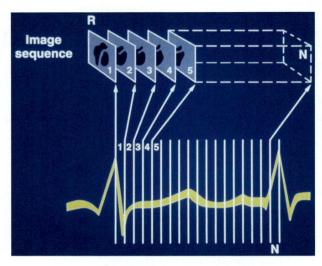

Fig. 1. Radionuclide ventriculography acquisition scheme. Like MRI, acquisition is gated to the R-wave of the electrocardiogram. Imaging continues until either preset times or preset photon counts are reached in each of three planar views. Temporal resolution is a function of the heart rate and the number of phases acquired (16–32 per R–R interval).

counts binned into each phase during acquisition, which is gated to the R-wave of the surface electrocardiogram (Fig. 1). Consequently,

$$\text{Temporal resolution} = \text{Heart rate/Number of phases}$$

and is generally on the order of 25–40 ms. This compares favorably with MRI cine methods. LVEF can be calculated by

$$\text{LVEF} = (\text{Diastolic counts} - \text{Systolic counts})/\text{Diastolic counts}$$

Another advantage of the method is that LVEF determination is far less dependent on myocardial edge detection. Because RVG is count based, the only manual manipulation is the drawing of a region of interest (ROI) that encompasses the LV. Images are generally not acquired tomographically, so the majority of the counts are centrally located (because the image is a two-dimensional display of a three-dimensional sphere). Errors on the edges of the image have less impact with a planar count-based approach. This contributes to the excellent reproducibility in comparison to other techniques *(2–9)* (Table 1).

Ventricular volumes are relative by this technique in contrast to MRI. Counts are translated to milliliters by obtaining a reference sample of blood from the patient, taping the tube to the gamma camera face, and counting the activity within it for a fixed period of time. End-systolic and end-diastolic volumes are obtained by

$$\text{Volume (mL)} = \text{ROI Counts in End-systole or}$$
$$\text{End-diastole/Counts per mL}$$
$$\text{in Reference sample} \qquad (1)$$

The problem with this method is that the in vivo counts are obtained through the interface of a chest wall (with resultant scatter and attenuation) and at a certain depth from the camera face; the reference tube counts are acquired through a glass tube at

Table 1
Reproducibility of Serial LVEF Determinations

Reference	Patients	Type	95% CI
RNA			
2	70	Normal	10
2	29	CHF	5
3	25	Post-MI	4
4	10	Normal	8
Echo			
5	19	Mixed	4
6	12	Normal	7–19
7	96	Mixed	5
MRI			
8	18	Normal	5
9	15	Normal	3.5
9	15	CHF	6

CI, confidence interval.

zero distance. For this reason, the volumes are only relative but highly reproducible in a specific patient as the chest wall barrier remains a constant.

There are disadvantages of the RVG method when compared to MR cine acquisitions. Most RVG exams are acquired in three planar acquisitions. Consequently, the technique is not tomographic. Regional wall motion is difficult to evaluate for this reason, and the technique is best used as a global measure of function. Some centers have explored tomographic RVG methods (10). With planar imaging, it is difficult to obtain uncontaminated views of individual chambers. This is particularly a problem for the right ventricle (RV), which limits its evaluation to subjective parameters. As with all conventional nuclear image methods, spatial resolution is low.

Despite the disadvantages, RVG has been shown to be a powerful prognosticator in patients with coronary artery disease. Most of the early work that established the link between LV function and outcome was established using the RVG (11,12). It has been coupled with supine bicycle exercise to provide both rest and stress LV function measures (possibly because of the reproducibility of the method) to risk stratify patients (13). With the advent of precutaneous coronary intervention (PCI) therapy, cardiac imaging became regional out of necessity. RVG did not have the spatial resolution to accommodate this need. It has fallen out of favor but remains an excellent tool for the assessment of global ventricular function.

With the advent of Tc 99m perfusion tracers for single photon emission computed tomographic (SPECT) studies (sestamibi, tetrofosmin), the radionuclide ventriculogram had some resurgence in the form of a first-pass study. The earliest assessments of LV function with radionuclide tracers were first-pass studies (14), and it remains an excellent technique to assess both ventricles for global function. This method does not provide the count statistics that an equilibrium red cell-labeled study does, but it has been shown to be accurate (15). It has the advantage of assessing the RV without contamination from other chambers (Fig. 2). Tc 99m perfusion tracers can be used to acquire a first-pass study if injected at a sufficient dose for the rest of the study (16). Regional wall motion assessment is not feasible, however.

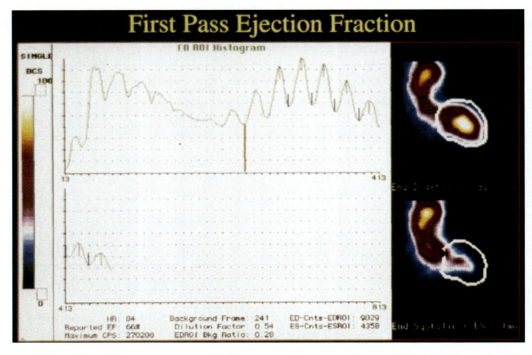

Fig. 2. First-pass Tc 99m sestamibi acquisition from a resting scan of a 2-days protocol (30 mCi injected). A multicrystal camera dedicated to first-pass imaging was used for this study. The time–activity curve is from a ventricular ROI, so the bolus can be seen to traverse the RV phase and LV phase separately. This allows for the measure of an uncontaminated RV ejection fraction.

Gated SPECT Functional Imaging

The Tc 99m-based perfusion scans have significantly higher count activity compared to those performed with Tl 201. This is because of higher photon energy of technetium combined with its shorter half-life (which allows for larger doses to be given). Because of the improved count statistics, gating of the image through the cardiac cycle became a possibility (17). For gating to provide a reliable assessment of ventricular volumes, each image that makes up the "cine" has to have adequate counts to generate a recognizable image for each phase of the cardiac cycle.

Most SPECT gated acquisitions divide the R–R interval into eight phases. Each phase has one-eighth the count statistics of an ungated image acquired for the same length of time. For thallium 201, this is perhaps too little activity to obtain reliable frames. The temporal resolution of gated SPECT floats with the R–R interval:

Temporal resolution = Heart rate/No. of Phases

More phases could be acquired through the cardiac cycle, but acquisition time would have to be prolonged to maintain adequate counts. This increases the potential for patient motion and subsequent artifacts. For a heart rate of 72 beats per minute, the temporal resolution for gated SPECT at eight phases is 104 ms. The spatial resolution is between 1 and 1.5 cm. This compares rather unfavorably to MRI cine imaging (Fig. 3).

The switch to a 1-day protocol for perfusion imaging with Tc 99m-based perfusion tracers had two effects on the assessment of LV function during a radionuclide perfusion

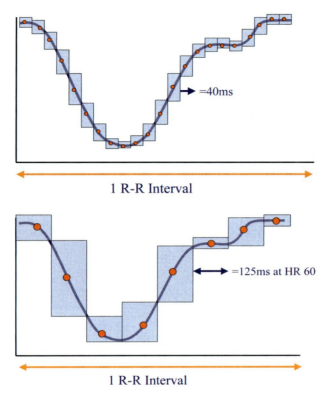

Fig. 3. Comparison of temporal resolution between steady-state free precession MRI (above) and gated SPECT (below). An LV filling curve across one R–R interval is shown for each technique. The superimposed rectangles represent the number of cardiac phases acquired for each technique (30 for MRI and 8 for gated SPECT). The width of the rectangle is the temporal resolution. The height of the rectangle reflects the degree of change in the LV filling curve that occurs during each specific phase. This is a measure of the motion that is averaged into each frame of the acquisition. Note that it is not possible to capture true end-systole by gated SPECT.

scan. First-pass studies became less feasible, and gated SPECT had to be done off the poststress acquisition instead of a pure rest determination. The first Tc 99m sestamibi image acquisition contaminates the second acquisition when performed in a time-frame significantly less than four half-lives (most protocols only pause 30–60 minutes between the rest and the stress acquisition). To minimize crosstalk, the first study must be acquired with a much lower radioactivity dose than the second study.

For a variety of reasons, it is best to do the rest scan first (18). Because it is difficult to do a first-pass acquisition during stress with a gamma camera, it must be acquired at rest. Unfortunately, the rest study is usually the low-dose study, which diminishes the accuracy of the first-pass study. Consequently, most assessment of LV function by Tc 99m perfusion imaging is a 30-minute poststress gated perfusion image.

The poststress acquisition of LV function is a hybrid between resting function and stress function. In the absence of pathology, this has few consequences. However, in the presence of ischemia, resting LV function is underestimated because of postischemic dysfunction (19). Although this may be useful information, the majority

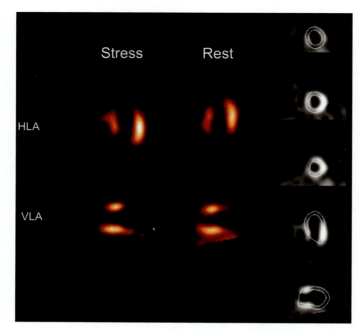

Fig. 4. A Tc 99m-gated SPECT study from a patient with a large prior infarction. There is cavity dilation and distortion poststress that is not evident on the rest image. The gated LVEF edge detection algorithm (third column of images) is applied to the poststress images because of the more favorable count statistics. Two points are illustrated: (1) The LVEF determination is likely going to be lower on the poststress image in the setting of significant ischemia. (2) Edge detection is going to be a problem for both sets of images because of the large areas devoid of counts from infarction.

of the prognostic information regarding LV function is based on resting function *(12)*. The presence of regional wall dysfunction may help detect this phenomenon, but there is no true rest scan to gauge whether the regional wall motion (RWM) is chronic or acute.

The impact of ischemia on ventricular geometry for calculation of LVEF is shown in Fig. 4. MRI can be equally affected if stress perfusion imaging is performed prior to LV function acquisitions, but the majority of stress studies currently involve vasodilation, which is less likely to cause ventricular stunning. The net effect is an overall slight underestimation of true LVEF, although this can be variable within individual patients *(25)*.

The correlation of SPECT and positron emission tomographic (PET) gated LV function with MRI-based measures is surprisingly good given the limited spatial and temporal resolution *(20–24)*. The underestimation of true LVEF because of the use of only eight cardiac phases by SPECT is well documented *(26,27)*. LV volumes can be underestimated when the LV cavity size is small. This is caused by the effects of photon scatter "filling in" the small cavity secondary to the close proximity of the ventricular walls to the center. This is particular problematic for end-systolic images in women *(27)*, with a resultant overestimation in LVEF (Fig. 5).

The spatial resolution issue is less clear. Figure 6 may help demonstrate why gated SPECT functions fairly well despite its physical limitations. This is an MRI steady-state free precession still frame at the acquisition matrix ($1.3 \times 1.3 \times 8$ mm) on the left and the same image displayed with a spatial resolution of 1 cm^3 (similar to the spatial

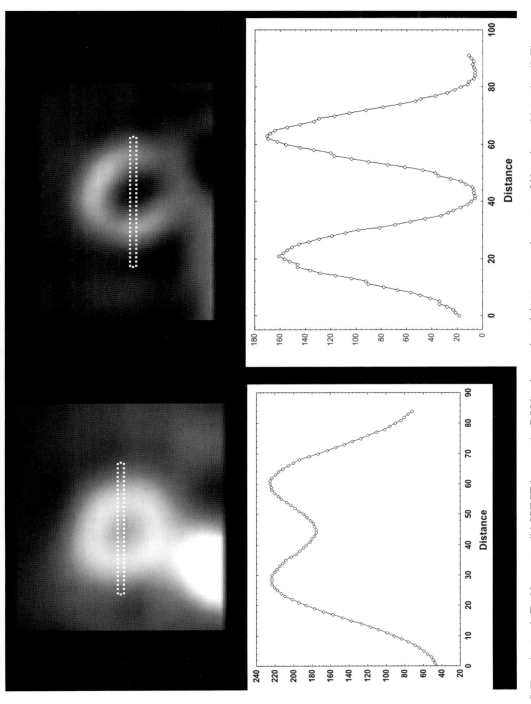

Fig. 5. Two short-axis Tc 99m sestamibi SPECT images. An ROI has been selected that traverses the septum, LV cavity, and lateral wall. The mean count profile under this linear area is plotted for each image. Note with the smaller cavity size (left) that the LV cavity is significantly "filled in." This translates to artifactually smaller LV cavity size from photon scatter to the more closely approximated LV walls. For larger ventricles (right), this is less of an issue.

383

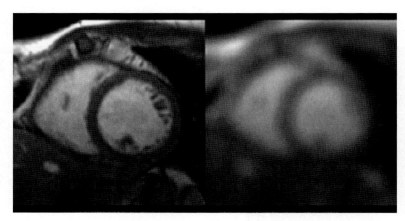

1.3x1.3mm res.   1cm res.

Fig. 6. A short-axis slice from a steady-state free precession MRI acquired with a matrix of 1.3 × 1.3 × 8 mm (left). The same image (right) has been reprocessed and filtered to a spatial resolution of 10 × 10 × 8 mm resolution. Despite the low resolution, edge detection is probably not significantly impacted for the calculation of LV volumes. The case is somewhat understated because cardiac motion and photon scatter are not accounted for in this hypothetical example.

resolution of SPECT). Although cardiac motion is not accounted for in this hypothetical figure, it does demonstrate that, despite the loss of detail, the myocardial wall edges are still discernable. It is not hard to imagine that an edge detection algorithm would function fairly well on such an image.

The incorporation of gated LV function within the SPECT acquisition has proven to be of dual benefit for SPECT imaging. Gating helps to determine the significance of perfusion defects—particularly those that are "fixed" by examining the regional wall motion—and it can stand alone as an assessment of global LV function. Although it may not be as pretty as an MR cine acquisition, it gets the job done and is prognostically significant *(28)*.

PERFUSION

SPECT perfusion tracers combined with exercise or pharmacological vasodilation remain the standard of care for assessing the myocardial circulation noninvasively. Advances in camera technology from the initial planar images have allowed the assessment of regional perfusion abnormalities. The two common tracers employed today are thallium–201 and Tc–99m sestamibi.

Thallium 201

Thalium 201 belongs to the same atomic family as potassium and is handled by the myocardial cell in the same manner as the K^+ ion. The main entry for Tl 201 is through Na/K^+ pump within the cell membrane. Consequently, it requires intact cellular integrity plus adenosine triphosphate. This allows the presence of uptake to confer cellular viability. Uptake is in proportion to blood flow up to about 2.5–3.0 mL/minute/g tissue *(29)*, beyond which uptake plateaus and becomes nonlinear with myocardial blood flow.

Thallium 201 is in equilibrium with the blood pool and will distribute according to this gradient. A single injection during stress can be used to acquire both the stress and rest perfusion images. Areas of hypoperfusion at rest appear to "redistribute" over time if the tissue is viable. This simply reflects a steeper concentration gradient out of the cell toward the blood pool in normal myocardium as the concentration of Tl 201 declines in the blood pool. Ischemic tissue has less Tl 201 to start and therefore less of a gradient over the blood pool. This results in decreased washout in relatively hypoperfused territories.

Thallium 201 is easily combined with stress testing, with acquisitions occurring 5–15 minutes from tracer injection. An early anterior planar view is valuable in determining lung uptake of the tracer. This has correlated fairly well with LVEDP *(30)*. Tomographic acquisition follows on completion of the anterior planar view. Thallium 201 has performed well clinically *(31)* in detecting coronary artery disease with an overall sensitivity of 90% and a specificity of 70% (pooled data). However, publication bias and verification bias need to be kept in mind when considering such studies. Results have been similar with either exercise stress or vasodilator stress.

Tc 99m Sestamibi

The Tc 99m-based tracers have two physical advantages over Tl 201: photon energy and half-life. The kilo electron volts of the Tc 99m photon is approximately double (140 keV) that of Tl 201. This markedly reduces photon attenuation and photon scatter, the two biggest issues with nuclear imaging. The half-life of 6 hours means a larger dose (usually tenfold higher) can be given to a patient without increasing the biological radiation exposure compared to Tl 201. Consequently, more photons are produced, with more of them reaching the camera face from their true source. The disadvantage is that the physiological equilibrium with the blood pool is lost, so separate rest and stress injections must be given, with some inevitable contamination of the second image from the first if given on the same day. Some centers avoid this issue by using Tl 201 rest imaging followed by Tc 99m stress imaging. The different physical properties of the tracers can make interpretation difficult, and there is still some crosstalk for the second acquisition. A Tc 99m sestamibi-gated SPECT example of a patient with ischemia and infarction within the same territory is shown in Fig. 7.

Both Tl 201 and Tc 99m sestamibi are relatively static perfusion tracers (Fig. 8). This has large impact. It means that imaging can be delayed until exercise is complete. The ability to perform exercise testing on patients with and without interpretable electrocardiograms provides a strong set of prognostic variables that have withstood the test of time *(32,33)*. MR currently has no static perfusion tracer, although preliminary work with manganese compounds has potential *(34,35)*.

When designing perfusion tracers, the key element is the linearity of the signal emitted in proportion to myocardial blood flow, which is impacted by the kinetics of uptake from the blood pool into the myocardium. Both Tl 201 and Tc 99m sestamibi have linear uptake with myocardial blood flow (MBF) up to flow rates of 2.5–3.0 mL/minute/g tissue *(29,36)*. The extraction efficiency of both tracers is high (about 92–95% of available tracer is extracted under rest conditions during the first pass through the myocardium). Consequently, signal intensity can be relied on as an accurate indicator of MBF under most flow rates encountered clinically except the upper levels of hyperemia.

Gadolinium-diethyltriaminepentaacetic acid uptake is a complex and not well understood phenomenon. Myocardial enhancement is the sum of the relaxed blood volume entering the vasculature and passing through as an intravascular tracer and the proportion of contrast that enters the interstitial space and is transiently retained. It is not wholly intravascular or efficiently extracted and retained by the

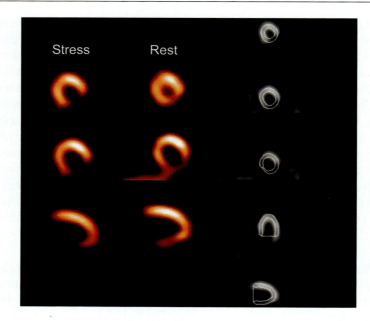

Fig. 7. A patient with ischemia and infarction in the inferolateral wall with known left circumflex artery disease. There is still abnormal but improved uptake of Tc 99m sestamibi on the rest as compared to the stress images. This likely coincides with subendocardial infarction in this territory with superimposed stress-induced ischemia. Consequently, sestamibi functions as both a perfusion and viability tracer simultaneously.

- *Static*
  - –Tracers stick and stay allowing delayed imaging-temporal resolution unimportant
  - –Imaging is static in nature
  - –Absolute MBF not possible w/o 100% extraction of tracer
- *Dynamic*
  - –Tracer does not stick anywhere so imaging has to coincide with injection during stress
  - –Imaging is dynamic in nature
  - –Temporal resolution (speed) important
  - –Absolute quantification difficult w/o 100% intravascular retention.

Fig. 8. The major differences between SPECT and MRI perfusion imaging.

myocardium. Further, the proportion of tracer that enters the myocardial interstitial space likely changes in relation to flow rate; low flow generates a higher proportion of contrast to enter the interstium, and high flow produces more of an intravascular effect *(37)* (see Fig. 9). Linearity between myocardial blood flow and raw signal intensity under these conditions is unlikely.

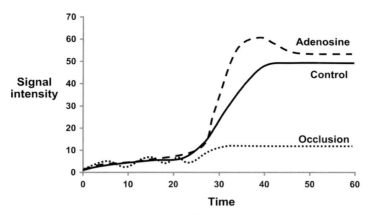

Fig. 9. MR perfusion time intensity curves obtained in an animal model of regional coronary occlusion or adenosine infusion *(37)*. Control zone curves are shown as well. Note that there is little additional signal enhancement with increasing MBF rates (adenosine zone MBF mean 2.3 mL/m/g) but the shape of the time intensity curve (TIC) changes and resembles more of an intravascular agent with an upslope, peak, and downslope.

Table 2
Clinical MRI Perfusion Studies: Comparison With Coronary Angiography

Reference	n	Sensitivity (%)	Specificity (%)	Accuracy (%)
40	84	88	90	89
41	25	86	84	85
42	30	93	60	—
43	34	90	83	87

For this reason, various modeling algorithms have been used to quantify MBF *(37–39)*. Simply measuring the magnitude of signal intensity increase only provides a rough estimate of MBF. To perform at a level comparable to the SPECT tracers, MR must develop a tracer such as sestamibi, which is efficiently extracted in proportion to MBF and retained in the myocardium, allowing stress outside the magnet. Early clinical studies using pharmacological stress have shown promising results using coronary angiography as the gold standard *(40–43)* despite these limitations (Table 2).

Determination of absolute MBF in milliliters per minute per gram of myocardium is possible by both PET and MRI techniques but not by SPECT. SPECT has too much photon attenuation and scatter to accurately relate tracer concentration in the myocardium to the signal intensity registered by the gamma camera. PET has the ability to measure MBF in quantitative terms because it is not hindered by compartment models (water is the only freely diffusible substance within the myocardium), and the high-energy dual photons reduce the impact of attenuation. Coincidence detection markedly reduces the issue of photon scatter.

The arterial input function is a bit of an issue because of the relatively low spatial resolution and the possibility of contamination from the LV myocardial wall. Generally, the myocardial response is related mathematically to the washout slope of the arterial input curve. A dynamic PET O15 water acquisition is shown in Fig. 10. Note the

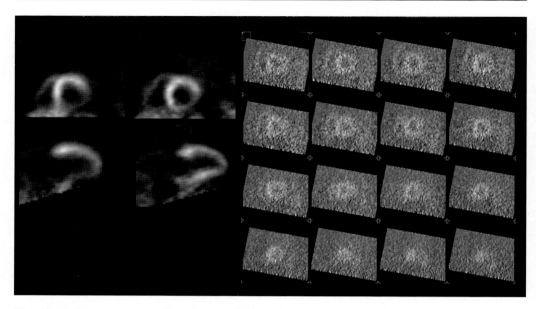

Fig. 10. Multiple short-axis slices from an O15 perfusion study during the myocardial enhancement phase. Although kinetic modeling is extremely favorable for this technique, physical characteristics are challenging.

overall poor resolution of the method, which detracts from its otherwise attractive kinetics. These images can be summed, however, to provide a more count-rich image for ROI determinations.

Despite the mentioned issues in the kinetics of Gd-diethyltriaminepentaacetic acid, estimation of absolute MBF is possible because of the exceptional physical imaging properties of MRI. As long as Gd concentration within the blood pool proximal to the coronary arteries does not become nonlinear with signal intensity from T_2* effects, the arterial input function curve can be clearly generated. The response (enhancement) of the myocardium can be quantified (37–39) in discrete segments of tissue (1–2 g). Whether these methods can be translated to clinical practice remains to be determined. An example of a first-pass MR quantitative perfusion acquisition is shown in Fig. 11.

VIABILITY

There are four methods in which nuclear imaging can be used to infer myocardial viability. These are tomographic wall motion, uptake imaging with Tl 201, uptake imaging with Tc 99m sestamibi, and static or dynamic uptake imaging with 18-fluorodeoxyglucose. Because wall motion has been discussed in this chapter, the focus is on the last three tracers.

A word must be said about the concept of viability. *Viability* means a cell or a territory of cells are alive. It does not mean that revascularization of viable tissue automatically confers an improvement in regional function (*see* Fig. 12). All reversible LV dysfunction must occur in viable tissue but not all viable tissue has the potential for reversible contractile dysfunction. Infarcts where there has been vessel recanalization and preserved subepicardial tissue will not improve further if there is not an element of severe ischemia producing hibernation or repetitive

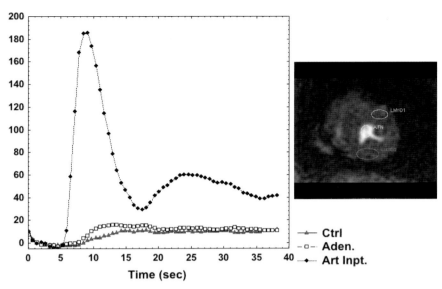

Fig. 11. MRI time intensity curves obtained from an animal model of regional hyperemia (adenosine infused down the left anterior descending [LAD] artery). The saturation recovery images were acquired every R-R interval. The LV blood pool provides the arterial input function; [Gd] = 0.025 mmol/kg. A control zone (CTRL) and an adenosine zone (aden.) are time intensity curves from two myocardial ROIs. Absolute flow is quantified by deconvolution of the arterial input function with the TIC, usually through a gamma variate fit using a filter function. Linearity of Gd concentration with signal intensity for the arterial input function is critical to the accuracy of the calculation. Note on this scale that there is little difference between the two myocardial ROI curves.

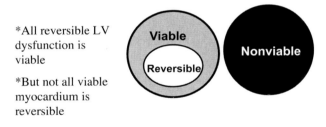

Fig. 12. The paradox of viability testing. All segments that demonstrate reversible contractile function are viable, but it does not follow that all viable segments will improve contractility with revascularization. Tests aimed solely at reversible LV dysfunction as the definition of viability will underestimate viability.

stunning. Also, cardiomyopathies are viable but will not improve with revascularization. A combination of resting ischemia and preserved viability is required for reversible LV dysfunction in most cases.

Thallium 201

Thallium 201 is inherently a viability tracer because of its dependence on the Na/K$^+$ pump and membrane integrity for uptake and equilibrium with the blood pool. Rest

Table 3
Noninvasive Test Performance for the Prediction of Reversible LV Dysfunction

Technique	+ Predictive value (%)	− Predictive value (%)	No. studies/patients
Stress Tl 201 (44)	76	59	14/420
Rest Tl 201 (44)	78	68	8/166
Reinjection Tl 210 (44)	83	80	5/82
18-FDG (PET) (44)	80	82	9/217
Delayed-enhancement cardiovascular MRI (45)	83	79	1/50
Dobutamine MRI (46,47)	81	57	2/43

imaging is preferred for viability assessment as the high-stress flows in the setting of ischemic heart disease only serve to widen the gradient gap between low-flow and high-flow territories. Uptake of Tl 201 is all that is required to confer some degree of viability.

A number of studies have examined the ability of Tl 201 to predict improvement in LV function following revascularization (*see* Table 3). Resting thallium has performed reasonably in this regard in comparison to other techniques (*44–47*). Clearly, below 50% of maximal activity, tissue is nonviable by this technique, but there is stepwise correlation with 18-fluorodeoxyglucose (18-FDG) uptake at higher values (*48*). When uptake is normal at rest, no further imaging is required. However, for persistent moderate and severe defects, delayed images are obtained at 4 hours and again at 24 hours if necessary. Occasionally, severe defects will show redistribution at 24 hours (*49*). However, the potential prolonged nature of the exam has been a disadvantage for rest thallium 201.

Tc 99m Sestamibi

Tc 99m sestamibi, like Tl 201, is both a viability agent and a flow tracer. Unlike Tl 201, however, it is not in equilibrium with the blood pool. It is trapped within mitochondria through a large electrostatic charge. In this manner, it functions more like a microsphere in that it sticks to a viable mitochondria and does not redistribute (*50*). This is fine as long as blood flow to the area in question is adequate. However, in low-flow states (which are possible with myocardial hibernation), the tracer will not be delivered in adequate amounts to assess viability. For this reason, sestamibi is a good indicator of viability when uptake is high, but all bets are off when the uptake is low (*51*).

18-Fluorodeoxyglucose

The natural substrate for cardiac metabolism is free fatty acids. Glucose is reserved for anaerobic metabolism. Imaging with 18-FDG is the gold standard for myocardial viability and can be accomplished using one of two strategies. The first method is to force glucose into the myocyte using insulin because glucose is not normally a part substrate for the myocardium. The 18-FDG molecule is metabolized in one step in the myocardial cell and then trapped as the deoxy portion of the molecule prevents further substrate utilization. Initial entry of 18-FDG into the myocyte can be accomplished using boluses of insulin and glucose, or as a constant infusion of both substances to maintain a steady uptake of glucose (insulin/glucose clamp). The advantage of this approach is that the entire myocardium is well visualized by high-count statistics and the abundance of high-energy dual 511-keV photons. The disadvantage is that selective

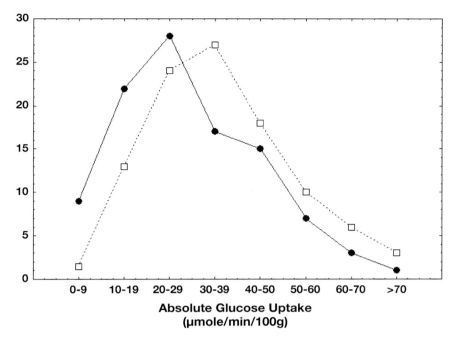

Fig. 13. Absolute 18-FDG uptake in patients with normal and dysfunctional (hypocontractile) segments from six European centers using a standardized insulin/glucose clamp technique *(37)*. The significant overlap of glucose utilization between the two segment types suggests that absolute values are not discriminative, and that normalized values for each patient should be used.

metabolic information may be lost. Imaging generally occurs after injection of the tracer, and relative concentrations of 18-FDG are displayed.

To provide more quantitative information on myocardial glucose utilization, investigators have performed dynamic 18-FDG scans by which the absolute myocardial utilization can be calculated with the aid of the arterial input function. This approach requires the patient to be in the scanner during the injection so that an arterial input function can be measured. An image of cellular metabolism is created, which is an attractive goal. Unfortunately, the separation of normal myocardium from myocardium with contractile dysfunction has not been clean (Fig. 13). There is considerable overlap of glucose utilization in normally contracting regions and dysfunctional regions *(52)*.

Because perfusion tracers are often part of a PET examination, the presence of ischemic tissue can be inferred from a resting perfusion defect combined with preserved 18-FDG uptake with an insulin-aided acquisition (Fig. 14). Despite the advantages in metabolic information, physical characteristics, and long experience, the performance of 18-FDG for predicting reversible LV dysfunction has not been superior to other, less-costly methods (*see* Table 3).

MAGNETIC RESONANCE IMAGING

Delayed-enhancement imaging by MRI has several advantages over the PET and SPECT methods. The two biggest are the improved resolution properties of the MR image and the ability to measure a positive image rather than a negative image (measuring what you cannot see). The advantages of spatial resolution are obvious and form

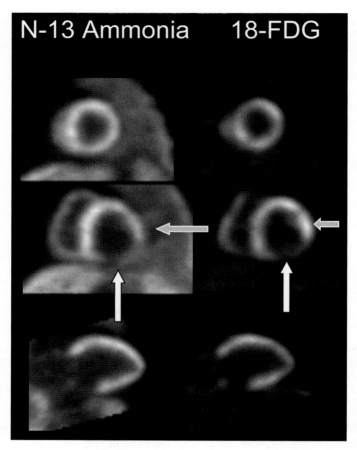

Fig. 14. An example of a combined N 13 ammonia scan (for perfusion, left) followed by an 18-FDG scan (for viability, right). The arrows show a matched defect (white arrow) and an area of mismatch: hypoperfusion and enhanced 18-FDG uptake (grey arrow). The coexistence of normal, infracted, and potentially hibernating tissue is often the case with patients with severe ischemic heart disease. The challenge is to gage the potential for benefit with revascularization within this mix.

the basis of prediction by MRI. The ability to resolve subendocardial infarction from transmural infarction is a key attribute of MRI. This is important as the lateral edges (extent) of an infarct are established early in the course *(53)*.

It is the degree of progression from subendocardium to subepicardium with time, which determines the impact of the infarct clinically. Only MRI can resolve this. There is a correlation, however, between the degree of transmurality of an infarct and the reduction in uptake activity on PET or SPECT from maximal activity *(54,55)*. Consequently, infarcts producing a reduction in counts below 50% of maximum are likely transmural, whereas reductions in the 70% range are likely only 50% through the wall by MRI (Fig. 15). There are a multitude of studies comparing SPECT or PET with viability imaging by delayed-enhancement MRI, with fairly comparable results *(56–59)*. Some are shown in Table 4.

The ability to quantify infarct size is possible with both SPECT and delayed-enhancementE MRI. Physical properties again favor MRI, however. The spatial resolution and ability to quantify a positive image produce temporal reproducibility infarct values

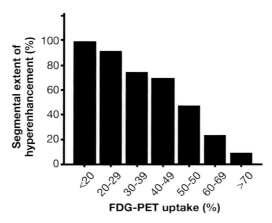

Fig. 15. 18-FDG uptake as a function of the degree of transmurality derived from delayed-enhancement MRI *(39)*. PET lacks the resolution to accurately quantify the degree of subendocardial infarction, but the information can be extrapolated from the relative reduction in counts in the infarct territory.

Table 4
Comparison of Infarct Size Measures Between Nuclear and MRI Methods

Reference	Methods	n	Difference 95% CI	Correlation measures	Missed infarcts
56	Tc 99m Sestamibi SPECT, DE MRI	33	±3%	R = 0.86	–
57	Tl 201 SPECT DE MRI	60	±9.8%	R = 0.73	20%
58	18-FDG SPECT, DE MRI	31	–	R = 0.91	11%
59	Tl 201 SPECT, DE MRI	38	–	R = 0.84	13%

CI, confidence interval; DE, delayed enhancement.

of 2.5% of the myocardial mass by MRI in both acute and chronic infarctions *(60,61)*. SPECT has reported reproducibility values of 6%, but these were acquired in a static phantom simply imaged twice rather than in vivo on separate days *(62)*. The sharp delineation of the edges of the infarct contributes to the reproducibility of the technique (Fig. 16). Viability imaging is about separating tissues. Consequently, a threshold must be selected based on some aspect of the image that reflects viability. Usually, this is a function of the signal intensity that a tracer generates (either positively or negatively) based on its distribution within the myocardium: the sharper the borders, the cleaner the cut.

Tc 99m sestamibi imaging has been used effectively in the past for infarct sizing *(63)*. Because of the lower resolution of SPECT image acquisition and the associated photon scatter, even in a severely transmural defect like the one shown *(64)*, the borders between viable and necrotic myocardium are sloped (Fig. 16). Because such thresholds are usually taken as a percentage of the maximal myocardial activity, they are subject to some variability by threshold choice and normalization zone. The depth at which a threshold is placed will alter the infarct size measure. MR viability imaging is a scatter-free high-resolution technique and is therefore relatively independent of the threshold value. With such sharp interfaces, reproducibility is not impacted by physical parameters. Automated quantitation programs may further improve consistency. However, most inexperienced observers could consistently trace an MR-derived infarct volume from Fig. 16.

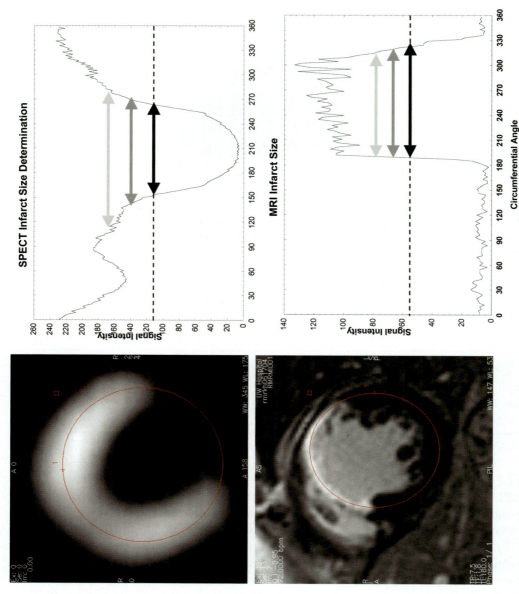

Fig. 16. Two short-axis midventricular images from separate patients who have suffered transmural myocardial infarction. The top row is data from a patient with inferolateral infarction (arrows) demonstrated by SPECT imaging with Tc 99m sestamibi, and the bottom row is a patient with anterior infarction demonstrated by MRI delayed-hyperenhanced imaging using an inversion recovery gradient sequence following gadolinium administration. The graphs on the right side represent a circumferential intensity profile from each image. The signal intensity along the thin circular ROI is plotted as a function of angle location. Note the inverted wavelike shape of the SPECT curve as compared to the delta-function-like appearance of the MR curve when the infarct is encountered. The shaded arrows represent 70% (light gray), 60% (dark gray), and 50% (black) threshold values of signal intensity for infarct size measurements (arrow width). There is more potential variability for SPECT determinations.

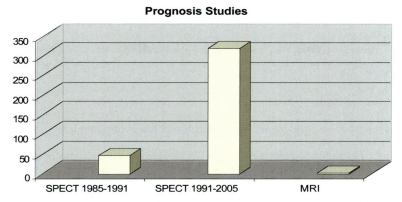

Fig. 17. Literature search for studies that have examined the prognostic capability for predicting event-free survival by modality. Note that it took a number of years before the prognostic literature for SPECT imaging to bloom.

A natural consequence of the physical differences between SPECT and MRI is the discrepancy in detecting small infarcts. Because the spatial resolution of SPECT is greater than the thickness of a normal myocardial wall, small, subendocardial defects are averaged with normal myocardium. This is termed a *partial volume effect*. A subendocardial defect by SPECT will produce a drop in signal (*see* Fig. 10), but it may not be enough to reach whatever threshold has been chosen to define pathology. This has been clearly documented in the literature *(65)*.

FUTURE DIRECTIONS

Figure 17 quantifies the prognostic literature for both nuclear imaging and SPECT in ischemic heart disease. MRI has a long way to go in this regard. Ultimately, it is the prognostication of a test that gives it clinical value. This will surely come for MRI for viability. The case is not so clear for perfusion imaging, for which exercise capacity is eliminated from the equation. Much work needs to be done in this field from both a contrast agent perspective and a prognosis perspective to be competitive with SPECT imaging. There is little doubt that MRI is now the gold standard for LV function measurement despite the lack of prognostic studies for this modality. The reproducibility of these measures is high and better than any other modality at present.

These two modalities will continue to cross paths in the future. This is most prone to occur in the field of molecular imaging. MRI clearly has the upper hand for imaging small events but lacks the biological coupling present for the PET and SPECT tracers. The field of MR should begin to turn efforts in the direction of biological tracer development.

REFERENCES

1. Clements IP, Brown ML, Smith HC. Radionuclide measurement of left ventricular volume. Mayo Clin Proc 1981;56:733–739.
2. Wackers FJ, Berger HJ, Johnstone DE, et al. Multiple gated cardiac blood pool imaging for left ventricular ejection fraction: validation of the technique and assessment of variability. Am J Cardiol 1979;43:1159–1166.

3. Slutsky R, Karliner J, Battler A, Pfisterer M, Swanson S, Ashburn W. Reproducibility of ejection fraction and ventricular volume by gated radionuclide angiography after myocardial infarction. Radiology 1979;132:155–159.
4. Upton MT, Palmeri ST, Jones RH, Coleman RE, Cobb FR. Assessment of left ventricular function by resting and exercise radionuclide angiocardiography following acute myocardial infarction. Am Heart J 1982;104:1232–1243.
5. Oberman A, Fan PH, Nanda NC, et al. Reproducibility of two-dimensional exercise echocardiography. J Am Coll Cardiol 1989;14:923–928.
6. Otterstad JE, Froeland G, St John Sutton M, Holme I. Accuracy and reproducibility of biplane two-dimensional echocardiographic measurements of left ventricular dimensions and function. Eur Heart J 1997;18:507–513.
7. Gottdiener JS, Livengood SV, Meyer PS, Chase GA. Should echocardiography be performed to assess effects of antihypertensive therapy? Test-retest reliability of echocardiography for measurement of left ventricular mass and function. J Am Coll Cardiol 1995;25:424–430.
8. Benjelloun H, Cranney GB, Kirk KA, Blackwell GG, Lotan CS, Pohost GM. Interstudy reproducibility of biplane cine nuclear magnetic resonance measurements of left ventricular function. Am J Cardiol 1991;67:1413–1420.
9. Grothues F, Smith GC, Moon JC, et al. Comparison of interstudy reproducibility of cardiovascular magnetic resonance with two-dimensional echocardiography in normal subjects and in patients with heart failure or left ventricular hypertrophy. Am J Cardiol 2002;90:29–34.
10. Sanchez-Ortiz GI, Wright GJ, Clarke N, Declerck J, Banning AP, Noble JA. Automated 3-D echocardiography analysis compared with manual delineations and SPECT MUGA. IEEE Trans Med Imaging 2002;21:1069–1076.
11. Miller TD, Taliercio CP, Zinsmeister AR, Gibbons RJ. Risk stratification of single or double vessel coronary artery disease and impaired left ventricular function using exercise radionuclide angiography. Am J Cardiol 1990;65:1317–1321.
12. White HD, Norris, RM, Brown MA, Brandt PW, Whitlock M. Wild CJ. Left ventricular end-systolic volume as the major determinant of survival after recovery from myocardial infarction. Circulation 1978;76:44–51.
13. Gibbons RJ, Zinsmeister AR, Miller TD, Clements IP. Supine exercise electrocardiography compared with exercise radionuclide angiography in noninvasive identification of severe coronary artery disease. Ann Intern Med 1990;112:743–749.
14. Port S, Cobb FR, Coleman RE, Jones RH. Effect of age on the response of the left ventricular ejection fraction to exercise. N Engl J Med 1980;303:1133–1137.
15. Olvey SK, Reduto LA, Stevens PM, Deaton WJ, Miller RR. First pass radionuclide assessment of right and left ventricular ejection fraction in chronic pulmonary disease. Effect of oxygen upon exercise response. Chest 1980;78:4–9.
16. Chareonthaitawee P, Christian TF, Miller TD, Hodge, DO, Gibbons RJ. The correlation of resting first pass left ventricular ejection fraction with resting infarct size: is ventricular function assessment always necessary? Am J Cardiol 1998;81:1281–1285.
17. Chua T, Kiat H, Germano G, et al. Gated technetium-99m sestamibi for simultaneous assessment of stress myocardial perfusion, postexercise regional ventricular function and myocardial viability. Correlation with echocardiography and rest thallium-201 scintigraphy. J Am Coll Cardiol 1994;23: 1107–1114.
18. Taillefer R, Primeau M, Costi P, Lambert R, Leveille J, Latour Y. Technetium-99m-sestamibi myocardial perfusion imaging in detection of coronary artery disease: comparison between initial (1-hour) and delayed (3-hours) postexercise images. J Nucl Med 1991;32:1961–1965.
19. Johnson LL, Verdesca SA, Aude WY, et al. Postischemic stunning can affect left ventricular ejection fraction and regional wall motion on post-stress gated sestamibi tomograms. J Am Coll Cardiol 1997;30:1641–1648.
20. Germano G, Kiat H, Kavanagh PB, et al. Recovery of regional left ventricular dysfunction from gated myocardial perfusion SPECT. J Nucl Med 1995;36:2138–2147.
21. Schaefer WM, Lipke CSA, Nowak B, et al. Validation of QGS and 4D-MSPECT for quantification of left ventricular volumes and ejection fraction from gated ^{18}F-FDG PET: comparison with cardiac MRI. J Nucl Med 2004;45:74–79.
22. Iskandrian AE, Germano G, VanDecker E, et al. Validation of left ventricular volume measurement by gated SPECT ^{99m}Tc-labeled sestamibi imaging. J Nucl Cardiol 1998;5:574–578.

23. Ioannidis JP, Trikalinos TA, Danias PG. Electocardiogram-gated single-photon emission computed tomography vs cardiac magnetic resonance imaging for the assessment of left ventricular volumes and ejection fraction: a meta-analysis. J Am Coll Cardiol 2002;39:2059–2068.

24. Rajappan K, Livieratos L, Camici PG, Pennell DJ. Measurement of ventricular volumes and function: a comparison of gated PET and cardiovascular magnetic resonance. J Nucl Med 2002;43:806–810.

25. Manrique A, Faraggi M, Vera P, et al. ^{201}Tl and ^{99m}Tc-MIBI gated SPECT in patients with large perfusion defects and left ventricular dysfunction: comparison with equilibrium radionuclide angiography. J Nucl Med 1999;40:805–809.

26. Persson E, Carlsson M, Palmer J, Pahlm O, Arheden H. Evaluation of left ventricular volumes and ejection fraction by automated gated myocardial SPECT vs cardiovascular magnetic resonance. Clin Physiol Funct Imaging 2005;25:135–141.

27. Kane GC, Hauser MF, Behrenbeck T, Miller TD, Gibbons RJ, Christian TF. The impact of gender on Tc-99m sestamibi gated left ventricular ejection fraction. Am J Cardiol 2002;89:1238–1241.

28. Travin MI, Heller GV, Johnson LL, et al. The prognostic value of ECG-gated SPECT imaging in patients undergoing stress Tc-99m sestamibi myocardial perfusion imaging. J Nucl Cardiol 2004;11:253–262.

29. Leppo JA, Okada RD, Strauss HW, Pohost GM. Effect of hyperaemia on thallium-201 redistribution in normal canine myocardium. Cardiovasc Res 1985;19:679–685.

30. Kushner FG, Okada RD, Kirshenbaum HD, Boucher CA, Strauss HW, Pohost GM. Lung thallium-201 uptake after stress testing in patients with coronary artery disease. Circulation 1981;63:341–347.

31. Mahmarian JJ. State of the art for coronary disease detection: thallium-201. In Zaret BL, Beller GA, eds. Nuclear cardiology: state of the art and future directions. St. Louis, MO: Mosby; 1999:237–272.

32. Kwok JM, Miller TD, Christian TF, Hodge DO, Gibbons RJ. Prognostic value of a treadmill exercise score in symptomatic patients with nonspecific ST-T abnormalities on resting ECG. JAMA 1999; 282:1047–1053.

33. Mark DB, Shaw L, Harrell FE Jr, et al. Prognostic value of a treadmill exercise score in outpatients with suspected coronary artery disease. N Engl J Med 1991;325:849–853.

34. Hu TC, Christian TF, Aletras AH, Taylor JL, Korestsky AP, Arai AE. Maganese enhanced MRI of normal and ischemic canine myocardium. Magn Reson Med 2005;54:196–200.

35. Natanzon A, Aletras AH, Hsu LY, Arai AE. Determining canine myocardial area at risk with manganese-enhanced MR imaging. Radiology 2005;236:859–866.

36. Glover DK, Ruiz M, Edwards NC, et al. Comparison between ^{201}Tl and ^{99m}Tc sestamibi uptake during adenosine-induced vasodilation as a function of coronary stenosis severity. Circulation 1995 Feb 1;91:813–820.

37. Christian TF, Rettmann DW, Aletras AH, et al. Absolute myocardial perfusion in canines measured using dual-bolus first-pass MR imaging. Radiology 2004;232:677–684.

38. Jerosch-Herold M, Wilke N, Stillman AE. Magnetic resonance quantification of the myocardial perfusion reserve with a Fermi function model for constrained deconvolution. Med Phys 1998;25:73–84.

39. Kroll K, Wilke N, Jerosch-Herold M, et al. Modeling regional myocardial flows from residue functions of an intravascular indicator. Am J Physiol 1996;271(4 pt 2):H1643–H1655.

40. Nagel E, Thouet T, Klein C, et al. Magnetic resonance perfusion measurements for the noninvasive detection of coronary artery disease. Circulation 2003;108:432–437; Epub July 14, 2003.

41. Ibrahim T, Nekolla SG, Schreiber K, et al. Assessment of coronary flow reserve: comparison between contrast-enhanced magnetic resonance imaging and positron emission tomography. J Am Coll Cardiol 2002;39:864–870.

42. Sensky PR, Samani NJ, Reek C, Cherryman GR. Magnetic resonance perfusion imaging in patients with coronary artery disease: a qualitative approach. Int J Cardiovasc Imaging 2002;18:373–383.

43. Al-Saadi N, Nagel E, Gross M, et al. Noninvasive detection of myocardial ischemia from perfusion reserve based on cardiovascular magnetic resonance. Circulation 2000;101:1379–1383.

44. Ling LH, Christian TF, Mulvagh SL, et al. Determining myocardial viability in chronic ischemic left ventricular dysfunction: a prospective comparison of rest–redistribution thallium 201 single–photon emission computed tomography, nitroalvcerin–dobutamine echocardiography, and intracoronary myocardial contrast echocardiography. Am Heart J 2006 Apr;151(4):882–9.

45. Kim RJ, Wu E, Rafael A, et al. The use of contrast-enhanced magnetic resonance imaging to identify reversible myocardial dysfunction. N Engl J Med 2000;343:1445–1453.

46. Uemura S, Sakuma H, Motoyasu M, et al. Thallium-201 SPECT and low-dose dobutamine stress cine MRI for predicting functional recovery of regional myocardial contraction in patients with myocardial infarction. J Cardiovasc Magn Reson 2004;6:697–707.

47. Gunning MG, Anagnostopoulos C, Knight CJ, et al. Comparison of ^{20}T1, ^{99m}Tc-tetrofosmin, and dobutamine magnetic resonance imaging for identifying hibernating myocardium. Circulation 1998;98:1869–1874.
48. Bonow RO, Dilsizian V, Cuocolo A, Bacharach SL. Identification of viable myocardium in patients with chronic coronary artery disease and left ventricular dysfunction. Comparison of thallium scintigraphy with reinjection and PET imaging with ^{18}F-fluorodeoxyglucose. Circulation 1992;86:1125–1137.
49. Wagdy H, Christian TF, Miller TD, Gibbons RJ. The value of 24 hours images after rest thallium injection. Nucl Med Commun 2002;23:629–637.
50. Piwnica-Worms D, Kronauge JF, Holman BL, Lister-James J, Davison A, Jones AG. Hexakis(carbomethoxyisopropylisonitrile) technetium(I), a new myocardial perfusion imaging agent: binding characteristics in cultured chick heart cells. J Nucl Med 1988;29:55–61.
51. Dilsizian V, Arrighi JA, Diodati JG, et al. Myocardial viability in patients with chronic coronary artery disease. Comparison of ^{99m}Tc-sestamibi with thallium reinjection and [18F] fluorodeoxyglucose. Circulation 1994;89:578–587.
52. Gerber BL, Ordoubadi FF, Wijns W, et al. Positron emission tomography using F-fluoro-deoxyglucose and euglycaemic hyperinsulinaemic glucose clamp: optimal criteria for the prediction of recovery of post-ischaemic left ventricular dysfunction. Results from the European Community Concerted Action Multicenter study on use of F-fluoro-deoxyglucose positron emission tomography for the detection of myocardial viability. Eur Heart J 2001;22:1691–1701.
53. Reimer KA, Jennings RB. The "wavefront phenomenon" of myocardial ischemic cell death. II. Transmural progression of necrosis within the framework of ischemic bed size (myocardium at risk) and collateral flow. Lab Invest 1979;40:633–644.
54. Kuhl HP, Beek AM, Van der Weert AP, et al. Myocardial viability in chronic ischemic heart disease comparison of contrast-enhanced magnetic resonance imaging with ^{18}F-fluorodeoxyglucose positron emission tomography. J Am Coll Cardiol 2003;41:1341–1348.
55. Giorgettie A, Pingitore A, Favilli B, et al. Baseline/postnitrate tetrofosmin SPECT for myocardial viability assessment in patients with postischemic severe left ventricular dysfunction: new evidence from MRI. J Nucl Med 2005;46:1285–1293.
56. Ibrahim T, Nekolla SG, Hornke M, et al. Quantitative measurement of infarct size by contrast-enhanced magnetic resonance imaging early after acute myocardial infarction: comparison with single-photon emission tomography using tc99m-sestamibi. J Am Coll Cardiol 2005;45:544–552.
57. Lund GK, Stork A, Saeed M, et al. Acute myocardial infarction: evaluation with first-pass enhancement and delayed enhancement MR imaging compared with ^{201}T1 SPECT imaging. Radiology 2004; 232:49–57; Epub May 27, 2004.
58. Klein C, Nekolla SG, Bengel FM, et al. Assessment of myocardial viability with contrast enhanced magnetic resonance imaging: comparison with positron emission tomography. Circulation 2002; 105:162–167.
59. Slomka PJ, Fieno D, Thomson L, et al. Automatic detection and size quantification of infarcts by myocardial perfusion SPECT: clinical validation by delayed-enhancement MRI. J Nucl Med 2005; 46:728–735.
60. Thiele H, Kappl MJE, Conradi S, Niebauer J, Hambrecht R, Schuler G. Reproducibility of chronic and acute infarct size measurement by delayed enhancement magnetic resonance imaging. J Am Coll Cardiol 2006 Apr 18;47(8):1641–5.
61. Mahrholdt H, Wagner A, Holly TA, Elliott MD, Bonow RO, Kim RJ. Reproducibility of chronic infarct size measurement by contrast-enhanced magnetic resonance imaging. Circulation 2002;106: 2322–2327.
62. O'Connor MK, Hammell T, Gibbons RJ. In vitro validation of a simple tomographic technique for estimation of percentage myocardium at risk using methoxyisobutyl isonitrile technetium 99m (sestamibi). Eur J Nucl Med 1990;17:69–76.
63. Miller TD, Hodge DO, Sutton JM, et al. Usefulness of Tc-99m sestamibi infarct size in predicting posthospital mortality following acute myocardial infarction. Am J Cardiol 1998;81:1491–1493.
64. Christian TF. Related articles links. No abstracts. Positively magnetic north. J Am Coll Cardiol 2006 Apr 18;47(8):1646–1648.
65. Wagner A, Marholdt H, Holly TA, et al. Contrast-enhanced MRI and routine single photon emission computed tomography (SPECT) perfusion imaging for detection of subendocardial myocardial infarcts: an imaging study. Lancet 2003;361:374–379.

19 Magnetic Resonance of Cardiomyopathies and Myocarditis

Hassan Abdel-Aty and Matthias G. Friedrich

CONTENTS

Cardiomyopathies (CMPs) include dilated cardiomyopathy (DCM), hypertrophic cardiomyopathy (HCM), restrictive cardiomyopathy (RCM), and arrhythmogenic right ventricular cardiomyopathy (ARVC) *(1)*. Other forms of acute and chronic nonischemic myocardial diseases have been detected, with stress-induced CMP and noncompaction CMP the most vividly discussed.

The diagnosis of CMPs used to be established by exclusion of other cardiovascular causes, and the specific type of CMP must be confirmed because it has great impact for therapy and prognosis; a specific cause could not be identified in many cases *(2)*. Therefore, the ability of cardiovascular magnetic resonance (CMR) to visualize function, morphology, and especially tissue abnormalities has significantly improved our understanding of CMP.

THE IMAGING APPROACH OF CARDIOMYOPATHY PATIENTS

Echocardiography is usually the first-line modality to assess patients with CMPs and will obviously retain this position because of its availability, lower cost, and relative ease. CMR is emerging as a crucial adjunct to echocardiography in three main areas: tissue characterization (discussed in a separate section); whenever accurate measurements

From: *Contemporary Cardiology: Cardiovascular Magnetic Resonance Imaging*
Edited by: Raymond Y. Kwong © Humana Press Inc., Totowa, NJ

of morphology and function are needed (e.g., for monitoring the effects of an intervention); and when echocardiography is unable to provide a clear answer (e.g., for cases ARVC or suspected infiltrative CMPs).

MORPHOLOGY AND FUNCTION

CMPs are characterized by specific alterations of ventricular and myocardial geometry or function. To assess volumes and mass, steady-state free precession (SSFP) gradient echo sequences are applied during a breath hold, with approximately 30 phases per heartbeat *(3,4)*. A stack of short-axis slices covering the entire left ventricle (LV) from the mitral plane to the apex can be considered the gold standard to assess LV volumes and mass *(5)*. We recommend including the trabeculae and papillary muscle as part of the myocardial mass; this may slightly increase the analysis time, but it provides more accurate measurements.

TISSUE CHARACTERIZATION

Although CMR offers more accurate assessment of function and morphology than most available imaging modalities, it is the versatile tissue characterization capabilities of CMR that entitled the modality its unique position in evaluating CMPs. The relaxation times T_1, T_2, and T^* are sensitive to even early changes in myocardial tissue composition. Such changes not only can be visually assessed as abnormal signal intensities but also can be accurately quantified by measuring myocardial relaxation times via techniques like T_1 mapping or T_2^* susceptometry *(6,7)* Particularly in infiltrative CMPs, CMR tissue characterization becomes a tool of special relevance. Iron deposition results in shortening of T_2^*, and amyloid deposition results in shortened T_1 times. This provides a noninvasive means to quantify disease burden and monitor its response to therapy.

The intravenous injection of gadolinium chelates further enhances the tissue characterization abilities of CMR. Gadolinium chelates generally act by shortening the T_1 relaxation time and hence brightening of the signal in areas where they accumulate.

By modulating the time window or the sequence used for image acquisition, three different tissue characteristics could be obtained. Tissue ischemia, as in some cases of HCM, can be assessed using first-pass perfusion imaging immediately after contrast injection *(8)*. Tissue hyperemia, as in acute myocarditis, can be assessed 3–4 minutes after contrast injection *(9)*, and myocardial fibrosis characterizing many CMPs (e.g., dilated or infiltrative CMP or HCM) can be visualized 10 minutes after contrast injection (late enhancement) *(10–12)*.

METABOLISM

Magnetic resonance spectroscopy (MRS) has generally relied on ^1H and ^{31}P and has been applied in several studies of CMP. Changes of high-energy phosphates as studied by ^{31}P MRS in CMP were reported for DCM *(13,14)* and HCM *(15)*. However, MRS remains an experimental approach for several reasons: ^1H MRS is limited by a strong signal from water-bound protons and difficulties in spectral interpretation, and ^{31}P MRS is limited by the weakness of the phosphorus signal. Thus, voxels must be sufficiently large to cover circumscribed myocardial regions, and spectra are often altered by blood or adjacent tissue (e.g., skeletal muscle). Furthermore, the information obtainable from an MRS study does not yet have a concrete place in the management strategy of CMP patients.

DILATED NONISCHEMIC CARDIOMYOPATHY

DCM is characterized by progressive LV dilation and deteriorated LV function. Diffuse myocardial fibrosis is a common finding in histopathological studies. Once thought to be simply idiopathic, there is mounting immunological, histochemical, and histopathological evidence establishing many links between the DCM and myocardial inflammation (16–20). Interestingly, the pattern of late enhancement often observed in DCM (10) is rather similar to the foci of late enhancement in myocarditis cases (21). It is assumed that—at least in some patients—inflammation may trigger the DCM process, perhaps in the genetically susceptible individuals.

Echocardiography is a standard tool and provides information on LV size and function, although the variability of two-dimensional results may limit its value. CMR has three main values in assessing patients with DCM. First, it can accurately differentiate nonischemic from ischemic DCM. In contrast to ischemic DCM, focal fibrosis in nonischemic DCM characteristically spares the subendocardial layers (10).

Second, CMR is able to overcome many of the limitations of echocardiographic assessment of ventricular function and volumes. The significantly lower inter- and intraobserver variability in CMR measurements allow better monitoring of response to medical intervention or disease progression (22,23).

Third, the unique ability of CMR to characterize myocardial tissue changes in DCM, particularly focal fibrosis, has provided novel insights into the etiological and risk assessment. Once considered simply idiopathic, the recognition of focal fibrosis in DCM in a pattern similar to that observed in myocarditis has provided another missing link between the two diseases, which confirms previous histopathological and immunohistochemical observations. Focal septal fibrosis in DCM, the so-called midwall sign, has been linked to ventricular arrhythmia (24), a main cause of sudden death in this patient population (Fig. 1). If these results were confirmed in large clinical trials, then CMR would be expected to play an important role in risk stratifying DCM patients.

ACUTE CARDIOMYOPATHIES

Acute Viral Myocarditis

Postmortem studies identified myocarditis as a cause of sudden cardiac death in about 20% of men under the age of 40 (25,26). Other studies detected evidence of myocardial inflammation in 1–9% of routine post-mortem examinations (27). The discrepancy between a relatively common postmortem finding and an infrequent clinical diagnosis suggests that the traditional methods of diagnosing the disease are inaccurate. Once considered the gold standard to diagnose the disease, the so-called Dallas criteria (28) are now generally considered inadequate to achieve this complex task, and a new set of criteria, including laboratory, immunological, histopathological, and imaging criteria, is currently awaited (29).

In contrast to ischemic syndromes in which the myocardial injury is focal, myocarditis often proceeds from a focal to a global pattern, and only about 30–40% of the patients would present with a focal, "visible" myocardial injury. Mild-to-moderate tissue inflammation may be present in extensive myocardial areas and thus not be readily apparent in a mere visual assessment.

Thus, a quantitative analysis of global signal intensity has a special role. As several studies have shown, the quantification of global myocardial signal intensity changes reflecting inflammation, especially edema, offers a high diagnostic accuracy to detect acute myocarditis *(21,30,31)*. Furthermore, the potential absence of visible foci implies that late-enhancement imaging in myocarditis *(32)*, which depends on suppressing a "normal" myocardial signal, would fail to detect any abnormality in many cases because there is no normal myocardium to suppress. Figure 2 shows tissue abnormalities as detected by CMR in a patient with acute myocarditis (Fig. 2).

We compared the diagnostic accuracy of different sequences to detect myocarditis and found that T_2 (edema) imaging offers the highest single-sequence accuracy, which can be improved if data from T_2 and early and late enhancement are combined *(21)*. As in cases of myocardial infarction *(33)*, late enhancement is unable to differentiate acute from chronic myocarditis lesions, which likely explains its lack of correlation with serum markers of acute injury *(32)*. This is even a more serious limitation in myocarditis compared to myocardial infarction because patients frequently experience multiple episodes, and the clinical presentation is usually vague even during the acute phase *(34)*.

Acute Reversible Cardiomyopathy

A recently recognized and interesting type of CMP is acute reversible stress-related CMP, also referred to as Tako Tsubo or apical ballooning CMP *(35–37)*. This condition mainly affects women who are subjected to an emotional stressor and is characterized by myocardial stunning that selectively affects the apical myocardium *(38)*. Biopsy invariably identifies acute interstitial inflammatory response *(39)*, which suggests that T_2 imaging, a marker of edema, may be positive in such cases. Indeed, we have consistently observed a high T_2 signal intensity pattern matching the distribution of LV dysfunction in these patients. Subendocardial late enhancement is characteristically absent *(38,39)*, which helps to differentiate the condition from acute myocardial infarction.

HYPERTROPHIC CARDIOMYOPATHY

HCM is a genetic disorder characterized by inappropriate symmetrical or asymmetrical myocardial hypertrophy with loss of diastolic function and possible dynamic systolic obstruction of the LV outflow tract *(40)*.

CMR is currently the accepted gold standard to quantify myocardial mass, but because HCM is mostly focal, wall thickness may be a more important parameter. Echocardiography is the modality of choice to measure wall thickness, and the two crucial wall thickness values (e.g., the 15- and 30-mm thicknesses to establish the diagnosis and predict sudden cardiac death, respectively) are echo based.

A report by Rickers et al. *(41)*, however, showed that the diagnosis of HCM was overlooked by echo in about 5% of the patients, mainly because of the limited ability to visualize the basal anterolateral segment. This limitation is easily overcome by the three-dimensional capabilities of CMR, by which the LV myocardium is covered in short-axis views from base to apex. Cine studies in the three-chamber (inflow-outflow) using SSFP sequences may allow detection of the turbulent jet during systolic left ventricular outflow tract (LVOT) obstruction. Care should be taken that visualization of turbulent jets is generally technical factor dependent. The same view allows the visualization of the systolic anterior motion of the anterior mitral valve leaflet, which may contribute significantly to the LVOT. Planimetry of the LVOT area using thin SSFP slices is a promising tool to quantify the obstruction in HCM *(42)*. Doppler studies remain the mainstay in this setting, but planimetry may provide a more stable measure of obstruction free from day-to-day variations or hemodynamic changes (43,44).

An array of reports demonstrated the presence of a distinctive pattern of irreversible myocardial injury in HCM (11,45,46). Intramural foci of late enhancement are frequently seen involving the interventricular septum, especially at the right ventricular (RV) insertion points, and appear to be associated with increased thickness, decreased thickening, and defective perfusion (8) (Fig. 3). The exact pathophysiological grounds of these foci are not clear. Some reports suggested they represent fibrosis (47); others suggested other mechanisms such as ischemia or inflammation. Importantly, however, the presence of late enhancement correlates with the traditional risk factors of the disease (45).

Septal artery embolization to reduce the thickness of the basal septum and hence relieve obstruction in HCM is emerging as an attractive management strategy (48,49). CMR has the ability to quantify the procedure-related acute and chronic injuries, particularly edema and irreversible injury via T_2 and late enhancement techniques, respectively (50), and to relate the tissue changes caused by focal and global procedure-related functional remodeling (51,52).

ARRHYTHMOGENIC RIGHT VENTRICULAR CARDIOMYOPATHY

ARVC is characterized by a progressive degeneration of the RV myocardium. The LV may be involved in some cases as well.

Axial and sagittal SSFP cine images covering the RV are key in evaluating patients with suspected ARVC. Visual analysis allows detection of regional wall motion abnormalities, aneurysms, segmental or global dilatation, and global hypokinesis (Fig. 4). Quantitative analysis allows parameters such as RV volumes and ejection fraction to be accurately measured (53–55).

There has been initial interest in the detection of fat within the RV myocardium as a sign of the disease (56). The premise was that fatty and fibrofatty infiltrations are disease characteristics. This premise, however, is challenged by technical as well as scientific confounders. Technically, fat suppression techniques often used to confirm the presence of fat do not consistently provide homogeneous and reliable fat suppression. But, even more importantly, the presence of fat in the RV wall is observed in a host of other RV disorders and even in some healthy individuals (57,58).

Accordingly, we believe that the CMR image acquisition and analysis strategies should avoid using fat imaging as a target to identify the disease. The fibrous component of the infiltration seems to provide a more interesting approach. Tandri et al. (59) were successfully able to visualize areas of late enhancement indicating myocardial fibrosis in a group of patients with ARVC. Larger-scale trials are awaited to confirm the clinical applicability of these findings.

Furthermore, two technical challenges need to be overcome. First, there is a need for fat-suppressed late-enhancement sequences because it may be impossible in some cases to separate the enhancing thin RV wall from surrounding fat. Second, identifying the optimal inversion time needed to null the signal from the RV myocardium may be more challenging than in the LV (60).

Only one case report demonstrated the presence of edema in the RV wall using T_2-weighted imaging in ARVC (61). Although this approach is promising, technical improvements in cavitary blood suppression have to be awaited to enable differentiating the thin-walled RV edema from the slow-flowing blood within the cavity.

RESTRICTIVE CARDIOMYOPATHY

Primary infiltration of the myocardium by fibrosis or other tissues leads to the rare entity of RCM, which is associated with a grave prognosis *(2)*. The condition is characterized by severe diastolic dysfunction, biatrial dilatation, normal or small LV size, and usually normal systolic function *(62)*. Atrial thrombi may occur in patients with this disease. The main differential diagnostic consideration is constrictive pericarditis, which must be excluded in a patient with suspected RCM. Late enhancement with fat suppression may offer an attractive tool to detect abnormal pericardial enhancement and thickening suggestive of pericardial inflammation.

CMR studies in RCM should focus on myocardial morphology and function, as well as on the exclusion of constrictive pericardial disease. Biatrial dilatation is easily visualized by means of a four-chamber view. MR volumetry of the enlarged atria is recommended by some authors *(63)*. A combined approach using contrast-enhanced and nonenhanced CMR techniques may be helpful in assessing atrial thrombi *(64,65)*. Concomitant mitral and tricuspid regurgitation should be noted.

INFILTRATIVE SECONDARY CARDIOMYOPATHIES AND ENDOMYOCARDIAL DISEASES

Infiltrative CMPs include sarcoidosis, amyloidosis, and hemochromatosis. The myocardium may be infiltrated in these systemic diseases, leading to impairment of function or conduction abnormalities. Compared with other forms of CMP, infiltrative myocardial disease was found to have a worse prognosis *(2)*. Because infiltration of the tissue is accompanied by changes of myocardial signal properties, CMR may become the most powerful diagnostic tool, although the specificity may be limited.

Sarcoidosis

Sarcoidosis is a condition from a granulomatous inflammation of unknown cause. Cardiac involvement is observed in up to 50% of patients with sarcoidosis, although only 5% present with symptoms suggestive of cardiac disease. Yet, cardiac involvement is the cause of death in up to two-thirds of patients with this condition *(66,67)*. Although CMR can easily detect wall motion abnormalities or myocardial aneurysms, the main strength of the technique in this setting is its ability to characterize myocardial inflammation. As with the case in acute myocarditis, the combination of early- (spin echo) and late-enhancement techniques together with T_2-weighted imaging provides the most comprehensive approach. Early contrast enhancement identifies global myocardial inflammation; late enhancement accurately detects areas of acute or chronic irreversible injury *(68–71)* (Fig. 5). T_2-weighted images identify both global and focal edema, a feature of acute but not of chronic inflammatory injury.

Amyloidosis

Infiltration of the heart by amyloid deposits is found in almost all cases of primary amyloidosis and in approximately one-fourth of familial amyloidosis. Diffuse myocardial thickness with impaired LV function is frequent, and this can be detected by echo or by CMR, but as with other infiltrative CMPs, the merits of CMR are related to tissue characterization. Amyloid tissue has short T_1 and T_2 relaxation times and shows altered wash-in and wash-out dynamics after gadolinium injection *(72)* *(see Fig. 6)*. Using these criteria, the diagnosis of cardiac amyloidosis can be established with a high accuracy that may even render biopsy unnecessary in some cases.

One important technical note in all infiltrative CMPs and particularly amyloid heart disease is the choice of the proper inversion time in late-enhancement sequences. Such choice is classically described as optimal-to-null normal myocardial signal, but in the setting of diffuse myocardial infiltration such normal myocardium may not be available. Hence, reliance on quantitative measures of relaxation times, although more time consuming and sometimes less attractive than visual assessment, appears to be more reliable in this setting.

Transplant Cardiomyopathy

The utilization of CMR to investigate transplant CMP has been extensively studied in animal models since the early days of CMR *(73–76)*. Technical improvements have significantly enhanced the CMR capabilities, but the concepts remain almost the same. Quantification of T_2 relaxation times as a marker of myocardial edema as a substantial feature of rejection offers an attractive approach.

The report from Marie et al. *(77)*, which included the largest transplant patient series studied with T_2 imaging, offered two novel insights. First, T_2 imaging was able to detect biopsy-defined moderate acute rejection with sensitivity and specificity of 89 and 70%, respectively. Second, and more important, T_2 findings were prognostic even in patients for whom disparity was observed between T_2 imaging and biopsy findings at baseline. T_2 imaging was shown to be the most powerful predictor of rejection occurring within 3 months of transplantation. Early contrast enhancement using spin echo sequences have also been successfully used to monitor rejection when the myocardial enhancement ratio was found to correlate with the degree of the histologically identified irreversible injury *(78)*. Myocardial perfusion reserve (stress to rest) calculated from first-pass myocardial perfusion appears to be a promising approach in identifying transplant arteriopathy *(79)*.

Hemochromatosis

Repeated transfusions in patients with thalassemia result in myocardial iron deposition in more than half of the patients. Heart failure related to iron deposition CMP remains the leading cause of death in this patient population.

Increased end-diastolic and stroke volumes, myocardial mass, and a reduction of end-systolic volume can all be observed in thalassemic patients. CMR seems well suited to evaluate myocardial function in this setting for two reasons. First, wall motion abnormalities are common, rendering echocardiographic measurements, which depend on geometric assumptions of the LV shape, can be potentially inaccurate. Second, echocardiography may not be the optimal choice if sequential LV function measurements are essential in suspected iron deposition CMP because the technique is limited by the relatively wide interobserver variability. Of particular importance is the fact that the ejection fraction in thalassemic patients may be higher than normal because of the associated hemodynamic changes, which again explains the need for an accurate and highly reproducible tool able to detect early and sequential changes in LV ejection fraction.

The introduction of T_2* "susceptometry" of the myocardium to measure its iron deposition burden has revolutionized disease management *(6)*. A single-slice, breath-hold gradient echo sequence with multiple "rising" echo times is the technique of choice to measure the T_2* value of the myocardium. Normal value is estimated to be 52 ± 16 ms, and thus a cutoff value of 20 ms (lower 95% confidence interval) was chosen to identify patients with reduced T_2* values; a T_2* less than 10 ms marks severe disease *(7,80–82)*. The premise is that iron deposition results in reduction of T_2* values because of its susceptibility effect.

Although T_2* correlates well with LV systolic function, neither seem to relate to the conventional parameters of assessing iron overload, such as liver iron content or serum ferritin. This dissociation between cardiac and extracardiac iron content appears to be caused by the slower (about sixfold) iron clearance from the heart compared to the liver and highlights the unreliability of liver biopsy to monitor myocardial iron deposition. T_2* measurements are now a key tool not only in identifying iron deposition but also in monitoring and comparing the effects of various iron-chelating therapies. The results of the first randomized trial to use T_2* as a primary end point have been reported *(83)*.

Endomyocardial Diseases

Endomyocardial fibrosis is related to two forms, one occurring in the tropics and one occurring in a temperate climate, termed Loffler's endocarditis. Both conditions lead to primarily posterobasal concentric wall thickening followed by extensive subendocardial fibrosis and frequent apical thrombus formation. Both ventricles may be affected. Progressive diastolic dysfunction and reduction of stroke volume are frequently encountered characteristics.

The morphological and functional features can be well visualized and quantified by CMR *(84,85)*. Late-enhancement images show the diffuse pattern of endocardial fibrosis. Differentiation from apical infarction is easy by visualization of the preserved (or increased) wall thickness and the V-shaped outer form of the apex in the long-axis views.

Noncompaction Cardiomyopathy

Noncompaction cardiomyopathy is an uncommon form of CMP that may be inherited as an autosomal dominant genotype *(86,87)*. Phenotypically, there is failure or arrest of compaction of the trabecular layer, a process that usually takes place from base to apex, from epicardium to endocardium, and septally to laterally *(88) (see Fig. 7)*. These considerations are helpful in predicting the most common morphological pattern of the disease.

CMR diagnosis is based on the identification of increased noncompacted-to-compacted myocardium at end-diastole; a ratio of 2.3 or more seems to offer high diagnostic accuracy *(89)*. Wall motion abnormalities and global systolic dysfunction or thrombi can also be encountered *(90)*.

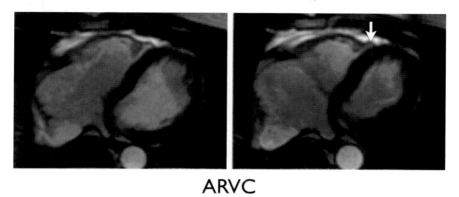

ARVC

Fig. 1. Arrythmogenic right ventricular cardiomyopathy (ARVC). Diastolic (left) and systolic (right) still frames from a cine study of the RV. The RV free wall is thinned with a small area of severe thinning, dyskinesis, and diastolic bulging, fulfilling the criterion of an aneurysm (arrow). The free wall is hypokinetic.

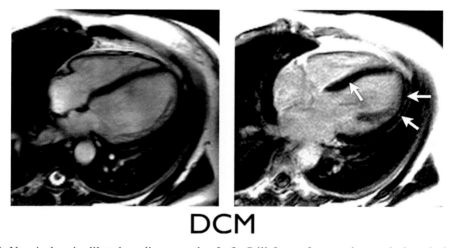

DCM

Fig. 2. Non-ischemic dilated cardiomyopathy. Left: Still frame from a cine study in a 4-chamber view. The LV is dilated. Right: Late enhancement study in the same orientation with a stripe-shaped area of high signal intensity in the basal septum and the lateral wall (arrow), often referred to as "midwall signal".

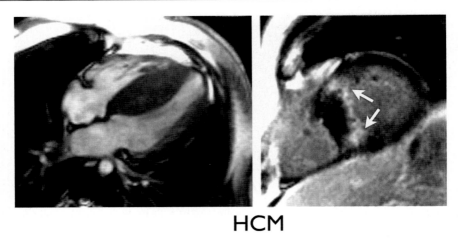

HCM

Fig. 3. Hypertrophic cardiomyopathy (HCM). Left: Systolic cine still frame in the four-chamber view. Right: Short-axis late-enhancement image. The septum is asymmetrically and markedly thickened. Foci of late enhancement (arrows) are seen within the interventricular septum at the insertion points of the RV as well as the subendocardial layer of the septum.

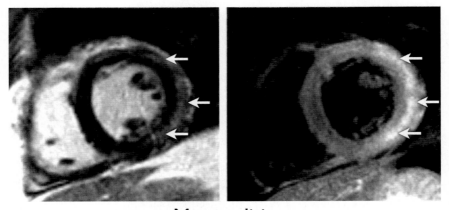

Myocarditis

Fig. 4. Acute myocarditis. Short-axis slices showing late enhancement (left) and corresponding triple inversion recovery T_2-weighted (right) images. A large subepicardial area of late enhancement is seen within the anterior, anterolateral, lateral, and inferolateral walls (arrows). High T_2 signal indicating edema is seen in the same locations, sparing the subendocardium as well and establishing the acute nature of the myocardial injury in this case (arrows).

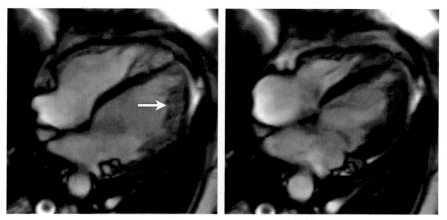

Non-compaction CMP

Fig. 5. Noncompaction cardiomyopathy. Diastolic (left) and systolic (right) still frames from a cine study in a four-chamber view. The compact myocardial wall gradually thins toward the apex, and a prominent network of interlacing trabeculae is seen in relation to the thinned areas, which were hypokinetic as well. The ratio of the noncompacted to the compacted myocardial wall in this case was 5 to 1.

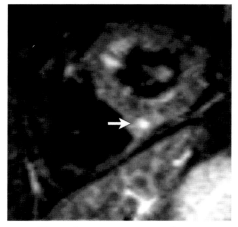

Cardiac sarcoidosis

Fig. 6. Cardiac sarcoidosis. Triple inversion recovery T_2-weighted image. Patchy areas of high T_2 signal indicating edema, consistent with sarcoid granulomas with a larger focus in the interventricular septum at the insertion point of the right ventricle (arrow).

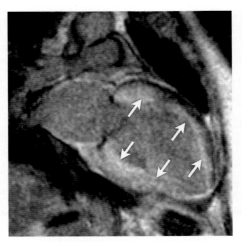

Cardiac amyloidosis

Fig. 7. Cardiac amyloidosis. Diffuse contrast enhancement is seen within the myocardium (arrows).

REFERENCES

1. Richardson P, McKenna W, Bristow M, et al. Report of the 1995 World Health Organization/International Society and Federation of Cardiology Task Force on the Definition and Classification of cardiomyopathies. Circulation 1996;93:841–842.
2. Felker GM, Thompson RE, Hare JM, et al. Underlying causes and long-term survival in patients with initially unexplained cardiomyopathy. N Engl J Med 2000;342:1077–1084.
3. Michaely HJ, Nael K, Schoenberg SO, et al. Analysis of cardiac function—comparison between 1.5 T and 3.0 T cardiac cine magnetic resonance imaging: preliminary experience. Invest Radiol 2006;41:133–140.
4. Alfakih K, Thiele H, Plein S, Bainbridge GJ, Ridgway JP, Sivananthan MU. Comparison of right ventricular volume measurement between segmented k-space gradient-echo and steady-state free precession magnetic resonance imaging. J Magn Reson Imaging 2002;16:253–258.
5. Bellenger NG, Burgess MI, Ray SG, et al. Comparison of left ventricular ejection fraction and volumes in heart failure by echocardiography, radionuclide ventriculography and cardiovascular magnetic resonance; are they interchangeable? Eur Heart J 2000;21:1387–1396.
6. Pennell DJ. T_2* magnetic resonance and myocardial iron in thalassemia. Ann N Y Acad Sci 2005; 1054:373–378.
7. Anderson LJ, Holden S, Davis B, et al. Cardiovascular T_2-star (T_2*) magnetic resonance for the early diagnosis of myocardial iron overload. Eur Heart J 2001;22:2171–2179.
8. Matsunaka T, Hamada M, Matsumoto Y, Higaki J. First-pass myocardial perfusion defect and delayed contrast enhancement in hypertrophic cardiomyopathy assessed with MRI. Magn Reson Med Sci 2003;2:61–69.
9. Friedrich MG, Strohm O, Schulz-Menger J, Marciniak H, Luft FC, Dietz R. Contrast media-enhanced magnetic resonance imaging visualizes myocardial changes in the course of viral myocarditis. Circulation 1998;97:1802–1809.
10. McCrohon JA, Moon JC, Prasad SK, et al. Differentiation of heart failure related to dilated cardiomyopathy and coronary artery disease using gadolinium-enhanced cardiovascular magnetic resonance. Circulation 2003;108:54–59.
11. Choudhury L, Mahrholdt H, Wagner A, et al. Myocardial scarring in asymptomatic or mildly symptomatic patients with hypertrophic cardiomyopathy. J Am Coll Cardiol 2002;40:2156–2164.
12. Bogaert J, Goldstein M, Tannouri F, Golzarian J, Dymarkowski S. Original report. Late myocardial enhancement in hypertrophic cardiomyopathy with contrast-enhanced MR imaging. AJR Am J Roentgenol 2003;180:981–985.
13. Neubauer S, Krahe T, Schindler R, et al. [31]P magnetic resonance spectroscopy in dilated cardiomyopathy and coronary artery disease. Altered cardiac high-energy phosphate metabolism in heart failure. Circulation 1992;86:1810–1818.

14. Neubauer S, Horn M, Cramer M, et al. Myocardial phosphocreatine-to-ATP ratio is a predictor of mortality in patients with dilated cardiomyopathy. Circulation 1997;96:2190–2196.
15. Jung WI, Sieverding L, Breuer J, et al. ^{31}P NMR spectroscopy detects metabolic abnormalities in asymptomatic patients with hypertrophic cardiomyopathy. Circulation 1998;97:2536–2542.
16. Pauschinger M, Chandrasekharan K, Schultheiss HP. Myocardial remodeling in viral heart disease: possible interactions between inflammatory mediators and MMP-TIMP system. Heart Fail Rev 2004;9:21–31.
17. Maisch B, Richter A, Sandmoller A, Portig I, Pankuweit S. Inflammatory dilated cardiomyopathy (DCMI). Herz 2005;30:535–544.
18. Kandolf R, Klingel K, Zell R, et al. Molecular pathogenesis of enterovirus-induced myocarditis: virus persistence and chronic inflammation. Intervirology 1993;35(1–4):140–151.
19. Brown CA, O'Connell JB. Myocarditis and idiopathic dilated cardiomyopathy. Am J Med 1995;99: 309–314.
20. Schultheiss HP, Kuhl U. Overview on chronic viral cardiomyopathy/chronic myocarditis. Ernst Schering Res Found Workshop 2006(55):3–18.
21. Abdel-Aty H, Boye P, Zagrosek A, et al. Diagnostic performance of cardiovascular magnetic resonance in patients with suspected acute myocarditis: comparison of different approaches. J Am Coll Cardiol 2005;45:1815–1822.
22. Strohm O, Schulz-Menger J, Pilz B, Osterziel KJ, Dietz R, Friedrich MG. Measurement of left ventricular dimensions and function in patients with dilated cardiomyopathy. J Magn Reson Imaging 2001;13:367–371.
23. Bellenger NG, Davies LC, Francis JM, Coats AJ, Pennell DJ. Reduction in sample size for studies of remodeling in heart failure by the use of cardiovascular magnetic resonance. J Cardiovasc Magn Reson 2000;2:271–278.
24. Nazarian S, Bluemke DA, Lardo AC, et al. Magnetic resonance assessment of the substrate for inducible ventricular tachycardia in nonischemic cardiomyopathy. Circulation 2005;112:2821–2825.
25. Drory Y, Turetz Y, Hiss Y, et al. Sudden unexpected death in persons less than 40 years of age. Am J Cardiol 1991;68:1388–1392.
26. Wesslen L, Ehrenborg C, Holmberg M, et al. Subacute bartonella infection in Swedish orienteers succumbing to sudden unexpected cardiac death or having malignant arrhythmias. Scand J Infect Dis 2001;33:429–438.
27. Saphir O. Acute myocarditis in sudden and unexpected death. Postgrad Med 1955;18:A-38–A-44.
28. Aretz HT. Myocarditis: the Dallas criteria. Hum Pathol 1987;18:619–624.
29. Baughman KL. Diagnosis of myocarditis: death of Dallas criteria. Circulation 2006;113:593–595.
30. Friedrich MG, Strohm O, Schulz-Menger JE, Marciniak H, Dietz R. Noninvasive diagnosis of acute myocarditis by contrast-enhanced magnetic resonance imaging. Proceedings of the ISMRM 6th Annual Meeting, Sydney 1998:912.
31. Laissy JP, Messin B, Varenne O, et al. MRI of acute myocarditis: a comprehensive approach based on various imaging sequences. Chest 2002;122:1638–1648.
32. Mahrholdt H, Goedecke C, Wagner A, et al. Cardiovascular magnetic resonance assessment of human myocarditis: a comparison to histology and molecular pathology. Circulation 2004;109:1250–1258.
33. Abdel-Aty H, Zagrosek A, Schulz-Menger J, et al. Delayed enhancement and T_2-weighted cardiovascular magnetic resonance imaging differentiate acute from chronic myocardial infarction. Circulation 2004;109:2411–2416.
34. Feldman AM, McNamara D. Myocarditis. N Engl J Med 2000;343:1388–1398.
35. Ishikawa K. "Takotsubo" cardiomyopathy. A syndrome characterized by transient left ventricular apical ballooning that mimics the shape of a bottle used for trapping octopus in Japan. Intern Med 2004;43: 275–276.
36. Ako J, Kozaki K, Yoshizumi M, Ouchi Y. Transient left ventricular apical ballooning without coronary artery stenosis: a form of stunning-like phenomenon? J Am Coll Cardiol 2002;39:741–742.
37. Abe Y, Kondo M. Apical ballooning of the left ventricle: a distinct entity? Heart 2003;89:974–976.
38. Sharkey SW, Lesser JR, Zenovich AG, et al. Acute and reversible cardiomyopathy provoked by stress in women from the United States. Circulation 2005;111:472–479.
39. Wittstein IS, Thiemann DR, Lima JA, et al. Neurohumoral features of myocardial stunning to sudden emotional stress. N Engl J Med 2005;352:539–548.
40. Maron BJ, McKenna WJ, Danielson GK, et al. American College of Cardiology/European Society of Cardiology clinical expert consensus document on hypertrophic cardiomyopathy. A report of the American College of Cardiology Foundation Task Force on Clinical Expert Consensus Documents and

the European Society of Cardiology Committee for Practice Guidelines. J Am Coll Cardiol 2003;42:1687–1713.

41. Rickers C, Wilke NM, Jerosch-Herold M, et al. Utility of cardiac magnetic resonance imaging in the diagnosis of hypertrophic cardiomyopathy. Circulation 2005;112:855–861.

42. Schulz-Menger J, Strohm O, Waigand J, Uhlich F, Dietz R, Friedrich MG. The value of magnetic resonance imaging of the left ventricular outflow tract in patients with hypertrophic obstructive cardiomyopathy after septal artery embolization. Circulation 2000;101:1764–1766.

43. Paz R, Jortner R, Tunick PA, et al. The effect of the ingestion of ethanol on obstruction of the left ventricular outflow tract in hypertrophic cardiomyopathy. N Engl J Med 1996;335:938–941.

44. Kizilbash AM, Heinle SK, Grayburn PA. Spontaneous variability of left ventricular outflow tract gradient in hypertrophic obstructive cardiomyopathy. Circulation 1998;97:461–466.

45. Moon JC, McKenna WJ, McCrohon JA, Elliott PM, Smith GC, Pennell DJ. Toward clinical risk assessment in hypertrophic cardiomyopathy with gadolinium cardiovascular magnetic resonance. J Am Coll Cardiol 2003;41:1561–1567.

46. Wilson JM, Villareal RP, Hariharan R, Massumi A, Muthupillai R, Flamm SD. Magnetic resonance imaging of myocardial fibrosis in hypertrophic cardiomyopathy. Tex Heart Inst J 2002;29:176–180.

47. Moon JC, Reed E, Sheppard MN, et al. The histologic basis of late gadolinium enhancement cardiovascular magnetic resonance in hypertrophic cardiomyopathy. J Am Coll Cardiol 2004;43:2260–2264.

48. Gietzen FH, Leuner CJ, Obergassel L, Strunk-Mueller C, Kuhn H. Role of transcoronary ablation of septal hypertrophy in patients with hypertrophic cardiomyopathy, New York Heart Association functional class III or IV, and outflow obstruction only under provocable conditions. Circulation 2002;106:454–459.

49. Sigwart U. Non-surgical myocardial reduction for hypertrophic obstructive cardiomyopathy. Lancet 1995;346:211–214.

50. Schulz-Menger J, Gross M, Messroghli D, Uhlich F, Dietz R, Friedrich MG. Cardiovascular magnetic resonance of acute myocardial infarction at a very early stage. J Am Coll Cardiol 2003;42:513–518.

51. van Dockum WG, Beek AM, ten Cate FJ, et al. Early onset and progression of left ventricular remodeling after alcohol septal ablation in hypertrophic obstructive cardiomyopathy. Circulation 2005;111:2503–2508.

52. van Dockum WG, ten Cate FJ, ten Berg JM, et al. Myocardial infarction after percutaneous transluminal septal myocardial ablation in hypertrophic obstructive cardiomyopathy: evaluation by contrast-enhanced magnetic resonance imaging. J Am Coll Cardiol 2004;43:27–34.

53. Tandri H, Friedrich MG, Calkins H, Bluemke DA. MRI of arrhythmogenic right ventricular cardiomyopathy/dysplasia. J Cardiovasc Magn Reson 2004;6:557–563.

54. Keller DI, Osswald S, Bremerich J, et al. Arrhythmogenic right ventricular cardiomyopathy: diagnostic and prognostic value of the cardiac MRI in relation to arrhythmia-free survival. Int J Cardiovasc Imaging 2003;19:537–543; discussion 545–537.

55. Bluemke DA, Krupinski EA, Ovitt T, et al. MR imaging of arrhythmogenic right ventricular cardiomyopathy: morphologic findings and interobserver reliability. Cardiology 2003;99:153–162.

56. Menghetti L, Basso C, Nava A, Angelini A, Thiene G. Spin-echo nuclear magnetic resonance for tissue characterisation in arrhythmogenic right ventricular cardiomyopathy. Heart 1996;76:467–470.

57. Tansey DK, Aly Z, Sheppard MN. Fat in the right ventricle of the normal heart. Histopathology 2005;46:98–104.

58. Basso C, Thiene G. Adipositas cordis, fatty infiltration of the right ventricle, and arrhythmogenic right ventricular cardiomyopathy. Just a matter of fat? Cardiovasc Pathol 2005;14:37–41.

59. Tandri H, Saranathan M, Rodriguez ER, et al. Noninvasive detection of myocardial fibrosis in arrhythmogenic right ventricular cardiomyopathy using delayed-enhancement magnetic resonance imaging. J Am Coll Cardiol 2005;45:98–103.

60. Desai MY, Gupta S, Bomma C, et al. The apparent inversion time for optimal delayed enhancement magnetic resonance imaging differs between the right and left ventricles. J Cardiovasc Magn Reson 2005;7:475–479.

61. Sen-Chowdhry S, Prasad SK, McKenna WJ. Arrhythmogenic right ventricular cardiomyopathy with fibrofatty atrophy, myocardial oedema, and aneurysmal dilation. Heart 2005;91:784.

62. Kushwaha SS, Fallon JT, Fuster V. Restrictive cardiomyopathy. N Engl J Med 1997;336:267–276.

63. Jarvinen VM, Kupari MM, Poutanen VP, Hekali PE. A simplified method for the determination of left atrial size and function using cine magnetic resonance imaging. Magn Reson Imaging 1996;14:215–226.

64. Barkhausen J, Hunold P, Eggebrecht H, et al. Detection and characterization of intracardiac thrombi on MR imaging. AJR Am J Roentgenol 2002;179:1539–1544.
65. Ohyama H, Hosomi N, Takahashi T, et al. Comparison of magnetic resonance imaging and transesophageal echocardiography in detection of thrombus in the left atrial appendage. Stroke 2003;34:2436–2439.
66. Yazaki Y, Isobe M, Hiroe M, et al. Prognostic determinants of long-term survival in Japanese patients with cardiac sarcoidosis treated with prednisone. Am J Cardiol 2001;88:1006–1010.
67. Sekiguchi M, Yazaki Y, Isobe M, Hiroe M. Cardiac sarcoidosis: diagnostic, prognostic, and therapeutic considerations. Cardiovasc Drugs Ther 1996;10:495–510.
68. Schulz-Menger J, Wassmuth R, Abdel-Aty H, et al. Patterns of myocardial inflammation and scarring in sarcoidosis as assessed by cardiovascular magnetic resonance. Heart 2006;92:399–400.
69. Vignaux O, Dhote R, Duboc D, et al. Detection of myocardial involvement in patients with sarcoidosis applying T_2-weighted, contrast-enhanced, and cine magnetic resonance imaging: initial results of a prospective study. J Comput Assist Tomogr 2002;26:762–767.
70. Smedema JP, Snoep G, van Kroonenburgh MP, et al. Evaluation of the accuracy of gadolinium-enhanced cardiovascular magnetic resonance in the diagnosis of cardiac sarcoidosis. J Am Coll Cardiol 2005;45:1683–1690.
71. Schulz-Menger J, Strohm O, Dietz R, Friedrich MG. Visualization of cardiac involvement in patients with systemic sarcoidosis applying contrast-enhanced magnetic resonance imaging. Magma 2000;11: 82–83.
72. Maceira AM, Joshi J, Prasad SK, et al. Cardiovascular magnetic resonance in cardiac amyloidosis. Circulation 2005;111:186–193.
73. Tscholakoff D, Aherne T, Yee ES, Derugin N, Higgins CB. Cardiac transplantations in dogs: evaluation with MR. Radiology 1985;157:697–702.
74. Lund G, Morin RL, Olivari MT, Ring WS. Serial myocardial T_2 relaxation time measurements in normal subjects and heart transplant recipients. J Heart Transplant 1988;7:274–279.
75. Doornbos J, Verwey H, Essed CE, Balk AH, de Roos A. MR imaging in assessment of cardiac transplant rejection in humans. J Comput Assist Tomogr 1990;14:77–81.
76. Sasaguri S, LaRaia PJ, Fabri BM, et al. Early detection of cardiac allograft rejection with proton nuclear magnetic resonance. Circulation 1985;72(3 pt 2):II231–II236.
77. Marie PY, Angioi M, Carteaux JP, et al. Detection and prediction of acute heart transplant rejection with the myocardial T_2 determination provided by a black-blood magnetic resonance imaging sequence. J Am Coll Cardiol 2001;37:825–831.
78. Almenar L, Igual B, Martinez-Dolz L, et al. Utility of cardiac magnetic resonance imaging for the diagnosis of heart transplant rejection. Transplant Proc 2003;35:1962–1964.
79. Muehling OM, Panse P, Jerosch-Herold M, et al. Cardiac magnetic resonance perfusion imaging identifies transplant arteriopathy by a reduced endomyocardial resting perfusion. J Heart Lung Transplant 2005;24:1122–1123.
80. Westwood M, Anderson LJ, Firmin DN, et al. A single breath-hold multiecho T_2* cardiovascular magnetic resonance technique for diagnosis of myocardial iron overload. J Magn Reson Imaging 2003;18:33–39.
81. Anderson LJ, Wonke B, Prescott E, Holden S, Walker JM, Pennell DJ. Comparison of effects of oral deferiprone and subcutaneous desferrioxamine on myocardial iron concentrations and ventricular function in β-thalassaemia. Lancet 2002;360:516–520.
82. Anderson LJ, Westwood MA, Holden S, et al. Myocardial iron clearance during reversal of siderotic cardiomyopathy with intravenous desferrioxamine: a prospective study using T_2* cardiovascular magnetic resonance. Br J Haematol 2004;127:348–355.
83. Pennell DJ, Berdoukas V, Karagiorga M, et al. Randomized controlled trial of deferiprone or deferoxamine in β-thalassemia major patients with asymptomatic myocardial siderosis. Blood. May 1 2006;107(9):3738–3744.
84. Celletti F, Fattori R, Napoli G, et al. Assessment of restrictive cardiomyopathy of amyloid or idiopathic etiology by magnetic resonance imaging. Am J Cardiol 1999;83:798–801, a710.
85. D'Silva SA, Kohli A, Dalvi BV, Kale PA. MRI in right ventricular endomyocardial fibrosis. Am Heart J 1992;123:1390–1392.
86. Wieneke H, Neumann T, Breuckmann F, et al. [Non-compaction cardiomyopathy]. Herz 2005;30: 571–574.
87. Vatta M, Mohapatra B, Jimenez S, et al. Mutations in Cypher/ZASP in patients with dilated cardiomyopathy and left ventricular non-compaction. J Am Coll Cardiol 2003;42:2014–2027.

88. Sedmera D, Pexieder T, Vuillemin M, Thompson RP, Anderson RH. Developmental patterning of the myocardium. Anat Rec 2000;258:319–337.
89. Petersen SE, Selvanayagam JB, Wiesmann F, et al. Left ventricular non-compaction: insights from cardiovascular magnetic resonance imaging. J Am Coll Cardiol 2005;46:101–105.
90. Petersen SE, Timperley J, Neubauer S. Left ventricular thrombi in a patient with left ventricular non-compaction in visualisation of the rationale for anticoagulation. Heart 2005;91:e4.

20 Assessment of Diastolic Function by Cardiac MRI

Bernard P. Paelinck and Hildo J. Lamb

CONTENTS

INTRODUCTION

Cardiac magnetic resonance imaging (MRI) techniques continue to change rapidly, and cardiac MRI is developing as an alternative noninvasive technique having the unique potential of three-dimensional function analysis with great accuracy and reproducibility. Advances in rapid cardiac MRI technology are making real-time imaging possible at approaching echocardiographic frame rates. Together with the increasing availability of cardiac MRI machines, cardiac MRI has the potential of a powerful and comprehensive tool for the analysis of heart function. In this chapter, the potential role of cardiac MRI in the evaluation of diastolic heart function is reviewed.

PHYSIOLOGY

During diastole, the myocardium loses its ability to generate force and shorten and returns to resting force and length. Relaxation is an energy-consuming process that starts when myofiber tension declines during late ejection *(1)*. Ventricular pressure further falls during isovolumic relaxation and early ventricular filling (Fig. 1). Relaxation is quantified by measuring the rate of ventricular pressure decay (time constant τ). Myocardial relaxation occurs because of the release of calcium from troponin C, detachment of the actin-myosin cross-bridges, and adenosine triphosphatase-induced calcium sequestration into the sarcoplasmatic reticulum. Besides active relaxation, passive viscoelastic properties contribute to diastolic dysfunction *(2)*.

From: *Contemporary Cardiology: Cardiovascular Magnetic Resonance Imaging*
Edited by: Raymond Y. Kwong © Humana Press Inc., Totowa, NJ

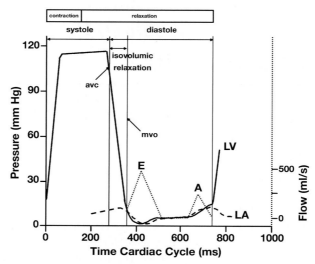

Fig. 1. Diagram showing the hemodynamic aspects of the cardiac cycle including systole and diastole: intracardiac pressures (full line displays LV pressure and dashed line indicates LA pressure, left *y*-axis) and transmitral flow (dashed diagram). Atrioventricular pressure gradient results in transmitral flow (dashed diagram, right *y*-axis). During isovolumic relaxation, which starts after closure of aortic valve and ends with opening of the mitral valve, LV pressure drops and LV volume remains constant. When LV pressure falls below LA pressure, the mitral valve opens, and rapid filling (early or E wave) occurs. During early diastole, LV pressure further decreases despite increasing LV volume, resulting in suction of blood toward the ventricle. Rapid filling continues until LA and LV pressures equalize. At the end of diastole, active contraction of the LA results in late filling (atrial or A wave). The cyclic interaction of myofilaments is subdivided in contraction and relaxation. LV, left ventricular; LA, left atrial; E, early transmitral flow; A, late transmitral flow; avc, aortic valve closure; mvo, mitral valve opening.

Diastolic dysfunction occurs when these processes are prolonged or incomplete. Diastolic dysfunction is an early marker of cardiac disease and precedes systolic dysfunction. It can occur in the presence or absence of symptoms and with normal or abnormal systolic function *(1)*.

The diagnosis of diastolic heart failure or heart failure with a normal or mildly reduced left ventricular (LV) ejection fraction has been challenging because the simultaneous presence of elevated heart pressures caused by increased resistance to ventricular filling (upward shift of the diastolic pressure–volume relationship) has to be demonstrated *(3,4)*. One-third of patients with congestive heart failure suffers from primary diastolic heart failure *(4)*.

Assessment of LV filling pressures is important for the interpretation of symptoms, optimization of unloading therapy, and prediction of prognosis in heart disease *(5)*. However, routine use of cardiac catheterization for the assessment of relaxation and demonstration of elevated filling pressures is not feasible. Therefore, noninvasive techniques have been developed to assess diastolic function. Although relaxation occurs mostly before ventricular filling starts (during the isovolumic period), noninvasive parameters of diastolic function are mostly derived from rates of ventricular inflow of blood (after mitral valve opening or when the relaxation process is almost completed). Consequently, the practice of these noninvasive parameters has been restricted by dependence on loading conditions, heart rate, and systolic function *(6)*. New, less load-dependent Doppler techniques are under evaluation *(7)*. Cardiac MRI techniques have specific advantages for assessing diastolic heart function.

TECHNIQUES

Cardiac MRI techniques have been used to assess diastolic function in different experimental and clinical settings. Each cardiac MRI technique has its own characteristics and its specific advantages to assess diastolic function: gradient echo (GRE) for evaluation of functional dimensions, phase contrast to measure flow, and myocardial tagging to assess regional dynamics *(8)*.

The greatest challenges in the acquisition of cardiac MRI movies or cine display have been cardiac motion from breathing and flow artifacts from myocardial and blood motion *(9)*.

Gradient Echo

GRE uses repetitive radio-frequency pulses gated to the electrocardiogram, which permits imaging at multiple phases of the cardiac cycle so that a cine display can be generated. By using the GRE sequence with very short echo times (approximately 2 ms) repeated at brief intervals (repetition time [TR] of approximately 10 ms) and a reduced flip angle (30–40°) and by acquiring multiple lines of image resolution per heartbeat for each phase, cine images could be generated during a breath hold. These techniques are known as segmented *k*-space imaging.

Breath-hold imaging has been the most widely used approach to avoid respiratory-related displacement of the heart. A temporal resolution of 15 ms or less can be achieved. This approach, however, assumes that cardiac motion is highly reproducible and does not vary from beat to beat, causing blurring of the images as seen in arrhythmias. New sequences yielding real-time acquisition eliminate the need for breath holding and facilitate the capture of beat-to-beat variation *(9)*.

Real-time dynamic imaging, or cardiac MRI "fluoroscopy," has developed into a robust way to avoid motion artifacts with numerous improvements in gradient hardware, novel *k*-space coverage, and new reconstruction techniques yielding a temporal resolution of up to 40 frames/second *(10)*. From these GRE-generated diastolic volumetric images, both global and regional ventricular filling can be analyzed *(11)*.

Phase Contrast

Quantitative measurements of velocities of moving structures and blood in any chosen direction can be measured by phase contrast MRI or MRI velocity mapping. The basic principle of this technique is the spin phase shift or the shift that magnetic spins of intravascular protons acquire when flowing along a magnetic field gradient relative to stationary spins. Subtraction of the magnetic resonance reference and the velocity-encoded images allows calculation of velocities of the myocardium and blood flow at specified sites in the heart.

Flow may be measured parallel in-plane or perpendicular through-plane to flow. Summation of flow at a given area throughout the cardiac cycle will yield flow during one heartbeat. The technique is accurate and has a wide dynamic range, allowing encoding of velocities from several millimeters per second to at least 10 m/second at high temporal resolution over the complete cardiac cycle *(10,12)* (e.g., enabling flow measurement of pulmonary vein, mitral and tricuspid valves). In addition, a slice-following technique is under clinical investigation; it corrects for through-plane motion *(13)*. Pressure gradients can be calculated using the modified Bernoulli equation *(10)*.

Analogous to flow velocities, phase contrast MRI allows measurement of tissue velocities or tissue MRI *(14)*. Plus, myocardial motion can be derived by integrating the myocardial velocities, enabling calculation of any local strain. In each myocardial voxel, myocardial strain rate can be quantified *(15)*.

Tagging

With tagged MRI, the myocardium is labeled ("tagged") by selective radio-frequency saturation prepulses in planes perpendicular to the imaging plane. Tags reveal the deformation and displacement of the myocardium on which they are placed. They appear as black lines (absence of signal from these protons) in a radial (measurement of torsion) *(16)* or a grid pattern (calculation of full strain field) *(17)* superimposed on the image. These tag lines persist for several hundreds of milliseconds. Myocardial tagging has been refined with the introduction of spatial modulation of magnetization (SPAMM), which wraps a saturation effect through three-dimensional space. Also, complementary spatial modulation of magnetization (CSPAMM) has significantly improved the signal-to-noise ratio by using a slice-following technique that compensates for through-plane motion in the original tagging technique. By spatial mapping of the distortion of the grid throughout the cardiac cycle, the technique allows accurate noninvasive analysis of any diastolic strain and three-dimensional motion (rotation, radial displacement, and translation) of the heart. Images can be obtained every 20 ms, yielding high temporal resolution *(18)*. Semiautomated and automated methods are under development for three-dimensional and quantitative analysis of myocardial strains *(19,20)*.

Spectroscopy

Finally, phosphorus 31 cardiac MRI spectroscopy has the ability to analyze ^{31}P cardiac MRI spectra and measure the ratio of myocardial phosphocreatine (PCr) and adenosine triphosphate (ATP) levels or PCr/ATP reflecting the energy status of tissue of the human heart in vivo *(21)*.

PARAMETERS FOR THE ASSESSMENT OF DIASTOLIC FUNCTION

The cardiac MRI techniques mentioned have been applied for the evaluation of both global and regional diastolic function: peak filling rate (PFR) and time-to-peak filling rate; flow mapping of mitral valve, pulmonary vein, and tricuspid valve; global and regional rotation, translation, and radial motion; endocardial vs epicardial motion. In addition, phosphorus 31 cardiac MRI spectroscopy measures the myocardial energy content necessary for the active energy-dependent process of myocardial relaxation (Table 1).

Ventricular Volume and Wall Thickness Curves

Time–volume curves generating from GRE images provide accurate assessment of global diastolic function. From the contours describing the endocardial and epicardial border of the myocardium, ventricular volumes can be measured from which area-vs-time curves of both ventricles can be calculated *(11)*. PFR can be determined from the maximal change of ventricular volume during the rapid-filling phase. Time to PFR is the time between end-systole and the time-point at which PFR occurs *(22,23)*. PFR can be expressed relative to the end-diastolic volume (PFR/EDV) and to stroke volume (PFR/SV).

Table 1
Techniques for the Assessment of Diastolic Function

Global diastolic function	
Transmitral and tricuspid flow	Phase contrast
Ventricular peak filling rate and time-to-peak filling rate	GRE
Myocardial metabolism	Spectroscopy
Regional diastolic function	
Wall-thinning dynamics	GRE
Myocardial strains	Tagging
Myocardial velocities	Phase contrast

GRE, gradient echo.

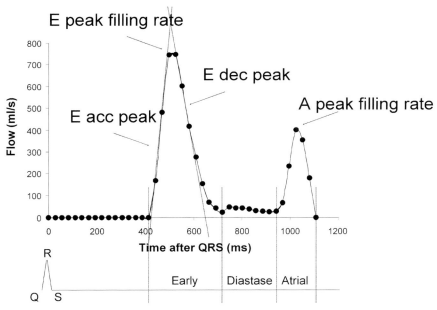

Fig. 2. Phase contrast MRI measurement of transmitral flow. In this example, 41 phases are acquired during 1100 ms, yielding a temporal resolution of 27 ms. E, early transmitral flow; A, late transmitral flow. Reprinted from ref. *8*, copyright 2002, with permission from Elsevier.

Analysis of GRE images allows measurement of other regional diastolic function parameters as peak rate of wall thinning and time-to-peak rate of wall thinning, which can be derived from Fourier filtered wall thickness curves *(24)*.

Transmitral and Tricuspid Velocity and Flow

Peak velocities of early (E) and late or atrial filling waves (A) through both mitral (Fig. 2) and tricuspid valves *(25–27)* and peak velocities of systolic, diastolic, and atrial reversal components of the pulmonary vein flow *(26)* have been measured accurately using phase contrast cardiac MRI velocity mapping in close agreement with Doppler data. A good correlation between velocity-based indexes and volumetric data has been demonstrated *(28)*. In addition, this technique is not restricted by poor acoustic windows *(29)* and

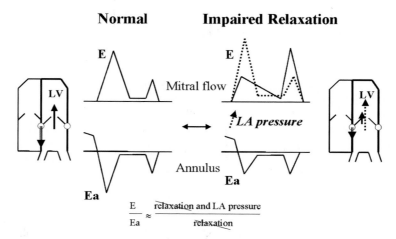

Fig. 3. Diagram showing mitral filling pattern, mitral annulus velocities, and corresponding four-chamber view during early diastole. Normal left ventricular (LV) diastole (left panel) is characterized by swift myocardial relaxation and elastic recoil. Therefore, normal transmitral flow is characterized by a prominent and rapid early (E) filling wave (arrow) caused by passive suction and by a diminutive late (A) atrial filling wave caused by atrial contraction. During diastole, there is a longitudinal expansion of the LV, resulting in a descent of the mitral annulus (open arrow) opposed to the relatively fixed apex. Because the velocity of the earliest diastolic motion of the mitral valve annulus (Ea) relates to the rate of myocardial relaxation, Ea is prominent in normal hearts. In heart disease myocardial relaxation is impaired. LV pressure falls slowly, reducing early transmitral driving pressure. This results in a decreased E (arrow) and, because of increased atrial preload, increased A (right panel). Because of decreased myocardial relaxation velocity, Ea is reduced (open arrow). With further progression of heart disease, impairment of LV compliance occurs, and LV filling becomes dependent on increased left atrial (LA) or filling pressure (dashed arrow). As a result, E increases. Therefore, the underlying impaired relaxation is masked. Because the pattern resembles the normal mitral filling pattern, it is called a pseudonormalized pattern. By combining E, which is dependent on both filling pressure and myocardial relaxation, with Ea, which is mainly dependent on myocardial relaxation, differentiation of a normal from a pseudonormal signal and better evaluation of filling pressures are possible. E, peak mitral velocity in early diastole; Ea, early diastolic tissue velocity. Reprinted from ref. *14*, copyright 2005, with permission from Elsevier.

allows reproducible alignment with jets of any orientation, avoiding echocardiographer-dependent difficulties in obtaining correct flow velocity profiles *(30)*.

Myocardial Velocities

By decreasing velocity encoding, phase contrast MRI velocity mapping allows measurement of myocardial velocities or tissue MRI *(14)*. The transmitral flow is not only dependent on left atrial (LA) pressure, but also affected by different degrees of LV elastic recoil, myocardial relaxation, and chamber and atrial compliance. As a result, the transmitral filling pattern is a dynamic phenomenon, and its use as a single parameter is restricted, especially in patients with LV hypertrophy *(31, 32)* and normal systolic function *(33)*. By normalizing phase contrast MRI-assessed early mitral velocity (E) for the influence of myocardial relaxation by combining E with tissue MRI-assessed early diastolic mitral septal tissue velocity (Ea), better estimation of LV filling pressure similar to Doppler is made possible *(14)* (Figs. 3 and 4). As early diastolic long-axis myocardial velocities have a significant effect on LV filling, they were found to correlate with the classical early filling parameters *(14,34)*. Velocity encoding of the myocardium in three

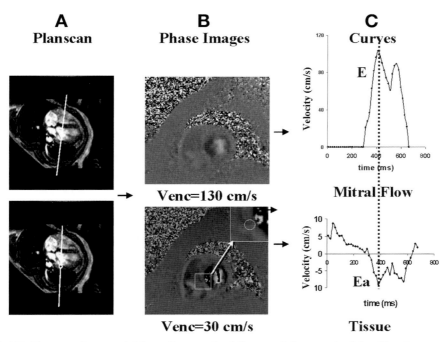

Fig. 4. (A) Planscan for acquisition of transmitral flow and tissue velocities. For the assessment of transmitral flow, a phase contrast MRI sequence was used with a velocity encoding of 130 cm/second. The center of the slice was positioned perpendicular to mitral inflow, at early diastole (upper panel). For the assessment of tissue MRI velocities, phase contrast MRI was repeated with a velocity encoding of 30 cm/second and the image slice positioned at two-thirds of the long axis, planned on early diastolic two- and four-chamber images, perpendicular to the interventricular septum (lower panel). **(B)** Velocity-encoded images for the assessment of transmitral flow (upper) and tissue velocities (lower). The tissue velocities are measured from a circular region of interest of 20 pixels in the posteroseptal region. **(C)** Velocity-vs-time curves. From these curves, peak mitral velocity in early diastole E = 103 cm/second, early diastolic posteroseptal tissue velocity Ea = 8.9 cm/second, and E/Ea = 11.6 cm/second were derived. Venc, velocity encoding; ROI, region of interest. Reprinted from ref. *14*, copyright 2005, with permission from Elsevier.

directions evaluates three-dimensional global and regional LV and RV motion throughout the whole cardiac cycle with a high spatial and temporal resolution *(35)*.

Myocardial Strains

Patterns of ventricular filling and flow only indirectly reflect diastolic myocardial function compared to patterns of myocardial wall motion. During diastole, the LV rotates (untwisting), translates, and extends radially. Segmental contribution to this complex motion is different: untwisting is opposite in basal (counterclockwise rotation when viewed from the apex) compared to apical (clockwise rotation) segments, and radial displacement is highest in the endocardial layer compared to the epicardial layer *(36)*. Untwisting or recoil of torsion is a largely isovolumic event. Therefore, the rate of recoil was shown to provide a noninvasive and preload-independent assessment of LV relaxation or τ *(37)*.

By measurement of the displacement of the tag lines, tagged MRI has the unique ability to quantify this complex myocardial deformation or strain not only globally but also regionally at different time-points during the cardiac cycle. Some investigators have calculated strains on the endocardial and epicardial surfaces *(36)* and strains

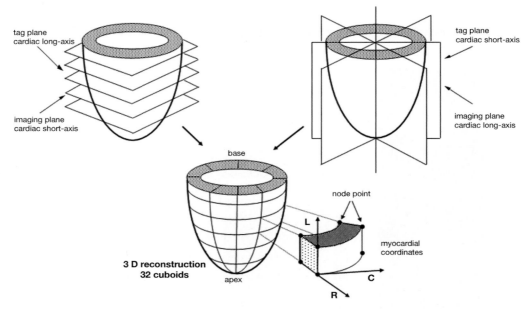

Fig. 5. MRI tagging and strain analysis. In each cuboid radial, circumferential and longitudinal strains can be measured. Reprinted from ref. *52*, copyright 2000, with permission from Elsevier.

originating from rotation of the apex relative to its base *(38)* (Fig. 5). When used in combination with dobutamine-tagged MRI, automated myocardial strain analysis might be a powerful tool in detecting early ischemia in different myocardial segments *(19)*.

Myocardial Energy Content

Myocardial relaxation is an active energy-dependent process. Phosphorus 31 cardiac MRI spectroscopy offers a unique opportunity to study the myocardial high-energy phosphate metabolism *(21)*. The ratio of levels of PCR and ATP or PCr/ATP reflecting the energy status of tissue have been associated with disturbed diastolic function *(39)*.

APPLICATIONS IN CARDIAC DISEASE

Assessment of diastolic heart function by cardiac MRI has been performed in numerous clinical settings, including hypertrophic cardiomyopathy, LV hypertrophy, coronary artery disease, and congenital heart disease (Table 2).

Hypertrophic Cardiomyopathy

Impaired diastolic filling results from myocyte hypertrophy and disarrangement, interstitial fibrosis, impaired inactivation and contraction loading, nonuniform temporal and regional distribution of load, and inactivation *(40)*. Because of prolongation of LV pressure decay, an upward shifting and flattening of the diastolic LV pressure–volume relation is seen *(40)*. Prolonged time to PFR and time–to–peak rate of wall thinning occur with underlying impaired relaxation. Nonuniform myocardial hypertrophy and fibrosis contribute to regional diastolic dysfunction. Regional heterogeneity in diastolic dysfunction is obvious from regionally prolonged time-to-peak wall thinning rate *(41)*.

Table 2
Applications in Cardiac Disease

Disease (reference)	Technique	Findings
HCM (41)	GRE	Impairment of regional relaxation
HCM (42)	Tagging	↓ Circumferential curvatures
HCM (43)	Tagging	↓ Early diastolic strain rates
HCM (44)	Spectroscopy	↓ PCr/ATP in symptomatic patients
HCM (45)	Spectroscopy	↓ PCr/ATP in asymptomatic patients
AS (28)	Phase contrast	Volumetric mitral flow correlates with Doppler
AS (48)	Phase contrast	Improvement of diastolic filling after valve replacement
AS (49)	Tagging	Prolonged and delayed untwisting
Hypertension (39)	Spectroscopy	↓ PCr/ATP correlates with impaired relaxation
Diabetes mellitus (50)	Phase contrast spectroscopy	Diastolic dysfunction is associated with ↓ PCr/ATP in asymptomatic patients
Previous MI (51)	Phase contrast	Early diastolic filling velocities correlate with Doppler
Previous MI (53)	Tagging	Nonuniform, delayed, and prolonged untwisting
CAD/previous MI (56)	GRE	↓ Early diastolic long-axis velocity
Fallot (60)	Phase contrast	Restrictive flow is associated with ↓ exercise
Mustard/Senning (59)	Phase contrast	Restrictive tricuspid flow
Fallot (58)	GRE	Impaired ventricular filling corrlates with exercise
RVPO (42)	Tagging	Strain heterogeneity
ARVD (62)	GRE	↓ Left and right ventricular peak filling rate

ARVD, arrhythmogenic right ventricular dysplasia; AS, aortic stenosis; ATP, adenosine triphosphate; CAD, coronary artery disease; GRE, gradient echo; HCM, hypertrophic cardiomyopathy; LVH, left ventricular hypertrophy; MI, myocardial infarction; PCr, phosphocreatine; RVPO, right ventricular pressure overload.

Analysis of the tagged images revealed marked changes in ventricular shape and function, displaying smaller circumferential curvatures (42) and reduced early diastolic strain rates in hypertrophied segments (43). Finally, phosphorus 31 MRI spectroscopy detected an altered myocardial high-energy phosphate metabolism in both symptomatic (44) and asymptomatic (45) patients with hypertrophic cardiomyopathy. The decrease in PCr/ATP ratio was also associated with the extent of hypertrophy (45). Possibly the lower myocardial energy content may contribute to relaxation abnormalities in hypertrophic hearts (39).

LV Hypertrophy

The LV responds to chronic pressure overload such as systemic hypertension and aortic valve stenosis by developing hypertrophy, with addition of new sarcomeres in parallel to existing ones to normalize wall tension *(46)*. Diastolic dysfunction occurs because of impaired relaxation together with a variable degree of altered passive viscoelastic properties *(47)*. Prolongation of the isovolumic relaxation is an early and sensitive marker of diastolic dysfunction and can be present in hypertensive patients even in the absence of structural myocardial dysfunction. Delayed and impaired myocardial relaxation is apparent from a depressed ratio of early LV filling to LA contribution (E/A < 1), which can be measured accurately by phase contrast MRI velocity mapping.

Delay and prolongation of diastolic untwisting as shown by MRI-tagged data may in part be responsible for the decrease in relaxation rate and diminished early diastolic filling velocity *(48)*. Prolongation of diastolic untwisting is present in pathological hypertrophy as found in the pressure-overloaded heart *(48)* and may be useful to differentiate physiological hypertrophy as found in athletes. In addition, pathological hypertrophy could potentially be distinguished from physiological hypertrophy by measuring the myocardial energy content. After aortic valve replacement, LV diastolic function improves, as apparent from transmitral volumetric flow parameters *(49)*.

Even in the absence of evident LV hypertrophy, impaired LV filling in hypertensive heart disease has been associated with a decreased PCr/ATP ratio or subnormal myocardial high-energy phosphate metabolism using phosphorus 31 MRI spectroscopy *(39)*. These data support the hypothesis that the lower content of myocardial PCr leads to an impaired relaxation in cardiomyocytes or diastolic dysfunction at the cellular level through impaired Ca^{2+} sequestration. Possibly these metabolic changes occur early in hypertension, even before changes in cardiac function become apparent *(39)*. Similar findings were found in normotensive and uncomplicated type 2 diabetes patients *(50)*.

Coronary Artery Disease: Ischemia and Previous Myocardial Infarction

Even at rest, impairment of diastolic function frequently occurs in ischemic heart disease. More pronounced abnormalities appear during acute ischemia. Diastolic dysfunction precedes systolic dysfunction and occurs as the earliest sign of myocardial ischemia (ischemic cascade). In patients with coronary artery disease and previous myocardial infarction, phase contrast MRI velocity mapping has been used accurately to measure mitral valve flow and shows close agreement with Doppler *(51)*.

Because of regional heterogeneity of myocardial function in coronary artery disease because of different degrees of ischemia, infarction, postinfarction LV shape changes or remodeling, myocardial stunning, and hibernation, various and complex changes in diastolic function have been recognized. MRI tagging has been used to assess three-dimensional strains in the postinfarcted remodeling LV. A reduction of systolic strains was observed in both the infarcted and—to a lesser extent—the remote regions *(52)*. The impact of these changes in ventricular shape and contraction on regional diastolic function and strains in the adjacent and remote myocardium needs further study.

In anterolateral infarction, diastolic untwisting was shown to be nonuniform, delayed, and prolonged *(53)*. Similar changes occur in hibernating myocardium *(36)* and transmural ischemia *(54)*. Although some authors found restoration of the untwisting motion *(54)*, others found persistent reduced strain rates despite complete functional recovery after reperfused myocardial infarction *(55)*. Less-sophisticated evaluation of regional diastolic function has been performed using phase contrast MRI in patients with previous myocardial infarction and angina. These data showed significantly reduced regional early diastolic long-axis myocardial velocities influencing LV filling *(56)*.

Congenital Heart Disease

Cardiac MRI is the primary imaging modality for the evaluation of physiology and function in corrected congenital heart disease *(57)*. The use of transthoracic echocardiography is often restricted because surgical scar, bone, or lung tissue may interfere with the acoustic window, and chest deformations may be present *(57)*. In addition, the study of the right ventricle is possible without any geometrical assumptions of its shape.

Phase contrast MRI velocity mapping of both tricuspid valve and pulmonary artery provides information on the diastolic filling pattern of the right ventricle in the presence of pulmonary regurgitation and allows the construction of a right ventricular time–volume curve *(58)*. Restrictive tricuspid flow patterns have been found using phase contrast MRI velocity mapping after a Mustard or Senning operation *(59)*. In arrhythmogenic right ventricular dysplasia, both regional and global right ventricular and LV PFRs are reduced *(60)*.

Right ventricular diastolic function after repair of congenital heart disease has major prognostic value. In patients who underwent primary repair of tetralogy of Fallot in infancy, reduced early diastolic filling fraction and reduced PFR derived from GRE-generated images were associated with pulmonary insufficiency and diminished exercise performance *(61)*. Restriction to right ventricular filling was identified by increased early tricuspid filling rate and decreased deceleration time together with diastolic forward pulmonary flow and accompanied with decreased exercise performance *(58)*. Pressure overload and secondary hypertrophy have been shown to affect right ventricular diastolic function. As diastolic filling abnormalities may precede systolic dysfunction, the assessment of postoperative diastolic ventricular performance may provide early information on the development of right ventricular dysfunction *(61)*.

Heterogeneity in local strains as shown by high circumferential and longitudinal septal flattening in right ventricular pressure overload have been found using three-dimensional tagged images *(42)*. In functionally single LVs (e.g., tricuspid atresia) after Fontan procedure, MR tagging could demonstrate a large regional strain dispersion. As systolic and diastolic functions are closely interrelated, an abnormal ventricular systolic twist impairs optimal storage of potential energy necessary for diastolic recoil and optimal diastolic filling *(62)*.

ASSESSMENT OF DIASTOLIC HEART FUNCTION IN CLINICAL PRACTICE

For the assessment of diastolic heart function, cine images are made using a GRE technique. Usually, a data set of 10–12 (depending on cardiac size) multiphase slices is acquired using breath holding ranging from several to about 20 seconds, depending essentially on available technique (one slice or multislice per breath hold, parallel acquisition technique, or not) and heart rate, the size of the image matrix (determines number of phase-encoding steps), together with aimed resolution and signal-to-noise ratio. Each slice can be imaged the same way using a tagging technique. Phase contrast MRI in an imaging plane perpendicular to flow direction (adjusted in three directions) can be performed for both atrioventricular valves. To avoid aliasing, one needs to chose a velocity sensitivity high enough (e.g., 130 cm/second for mitral valve). When using retrospective gating, acquisition time typically ranges from 3 to 4 minutes for each flow measurement. In addition, tissue MRI can be performed by decreasing velocity encoding (30 cm/second).

Data acquisition for a comprehensive cardiac MRI assessment of diastolic function typically includes a multislice short-axis cine data set of the ventricles and phase contrast flow velocity mapping of atrioventricular valves and requires about 30–45 minutes. Phosporus 31 cardiac MR spectroscopy necessitates a special surface coil. Total acquisition time for ^{31}P MR spectra is about 10 minutes *(39)*.

CONCLUSIONS

Cardiac MRI is a powerful noninvasive technique with the unique potential for three-dimensional analysis of diastolic function. Cardiac MRI quantifies both global and regional diastolic function with great accuracy and reproducibility, including analysis of diastolic velocity and volume flow, volumetric assessment of ventricular chamber volume, analysis of myocardial strains, and assessment of energy content.

ACKNOWLEDGMENT

Part of the manuscript for this chapter is reproduced from ref. *8*, copyright 2002, with permission from Elsevier.

REFERENCES

1. Zile MR, Brutsaert DL. New concepts in diastolic dysfunction and diastolic heart failure: part I: diagnosis, prognosis, and measurements of diastolic function. Circulation 2002;105:1387–1393.
2. Zile MR, Brutsaert DL. New concepts in diastolic dysfunction and diastolic heart failure: Part II: causal mechanisms and treatment. Circulation 2002;105:1503–1508.
3. Grossman W. Defining diastolic dysfunction. Circulation 2000;101:2020–2021.
4. Vasan RS, Benjamin EJ. Diastolic heart failure—no time to relax. N Engl J Med 2001;344:56–59.
5. Stevenson LW. Tailored therapy to hemodynamic goals for advanced heart failure. Eur J Heart Fail 1999;1:251–257.
6. Appleton CP, Firstenberg MS, Garcia MJ, Thomas JD. The echo-Doppler evaluation of left ventricular diastolic function: a current perspective. Cardiol Clin 2000;18:513–546.
7. Nagueh SF, Middleton KJ, Kopelen HA, Zoghbi WA, Quinones MA. Doppler tissue imaging: a noninvasive technique for evaluation of left ventricular relaxation and estimation of filling pressures. J Am Coll Cardiol 1997;30:1527–1533.
8. Paelinck BP, Lamb HJ, Bax JJ, Van der Wall EE, de Roos A. Assessment of diastolic function by cardiovascular magnetic resonance. Am Heart J 2002;144:198–205.
9. Reeder SB, Faranesh AZ. Ultrafast pulse sequence techniques for cardiac magnetic resonance imaging. Top Magn Reson Imaging 2000;11:312–330.
10. Pettigrew RI, Oshinski JN, Chatzimavroudis G, Dixon WT. MRI techniques for cardiovascular imaging. J Magn Reson Imaging 1999;10:590–601.
11. van der Geest RJ, Reiber JH. Quantification in cardiac MRI. J Magn Reson Imaging 1999;10:602–608.
12. Szolar DH, Sakuma H, Higgins CB. Cardiovascular applications of magnetic resonance flow and velocity measurements. J Magn Reson Imaging 1996;1:78–89.
13. Kozerke S, Scheidegger MB, Pedersen EM, Boesiger P. Heart motion adapted cine phase-contrast flow measurements through the aortic valve. Magn Reson Med 1999;42:970–978.
14. Paelinck BP, de Roos A, Bax JJ, et al. Feasibility of tissue magnetic resonance imaging: a pilot study in comparison with tissue Doppler imaging and invasive measurement. J Am Coll Cardiol 2005;45:1109–1016.
15. WedeenVJ. Magnetic resonance imaging of myocardial kinematics: technique to detect, localize, and quantify the strain rates of the active human myocardium. Magn Reson Med 1992;27:52–67.
16. Zerhouni EA, Parish DM, Rogers WJ, Yang A, Shapiro EP. Human heart: tagging with MR imaging–a method for non-invasive assessment of myocardial motion. Radiology 1988;169:59–63.
17. Axel L, Dougherty L. MR imaging of motion with spatial modulation of magnetization. Radiology 1989;171:841–845.
18. Fischer SE, McKinnon GC, Scheidegger MB, Prins W, Meier D, Boesiger P. True myocardial motion tracking. Magn Reson Med 1994;31:401–413.

19. Garot J, Bluemke DA, Osman NF, et al. Fast determination of regional myocardial strain fields from tagged cardiac images using harmonic phase MRI. Circulation 2000;101:981–988.
20. Declerck J, Denney TS, Ozturk C, O'Dell W, McVeigh ER. Left ventricular motion reconstruction from planar tagged MR images: a comparison. Phys Med Biol 2000;45:1611–1632.
21. Bottomley PA. Noninvasive study of high-energy phosphate metabolism in human heart by depth-resolved ^{31}P-NMR spectroscopy. Science 1985;229:769–772.
22. Suzuki J, Caputo GR, Masui T, Chang JM, O'Sullivan M, Higgins CB. Assessment of right ventricular diastolic and systolic function in patients with dilated cardiomyopathy using cine magnetic resonance imaging. Am Heart J 1991;122:1035–1040.
23. Fujita N, Hartiala J, O'Sullivan M, et al. Assessment of left ventricular diastolic function in dilated cardiomyopathy with cine magnetic resonance imaging: effect of an angiotensin converting enzyme inhibitor, benzepril. Am Heart J 1993;125:171–178.
24. Lamb HJ, Singleton RR, van der Geest RJ, Pohost GM, de Roos A. MR imaging of regional cardiac function: low-pass filtering of wall thickness curves. Magn Reson Med 1995;34:498–502.
25. Mohiaddin RH, Gatehouse PD, Henien M, Firmin DN. Cine MR Fourier velocimetry of blood flow through cardiac valves: comparison with Doppler echocardiography. J Magn Reson Imaging 1997;7:657–663.
26. Hartiala JJ, Mostbeck GH, Foster E, et al. Velocity-encoded cine MRI in the evaluation of left ventricular diastolic function. Measurement of mitral valve and pulmonary vein flow velocities and flow volume across the mitral valve. Am Heart J 1993;125:1054–1066.
27. Kayser HWM, Stoel BC, van der Wall EE, van der Geest RJ, de Roos A. MR velocity mapping of tricuspid flow: correction for through-plane motion. J Magn Reson Imaging 1997;7:669–673.
28. Hartiala JJ, Foster E, Fujita N, et al. Evaluation of left atrial contribution to left ventricular filling in aortic stenosis by velocity-encoded cine MRI. Am Heart J 1994;127:593–600.
29. Kasprzak JD, Paelinck B, Ten Cate FJ, et al. Comparison of native and contrast-enhanced harmonic echocardiography for visualization of left ventricular endocardial border. Am J Cardiol 1999;83:211–217.
30. Fyrenius A, Wigstrom L, Bolger AF, et al. Pitfalls in Doppler evaluation of diastolic function: insights from three-dimensional magnetic resonance imaging. J Am Soc Echocardiogr 1999;12:817–826.
31. Nishimura RA, Appleton CP, Redfield MM, Ilstrup DM, Holmes DR Jr, Tajik AJ. Noninvasive Doppler echocardiographic evaluation of left ventricular filling pressures in patients with cardiomyopathies: a simultaneous Doppler echocardiographic and cardiac catheterization study. J Am Coll Cardiol 1996;28:1226–1233.
32. Nagueh SF, Lakkis NM, Middleton KJ, Spencer WH 3rd, Zoghbi WA, Quinones MA. Doppler estimation of left ventricular filling pressures in patients with hypertrophic cardiomyopathy. Circulation 1999;99:254–261.
33. Yamamoto K, Nishimura RA, Chaliki HP, Appleton CP, Holmes DR Jr, Redfield MM. Determination of left ventricular filling pressure by Doppler echocardiography in patients with coronary artery disease: critical role of left ventricular systolic function. J Am Coll Cardiol 1997;30:1819–1826.
34. Karwatowski SP, Mohiaddin RH, Yang GZ, et al. Assessment of regional left ventricular long-axis motion with MR velocity mapping in healthy subjects. J Magn Reson Imaging 1994;4:151–155.
35. Kayser HWM, van der Geest RJ, van der Wall EE, Duchateau C, de Roos A. Right ventricular function in patients after acute myocardial infarction assessed with phase contrast MR velocity mapping encoded in three directions. J Magn Reson Imaging 2000;11:471–475.
36. Rademakers FE, Rogers WJ, Guier WH, et al. Relation of regional cross-fiber shortening to wall thickening in the intact heart. Three-dimensional strain analysis by NMR tagging. Circulation 1994;89:1174–1182.
37. Dong SJ, Hees PS, Siu CO, Weiss JL, Shapiro EP. MRI assessment of LV relaxation by untwisting rate: a new isovolumic phase measure of τ. Am J Physiol Heart Circ Physiol 2001;281:2002–2009.
38. Fogel MA, Weinberg PM, Hubbard A, Haselgrove J. Diastolic biomechanics in normal infants utilizing MRI tissue tagging. Circulation 2000;102:218–224.
39. Lamb HJ, Beyerbacht HP, van der Laarse A, et al. Diastolic dysfunction in hypertensive heart disease is associated with altered myocardial metabolism. Circulation 1999;99:2261–2267.
40. Pak PH, Maughan WL, Baughman KL, Kass DA. Marked discordance between dynamic and passive diastolic pressure-volume relations in idiopathic hypertrophic cardiomyopathy. Circulation 1996;94:52–60.

41. Yamanari H, Kakishita M, Fujimoto Y, et al. Regional myocardial perfusion abnormalities and regional myocardial early diastolic dysfunction in patients with hypertrophic cardiomyopathy. Heart Vessels 1997;12:192–198.

42. Petrank YF, Dong SJ, Tyberg J, Sideman S, Beyar R. Regional differences in shape and load in normal and diseased hearts studied by three dimensional tagged magnetic resonance imaging. Int J Card Imaging 1999;15:309–321.

43. Rademakers FE, Buchalter MB, Rogers WJ, et al. Dissociation between left ventricular untwisting and filling. Accentuation by catecholamines. Circulation 1992;85:1572–1581.

44. De Roos A, Doornbos J, Luyten PR, et al. Cardiac metabolism in patients with dilated and hypertrophic cardiomyopathy: assessment with proton-decoupled P-31 MR spectroscopy. J Magn Reson Imaging 1992;2:711–719.

45. Jung WI, Sieverding L, Breuer J, et al. ^{31}P NMR spectroscopy detects metabolic abnormalities in asymptomatic patients with hypertrophic cardiomyopathy. Circulation 1998;97:2536–2542.

46. Stuber M, Scheidegger MB, Fischer SE, et al. Alterations in the local myocardial motion pattern in patients suffering from pressure overload due to aortic stenosis. Circulation 1999;100:361–368.

47. Mandinov L, Eberli FR, Hess OM. Diastolic heart failure. Cardiovasc Res 2000;45:813–825.

48. Nagel E, Stuber M, Burkhard B, et al. Cardiac rotation and relaxation in patients with aortic valve stenosis. Eur Heart J 2000;21:582–589.

49. Lamb HJ, Beyerbacht HP, de Roos A, et al. Left ventricular remodelling early after aortic valve replacement: differential effects on diastolic function in aortic valve stenosis and aortic regurgitation. J Am Coll Cardiol 2002;40:2182–2188.

50. Diamant M, Lamb HJ, Groeneveld Y, et al. Diastolic dysfunction is associated with altered myocardial metabolism in asymptomatic normotensive patients with well-controlled type 2 diabetes mellitus. J Am Coll Cardiol 2003;42:328–335.

51. Karwatowski SP, Brecker SJD, Yang GZ, Firmin DN, Sutton MS, Underwood SR. Mitral valve flow measured with cine MR velocity mapping in patients with ischemic heart disease: comparison with Doppler echocardiography. J Magn Reson Imaging 1995;5:89–92.

52. Bogaert J, Bosmans H, Maes A, Suetens P, Marchal G, Rademakers FE. Remote myocardial dysfunction after acute anterior myocardial infarction: impact of left ventricular shape on regional function. J Am Coll Cardiol 2000;35:1525–1534.

53. Nagel E, Stuber M, Lakatos M, Scheidegger MB, Boesiger P, Hess OM. Cardiac rotation and relaxation after anterolateral myocardial infarction. Coron Artery Dis 2000;10:261–267.

54. Kroeker CA, Tyberg JV, Beyar R. Effects of ischemia on left ventricular apex rotation. An experimental study in anaesthetized dogs. Circulation 1995;92:3539–3548.

55. Azevedo CF, Amado LC, Kraitchman DL, et al. Persistent diastolic dysfunction despite complete systolic functional recovery after reperfused acute myocardial infarction demonstrated by tagged magnetic resonance imaging. Eur Heart J 2004;25:1419–1427.

56. Karwatowski SP, Brecker SJD, Yang GZ, Firmin DN, St John Sutton M, Underwood SR. A comparison of left ventricular myocardial velocity in diastole measured by magnetic resonance and left ventricular filling measured by Doppler echocardiography. Eur Heart J 1996;17:795–802.

57. Roest AA, Helbing WA, van der Wall EE, de Roos A. Postoperative evaluation of congenital heart disease by magnetic resonance imaging. J Magn Reson Imaging 1999;10:656–666.

58. Helbing WA, Niezen RA, Le Cessie S, van der Geest RJ, Ottenkamp J, de Roos A. Right ventricular diastolic function in children with pulmonary regurgitation after repair of tetralogy of Fallot: volumetric evaluation by magnetic resonance velocity mapping. J Am Coll Cardiol 1996;28:1827–1835.

59. Rebergen SA, Helbing WA, van der Wall EE, Maliepaard C, Chin JG, de Roos A. MR velocity mapping of tricuspid flow in healthy children and in patients who have undergone Mustard or Senning repair. Radiology 1995;194:505–512.

60. Bomma C, Dalal D, Tandri H, et al. Regional differences in systolic and diastolic function in arrhythmogenic right ventricular dysplasia/cardiomyopathy using magnetic resonance imaging. Am J Cardiol 2005;95:1507–1511.

61. Singh GK, Greenberg SB, Yap YS, Delany DP, Keeton BR, Monro JL. Right ventricular function and exercise performance late after primary repair of tetralogy of Fallot with the transannular patch in infancy. Am J Cardiol 1998;81:1378–1382.

62. Fogel MA, Weinberg PM, Gupta KB, et al. Mechanics of the single left ventricle. A study in ventricular-ventricular interaction II. Circulation 1998;98:330–338.

21 Cardiac and Pericardial Tumors

Maung M. Khin and Raymond Y. Kwong

CONTENTS

BENIGN TUMORS
MALIGNANT TUMORS
NONNEOPLASTIC CARDIAC MASSES
CONCLUSION
REFERENCES

Primary cardiac and pericardial tumors are rare and affect patients of all ages. Primary cardiac tumors have a reported incidence between 0.0017 and 0.19% in autopsy series *(1)*. Approximately 75% of all cardiac tumors are benign histologically, and the remainder are malignant. Approximately half (52%) of the benign cardiac tumors are myxomas, which account for the most frequent primary cardiac tumor. Other less-common benign tumors include papillary fibroelastomas (16%), lipomas (16%), hemangiomas (6%), fibromas (3%), and rhabdomyomas (1%). Less frequently, teratomas, neurofibromas, lymphangiomas, cystic tumors of the atrioventricular node, endocrine tumors (paraganglioma), and histiocytoid tumors comprise the rest of benign tumors *(2,3)*.

Almost all malignant cardiac tumors (about 95%) are sarcomas, which represent the second most common primary cardiac tumor after myxoma. Sarcomas derive from mesenchyme and therefore may display a wide variety of morphological types, including angiosarcoma (28%); rhabdomyosarcoma (11%); fibrosarcoma (8%); osteosarcoma (7%); malignant fibrous histiocytoma (6%); leiomyosarcoma (5%); and myxosarcoma (3%); other sarcomas comprised of liposarcomas, synovial, and neurogenic sarcomas (14%) and undifferentiated sarcomas (12%). Lymphomas (5%) account for the remaining primary malignant cardiac tumors *(4,5)*. Benign tumors, rhabdomyomas, and fibromas and their malignant counterparts rhabdomyosarcomas and fibrosarcomas are more common in childhood and infancy *(5)*. Common pericardial tumors that affect the heart include benign teratomas and malignant mesotheliomas. Patients with primary cardiac tumor present with a wide range of symptoms that can simulate more common cardiac diseases. Patients with cardiac tumors often present with signs and symptoms of heart failure because of mechanical obstruction to filling or outflow, valvular dysfunction, interference with systolic function because of impaired contractility, and diastolic dysfunction caused by restrictive physiology. Arrhythmias ranging from conduction disturbances to supraventricular and ventricular tachyarrhythmia can occur depending

From: *Contemporary Cardiology: Cardiovascular Magnetic Resonance Imaging*
Edited by: Raymond Y. Kwong © Humana Press Inc., Totowa, NJ

on the location of the intracavitary or intramural tumors. Embolic phenomena are frequent, and dramatic events result from embolization of tumor fragments or thrombi from the surface of the intracavitary tumors *(5,6)*.

The clinical presentation is determined mostly by location, size, texture, rate of growth, and invasiveness of the tumor. Pericardial lesions may present as pericardial effusion. A rapidly developing pericardial effusion that leads to pericardial tamponade or a pericardial constriction from large pericardial involvement should cause suspicion of pericardial tumor *(7)*.

Metastases to the heart and pericardium are more common than primary cardiac tumors and are generally associated with a poor prognosis, primarily related to advanced stage of primary malignancy. Local invasion by surrounding tumor is usually limited to the pericardium. Common secondary metastases include lung cancer, breast cancer, melanoma, and lymphoma.

Advances in cardiac imaging greatly facilitate the diagnosis and management of cardiac tumors. Although transthoracic echocardiography is useful in the initial evaluation for screening, cardiovascular magnetic resonance (CMR) imaging and computed tomography (CT) provide additional information about the morphology, location, and extent of a cardiac neoplasm. Similar to CT in defining the pericardium, great vessels, extracardiac diseases, and metastases, CMR has advantages in superior spatial resolution, multiplanar imaging, characterization of tumor tissue, visualization of tumor perfusion, and differential enhancement of tumor with gadolinium relative to the surrounding normal myocardium *(8)*.

BENIGN TUMORS

Myxoma

Cardiac myxomas is the most common primary tumor of the heart and represent approximately 50% of benign tumors in adult but are a less-common benign tumor (17%) in children *(9)*. Originating from the subendocardial layer of primitive mesenchymal cells, myxomas usually grow into the cardiac chamber. Approximately 75% of myxomas are found in the left atrium, 15–20% in the right atrium, and rarely (5%) in the right or left ventricle. Most myxomas attach to the region of fossa ovalis of the interatrial septum *(10)*.

CLINICAL MANIFESTATIONS

Myxomas can affect patients from a wide age range (mean age of presentation is 50 years), with a female predominance (two-thirds) *(11,12)*. Most patients present with one or more of the triad of intracardiac obstruction, embolism, and constitutional symptoms *(13,14)*. Nearly 70% of patients with left atrial myxomas have symptoms of heart failure and syncope, which may be positional as a result of tumor obstruction to left ventricular inflow and regurgitation of mitral valve *(14,15)*. Right atrial myxomas may obstruct the tricuspid valve and cause symptoms of right-sided heart failure *(10,14)*.

Embolic phenomena are the second most common manifestation of cardiac myxoma, occurring in approximately 30–40% of patients *(12,14)*. Cerebral emboli are represented in two-thirds of patients and cause transient ischemic attacks, strokes, or seizures; half of them have peripheral limb emboli *(16)*. Polypoid, friable, and villous tumors are more likely to embolize *(10,16)*.

Rarely, infected left atrial myxoma may mimick those of infective endocarditis *(17,18)*. Nonspecific constitutional symptoms, fever, arthralgias, Raynaud's phenomenon, and an elevated erythrocyte sedimentation rate might initially be mistaken for collagen-vascular disease. Cardiac arrhythmias, including atrial fibrillation and flutter, have been reported in approximately 20% of all patients with cardiac myxomas *(11,15)*. Small myxomas give fewer symptoms than larger (>5 cm) tumors. Approximately 20% of patients with cardiac myxoma are asymptomatic *(19,20)*. Physical findings, usually on auscultation, include mitral systolic murmur, diastolic murmur, and occasionally characteristic tumor plop *(11,20)*.

Two types of cardiac myxomas have been described. The more common, nonfamilial type of sporadic myxomas (93%) tend to be solitary in the left atrium, with a low potential for regrowth after surgical excision *(21,22)*. The second, less-common familial type (7%) often assumes an atypical location (left atrium ~50%, right atrium ~40%, ventricles ~10%), are multicentric (45%), are more likely to regrow after surgical excision (12–22%), and can be associated with dermatological and endocrine abnormalities (20%), including the Carney complex. The familial type tends to present earlier (mean age 20 years) and is more common in males. However, myxomas in both groups are histologically indistinguishable *(21,22)*.

The Carney complex is an autosomal-dominant, inherited disorder in which cardiac myxomas occur in association with cutaneous and mammary myxomas; spotty skin pigmentation; endocrine overactivity (Cushing syndrome, sexual precocity, and acromegaly); psammomatous melanotic schwannoma; primary pigmented nodular adrenal disease; and testicular neoplasms, particularly large-cell calcifying Sertoli cell tumor. Two-thirds of patients with the Carney complex have coexisting cardiac myxoma, which represents a potentially serious but treatable component of the syndrome *(22)*.

PATHOLOGICAL FINDINGS

Cardiac myxomas often appear as endocardial masses attached to the endocardium by a broad-based or pedunculated stalk (approximately one-fourth are sessile) without underlying tissue infiltration. They can be firm and lobular, myxoid and gelatinous, or friable and irregular. Cut sections of tumors typically have a variegated appearance, occasionally with gritty calcified areas *(23)*.

DIAGNOSTIC IMAGING FEATURES

Radiological evidence of mitral valve dysfunction or obstruction can be seen as left atrial enlargement and pulmonary venous hypertension with pulmonary vascular redistribution and interstitial edema *(24)*. In addition to diagnosis of cardiac myxoma, transthoracic echocardiography can be used to evaluate associated valvular regurgitation or stenosis by cardiac Doppler. Transesophageal echocardiography provides a more detailed structure, attachment, and mobility, particularly in small atrial tumors *(25,26)*.

CMR with cine gradient echo imaging demonstrates tumors as spherical or ovoid lobular masses of heterogeneous signal intensity with the attachment to the endocardial surface in multiplanar views. On T_1-weighted images, the majority of myxomas are isointense relative to the adjacent myocardium. Heterogeneous enhancement with gadolinium is typical and is thought to result from the cellular matrix or inflammation within the tumors, whereas nonenhancing areas likely represent cysts or necrosis *(8,27)*.

Myxomatous components appear low in signal intensity on T_1- and high on T_2-weighted magnetic resonance (MR) images, possibly owing to abundant polysaccharide-rich ground substance in the lesion. Tumor calcification manifests as low signal intensity, and subacute hemorrhage displays high signal intensity on both T_1- and T_2-weighted images *(28)*. Fresh hemorrhage has intermediate-to-low signal intensity on T_1- and low signal intensity on T_2-weighted images *(29)*. Cine gradient echo imaging studies are helpful in demonstrating tumor motion and prolapse across the atrioventricular valve. Myxomas usually become dark on T_2*-weighted gradient echo imaging, probably because of the magnetic susceptibility effects of the high iron content of these lesions *(27)* (Table 1).

TREATMENT

Successful surgical excision portends an excellent long-term prognosis and a low risk of recurrence *(14,30)*. The tumor recurrence is likely related to the development of unsuspected multifocal myxomas rather than an inadequate surgical excision because only about one-third of resected lesions recur *in situ (31)*. Because of the risk of recurrence, especially in the group of patients with familial atypical myxomas, postoperative serial follow-up imaging is necessary *(21,30)*.

Papillary Fibroelastoma

CLINICAL MANIFESTATIONS

Papillary fibroelastoma is the second most common primary benign cardiac neoplasm. It affects men and women equally, and the average age at detection is 60 years. These benign endocardial papillomas predominantly affect the cardiac valves and account for approximately three-fourths of all cardiac valvular tumors *(32,33)*. Although most papillary fibroelastomas are found incidentally, affected patients may present with chest pain, transient ischemic attacks or stroke, dyspnea, or sudden death secondary to obstruction of the coronary ostia or embolization.

PATHOLOGICAL FINDINGS

Gelatinous masses with a characteristic "sea anemone" appearance are produced by multiple narrow branching papillary fronds (best seen by immersing the tumor in water). Although papillary fibroelastomas are found mainly on the aortic or mitral valves, away from the valvular free edges, they may also occur on the endocardial surfaces of the atria or ventricles. They are usually solitary lesions that measure 1 cm or less in diameter and attach to the endocardial surface by a pedicle.

DIAGNOSTIC IMAGING FEATURES

Most papillary fibroelastomas are discovered with echocardiography, which usually demonstrates a small (<1.5 cm), mobile, pedunculated, homogeneous valvular or endocardial mass that flutters or prolapses with cardiac motion. A characteristic shimmer or vibration at the tumor-blood interface, ascribed to the fingerlike projections of the tumor, has been described and is best appreciated on transesophageal echocardiography *(33)*. Occasionally, a stippled pattern is demonstrated on the surface of the tumor and correlates with its papillary surface projections *(34)*. Valvular dysfunction is usually not an associated finding.

Transthoracic echocardiography has a reported sensitivity of 62% and transesophageal echocardiography a sensitivity of 77% in one series *(35)*. Typically, these tumors are not well seen on CT because of limited assessment of the motion of the tumor. CMR imaging usually demonstrates a mass on a valve leaflet or on the endocardial surface of the affected cardiac chamber. Valvular papillary fibroelastomas can result in turbulence of blood flow, which may be demonstrated on cine gradient echo imaging *(36)*.

TREATMENT

Treatment is with simple surgical excision with possible leaflet repair or valve replacement. Recurrence after surgical resection has not been reported *(32,34)*.

Rhabdomyoma

CLINICAL MANIFESTATIONS

Cardiac rhabdomyomas are more common cardiac benign tumors in infants and children (up to 90%) and usually are discovered in infancy *(37)*. The majority of rhabdomyomas are associated with tuberous sclerosis complex. Nearly 50% of infants with tuberous sclerosis complex have associated rhabdomyomas *(38)*. The remainder of these tumors occurs sporadically or in association with congenital heart disease. Affected individuals are mostly asymptomatic, and the tumors may be detected in utero because of nonimmune fetal hydrops and fetal death. Other presenting features include tachyarrhythmias, murmurs, and heart failure.

PATHOLOGICAL FINDINGS

Tumors are firm, white, well-circumscribed, lobulated intramural nodules that occur anywhere in the myocardium (but are more common in the ventricles). They may appear as numerous miliary nodules measuring less than 1 mm in diameter (termed *rhabdomyomatosis*). An average size of tumor is 3–4 cm but it may measure up to 10 cm, especially in sporadic cases *(23)*.

DIAGNOSTIC IMAGING FEATURES

At echocardiography, tumors are seen as solid hyperechoic masses, usually in the ventricular myocardium or ventricular septum and possibly protruding into and deforming the cardiac chambers *(39)*. When the lesions are small and multiple, diffuse myocardial thickening is the only finding on echocardiography *(32)*. However, CMR may allow better definition of tumor margins and may help demonstrate individual lesions. Tumors have signal intensity that is similar to that of the adjacent myocardium on T_1-weighted images and display relatively increased signal intensity on T_2-weighted images *(40)* (Table 1) The CMR assessment of these tumors can be extremely helpful when aggressive life-saving surgical resection is considered *(41)*.

TREATMENT

Because the majority of cardiac rhabdomyomas regress spontaneously, surgery is not routinely required. Tumors regress in size, number, or both in most patients aged younger than 4 years and less so in older patients *(42)*. However, patients with life-threatening symptoms, usually those secondary to left ventricular outflow tract obstruction or refractory arrhythmias, respond well to surgical excision *(43,44)*.

Fibroma

CLINICAL MANIFESTATIONS

Cardiac fibroma is more common in children, one-third of whom are under 1 year of age, with the rest up to 56 years of age at the time of presentation (the mean age of presentation is 13 years). However, approximately 15% of cardiac fibromas occur in adolescents and adults *(45)*. There is an increased risk of cardiac fibroma in patients with Gorlin (basal cell nevus) syndrome, which is characterized by multiple nevoid basal cell carcinomas of the skin, jaw cysts, and bifid ribs. Cardiac fibromas occur in

Table 1
Features of Primary Benign Cardiac Tumors

Type and percentage in adults	Common population	Age associated features	Location of tumor	Type and Morphologic features	Echo features	CT feature	CMR feature
Myxoma (52%)	Younger adults (30–60 years)	Carney complex	Interatrial septum at fossa ovalis Left atrium	Gelatinous, heterogeneous with calcification, hemorrhage, or necrosis	Mobile tumor with narrow stalk Heterogeneous with hypo and hyperechoic foci	Heterogeneous, low attenuation Occasionally with calcification	T_1: Isointense with areas of hypo- and hyperintensity T_2: Hyperintense MDE: Heterogeneous enhancement
Papillary fibroelastoma (16%)	Middle-aged Elderly	None	Cardiac valves	Small (<1 cm), frondlike, narrow stalk calcification rare No hemorrhage or necrosis	Mobile mass with short pedicle and "shimmering" edges	Difficult to see small intracavitary tumor	Difficult to see small intracavitary tumor
Lipomas (16%)	Any age	A few cases associated with tuberous sclerosis	Pericardial space Left ventricle Right ventricle Inter-atrial septum	Very large, broad-based No calcification, hemorrhage, or necrosis	Hypoechoic in pericardial space Echogenic in a cardiac chamber	Homogeneous fat attenuation (low attenuation)	T_1: Hyperintense, homogeneous Hypointense with fat saturation T_2: Hyperintense MDE: No enhancement
Fibroma (3%)	Infants Children Young adults	Gorlin syndrome	Ventricle	Large, intramural intramural Calcification common No hemorrhage	Intramural, calcified	Low attenuation calcified	T_1: Iso or hyperintense T_2: Hypointense MDE: Heterogeneous enhancement

Tumor (%)	Age	Association	Location	Morphology	Echocardiography	CT	MRI
Rhabdomyomas (1%)	Children	Associated with tuberous sclerosis (50%)	Left ventricle Right ventricle Inter-ventricular septum	Lobulated intramural nodules (3–4 cm) Numerous miliary nodules (1 mm)	Multiple small, lobulated hyperechoic intramural masses	Difficult to see because density of tumor is similar to myocardium	T1: Isointense homogeneous T2: Hyperintense MDE: nonspecific
Hemangiomas (6%)	All ages	Kasabach-Merritt syndrome Multiple systemic hemangiomas	Left ventricle Right ventricle Interventricular septum	Sessile or polypoid subendocardial nodule (2–4 cm)	Hyperechoic	Heterogeneous Calcification	T1: Isointense T2: Hyperintense MDE: Marked enhancement
Teratomas (1%)	Infants Children	Pericardial effusion and tamponade Fetal hydrops	Pericardium Right atrium Right ventricle Interatrial or inter-ventricular septum	Lobulated with multiple cystic cavities	Very heterogeneous Pericardial effusion	Very heterogeneous	Very heterogeneous
Paraganglioma (<5%)	Young adults	Sporadic Paragangliomas in other locations	Left atrium Coronary arteries Aortic root	Broad based, infiltrative, or circumscribed Hemorrhage or necrosis	Echogenic, relatively immobile	Low attenuation	T1: Isointense or hypointense T2: Hyperintense MDE: Marked enhancement
Lymphangioma (<5%)	Infants Children	Associated with other lymphangioma	Pericardial space	Large, cystic No calcification, hemorrhage or necrosis	Heterogeneous, septated, hypoechoic	Heterogeneous, septated	T1: Heterogeneous T2: Hyperintense MDE: Heterogeneous enhancement

*T_1 = T_1-weighted images; T_2 = T_2-weighted images; MDE = myocardial delayed enhancement.

fewer than 14% of these patients *(46)*. Common clinical manifestations in patients with cardiac fibromas are heart failure, arrhythmias, and sudden death. The most common cause of death from this tumor is arrhythmia, considered to be caused by invasion or compression of the cardiac conduction system. One-third of patients are asymptomatic, and their tumors are discovered because of a cardiac murmur detected during physical examination or at chest radiography. Embolic sequelae are not a feature of cardiac fibromas.

PATHOLOGICAL FINDINGS

Fibromas are round, bulging, well-circumscribed tumors located within the ventricular myocardium, often extending into or even obliterating the chamber lumen. Tumors are always single and range in size from 2 to 10 cm. Cut sections of cardiac fibromas reveal firm or rubbery masses without cysts, hemorrhage, or necrosis. They may display well-circumscribed or infiltrating margins. Tumor calcification is common, may be multifocal, and is occasionally evident at pathological examination *(45)*.

DIAGNOSTIC IMAGING FEATURES

Cardiomegaly is the most frequently observed radiographic abnormality. When the tumor involves the ventricular free wall, a focal cardiac bulge or contour abnormality may also be seen. Radiographic evidence of intramural calcification (approximately 25% of cases) suggests cardiac fibroma as the prospective diagnosis *(47)*. Echocardiography reveals an echogenic mass that may display heterogeneous echogenicity. Multifocal, central tumor calcifications are occasionally identified. The affected myocardium is usually hypokinetic *(45)*.

CT usually demonstrates a heterogeneous mural mass and has a high sensitivity for the detection of tumoral calcification. These lesions typically enhance homogeneously or heterogeneously after intravenous administration of contrast material. An associated pericardial effusion may be seen but is not a predominant feature *(45)*.

CMR reveals tumor as a discrete mural mass or focal myocardial thickening. The lesion appears isointense (Fig. 1A) to hyperintense relative to myocardium on T_1-weighted and hypointense on T_2-weighted images, which are characteristic findings of fibrous tissue. After gadolinium administration, fibroma typically demonstrates marked contrast enhancement because of high per voxel accumulation of gadolinium in fibrous tissues (Fig. 1B,C). However, on first-pass perfusion, fibroma usually does not enhance because of low tissue vascularity.

TREATMENT

For symptomatic patients with cardiac fibroma, surgical excision usually gives satisfactory results. Patients with extensive tumors that are not entirely resectable can benefit from partial tumor excision *(48)*. The surgical outcome is less favorable in patients with large masses, severe heart failure at initial presentation, or recurrent arrhythmias in the neonatal period or early infancy *(49)*. Tumors may remain stable in size for years or may even regress *(45)*. Recurrence of tumor after surgery is rare *(47)*.

Hemangioma

CLINICAL MANIFESTATIONS

Cardiac hemangiomas are rare benign vascular tumors that account for approximately 5–10% of benign cardiac tumors. All age groups are affected. The majority of affected

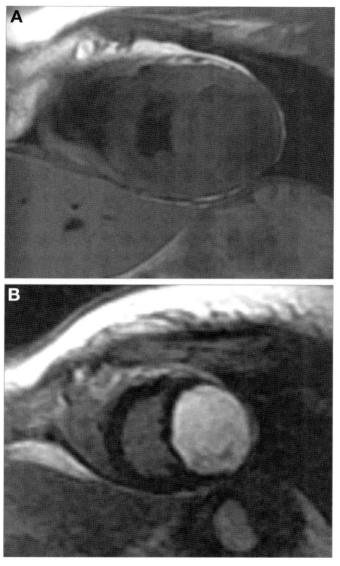

Fig. 1. *(Continued)*

patients are asymptomatic, and tumors are discovered incidentally *(23)*. In symptomatic patients, the most common presenting symptoms are dyspnea on exertion, heart failure, chest pain, pericarditis, pericardial effusion (which may be hemorrhagic), arrhythmias, syncope, and sudden death. Cardiac hemangiomas can occur in the clinical setting of Kasabach-Merritt syndrome, which is characterized by multiple systemic hemangiomas associated with recurrent thrombocytopenia and consumptive coagulopathy.

PATHOLOGICAL FINDINGS

Cardiac hemangiomas can occur in any chamber but more commonly are found in the lateral wall of the left ventricle, the anterior wall of the right ventricle, and the interventricular septum. They may be predominantly intramural or endocardial

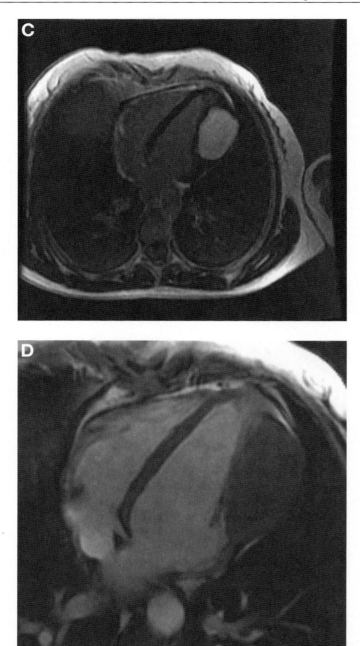

Fig. 1. *(Continued)*   A 33-years-old woman was referred for CMR imaging to further assess a left ventricular mass found on echocardiography. Her past medical history was remarkable for multiple basal cell carcinomas and surgical resection for odontogenic cysts. (**A**) CMR T_1-weighted spin echo imaging, short-axis slice at the level of midventricle demonstrates a tumor on lateral wall of left ventricle projecting into the cavity and partially obliterating the left ventricle. Signal intensity of the tumor is similar to surrounding myocardium (isointense). On myocardial delayed-enhancement CMR imaging, (**B**) short-axis slice and (**C**) long-axis slice revealed marked hyperenhancement of tumor on delayed images caused by fibrous tissue in the tumor. (**D**) Cine steady state free precession (SSFP) CMR images, four chamber view demonstrates the tumor occupying the whole lateral wall of the left ventricle interfering with contractile function of the left ventricle (*see* movie on CD-Rom).

based. Intramural hemangiomas are often poorly circumscribed, spongy masses that appear variably hemorrhagic or congested. Endocardial-based hemangiomas are well-circumscribed, variably myxoid, soft masses *(50)*.

DIAGNOSTIC IMAGING FEATURES

Cardiac hemangiomas are hyperechoic lesions at echocardiography. On unenhanced CT, tumors are heterogeneous but are intensely enhanced with contrast CT. These tumors typically demonstrate intermediate signal intensity on T_1-weighted CMR images and become hyperintense on T_2-weighted images *(51)*. An inhomogeneous hyperintense enhancement has been observed after gadolinium administration. First-pass perfusion CMR imaging may demonstrate enhancement indicating a high tumor vascularity, which is characterized by a vascular blush on coronary angiography, particularly in the capillary and arteriovenous types of hemangiomas. Cavernous hemangiomas have large vascular spaces with slow flow and therefore do not typically enhance at angiography *(52)*.

TREATMENT

Surgical resection is the treatment of choice for symptomatic cardiac hemangioma, and the long-term outcome of those patients treated surgically is excellent. Spontaneous regression of a cardiac hemangioma has been reported *(53)*. Therefore, surgery is primarily reserved for extensive symptomatic hemangiomas.

Lipoma

CLINICAL MANIFESTATIONS

Cardiac lipomas are rare benign neoplasms composed of adipose tissue. These tumors are typically found in adult patients but can affect patients of all ages. Although they usually do not cause symptoms, intracavitary lesions can manifest with dyspnea secondary to blood flow obstruction. In addition, involvement of the cardiac conduction system may result in arrhythmias.

PATHOLOGICAL FINDINGS

Lipomas are circumscribed, spherical, or elliptical masses of homogeneous yellow fat. Although nearly all cardiac lipomas are epicardial lesions occurring at any site on the atrial or ventricular surfaces, they may also occur in endocardial or myocardial locations. Most reported cases of cardiac lipomas are described as single lesions; however, multiple lipomas have been reported in patients with congenital heart defects, tuberous sclerosis, and rarely in an otherwise normal heart.

DIAGNOSTIC IMAGING FEATURES

Cardiomegaly (globular heart) is the most frequent radiographic finding in patients with cardiac lipoma. Echocardiographic appearance of lipomas varies with their location. Lipomas in the pericardial space may be completely hypoechoic, partly hypoechoic, or completely echogenic *(54,55)*, whereas intracavitary lipomas are typically homogeneous and hyperechoic *(56)*.

CT imaging is based on the findings of fat attenuation; lipomas appear as predominantly homogeneous masses with smooth contour but may display internal soft tissue septa or scattered strands of tissue with higher attenuation. CMR is useful for making a tissue-specific diagnosis by signal intensity characteristics of fat. Similar to subcutaneous fat, lipomas exhibit bright signal on T_1-weighted images and slightly decreased signal intensity on T_2-weighted images. The characteristic feature of lipoma is that signal intensity of tumor decreases with fat saturation sequence. The relationship of coronary arteries to the mass can also be evaluated with CMR preoperatively for planning and determining resectability of tumor *(57)*.

TREATMENT

The outcomes of cardiac lipomas treated surgically are generally good *(58)*. However, surgical resection may not be possible for lipomas that encase or displace the coronary arteries or deeply infiltrate the myocardium. Cardiac lipoma can be enormous to encase and compress the heart, resulting in severe cardiopulmonary compromise and death *(59)*. On the other hand, it can be asymptomatic and grow slowly over several years of follow-up *(57)*.

Paraganglioma

CLINICAL MANIFESTATIONS

Cardiac paragangliomas are extremely rare tumors that arise from intrinsic cardiac paraganglial cells, which are predominantly located within the atria. The majority present in adults, with the mean age of 40 years (18–85 years). Cardiac paragangliomas produce catecholamine in the majority of patients and manifest with arterial hypertension, headache, palpitations, and flushing (typical symptoms of pheochromocytoma). The biochemical laboratory abnormalities that lead to the diagnosis of a paraganglioma include elevated levels of urinary norepinephrine, vanillylmandelic acid, and total metanephrine or plasma norepinephrine and epinephrine *(60)*. Association with paragangliomas in other locations such as carotid body, adrenal gland, bladder, and para-aortic areas occurs in 20% of patients with cardiac paragangliomas. Approximately 5% of patients have osseous metastases.

PATHOLOGICAL FINDINGS

Cardiac paragangliomas are large, poorly circumscribed masses typically located on the epicardial surface of the base of the heart in the roof of the left atrium. Less-common locations include the atrial cavity, interatrial septum, and, rarely, the ventricles.

DIAGNOSTIC IMAGING FEATURES

After initial biochemical diagnosis of paragangliomas has been made, evaluation of paragangliomas usually follows with abdominal CT or MR imaging. If these studies fail to reveal a typical adrenal pheochromocytoma, I 131 MIBG (iodine 131 metaiodobenzylguanidine) scintigraphy is used to localize the occult lesion because catecholamine-producing tumors actively take up the radiotracer and store it in cate-cholamine granules. The I 131 MIBG can be used for total body imaging with a sensi-tivity of approximately 90% *(61,62)*. Cardiac paraganglioma located in the roof of the left atrium are usually seen as a middle mediastinal mass that splays the carina or sim-ulates left atrial enlargement on chest radiography *(63)*.

Cardiac paragangliomas are isoattenuating with adjacent structures on unenhanced CT scans. CT with contrast markedly enhances tumors; however, premedication with α- and β- blockers may be necessary because the intravenous administration of con-trast material can trigger a hypertensive crisis in patients with these tumors *(64)*. The central areas of low attenuation representing necrosis are observed in approximately half of these lesions.

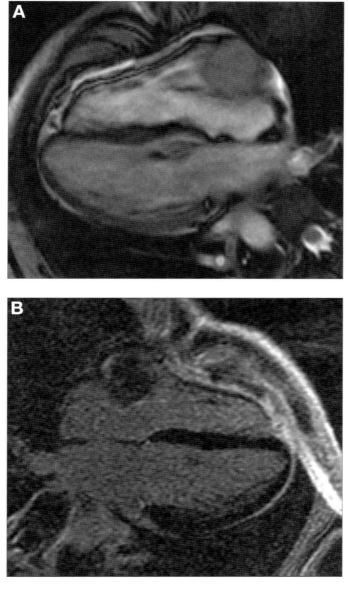

Fig. 2. *(Continued)*

Calcification of tumor can also be identified. CMR imaging typically demonstrates a mass that is iso- or hypointense on T_1-weighted and hyperintense on T_2-weighted images. Contrast hyperenhancement of tumor on delayed images reflects increased vascularity of these tumors *(63)* (Fig. 2B). The location of the mass and its relationship to the pericardium and myocardium are usually clearly demonstrated *(64)* (Fig. 2A). In addition, the relationship of the coronary arteries to the mass, including the blood supply to this highly vascular tumor, on coronary angiography is useful in the preoperative assessment of these patients *(65)*.

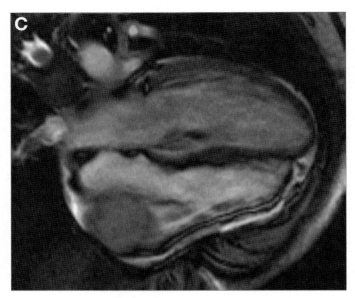

Fig. 2. *(Continued)*   A 37-years-old female presented with headache, nausea, and vomiting. CMR imaging clearly demonstrates the mass. (**A**) Steady-state free precession (SSFP) gradient echo CMR, long-axis slice, four-chamber view shows the tumor localized to the right atrioventricular groove beneath the visceral pericardium. Dynamic cine CMR imaging revealed the movement of the tumor with the atrioventricular groove. On myocardial delayed-enhancement CMR imaging, (**B**) long-axis slice displays enhancement of tumor at the peripheral rim. Additional biochemical test and subsequent biopsy confirmed cardiac paraganglioma arising from atrioventricular groove with evidence of production of catecholamine. (**C**) Cine SSFP CMR four chamber view revealed cine CMR imaging revealed the movement of the tumor with tricuspid annular ring suggest tumor originates from neurovascular gurdle in atrioventricular groove. The tumor grew into the right atrial cavity and partial obstruction of the right ventricular inflow is also noted. (*See* movie on CD-Rom.)

TREATMENT

Surgical excision of cardiac paragangliomas is usually successful and provides complete symptomatic relief. Surgical risks particular to cardiac paragangliomas include hypertensive crisis from intraoperative manipulation of the tumor and fatal hemorrhage because of the high vascularity of these lesions. Cardiopulmonary bypass isolates the heart from the systemic circulation and allows safe manipulation and dissection of the tumor. Because paragangliomas may be infiltrative lesions, extensive resection of the atrial wall may be required for complete excision *(66,67)*.

Teratoma

CLINICAL MANIFESTATIONS

Teratoma is a benign germ cell tumor that contains all three elements of germ cell layers, occurs in the pericardium, and attaches to the root of the aorta or the pulmonary trunk. Infants and children are affected and present with respiratory distress and cyanosis secondary to pericardial tamponade and compression of right-sided vascular structures such as aortic root, superior vena cava, pulmonary artery, and right atrium *(68,69)*.

Teratomas may be discovered on prenatal ultrasound examinations, which typically show an intrapericardial, multilocular cystic mass associated with pericardial effusion.

An affected fetus may present with ascites, pleural effusions, subcutaneous edema, and polyhydramnios (typical findings of fetal hydrops) *(70)*. Pericardial tamponade is a common cause of fetal death in affected individuals *(71)*.

PATHOLOGICAL FINDINGS

Teratomas usually present as right-sided masses, which typically connect to one of the great vessels via a pedicle. Most teratomas of the heart lie within the pericardial sac or, rarely, in the myocardium. Cross sections of these lesions reveal bosselated appearance with multiple cysts (ranging from a few millimeters to several centimeters) and intervening solid tissue between the cystic areas. The tumors can be large and are almost always associated with a pericardial effusion *(72)*.

DIAGNOSTIC IMAGING FEATURES

Chest radiography of affected patients typically demonstrates an enlarged cardiomediastinal silhouette and calcified teeth, when present *(70)*. Echocardiography demonstrates a heterogeneous and complex multilocular cystic mass in the pericardium, typically located on the right side of the heart, which may encase or compress the heart and the great vessels. Pericardial effusion is a frequently associated finding *(73)*.

On CMR and CT, teratomas usually demonstrate a large mass of heterogeneous signal intensity with areas of fat, cysts, soft tissue, calcification, and so on. The relationship of the tumor to the normal myocardium, great vessels, and other mediastinal structures can be better identified on CMR imaging *(69)*.

TREATMENT

With early diagnosis, curative surgical excision offers good prognosis. A resection of tumor also brings immediate relief of symptoms. Intrapericardial teratoma with pericardial tamponade is a life-threatening lesion, which usually requires emergent therapy with pericardiocentesis or surgical intervention *(68,71)*.

MALIGNANT TUMORS

Approximately 95% of all malignant tumors are sarcomas, making these tumors the second most common primary cardiac tumor after myxomas in overall frequency. Lymphomas account for the remaining 5% of primary malignant cardiac tumors.

Sarcomas

Sarcomas affecting the heart are more common among malignant mesenchymal tumors. The most common primary malignant cardiac tumors are angiosarcoma, fibrosarcoma, undifferentiated sarcoma, malignant fibrous histiocytoma, leiomyosarcoma, and osteosarcoma. Approximately 10% of surgically resected cardiac tumors are primary sarcomas. Although the majority of angiosarcomas occur in the right atrium, the other tumors more commonly affect the left atrium *(4)*.

CLINICAL MANIFESTATIONS

Cardiac sarcomas commonly affect middle-aged adults. Patients with leiomyosarcoma typically present 5–10 years earlier than those with other cardiac sarcomas. Angiosarcoma and osteosarcoma are approximately twice as common in men, and there is a slight female preponderance in patients with malignant fibrous histiocytoma. The majority of patients with cardiac sarcoma present with cardiopulmonary symptoms with a mean duration of approximately 5 months *(23)*.

The cardiac findings are determined primarily by the location of the tumor and by the extent of intracavitary obstruction *(4)*. The major presenting symptom is unexplained dyspnea with evidence of right-sided heart failure. Obstruction of the superior and inferior vena cava can result in congestion of upper and lower extremities. Precordial pain occurs in one-fourth of patients with sarcomas. Sarcomas commonly extend into the pericardial space and produce pericardial effusions, typically hemorrhagic and with or without tamponade physiology, and are seen in one-fourth of patients. In primarily intramural tumors, arrhythmias, conduction disturbances, and sudden death can occur.

With superior noninvasive imaging facilitating earlier diagnosis, cardiac sarcomas in general are diagnosed at the time of presentation without evidence of distant metastasis. Primary cardiac sarcomas most commonly metastasize to the lungs but also to lymph nodes, bone, liver, brain, bowel, spleen, adrenal glands, pleura, diaphragm, kidneys, thyroid, and skin *(74)*. Among cardiac sarcomas (95% of primary malignant cardiac tumors), cardiac angiosarcomas represent majority (approximately 30%) and other sarcomas of different mesenchymal origin represent minority (Table 2).

Because approximately 80% of cardiac angiosarcomas occur in the right atrium and involve the pericardium, symptoms from right-sided heart inflow obstruction or cardiac tamponade are common. The location and degree of invasiveness of these lesions makes them less likely to be confused clinically with myxomas.

Because of its right sided location and invasiveness, majority of angiosarcomas have metastases at the time of presentation. The *in utero* occurrence of a right atrial angiosarcoma that manifested with a pericardial effusion has been reported *(75)*. Cardiac sarcomas that typically affect the left atrium are malignant fibrous histiocytoma, osteosarcoma, and leiomyosarcoma. Affected patients present with symptoms of mitral valve obstruction, most commonly dyspnea and heart failure. Although the point of tumor attachment is usually not at the fossa ovalis, these sarcomas are often clinically mistaken for myxomas *(4,76)*.

PATHOLOGICAL FINDINGS

The pathological features of cardiac sarcomas may range from endocardial-based lesions similar to myxoma to large, infiltrative tumors. The majority of these are large, invasive masses at the time of diagnosis. Angiosarcomas are generally large, grossly hemorrhagic, multilobular, right atrial masses that spread along the epicardial surface, replace the right atrial wall, and may protrude into or fill the adjacent cardiac chambers. Cross sections of cardiac sarcomas are typically firm and heterogeneous, but the myofibroblastic tumors may be homogeneous *(4,23)*. (Table 2).

DIAGNOSTIC IMAGING FEATURES

The most common radiographic finding in patients with cardiac sarcoma is cardiomegaly. Other findings include heart failure, pleural effusion, focal cardiac mass, pulmonary consolidation, and pericardial effusion. The radiographic findings of left atrial sarcomas can mimic those of left atrial myxoma because of their location *(77)*. Echocardiography usually demonstrates cardiac sarcomas as intracavitary lesions, intramural mass, calcification, or pericardial effusion, depending on the type of cardiac sarcomas (Table 2).

CT is helpful in the evaluation of cardiac sarcomas as it demonstrates the broad-based tumor attachment; myocardial, pericardial, and mediastinal invasion; as well as extension into the great vessels and pulmonary metastases, when present. Angiosarcomas have been described as highly vascular right atrial tumors with pericardial extension. The pericardial space may be obliterated with hemorrhagic, necrotic tumor debris, which

Table 2
Features of Primary Malignant Cardiac Tumors

Type and percentage of malignant tumor in adult	Common population age	Location of tumor	Morphologic features	Echo features	CT feature	CMR feature
Angiosarcoma (30%)	30–50 years M: F = 3:1	Right atrium	Intracavitary and polypoid or diffuse and infiltrative, with involvement of the pericardium Heterogeneous with areas of hemorrhage & necrosis	Mass protruding into right atrium Pericardial effusion	Low attenuation	T_1: Isotense, with hyperintense focal areas (cauliflower appearance) T_2: Isointense, heterogeneous MDE: Linear areas of enhancement (sunray appearance)
Rhabdomyosarcoma (10%)	Most common malignacy in infant & children	Any chamber	Polypoid extension into the cardiac chamber or Nodular involvement pericardium	Mass into cavity Nodule into pericardium More likely to involve valve	Smooth or irregular Low attenuation	T_2: Isointense, T_2: Isointense, heterogeneous MDE: central non-enhanced area (cyst or central necrosis)
Undifferentiated Sarcoma (10–15%)	Variable	Left atrium	Possible pericardial origin, infiltrative or mass like appearance	Discrete myocardial mass Interacavitary lesion	Large, irregular Low attenuation	T_1: Isointense T_2: Isointense, MDE: Nonspecific
Leimyosarcoma (5%)	30 seconds	Left atrium	Sessile, gelatinous mass	Mass from posterior wall of left atrium May involve pulmonary vein or mitral valve	Low attenuation	T_1: Isointense T_2: Hyperintense, MDE: Nonspecific
Fibrosarcoma (5–10%)	Variable	Left atrium	Lobulated and gelatinous mass Heterogeneous with areas of hemorrhage & necrosis Possible pericardial origin	Extensive infiltration of the heart Mass may obliterate entire chamber or spread to pericardium	Low attenuation	T_1: Isointense T_2: Hyperintense, heterogeneous MDE: Central non-enhanced area

(Continued)

445

Table 2 (*Continued*)

Type and percentage of malignant tumor In adult	Common population age	Location of tumor	Morphologic features	Echo features	CT feature	CMR feature
Osteosarcoma (5–10%)	Variable	Left atrium	Broad base attachment to posterior atrial wall	Heavily calcified mass	Low attenuation with dense Calcification	T_1: Hyperintense T_2: Hyperintense MDE: Heterogenous enhancement
Liposarcoma (2%)	Variable	Left atrium or right atrium	Large, Multilobulated nodules Areas of hemorrhage and necrosis	Multilobulated nodules in atria, ventricles or pericardium Pericardial effusion	Low attenuation	Infiltrative and heterogeneous Variable intensity on T_1
Lymphoma (5%)	Median age = 64 years M:F=3:1	Right atrium	Homogenious nodule Multifocal commonly Extend into pericardium	Hypoechoic masses Pericardial effusion	Low attenuation or isoattenuation Heterogeneous	T_1: Isointense to hypointense T_2: Isointense or hyperintense MDE: Heterogeneous enhancement

446

may appear on CT as pericardial effusion or thickening, and tumor mass may appear as low attenuation areas *(78)*.

CMR imaging is mainly used for ultimate evaluation of cardiac sarcomas, which appear as large, heterogeneous, broad-based masses that frequently occupy most of the affected cardiac chamber or multiple chambers (Fig. 3). Pericardial and extracardiac invasion, valvular destruction, tumor necrosis, and metastases are often seen and are all characteristic features of malignant lesions. Pericardial invasion is characterized by disruption, thickening, or nodularity. Cardiac sarcomas enhance heterogeneously, with nonenhancing areas typically corresponding to necrosis *(79,80)*.

CMR typically demonstrates cardiac angiosarcomas as large, heterogeneous, invasive right atrial masses, frequently with extensive pericardial involvement and hemorrhagic pericardial effusion. Because of their propensity toward hemorrhage and necrosis, angiosarcomas typically have heterogeneous signal intensity on MR images *(81)*. Areas of increased signal intensity on T_1-weighted images may be focal or peripheral and are thought to represent blood products *(82)* (Fig. 4). Local nodular areas of increased signal intensity interspersed within areas of intermediate signal intensity on T_1- and T_2-weighted images have been described as having a "cauliflower" appearance *(77)*. Signal intensity of the majority of sarcomas is heterogeneous, with intermediate intensity (isointensity) on T_1-weighted images, higher signal intensity (hyperintensity) on T_2-weighted images, and variable enhancement on delayed myocardial enhancement imaging (Table 2).

TREATMENT

Primary cardiac sarcomas are highly aggressive lesions that are uniformly fatal, with a mean survival of 3 months to 1 years, although survivals of over 4 years have also been reported *(4)*. Pathological features that predict a better prognosis include tumor origin in the left atrium, low mitotic count, absence of necrosis, and absence of metastases at the time of diagnosis *(48)*. Aggressive surgery offers significant palliation of symptoms (caused by valvular and vascular obstruction) and improves survival *(74)*. Local recurrence and metastasis occur frequently and as early as 1 years, even after complete tumor excision *(83)*. Heart transplantation has been performed in some patients with unresectable cardiac sarcoma with satisfactory results *(84,85)*. Chemotherapy and radiation therapy have not proved beneficial for the treatment of affected patients *(74)*. Death in these patients usually results from postoperative complications, cardiopulmonary failure from progressive tumor growth, and metastatic disease *(4)*.

Primary Cardiac Lymphoma

CLINICAL MANIFESTATIONS

Primary cardiac lymphomas are typically of the non-Hodgkin type. These tumors primarily involve the heart or pericardium at the time of diagnosis, without evidence of extracardiac lymphoma *(23)*. Although 16–28% of patients with disseminated lymphoma have cardiac involvement, primary cardiac lymphoma is rare *(86)*. The incidence has increased in immunocompromised patients, particularly in association with immunosuppression from acquired immunodeficiency syndrome and solid organ transplant. Primary cardiac lymphoma should be suspected clinically when these patients present with cardiac complaints *(87,88)*. In immunocompetent patients, the median age of presentation is 64 years, and the male-to-female ratio is 3:1 *(86)*. They may present as nonspecific

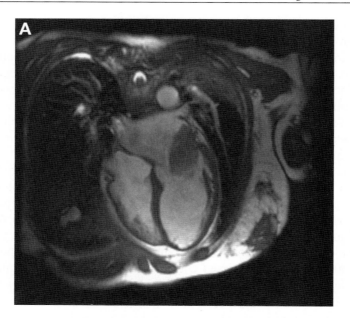

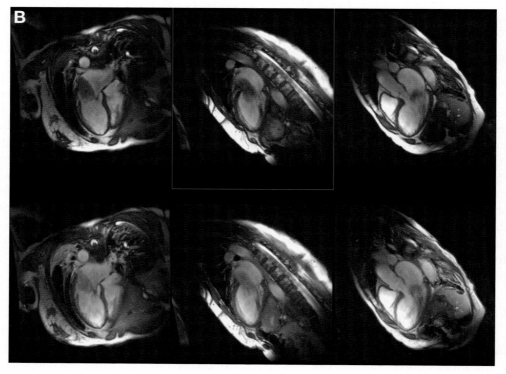

Fig. 3. A 55-years-old woman with a remote history of mesothelioma treated with combined surgery and chemotherapy and radiation therapy presented with atypical chest pain and was found to have a large left atrial mass. SSFP gradient echo CMR long-axis view (Figure 3A) shows a solid mobile mass attached to the atrial surface of the mitral annulus. Dynamic cine SSFP gradient echo (Figure 3B). Upper panel: before gadolinium and lower panel: after gadolinium administration) (*see* movie on CD-Rom.) demonstrate partial obstruction of mitral inflow with mobility of tumor across the mitral valve. Subsequent histopathology of resected tumor revealed poorly differentiated sarcoma.

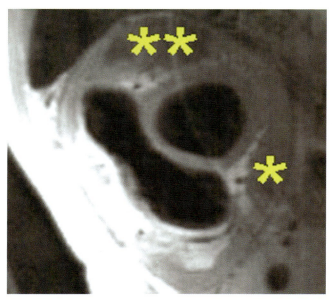

Fig. 4. CMR T_1-weighted spin echo imaging, short-axis slice demonstrates pericardial angiosarcoma as heterogeneous signal intensity; a tumor in the pericardium seen as a rim of increased signal intensity represents blood product, and areas of low signal intensity (shown in asterisks) reflect necrosis. Histopathology of the lesion revealed spindle cell angiosarcoma.

systemic symptoms, shortness of breath, chest pain, arrhythmia, superior vena cava obstruction, and cardiac tamponade.

PATHOLOGICAL FINDINGS

Cardiac lymphoma manifests with multiple firm, white nodular masses. These tumors are typically described as having a fish-flesh, homogeneous appearance, although foci of necrosis may occur. The areas most often affected by primary cardiac lymphoma are the right atrium, followed by the right ventricle, left ventricle, left atrium, atrial septum, and ventricular septum. Although tumors are confined to the atria, pericardium, and coronary arteries, more than one cardiac chamber is involved in over 75% of cases. Contiguous invasion of the pericardium is typical. Pericardial effusion, when present, is usually massive. Cytological analysis of pericardial fluid has reported sensitivities ranging from 14 to 67% *(86)*. Because transvenous endomyocardial biopsy has a sensitivity of only 50%, open biopsy of affected cardiac tissue through exploratory thoracotomy was required in many patients for definitive diagnosis *(86)*.

DIAGNOSTIC IMAGING FEATURES

Chest radiography of patients with primary cardiac lymphoma usually demonstrates cardiomegaly, pericardial effusion, and signs of heart failure. Echocardiography typically demonstrates hypoechoic myocardial masses in the right atrium or ventricle with an associated pericardial effusion.

At CT, cardiac lymphomas are hypoattenuating or isoattenuating relative to the myocardium and demonstrate heterogeneous enhancement after intravenous administration of contrast material *(89)*. CMR imaging demonstrates poorly marginated and heterogeneous lesions, which are isointense to slightly hypointense relative to myocardium on T_1-weighted MR images and isointense or hyperintense on proton density and T_2-weighted images. Delayed images after gadolinium administration revealed a heterogeneous pattern of enhancement.

TREATMENT

Most primary cardiac lymphomas are either diagnosed at autopsy or are fatal soon after diagnosis. However, early diagnosis and institution of chemotherapy may result in remission of disease, palliation of pain, and longer survival. Although the long-term prognosis is almost universally dismal, tumor debulking surgery may be an effective palliative procedure *(90)*. The median survival of patients with cardiac lymphomas without treatment is less than 1 month. Patients treated with chemotherapy or radiation have median survivals on the order of 1 years *(86)*. Patients may deteriorate immediately after initiation of therapy because of rapid intramural tumor lysis, which causes congestive heart failure, arrhythmias, and even cardiac rupture *(90,91)*. Isolated cases of complete remission after autologous stem cell transplant have been reported.

Pericardial Mesothelioma

Pericardial mesothelioma is a malignant neoplasm that primarily arises from the mesothelial cells of the pericardium. Although 50% of all primary pericardial tumors are pericardial mesotheliomas, they represent less than 1% of all malignant mesotheliomas *(23,92)*.

CLINICAL MANIFESTATIONS

Patients with pericardial mesotheliomas range widely in age, and a 2:1 male-to-female ratio is evident. Patients with diffuse pericardial involvement may present with symptoms and signs that mimic pericarditis, pericardial constriction, or cardiac tamponade. Patients with advanced tumors may present with symptoms and signs of widespread metastases. There appears to be some causal association with asbestos exposure *(23)*.

PATHOLOGICAL FINDINGS

Pericardial mesotheliomas typically form multiple pericardial masses that coalesce and obliterate the pericardial space. Cut sections of the masses are firm, white, and homogeneous. Although slight infiltration of the outer epicardium may occur, myocardial invasion is rare *(23)*.

DIAGNOSTIC IMAGING FEATURES

Chest radiography usually reveals cardiomegaly with evidence of pericardial effusion, an irregular cardiac contour, or diffuse mediastinal enlargement. CT demonstrates irregular, diffuse pericardial thickening and pericardial effusion *(93)*. CMR imaging also shows cardiac encasement by a soft tissue pericardial mass, as well as an associated pericardial effusion or evidence of pericardial constriction *(94)* (Fig. 5).

TREATMENT

Surgery combined with radiation therapy may be palliative, but the prognosis of all patients (even those who are treated) is extremely poor, with survival of 6 months to 1 year after diagnosis (the median survival from the onset of symptoms is 6 months) *(23,92)*.

Malignant Metastatic Tumors

Secondary metastatic tumors are far more frequent than are the primary cardiac tumors by at least a 30:1 ratio *(95)*. Carcinoma of the lung is the most commonly

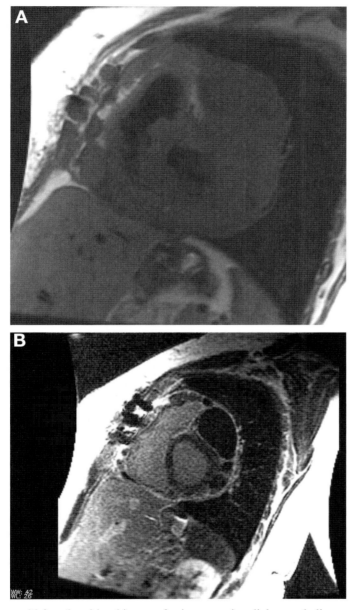

Fig. 5. A 49-years-old female with a history of primary pericardial mesothelioma, status post peri-cardiectomy, presented with recurrence. (**A**) CMR, short-axis view, displays tumor anterior and anterolateral to the left ventricle, isointense on T_1-weighted spin echo (Fig. 5A). (**B**) However, tumor does not enhance after gadolinium administration on myocardial delayed images (Fig. 5B). Histopathology of the resected mass revealed malignant mesothelioma.

encountered metastatic tumor at autopsy, with cancer of the breast, followed by lym-phoma and leukemia, as the next leading causes. Regarding frequency of metastases, however, melanoma has the highest frequency of metastases to the heart, followed by malignant germ cell tumor, leukemia, lymphoma, cancer of the lung, and then the vari-ous sarcomas *(23)*.

The distinction between primary and secondary cardiac tumors is usually easily made on clinical grounds because almost all cardiac metastases manifest in patients with known noncardiac primary malignant tumors, frequently in association with widespread systemic disease. However, in some cases, especially in patients with sarcoma and lymphoma, the diagnosis of primary cardiac tumor may be made at autopsy through exclusion of another primary tumor elsewhere. The pericardium, including the epicardium (visceral layer of the pericardium) is by far the most commonly affected site. The myocardium can be involved through direct tumor extension from the pericardium. However, malignant melanoma may result in diffuse myocardial involvement through hematogenous spread. Only about 5% of cardiac metastases are endocardial or intracavitary lesions (7,23).

Metastatic tumors classically involve, in descending order of frequency, the heart and pericardium by one of four pathways: hematogenous spread, retrograde lymphatic extension, direct invasion, or transvenous extension. Hematogenous (embolic) spread to the heart is commonly seen with systemic tumors such as malignant melanoma, lymphoma, leukemia, and sarcoma. Lymphatic spread of tumors is particularly frequent with carcinoma of the bronchus and the breast and mediastinal lymphomas. Frequently, lung cancer, breast cancer, and mediastinal tumors invade directly into pericardium and myocardium. Transvenous extension occurs occasionally via the inferior vena cava in cases with renal or hepatic tumors and via superior vena cava in cases with lung cancer (4).

Diagnosis can be suspected whenever cardiac manifestations occur in a patient diagnosed with a primary tumor in a noncardiac organ or tissue. The development of cardiac enlargement, tachycardia, arrhythmias, or heart failure in the presence of neoplasm elsewhere in the body is highly suggestive of cardiac metastases. By the time metastatic tumor is in the heart, it usually indicates that widespread metastases have occurred in a number of body organs. On rare occasion, cardiac involvement may be the first or only expression of a noncardiac primary neoplasm. The most common sign is tamponade (96). Direct invasion of the heart via the vena cava or pulmonary veins may lead to obstruction of an atrioventricular valve and to pulmonary or systemic emboli or both (97–99).

Carcinoma of the lung and carcinoma of the breast tend to invade the parietal pericardium and then the visceral pericardium, leading to myocardial constriction, pericardial effusion, or both. Another common presentation of cancer of the lung is invasion of the pulmonary veins within the lung, with spread of the cancer within the lumen of the pulmonary veins into the left atrium. From there, the cancer in turn can continue into the mitral orifice, sometimes causing mitral valvular obstruction (100,101). Metastatic cancer from the lung to the adrenal gland also may extend into the inferior vena cava and then into the right side of the heart (similar to primary adrenal or renal cancer) (102). Cancer of the lung or breast surrounding the main right or left pulmonary artery can lead to pulmonary arterial obstruction (103).

Melanoma has the highest frequency of metastases to the heart. The metastases may be anywhere in the heart; usually, melanotic metastases invade the walls of all four cardiac chambers, the epicardium, and the endocardium (104,105). The cancers in these patients are in so many organs that the presence of the neoplasm in the heart is almost incidental. Resection of an intracardiac melanoma has been accomplished (106).

Leukemia commonly invades the heart (107). Extensive hemorrhages into the myocardial walls and into the endocardium and epicardium were commonly found in patients with fatal leukemia of various types. Leukemic infiltration between myocardial cells is common and sometimes leads to gross deposits of leukemic cells within the heart. A few patients with leukemia present with pericardial effusion, which is usually hemorrhagic. Large calcific deposits in the right side of the heart have been reported *(108)*.

Lymphoma also has a high frequency of metastases to the heart. Nearly 25% of patients with lymphomas of various types have lymphoma involving the epicardium, myocardium, endocardium, or combinations. In contrast to leukemic involvement, the lymphomatous deposits are usually grossly discernible *(109,110)*.

CLINICAL MANIFESTATIONS

Metastatic involvement of the heart and pericardium may go unrecognized until autopsy. Secondary tumor involvement of the heart may be recognized as a pathological finding without clinical manifestations. More often, however, such involvement is symptomatic; on rare occasions, it may be the first or only expression of a remote primary tumor.

Pericardial involvement is often first manifested by pleuritic chest pain. Impairment of cardiac function occurs in approximately 30% of patients and is usually attributable to pericardial effusion *(111)*. The clinical presentation includes shortness of breath, which may be out of proportion to radiographic findings in patients with pericardial effusion or may be the result of associated pleural effusion *(112)*. Patients may also present with cough, anterior thoracic pain, pleuritic chest pain, or peripheral edema. Pericardial effusion often, but not always, is bloody, may result in progressive cardiac enlargement on roentgenogram with symptoms and signs of cardiac tamponade, and may be the first manifestation of a cardiac malignancy *(113)*. The association of large quantities of pericardial fluid with tumor encasing the heart frequently results in persistent cardiac constriction, even after the fluid is withdrawn by pericardiocentesis *(114)*.

Arrhythmia in patients with cardiac metastases is usually the result of concomitant factors such as hypoxemia, altered electrolyte concentrations, or anemia; however, arrhythmia can be secondary to tumor involving autonomic fibers or coronary arteries. Arrhythmia is the most prevalent manifestation of myocardial involvement by metastatic tumors. The sudden occurrence of an arrhythmia in a patient with a known malignancy suggests the possibility of metastatic involvement of the myocardium. The type of arrhythmia produced depends on the size of the tumor and its location relative to the conduction system of the heart. Atrial arrhythmias are common, probably because the atrium has less mobility and hence is invaded more often. Atrial flutter and fibrillation are frequent, and a patient with either one may be unusually resistant to conventional therapy. Ventricular extrasystoles and even serious ventricular arrhythmias may accompany invasion of a tumor into the myocardium. Conduction disturbances and complete heart block have been reported *(115,116)*.

Widespread myocardial involvement by tumor invasion or obstruction of the cardiac lymphatic drainage system may cause congestive failure. Myocardial damage and heart failure may also result from some of the chemotherapeutic agents used in the treatment of patients with neoplastic diseases, and combined radiotherapy and chemotherapy may synergistically increase cardiac damage *(117)*. In patients with malignant tumor, angina or myocardial infarction may result from concomitant atherosclerosis, coronary occlusion by tumor embolization, or external coronary compression by the tumor, as well as from coronary fibrosis or accelerated atherogenesis in patients who have received radiation to the mediastinum *(118)*. Hepatocellular carcinoma *(119)* and uterine leiomyomatosis *(120)* along the inferior vena cava and into the right atrium can present as an intracavitary obstructive mass. Leiomyosarcoma may be primary in the vena cava, most often the inferior, and extend directly into the heart *(121,122)* (Fig. 6).

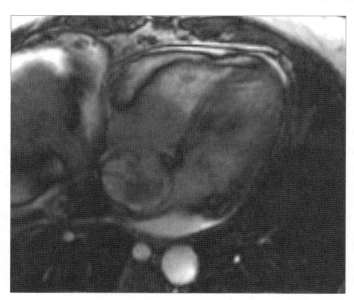

Fig. 6. A 53-years-old presented with right lower extremity edema was found to have leiomyosarcoma of the inferior vena cava. CMR SSFP long-axis four-chamber view shows tumor extending into the right atrium and right ventricle. (see movie on CD-Rom.)

Intracavitary metastases or an expanding myocardial tumor may progressively obliterate a cardiac chamber or result in a valvular obstruction and, rarely, may produce fever of unknown origin. Right atrial and tricuspid obstruction by an intracavitary mass can mimic pericardial constriction from tumor invasion or from previous intensive radiotherapy to the mediastinum *(123,124)*. Systemic or pulmonary emboli, so common with primary tumors of the heart, are uncommon with secondary tumors.

DIAGNOSTIC FEATURES

Intracavitary metastatic tumors, pericardial masses, and pericardial effusion are usually detected on echocardiographic imaging of the heart; however, right-sided intracavitary thrombi may mimic primary or secondary tumors *(125,126)*. CT offers excellent contrast resolution, which allows differentiation between tumor and myocardium. CT imaging facilitates identification of pericardial effusion and intracavitary and pericardial masses *(127,128)*. CMR provides a global view of cardiac anatomy and plays an important role in the diagnosis and evaluation of both primary and secondary tumors of the heart, providing information about the location, extent, and attachment of the tumor *(129,130)*. The distinction among tumor, thrombus, or blood flow artifact can be made more readily with CMR imaging than with CT. Signal intensities at CMR imaging may also help tissue characterization in some cases. For example, most cardiac tumors are of low signal intensity on T_1-weighted images (in an exception to other tumors, melanoma appears bright on T_1-weighted images, an effect attributed to paramagnetic metals bound by melanin) *(131–133)* and are brighter on T_2-weighted images *(134)*. Most malignant disease enhances after administration of gadolinium-diethyltriaminepentaacetic acid *(8)*.

The diagnosis of malignant pericardial effusion is made by pericardiocentesis, pericardioscopy, or both. Results of cytological studies are positive in 80–90% of patients with malignant pericardial effusions *(135)*. Pericardioscopy performed during surgical drainage procedures has enabled visual diagnoses and guided biopsies of suspicious areas *(136)*. The results of endomyocardial biopsy may contribute to the diagnosis in some cases *(137,138)*.

TREATMENT

Depending on the cytological subtype and radiosensitivity of the tumor, radiation to the cardiac area, with or without systemic chemotherapy, is the treatment of choice. Pericardiocentesis not only may afford prompt symptomatic relief from cases of cardiac tamponade but also provides a definitive cytological diagnosis for therapy. Malignant pericardial effusion usually recurs rapidly after pericardiocentesis.

Other therapeutic options include surgical creation of a pericardial window, pericardial sclerosis by intrapericardial administration of fluorouracil, radioactive gold (nitrogen mustard), and tetracycline *(139,140)*. Patients with myocardial infiltration by tumor also respond to radiation therapy and systemic chemotherapy. Heart block is treated with temporary or permanent electronic pacing as conditions dictate.

Surgical removal of intracavitary obstructing secondary tumors may ameliorate symptoms and prolong survival. CMR plays an important role in characterizing the three-dimensional extent and tissue attachment of cardiac tumors, which can help plan the surgical approach aimed at either complete removal or palliative debulking of a tumor mass.

NONNEOPLASTIC CARDIAC MASSES

Lipomatous Hypertrophy of the Interatrial Septum

Lipomatous hypertrophy of the interatrial septum is a hamartoma consisting of fatty deposition in the interatrial septum caused by an increased number of adipocytes (hyperplasia). They most commonly occur in female, obese (the thickness of the septum correlates with body weight and the thickness of adipose tissue surrounding the heart) elderly (over 50 years of age) patients *(141)*. Clinically, there is a high incidence of atrial arrhythmias, correlating with the degree of hypertrophy. Massive lipomatous hypertrophy can cause obstruction of the superior vena cava.

Pathologically, in contrast to true lipomas, lipomatous hypertrophy consists of a nonencapsulated accumulation of mature and fetal adipose tissue and atypical cardiac myocytes within the interatrial septum *(142)*. Lipomatous hypertrophy classically involves the anterior or superior portion of the interatrial septum, spares the fossa ovalis, and protrudes into the right atrium. On average, the septum is thickened up to 2.5 cm (the septum is usually >1 cm thick, and the upper limit of normal is generally considered 2 cm); however, tumors up to 10 cm in diameter have been described.

Lipomatous hypertrophy is easily seen on echocardiography as a highly echogenic, bilobed septal mass that spares the fossa ovalis. CT and CMR display tissue signal characteristics similar to subcutaneous fat (Fig. 7A). Similar to lipomas, lipomatous hypertrophy of the interatrial septum on CMR reveals bright signal on T_1-weighted images (Fig. 7B.) and slightly decreased signal intensity on T_2-weighted images. The signal intensity of the mass decreases with fat saturation sequence (Fig. 7C) *(143)*. Surgical resection of lipomatous hypertrophy of the septum is usually performed only in the setting of superior vena cava obstruction or clinically significant arrhythmias *(144)*. The nonneoplastic nature of these lesions permits performing incomplete resections that restore normal hemodynamics *(145)* (Fig. 7).

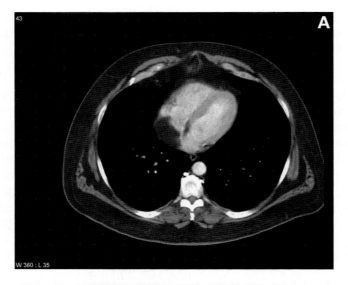

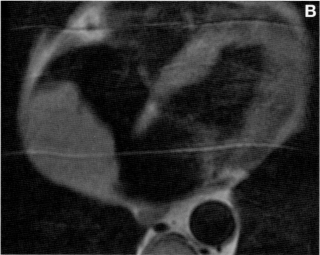

Fig. 7. *(Continued)*

Thrombus

Thrombus within an intracardiac cavity may be indistinguishable from intracavitary cardiac tumor. Thrombus is most commonly in the left atrium and left atrium appendage, especially in the patients with atrial fibrillation, or in the left ventricle in the patients with severe left ventricle dysfunction. It can also be found in the right side of the heart, usually in association with *in situ* catheters in the right ventricle and right atrium or its major draining veins. Right atrial thrombus may grow larger to become multilobular and mimic right atrial myxoma (Fig. 5).

On CMR imaging, the signal intensity of thrombus may vary depending on the age of the thrombus. Acute thrombus will appear bright on both T_1- and T_2-weighted images, whereas subacute thrombus will appear bright on T_1-weighted images with

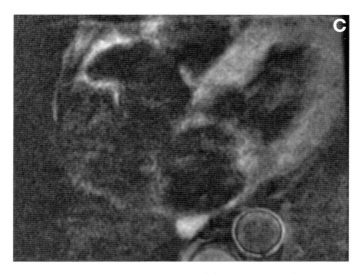

Fig. 7. *(Continued)*   A 61-years-old male presented with presyncope. (CT on top and CMR on bottom) (**A**) CT with contrast, axial view revealed the mass of fat attenuation in the right atrium, similar to subcutaneous fat. On CMR double inversion recovery spin echo imaging, axial view demonstrates a mass in the right atrium occupying the upper interatrial septum and partially obstructing the superior vena cava. The mass displays slight increase in intensity compared to surrounding tissue on images without fat saturation (**B**) in comparison with fat saturation images below, in which areas of fat (mass and epicardial fat) are decreased in signal intensity. (**C**) Bright signal intensity of the mass on T_1-weighted images suggests adipose tissue. Subsequent surgical resection and histopathology revealed lipomatous hypertrophy of the interatrial septum, measuring up to 7.6 cm in the largest diameter.

low signal intensity areas on T_2-weighted images because of the paramagnetic effect of methemoglobin and shortening of the T_2 relaxation times. Chronic organized thrombus will have low signal intensity on both T_1- and T_2-weighted images because of depleted water with or without calcification of the thrombus.

Gadolinium contrast is useful for differentiating thrombus from tumors. The thrombus typically does not enhance, but there is some evidence to suggest that organized thrombus may show some delayed enhancement, whereas the tumors usually enhance on delayed images *(146)*. Although dynamic cine CMR gradient echo imaging is also useful to detect larger thrombus and vegetation, small, highly mobile thrombus or vegetation may be missed because of lower temporal resolution compared to echocardiography (Figs. 8–10).

Pericardial Cyst

Pericardial cysts are congenital in origin and are usually found at the right cardiophrenic angle, although they may occur anywhere in the mediastinum. They are unilocular and contain water-based fluid without internal septa. The patients are usually asymptomatic, and the cysts are discovered incidentally on chest radiography, echocardiography, or CT. They usually demonstrate the MR imaging characteristics of simple fluid and do not enhance after contrast material administration. They occasionally may contain relatively proteinaceous fluid and thus may have high signal intensity on both T_1-weighted images and T_2-weighted images.

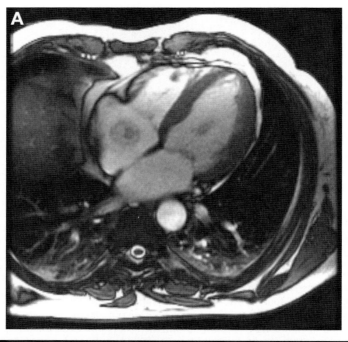

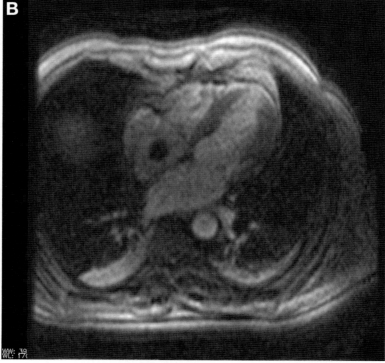

Fig. 8. A 47-year-old male with squamous cell carcinoma of the tongue status postchemotherapy with portacath *in situ* presented with transient monocular blindness. CMR SSFP four-chamber view (**A**) revealed highly mobile mass in the right atrium. The first-pass perfusion with gadolinium long-axis view (*see* movie on CD-Rom) (**B**) demonstrates the mobile mass between flowing contrast in the right atrium (*see* movie on CD-Rom).

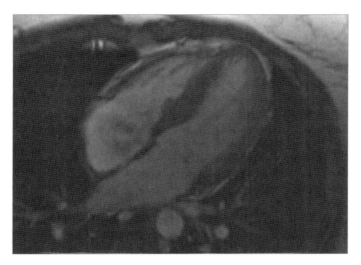

Fig. 9. A 25-years-old female with demyelinating syndrome had a large right atrial mass on echocardiography. On CMR, SSFP long-axis view revealed multilobular mass in right atrium with characteristics similar to of myxoma. Surgical removal and histopathology revealed multiple thrombi in various stages of organization (*see* movie on CD- Rom.)

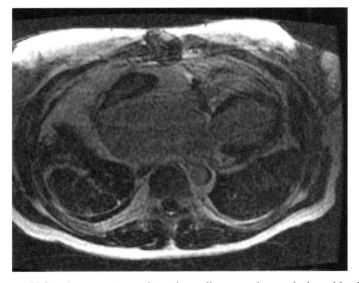

Fig. 10. A 47-years-old female, status postorthotopic cardiac transplant and tricuspid valve repair, had a mass attached to the anterior wall of the right atrium on routine echocardiography. Myocardial delayed CMR images revealed nonenhanced mass with central enhancement suggest organizing thrombus.

Bronchogenic Cyst

Bronchogenic cysts are again congenital in origin, arising from the bronchopulmonary foregut. They typically are located in the region of the carina, and the majority are asymptomatic. The cysts are lined with secretory respiratory epithelium, and the cystic fluid is composed of a mixture of water and proteinaceous mucus. Hemorrhage and calcification within the cyst can also occur *(147)*. Cysts typically demonstrate heterogeneous signal intensity on T_1-weighted images and high signal intensity on T_2-weighted images *(148)*. So-called fluid-fluid levels caused by layering of water on denser proteinaceous material have also been described *(149)*.

CONCLUSION

Differential diagnosis of cardiac and pericardial tumors includes neoplastic diseases as well as nonneoplastic diseases. Primary neoplastic diseases are summarized in Tables 1 (primary benign cardiac tumors) and 2 (primary malignant cardiac tumors). The primary cardiac and pericardial tumors must be differentiated from secondary involvement of the heart by metastatic cancers and other nonneoplastic conditions, such as intracardiac thrombus pericardial cyst and lipomatous hypertrophy of the inter-atrial septum.

The differential diagnosis can be narrowed down by correlating clinical presentation, distinctive clinical features, demographics, and relevant laboratory findings in association with imaging characteristics of the tumors. The diagnosis can usually be reached by using different imaging modalities, in particular by assessing the location of tumors, specific site of involvement (intracavitary, endocardial, myocardial, epicardial, or pericardial), morphology of the lesion, and imaging findings associated with the lesions. Primary cardiac and pericardial tumors are clinically significant lesions, with potential life-threatening sequelae that affect patients of all ages. The clinical features and laboratory findings usually lead to a clinical suspicion to a diagnosis of primary cardiac and pericardial tumors. However, different imaging modalities are often necessary in approaching the final diagnosis. The detection and characterization of the tumor is critical because most benign tumors are curable, and the early diagnosis of malignancy dictates therapeutic cure or palliation depending on the stage of cancer.

Initial imaging with radiography is helpful in screening. CT and CMR imaging are complementary to echocardiography in differentiating primary cardiac and pericardial tumors from metastatic tumors and nonneoplastic conditions. CMR imaging is especially useful for evaluation of primary cardiac neoplasm. Tumor location, morphological features, and tissue characteristics, including the presence of calcification, fat, fibrous tissue, hemorrhage, and cystic change, may help refine the radiological differential diagnosis. Invasive behavior is a feature of malignant lesions. CMR imaging is helpful in defining mass for biopsies, which will lead to histopathological diagnosis and in guiding therapeutic strategies, which may be curative or palliative to related pathological findings.

REFERENCES

1. Reynen K. Frequency of primary tumors of the heart. Am J Cardiol 1996;77:107.
2. Goodwin JF. The spectrum of cardiac tumors. Am J Cardiol 1968;21:307–314.
3. Silverman NA. Primary cardiac tumors. Ann Surg 1980;191:127–138.
4. Burke AP, Cowan D, Virmani R. Primary sarcomas of the heart. Cancer 1992;69:387–395.
5. Zipes DP, Libby P, Bonow RO, Braunwald E. Braunwald's heart disease; a textbook of cardiovascular medicine. In: Sabitine MS, Colucci WS, Schoen FJ, eds. Primary tumors of the heart. New York: Elsevier; 2005:1741–1755.
6. Perchinsky MJ, Lichtenstein SV, Tyers GF. Primary cardiac tumors: 40 years' experience with 71 patients. Cancer 1997;79:1809–1815.
7. Roberts WC. Primary and secondary neoplasms of the heart. Am J Cardiol 1997;80:671–682.

8. Funari M, Fujita N, Peck WW, Higgins CB. Cardiac tumors: assessment with Gd-DTPA enhanced MR imaging. J Comput Assist Tomogr 1991;15:953–958.

9. Arciniegas E, Hakimi M, Farooki ZQ, Truccone NJ, Green EW. Primary cardiac tumors in children. J Thorac Cardiovasc Surg 1980;79:582–591.

10. Burke AP, Virmani R. Cardiac myxoma. A clinicopathologic study. Am J Clin Pathol 1993; 100:671–680.

11. Premaratne S, Hasaniya NW, Arakaki HY, Mugiishi MM, Mamiya RT, McNamara JJ. Atrial myxomas: experiences with 35 patients in Hawaii. Am J Surg 1995;169:600–603.

12. Moriyama Y, Saigenji H, Shimokawa S, Toyohira H, Taira A. The surgical treatment of 30 patients with cardiac myxomas: a comparison of clinical features according to morphological classification. Surg Today 1994;24:596–598.

13. Reynen K. Cardiac myxomas. N Engl J Med 1995;333:1610–1617.

14. Bjessmo S, Ivert T. Cardiac myxoma: 40 years' experience in 63 patients. Ann Thorac Surg 1997;63:697–700.

15. Markel ML, Waller BF, Armstrong WF. Cardiac myxoma. A review. Medicine (Baltimore) 1987;66: 114–125.

16. Pinede L, Duhaut P, Loire R. Clinical presentation of left atrial cardiac myxoma. A series of 112 consecutive cases. Medicine (Baltimore) 2001;80:159–172.

17. Rajpal RS, Leibsohn JA, Liekweg WG, et al. Infected left atrial myxoma with bacteremia simulating infective endocarditis. Arch Intern Med 1979;139:1176–1178.

18. Revankar SG, Clark RA. Infected cardiac myxoma. Case report and literature review. Medicine (Baltimore) 1998;77:337–344.

19. Aldridge HE, Greenwood WF. Myxoma of the left atrium. Br Heart J 1960;22:189–200.

20. Heath D. Pathology of cardiac tumors. Am J Cardiol 1968;21:315–327.

21. McCarthy PM, Piehler JM, Schaff HV, et al. The significance of multiple, recurrent, and "complex" cardiac myxomas. J Thorac Cardiovasc Surg 1986;91:389–396.

22. Carney JA, Gordon H, Carpenter PC, Shenoy BV, Go VL. The complex of myxomas, spotty pigmentation, and endocrine overactivity. Medicine (Baltimore) 1985;64:270–283.

23. Burke A, Virmani R. Atlas of tumor pathology. Tumors of the heart and great vessels. Washington, DC: Armed Forces Institute of Pathology; 1996.

24. Steiner RE. Radiologic aspects of cardiac tumors. Am J Cardiol 1968;21:344–356.

25. Freedberg RS, Kronzon I, Rumancik WM, Liebeskind D. The contribution of magnetic resonance imaging to the evaluation of intracardiac tumors diagnosed by echocardiography. Circulation 1988;77:96–103.

26. DePace NL, Soulen RL, Kotler MN, Mintz GS. Two dimensional echocardiographic detection of intraatrial masses. Am J Cardiol 1981;48:954–960.

27. Matsuoka H, Hamada M, Honda T, et al. Morphologic and histologic characterization of cardiac myxomas by magnetic resonance imaging. Angiology 1996;47:693–698.

28. de Roos A, Weijers E, van Duinen S, van der Wall EE. Calcified right atrial myxoma demonstrated by magnetic resonance imaging. Chest 1989;95:478–479.

29. Masui T, Takahashi M, Miura K, Naito M, Tawarahara K. Cardiac myxoma: identification of intratumoral hemorrhage and calcification on MR images. AJR Am J Roentgenol 1995;164:850–852.

30. Larsson S, Lepore V, Kennergren C. Atrial myxomas: results of 25 years' experience and review of the literature. Surgery 1989;105:695–698.

31. Castells E, Ferran V, Octavio de Toledo MC, et al. Cardiac myxomas: surgical treatment, long-term results and recurrence. J Cardiovasc Surg (Torino) 1993;34:49–53.

32. Edwards FH, Hale D, Cohen A, Thompson L, Pezzella AT, Virmani R. Primary cardiac valve tumors. Ann Thorac Surg 1991;52:1127–1131.

33. Klarich KW, Enriquez-Sarano M, Gura GM, Edwards WD, Tajik AJ, Seward JB. Papillary fibroelastoma: echocardiographic characteristics for diagnosis and pathologic correlation. J Am Coll Cardiol 1997; 30:784–790.

34. Shahian DM, Labib SB, Chang G. Cardiac papillary fibroelastoma. Ann Thorac Surg 1995;59:538–541.

35. Sun JP, Asher CR, Yang XS, et al. Clinical and echocardiographic characteristics of papillary fibroelastomas: a retrospective and prospective study in 162 patients. Circulation 2001;103: 2687–2693.

36. al-Mohammad A, Pambakian H, Young C. Fibroelastoma: case report and review of the literature. Heart 1998;79:301–304.

37. Beghetti M, Gow RM, Haney I, Mawson J, Williams WG, Freedom RM. Pediatric primary benign cardiac tumors: a 15-years review. Am Heart J 1997;134:1107–1114.

38. Smith HC, Watson GH, Patel RG, Super M. Cardiac rhabdomyomata in tuberous sclerosis: their course and diagnostic value. Arch Dis Child 1989;64:196–200.
39. Aideyan UO, Zaleski CG, Rodriguez MM. Pediatric case of the day. Cardiac rhabdomyoma. Radiographics 1997;17:805–807.
40. Christophe C, Bartholome J, Blum D, et al. Neonatal tuberous sclerosis. US, CT, and MR diagnosis of brain and cardiac lesions. Pediatr Radiol 1989;19:446–448.
41. Berkenblit R, Spindola-Franco H, Frater RW, Fish BB, Glickstein JS. MRI in the evaluation and management of a newborn infant with cardiac rhabdomyoma. Ann Thorac Surg 1997;63:1475–1477.
42. Nir A, Tajik AJ, Freeman WK, et al. Tuberous sclerosis and cardiac rhabdomyoma. Am J Cardiol 1995;76:419–421.
43. Bosi G, Lintermans JP, Pellegrino PA, Svaluto-Moreolo G, Vliers A. The natural history of cardiac rhabdomyoma with and without tuberous sclerosis. Acta Paediatr 1996;85:928–931.
44. Smythe JF, Dyck JD, Smallhorn JF, Freedom RM. Natural history of cardiac rhabdomyoma in infancy and childhood. Am J Cardiol 1990;66:1247–1249.
45. Burke AP, Rosado-de-Christenson M, Templeton PA, Virmani R. Cardiac fibroma: clinicopathologic correlates and surgical treatment. J Thorac Cardiovasc Surg 1994;108:862–870.
46. Vidaillet HJ Jr. Cardiac tumors associated with hereditary syndromes. Am J Cardiol 1988;61:1355.
47. Parmley LF, Salley RK, Williams JP, Head GB 3rd. The clinical spectrum of cardiac fibroma with diagnostic and surgical considerations: noninvasive imaging enhances management. Ann Thorac Surg 1988;45:455–465.
48. Tazelaar HD, Locke TJ, McGregor CG. Pathology of surgically excised primary cardiac tumors. Mayo Clin Proc 1992;67:957–965.
49. Yamaguchi M, Hosokawa Y, Ohashi H, Imai M, Oshima Y, Minamiji K. Cardiac fibroma. Long-term fate after excision. J Thorac Cardiovasc Surg 1992;103:140–145.
50. Burke A, Johns JP, Virmani R. Hemangiomas of the heart. A clinicopathologic study of ten cases. Am J Cardiovasc Pathol 1990;3:283–290.
51. Brodwater B, Erasmus J, McAdams HP, Dodd L. Case report. Pericardial hemangioma. J Comput Assist Tomogr 1996;20:954–956.
52. Newell JD 2nd, Eckel C, Davis M, Tadros NB. MR appearance of an arteriovenous hemangioma of the interventricular septum. Cardiovasc Intervent Radiol 1988;11:319–321.
53. Palmer TE, Tresch DD, Bonchek LI. Spontaneous resolution of a large, cavernous hemangioma of the heart. Am J Cardiol 1986;58:184–185.
54. Doshi S, Halim M, Singh H, Patel R. Massive intrapericardial lipoma, a rare cause of breathlessness. Investigations and management. Int J Cardiol 1998;66:211–215.
55. King SJ, Smallhorn JF, Burrows PE. Epicardial lipoma: imaging findings. AJR Am J Roentgenol 1993;160:261–262.
56. Kamiya H, Ohno M, Iwata H, et al. Cardiac lipoma in the interventricular septum: evaluation by computed tomography and magnetic resonance imaging. Am Heart J 1990;119:1215–1217.
57. Hananouchi GI, Goff WB 2nd. Cardiac lipoma: 6-years follow-up with MRI characteristics, and a review of the literature. Magn Reson Imaging 1990;8:825–828.
58. Sankar NM, Thiruchelvam T, Thirunavukkaarasu K, Pang K, Hanna WM. Symptomatic lipoma in the right atrial free wall. A case report. Tex Heart Inst J 1998;25:152–154.
59. Ashar K, van Hoeven KH. Fatal lipoma of the heart. Am J Cardiovasc Pathol 1992;4:85–90.
60. Heufelder AE, Hofbauer LC. Greetings from below the aortic arch! The paradigm of cardiac paraganglioma. J Clin Endocrinol Metab 1996;81:891–895.
61. Conti VR, Saydjari R, Amparo EG. Paraganglioma of the heart. The value of magnetic resonance imaging in the preoperative evaluation. Chest 1986;90:604–606.
62. Shapiro B, Copp JE, Sisson JC, Eyre PL, Wallis J, Beierwaltes WH. Iodine-131 metaiodobenzylguanidine for the locating of suspected pheochromocytoma: experience in 400 cases. J Nucl Med 1985;26: 576–585.
63. Hamilton BH, Francis IR, Gross BH, et al. Intrapericardial paragangliomas (pheochromocytomas): imaging features. AJR Am J Roentgenol 1997;168:109–113.
64. Fisher MR, Higgins CB, Andereck W. MR imaging of an intrapericardial pheochromocytoma. J Comput Assist Tomogr 1985;9:1103–1105.
65. Cane ME, Berrizbeitia LD, Yang SS, Mahapatro D, McGrath LB. Paraganglioma of the interatrial septum. Ann Thorac Surg 1996;61:1845–1847.
66. Orringer MB, Sisson JC, Glazer G, et al. Surgical treatment of cardiac pheochromocytomas. J Thorac Cardiovasc Surg 1985;89:753–757.

67. Aravot DJ, Banner NR, Cantor AM, Theodoropoulos S, Yacoub MH. Location, localization and surgical treatment of cardiac pheochromocytoma. Am J Cardiol 1992;69:283–285.

68. Seguin JR, Coulon P, Huret C, Grolleau-Roux R, Chaptal PA. Intrapericardial teratoma in infancy: a rare disease. J Cardiovasc Surg (Torino) 1986;27:509–511.

69. Beghetti M, Prieditis M, Rebeyka IM, Mawson J. Images in cardiovascular medicine. Intrapericardial teratoma. Circulation 1998;97:1523–1524.

70. Cyr DR, Guntheroth WG, Nyberg DA, Smith JR, Nudelman SR, Ek M. Prenatal diagnosis of an intrapericardial teratoma. A cause for nonimmune hydrops. J Ultrasound Med 1988;7:87–90.

71. Tollens T, Casselman F, Devlieger H, et al. Fetal cardiac tamponade due to an intrapericardial teratoma. Ann Thorac Surg 1998;66:559–560.

72. Aldousany AW, Joyner JC, Price RA, Boulden T, Watson D, DiSessa TG. Diagnosis and treatment of intrapericardial teratoma. Pediatr Cardiol 1987;8:51–53.

73. Uzun O, Dickinson DF, Watterson KG. Acute tamponade in a newborn infant caused by a massive cystic teratoma. Heart 1996;76:188.

74. Putnam JB Jr, Sweeney MS, Colon R, Lanza LA, Frazier OH, Cooley DA. Primary cardiac sarcomas. Ann Thorac Surg 1991;51:906–910.

75. Rosenkranz ER, Murphy DJ Jr. Diagnosis and neonatal resection of right atrial angiosarcoma. Ann Thorac Surg 1994;57:1014–1015.

76. Laya MB, Mailliard JA, Bewtra C, Levin HS. Malignant fibrous histiocytoma of the heart. A case report and review of the literature. Cancer 1987;59:1026–1031.

77. Kim EE, Wallace S, Abello R, et al. Malignant cardiac fibrous histiocytomas and angiosarcomas: MR features. J Comput Assist Tomogr 1989;13:627–632.

78. Rettmar K, Stierle U, Sheikhzadeh A, Diederich KW. Primary angiosarcoma of the heart. Report of a case and review of the literature. Jpn Heart J 1993;34:667–683.

79. Araoz PA, Eklund HE, Welch TJ, Breen JF. CT and MR imaging of primary cardiac malignancies. Radiographics 1999;19:1421–1434.

80. Siripornpitak S, Higgins CB. MRI of primary malignant cardiovascular tumors. J Comput Assist Tomogr 1997;21:462–466.

81. Mader MT, Poulton TB, White RD. Malignant tumors of the heart and great vessels: MR imaging appearance. Radiographics 1997;17:145–153.

82. Bruna J, Lockwood M. Primary heart angiosarcoma detected by computed tomography and magnetic resonance imaging. Eur Radiol 1998;8:66–68.

83. Antunes MJ, Vanderdonck KM, Andrade CM, Rebelo LS. Primary cardiac leiomyosarcomas. Ann Thorac Surg 1991;51:999–1001.

84. Kakizaki S, Takagi H, Hosaka Y. Cardiac angiosarcoma responding to multidisciplinary treatment. Int J Cardiol 1997;62:273–275.

85. Harlamert HA, Moulton JS, Lewis W. Images in cardiovascular medicine. Primary malignant fibrous histiocytoma of the heart treated with orthotopic heart transplantation. Circulation 1998; 97:703–704.

86. Ceresoli GL, Ferreri AJ, Bucci E, Ripa C, Ponzoni M, Villa E. Primary cardiac lymphoma in immunocompetent patients: diagnostic and therapeutic management. Cancer 1997;80:1497–1506.

87. Curtsinger CR, Wilson MJ, Yoneda K. Primary cardiac lymphoma. Cancer 1989;64:521–525.

88. Holladay AO, Siegel RJ, Schwartz DA. Cardiac malignant lymphoma in acquired immune deficiency syndrome. Cancer 1992;70:2203–2207.

89. Dorsay TA, Ho VB, Rovira MJ, Armstrong MA, Brissette MD. Primary cardiac lymphoma: CT and MR findings. J Comput Assist Tomogr 1993;17:978–981.

90. Chim CS, Chan AC, Kwong YL, Liang R. Primary cardiac lymphoma. Am J Hematol 1997;54:79–83.

91. Beckwith C, Butera J, Sadaniantz A, King TC, Fingleton J, Rosmarin AG. Diagnosis in oncology. Case 1: primary transmural cardiac lymphoma. J Clin Oncol 2000;18:1996–1997.

92. Kaul TK, Fields BL, Kahn DR. Primary malignant pericardial mesothelioma: a case report and review. J Cardiovasc Surg (Torino) 1994;35:261–267.

93. Yilling FP, Schlant RC, Hertzler GL, Krzyaniak R. Pericardial mesothelioma. Chest 1982;81:520–523.

94. Gossinger HD, Siostrzonek P, Zangeneh M, et al. Magnetic resonance imaging findings in a patient with pericardial mesothelioma. Am Heart J 1988;115:1321–1322.

95. Lam KY, Dickens P, Chan AC. Tumors of the heart. A 20-years experience with a review of 12,485 consecutive autopsies. Arch Pathol Lab Med 1993;117:1027–1031.

96. Adenle AD, Edwards JE. Clinical and pathologic features of metastatic neoplasms of the pericardium. Chest 1982;81:166–169.

97. MacLowry JD, Roberts WC. Metastatic choriocarcinoma of the lung. Invasion of pulmonary veins with extension into the left atrium and mitral orifice. Am J Cardiol 1966;18:938–941.

98. Labib SB, Schick EC Jr, Isner JM. Obstruction of right ventricular outflow tract caused by intracavitary metastatic disease: analysis of 14 cases. J Am Coll Cardiol 1992;19:1664–1668.

99. Domanski MJ, Cunnion RE, Fernicola DJ, Roberts WC. Fatal cor pulmonale caused by extensive tumor emboli in the small pulmonary arteries without emboli in the major pulmonary arteries or metastases in the pulmonary parenchyma. Am J Cardiol 1993;72:233–234.

100. Onuigbo WI. Direct extension of cancer between pulmonary veins and the left atrium. Chest 1972;62:444–446.

101. Weg IL, Mehra S, Azueta V, Rosner F. Cardiac metastasis from adenocarcinoma of the lung. Echocardiographic-pathologic correlation. Am J Med 1986;80:108–112.

102. Kadir S, Coulam CM. Intracaval extension of renal cell carcinoma. Cardiovasc Intervent Radiol 1980;3:180–183.

103. Waller BF, Fletcher RD, Roberts WC. Carcinoma of the lung causing pulmonary arterial stenosis. Chest 1981;79:589–591.

104. Glancy DL, Roberts WC. The heart in malignant melanoma. A study of 70 autopsy cases. Am J Cardiol 1968;21:555–571.

105. Waller BF, Gottdiener JS, Virmani R, Roberts WC. The "charcoal heart"; melanoma to the cor. Chest 1980;77:671–676.

106. Chen RH, Gaos CM, Frazier OH. Complete resection of a right atrial intracavitary metastatic melanoma. Ann Thorac Surg 1996;61:1255–1257.

107. Roberts WC, Bodey GP, Wertlake PT. The heart in acute leukemia. A study of 420 autopsy cases. Am J Cardiol 1968;21:388–412.

108. Waller BF, Roberts WC. Systolic clicks caused by rocks in the right heart chambers. Am Heart J 1981;102:459–460.

109. Roberts WC, Glancy DL, DeVita VT Jr. Heart in malignant lymphoma (Hodgkin's disease, lymphosarcoma, reticulum cell sarcoma and mycosis fungoides). A study of 196 autopsy cases. Am J Cardiol 1968;22:85–107.

110. McDonnell PJ, Mann RB, Bulkley BH. Involvement of the heart by malignant lymphoma: a clinicopathologic study. Cancer 1982;49:944–951.

111. Thurber DL, Edwards JE, Achor RW. Secondary malignant tumors of the pericardium. Circulation 1962;26:228–241.

112. Quraishi MA, Costanzi JJ, Hokanson J. The natural history of lung cancer with pericardial metastases. Cancer 1983;51:740–742.

113. el Allaf D, Burette R, Pierard L, Limet R. Cardiac tamponade as the first manifestation of cardiothoracic malignancy: a study of 10 cases. Eur Heart J 1986;7:247–253.

114. Kutalek SP, Panidis IP, Kotler MN, Mintz GS, Carver J, Ross JJ. Metastatic tumors of the heart detected by two-dimensional echocardiography. Am Heart J 1985;109:343–349.

115. Sheldon R, Isaac D. Metastatic melanoma to the heart presenting with ventricular tachycardia. Chest 1991;99:1296–1298.

116. Redwine DB. Complete heart block caused by secondary tumors of the heart. Case report and review of literature. Tex Med 1974;70:59–64.

117. Kopelson G, Herwig KJ. The etiologies of coronary artery disease in cancer patients. Int J Radiat Oncol Biol Phys 1978;4:895–906.

118. Virmani R, Khedekar RR, Robinowitz M, McAllister HA Jr. Tumor embolization in coronary artery causing myocardial infarction. Arch Pathol Lab Med 1983;107:243–245.

119. Fujisaki M, Kurihara E, Kikuchi K, Nishikawa K, Uematsu Y. Hepatocellular carcinoma with tumor thrombus extending into the right atrium: report of a successful resection with the use of cardiopulmonary bypass. Surgery 1991;109:214–219.

120. Nakayama Y, Kitamura S, Kawachi K, Kawata T, Fukutomi M, Hasegawa J, Morita R. Intravenous leiomyomatosis extending into the right atrium. Cardiovasc Surg 1994;2:642–645.

121. Griffin AS, Sterchi JM. Primary leiomyosarcoma of the inferior vena cava: a case report and review of the literature. J Surg Oncol 1987;34:53–60.

122. Peh WC, Cheung DL, Ngan H. Smooth muscle tumors of the inferior vena cava and right heart. Clin Imaging 1993;17:117–123.

123. Birmingham CL, Peretz DI. Metastatic carcinoma presenting as obstruction to the right ventricular outflow tract. Report of a case and review of the literature. Am Heart J 1979;97:229–232.

124. Bartels P, O'Callaghan WG, Peyton R, Sethi G, Maley T. Metastatic liposarcoma of the right ventricle with outflow tract obstruction: restrictive pathophysiology predicts poor surgical outcome. Am Heart J 1988;115:696–698.

125. Van Osdol KD, Hall RJ, Warda M, Massumi A, Klima T. Right ventricular thrombus: clinical and diagnostic features. Tex Heart Inst J 1983;10:359–364.

126. Heitzman M, Gibson TC, Tabakin BS. A right-sided cardiac mass. Right atrial thrombus. Arch Intern Med 1984;144:1813–1815.

127. Watts FB Jr, Zingas AP, Das L, Cushing BA. Computed tomographic diagnosis of an intracardiac metastasis from osteosarcoma. J Comput Tomogr 1983;7:271–272.

128. Wolverson MK, Grider RD, Sundaram M, Heiberg E, Johnson F. Demonstration of unsuspected malignant disease of the pericardium by computed tomography. J Comput Tomogr 1980;4:330–333.

129. Salcedo EE, Cohen GI, White RD, Davison MB. Cardiac tumors: diagnosis and management. Curr Probl Cardiol 1992;17:73–137.

130. Emmot WW, Vacek JL, Agee K, Moran J, Dunn MI. Metastatic malignant melanoma presenting clinically as obstruction of the right ventricular inflow and outflow tracts. Characterization by magnetic resonance imaging. Chest 1987;92:362–364.

131. Enochs WS, Petherick P, Bogdanova A, Mohr U, Weissleder R. Paramagnetic metal scavenging by melanin: MR imaging. Radiology 1997;204:417–423.

132. Yoshioka H, Itai Y, Niitsu M, et al. Intramuscular metastasis from malignant melanoma: MR findings. Skeletal Radiol 1999;28:714–716.

133. Mousseaux E, Meunier P, Azancott S, Dubayle P, Gaux JC. Cardiac metastatic melanoma investigated by magnetic resonance imaging. Magn Reson Imaging 1998;16:91–95.

134. Fujita N, Caputo GR, Higgins CB. Diagnosis and characterization of intracardiac masses by magnetic resonance imaging. Am J Card Imaging 1994;8:69–80.

135. Meyers DG, Bouska DJ. Diagnostic usefulness of pericardial fluid cytology. Chest 1989;95:1142–1143.

136. Millaire A, Wurtz A, de Groote P, Saudemont A, Chambon A, Ducloux G. Malignant pericardial effusions: usefulness of pericardioscopy. Am Heart J 1992;124:1030–1034.

137. Hanley PC, Shub C, Seward JB, Wold LE. Intracavitary cardiac melanoma diagnosed by endomyocardial left ventricular biopsy. Chest 1983;84:195–198.

138. Gosalakkal JA, Sugrue DD. Malignant melanoma of the right atrium: antemortem diagnosis by transvenous biopsy. Br Heart J 1989;62:159–160.

139. Maher EA, Shepherd FA, Todd TJ. Pericardial sclerosis as the primary management of malignant pericardial effusion and cardiac tamponade. J Thorac Cardiovasc Surg 1996;112:637–643.

140. Shepherd FA, Morgan C, Evans WK, Ginsberg JF, Watt D, Murphy K. Medical management of malignant pericardial effusion by tetracycline sclerosis. Am J Cardiol 1987;60:1161–1166.

141. Shirani J, Roberts WC. Clinical, electrocardiographic and morphologic features of massive fatty deposits ("lipomatous hypertrophy") in the atrial septum. J Am Coll Cardiol 1993;22:226–238.

142. Prior JT. Lipomatous hypertrophy of cardiac interatrial septum. A lesion resembling hibernoma, lipoblastomatosis and infiltrating lipoma. Arch Pathol 1964;78:11–15.

143. Pochis WT, Saeian K, Sagar KB. Usefulness of transesophageal echocardiography in diagnosing lipomatous hypertrophy of the atrial septum with comparison to transthoracic echocardiography. Am J Cardiol 1992;70:396–398.

144. Zeebregts CJ, Hensens AG, Timmermans J, Pruszczynski MS, Lacquet LK. Lipomatous hypertrophy of the interatrial septum: indication for surgery? Eur J Cardiothorac Surg 1997;11:785–787.

145. Breuer M, Wippermann J, Franke U, Wahlers T. Lipomatous hypertrophy of the interatrial septum and upper right atrial inflow obstruction. Eur J Cardiothorac Surg 2002;22:1023–1025.

146. Paydarfar D, Krieger D, Dib N, et al. In vivo magnetic resonance imaging and surgical histopathology of intracardiac masses: distinct features of subacute thrombi. Cardiology 2001;95:40–47.

147. Mendelson DS, Rose JS, Efremidis SC, Kirschner PA, Cohen BA. Bronchogenic cysts with high CT numbers. AJR Am J Roentgenol 1983;140:463–465.

148. Nakata H, Egashira K, Watanabe H, et al. MRI of bronchogenic cysts. J Comput Assist Tomogr 1993;17:267–270.

149. Lyon RD, McAdams HP. Mediastinal bronchogenic cyst: demonstration of a fluid-fluid level at MR imaging. Radiology 1993;186:427–428.

22 Assessing Pericardial Disease by CMR

Mouaz Al-Mallah and Raymond Y. Kwong

NORMAL PERICARDIUM AND PERICARDIAL SINUSES

The pericardium consists of the parietal and visceral layers separated by 15–30 mL of serous fluid. The serous visceral layer envelops the heart and several centimeters of the proximal great vessels, where it reflects to form the fibrotic, outer parietal layer. The normal pericardium serves such functions as reducing motion friction between the heart and surrounding structures, maintaining diastolic pressures by confining diastolic expansion of thin-walled cardiac chambers, constraining the bulk cardiac motion in the middle mediastinum, and limiting the spread of infection from the mediastinal structures. However, it is not necessary for normal cardiac function, as shown by patients with a surgically or congenitally absent pericardium.

The normal visceral pericardium is too thin to be visible by any imaging techniques. Magnetic resonance (MR) imaging provides excellent visualization of the pericardium in most patients. Normal parietal pericardium, however, appears as a low-intensity circumferential layer that often lies between high-intensity mediastinal fat and epicardial fat or intermediate-intensity myocardium on T_1-weighted (T_1W) spin echo cardiovascular magnetic resonance (CMR) imaging (Fig. 1).

Pathological studies revealed that normal human parietal pericardium is 0.5–1 mm thick *(1)* and is most prominent adjacent to the right ventricular free wall and the inferior and apical aspect of the left ventricle. Discrimination of the pericardium from the myocardium on radiologic images requires the presence of epicardial fat or pericardial fluid. Because of partial volume averaging, cardiac motion, inclusion of pericardial fluid, and chemical shift artifact, normal parietal pericardium may appear as thick as 4 mm on T_1W spin echo CMR. The low signal intensity of the pericardium on T_1W spin echo imaging is attributable to the fibrous component of the pericardium in combination with a small quantity of adherent pericardial fluid.

From: *Contemporary Cardiology: Cardiovascular Magnetic Resonance Imaging*
Edited by: Raymond Y. Kwong © Humana Press Inc., Totowa, NJ

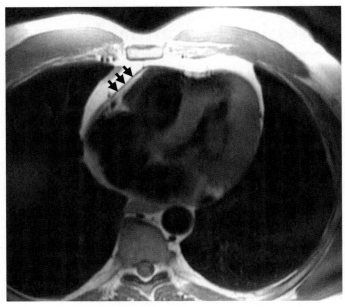

Fig. 1. The low signal intensity pericardium is commonly seen between the high signal intensity mediastinal fat and the epicardial fat on T_1W spin echo CMR imaging.

The superior aspect of the pericardial sac wraps around the great vessels and forms several pericardial sinuses, which are often mistaken for abnormality on CMR and computed tomography (CT) (Fig. 2). The transverse sinus of pericardium lies dorsal to the ascending aorta and may be mistaken for aortic dissection or lymphadenopathy. The superior pericardial recess, a curvilinear space adjacent to the right wall of the ascending aorta, may be mistaken for an aortic dissection or a mediastinal mass. The oblique sinus of pericardium, which is situated behind the left atrium, may be misinterpreted as esophageal lesions or bronchogenic cysts. Knowledge of these structures helps distinguish normal structures from pathological structures.

AN OVERVIEW OF PERICARDIAL IMAGING

The wide availability and portability of echocardiography, lack of ionizing radiation, and low cost make echocardiography most often the initial test in the evaluation of the pericardium, especially in patients suspected of having pericardial effusion or tamponade. Two-dimensional (2D) cine imaging and Doppler assessment are extremely useful for detecting pericardial effusion and any physiological evidence of cardiac tamponade in unstable patients. However, it is difficult to evaluate with echocardiography in the absence of pericardial effusion as it may have echogenicity similar to the surrounding tissues. 2D cine echocardiography is not accurate in quantifying the thickness of the pericardium or in viewing the entire pericardium or loculated pericardial effusion because of a limited acoustic window. It also cannot assess the nature of a pericardial mass or effusion because of a relative lack of tissue contrast. In addition, loculated effusions, especially those in anterior locations, can be difficult to detect with echocardiography. It is inferior to other the imaging modalities in sizing

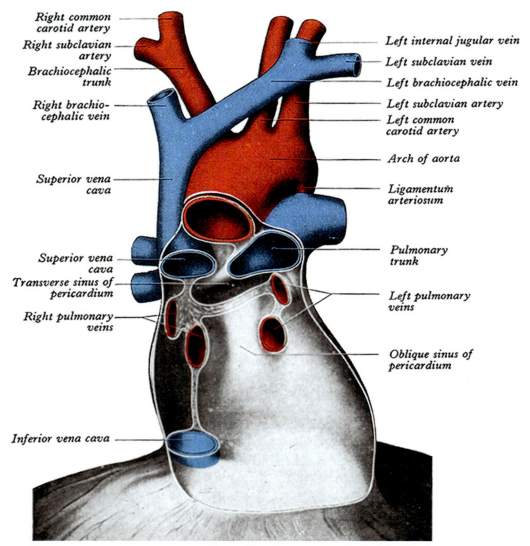

Fig. 2. The major pericardial sinuses. Illustration shows the location of the transverse and oblique pericardial sinuses. (From ref. *15.*)

loculated pericardial effusion, differentiating pericardial or epicardial fat pad from pericardial effusions, detecting regional or diffuse pericardial thickening, and characterizing the content of the pericardial mass or fluid. More important, the technique is operator dependent.

In contrast to echocardiography, CT can assess pericardial thickness of the whole heart at high spatial resolution. The thickness of the normal pericardium is less than 2 mm by CT techniques. CT can visualize pericardial calcifications—a finding indicative of constrictive pericarditis in patients with coexisting constrictive physiological features. Contrast enhancement is useful to help delineate blood vessels and the blood-filled cardiac chamber cavities from the myocardium. It requires less time than echocardiography and CMR.

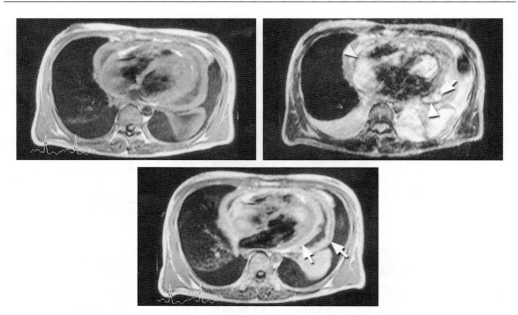

Fig. 3. Top: T_1W images show pericardial thickening with a signal intensity equal to the myocardium. Middle: T_2W image demonstrates low-intensity lesions at the inner surface of the thickened pericardium (arrowheads). Linear low signals are also depicted in the pericardial effusion (arrow). Bottom: Gadolinium-enhanced MRI demonstrates uniform, tramline like enhancement of the thickened parietal and visceral pericardia (arrow).

CT, however, involves the use of intravenously administered iodinated contrast material and ionizing radiation. If performed without electrocardiographic (ECG) gating, CT may lead to cardiac motion artifacts, which limit evaluation of pericardial thickness. Pretreatment with β-adrenergic blockers may be required in some cases to improve visualization of the pericardium. Another limitation of CT imaging of the pericardium is difficulty in differentiating highly proteinaceous or exudative pericardial effusion from thickened pericardial tissue.

CMR offers distinct advantages because of unrestricted imaging field, superior tissue contrast, and high spatial resolution. Having a wider field of view, CMR allows the examination of the entire chest and detection of the associated abnormalities in the mediastinum and lungs. Soft tissue contrast on CMR images is superior to that on echocardiograms. CMR can provide excellent anatomic delineation of pericardial thickness as well as characterize findings that reflect constrictive physiology.

CMR imaging can be acquired in any arbitrary scan planes for the depiction of pericardial thickness without the need for iodinated contrast material, ionizing radiation, or image reconstruction. Typically, a combination of T_1W and T_2-weighted (T_2W) sequences and cine gradient echo image in matching slice locations can provide complementary information regarding pericardial structure, fluid flow, and content of the pericardial effusion. Off-label use of intravenously injected gadolinium-DTPA (diethyltriaminepentaacetic acid) has been reported to enhance the pericardium secondary to inflammation of the pericardium (Figs. 3–5) *(2–4)*.

The use of the T_2/T_1-weighted steady-state free precession (SSFP) gradient echo cine MR imaging produces high signal-to-noise ratio motion images, which allows

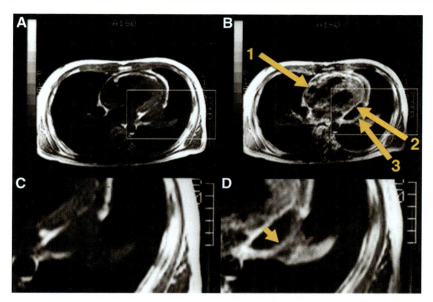

Fig. 4. (A) T_1W transverse MR image shows expansion of low-intensity band consistent with the pericardial effusion and thickened pericardium. **(B)** Gd-DTPA enhances the involved visceral pericardium (arrow 2), parietal pericardium (arrow 3) and adhered pericardium (arrow 1). The thickness of pericardium (arrowhead) is 6 mm **(D)**. **(C)** Close-up view of panel A; **(D)** Close-up view of panel B.

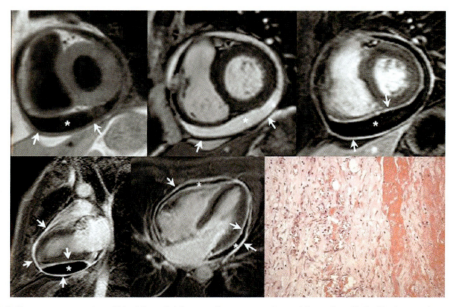

Fig. 5. Inflammatory pericarditis (chronic) in a patient presenting with pericardial effusion and pyrexia of unknown origin On short-axis spin echo MRI (upper left) and cine MRI (upper middle), a moderate pericardial effusion (asterisks) and thickened pericardial layers (arrows) are well seen. Late-enhancement cardiac MRI (remaining three images) shows strong enhancement of both thickened pericardial layers. Note the better differentiation between the pericardial layers (arrows) and fluid (asterisks) on the late-enhancement images than on the conventional spin echo MRI image. Histology (400×) shows thickened pericardium with young, vascularized granulation tissue and large amounts of fibrin (red areas).

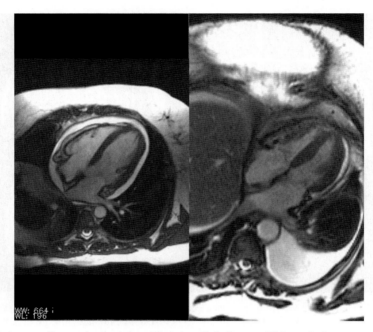

Fig. 6. SSFP cine gradient echo imaging of pericardial disease. This technique provides structural information regarding pericardial thickness, pericardial effusion, pericardial adhesions, and evidence of pericardial constriction without the need for contrast agent. On the left is a patient with pericarditis without clinical signs and symptoms of pericardial constriction. The SSFP cine imaging demonstrates moderate-size pericardial effusion but normal pericardial thickness. On the right, a patient with a remote history of pericarditis presents with recurrent lower extremity edema. SSFP imaging demonstrates marked thickened pericardium (most thickened adjacent to the right ventricle) and physiological signs of pericardial constriction, including paradoxical diastolic motion of the interventricular septum, biatrial enlargement, and hepatic fluid congestion (*see* figure 6 movie in CD).

pericardial thickness, pericardial effusion flow, pericardial adhesions, and structural changes from pericardial constriction to be readily determined without the use of contrast agents *(5)* (Fig. 6). The technique is not operator dependent. A disadvantage of CMR is the requirement for cardiac gating, which requires a critical number of regular heartbeats during a single breath hold to produce a high-quality image. The presence of supraventricular arrhythmias, including atrial fibrillation, which is common in pericardial diseases, often deteriorates imaging quality of CMR, although diagnostic-quality study is possible in most cases.

PERICARDIAL EFFUSION

There is normally less than 50 mL fluid in the pericardial sac. Accumulation of more than 50 mL fluid is abnormal and may lead to homodynamic deterioration depending on the rate of fluid accumulation. Echocardiography is almost always the first imaging tool used to diagnose, evaluate, and assess pericardial effusion. Echocardiography is both sensitive and specific in detecting even a small amount of pericardial effusion. The portability of the echo machine, lack of ionizing radiation, and low cost make echocardiography the test of choice to detect pericardial effusions, especially in unstable patients with physiologically significant cardiac tamponade. CMR, however, can provide more in-depth characterization of the pericardial diseases than echocardiography in hemodynamically stable patients.

CMR is better than echocardiography in detecting loculated effusions, especially those in the anterior and superior locations because of a wider field of view. When imaging patients with large pericardial effusion, special attention should be given to the gating process. These patients might have low voltage of the QRS complex and electrical alternans (varying size of the QRS complex reflecting a physical resonant swinging of the heart within the expanded pericardial space). These two phenomena may affect the gating and result in suboptimal images.

Cine SSFP CMR is extremely sensitive to even a small amount of pericardial effusion and can quantify the size of the effusion by volumetric technique better than echocardiography. Semiquantitatively, a dimension of more than 5 mm of pericardial fluid anterior to the right ventricle has been classified as moderate in size. When viewed in cine gradient echo magnetic resonance imaging (MRI), pericardial effusions usually demonstrate fluid mobility and changes in the regional dimension of the pericardial sac throughout the cardiac cycle, which is often helpful in distinguishing pericardial effusions from epicardial fat pad.

The ability of CMR to characterize the composition of the pericardial fluid is perhaps the most distinct advantage of CMR in imaging pericardial effusion compared to echocardiography and CT. Transudative pericardial effusions typically are related to decreased drainage caused by increased venous pressure, such as in congestive heart failure, lymphatic obstruction, or decreased serum osmolality as in a hypoproteinemic state, and have low cellular and protein content. In contrast, exudative, including hemorrhagic, effusions have high cellular content and are often related to injury (from trauma or myocardial infarction); myocardial or great vessel rupture; neoplasm (carcinoma of lung or breast, lymphoma); infection (bacterial, viral, or tuberculous); and inflammation (vasculitis/connective tissue disease). However, the exudates-vs-transudate characterization in different pericardial pathology may be obscured by the rate of pericardial fluid reabsorption (6).

Because of cardiac motion and flow effects, small effusions often have low signal intensity on spin echo imaging regardless of effusion type and can be difficult to characterize. Moderate-to-large transudative effusions have a relatively long T_1 because of few cells and low protein content and therefore usually have low signal intensity on T_1W spin echo imaging. Exudative or hemorrhagic effusions have high cellular and protein content; consequently, they have a relatively short T_1 and therefore a medium or high signal on T_1W spin echo (Figs. 7 and 8).

The T_2 and T_2* magnetic property from the formation of methemoglobin in hemorrhage has been used in detecting and defining the relative age of a hemorrhagic pericardial effusion. In general, T_2W spin echo is more reliable than gradient echo because it is less affected by cardiac motion. Acute hematomas demonstrate homogeneous high signal intensity, whereas subacute hematomas that are 1–4 weeks old typically show heterogeneous signal intensity, with patchy areas of high signal intensity on both T_1W and T_2W images (Fig. 9). Chronic organized hematomas may show a dark peripheral rim and low signal intensity internal foci that may represent calcification, fibrosis, or hemosiderin deposition (Fig. 10) (7). Chylous effusions have a short T_1 because of proteinaceous content and therefore appear bright on T_1W spin echo. With longer time for T_1 recovery, chylous effusions often appear to have even higher signal on T_2W spin echo than the T_1W spin echo imaging (Fig. 11).

	T1W Fast Spin-Echo	T2W Fast Spin-Echo
Transudative	Low	High
Exudative	Medium	High
Proteinaceous	High	Very High
Hemorrhagic (acute)	Homogeneous, High	Homogeneous, Low
Hemorrhagic (subacute or chronic)	Heterogeneous, Variable Intensities	Heterogeneous, subacute hemorrhage may show variable intensities. Chronic organized hematoma may become homogeneously dark.

Fig. 7. Characterization of the composition of moderate- to large-size pericardial effusions by CMR.

In common with echocardiography, MR can provide useful functional data, with cine images able to demonstrate right-sided chamber collapse in diastole, a useful early signal in the diagnosis of cardiac tamponade. This is best seen in short-axis cine images at the midventricular level.

Because most or the entire chest is evaluated during CMR imaging of the pericardium, associated abnormalities in the mediastinum and lungs also may be detected during the examination. When a large effusion is associated with an irregularly thickened pericardium or pericardial nodularity, malignancy should be suspected. In addition, MRI is superior to CT in differentiating thickened pericardium from fluid.

CONSTRICTIVE PERICARDITIS

Patients with constrictive pericarditis frequently present with symptoms of heart failure, such as dyspnea, orthopnea, and fatigue and occasionally may present with liver enlargement and ascites. At present, constrictive pericarditis in the Western nations is most frequently idiopathic or caused by cardiac surgery or radiation treatment to the mediastinum (Fig. 12). Pericardial constriction results from progressive pericardial fibrosis, which leads to sudden impaired filling of either the right or both ventricles during midlate diastole.

Transthoracic echocardiography is routinely the first test performed for the evaluation of myocardial function in patients with symptoms of constrictive physiology. However, it is not accurate in visualizing pericardial thickening. Transesophageal echocardiography is limited by the limited field of view.

Cardiac CT is widely accepted for imaging pericardial thickness and pericardial calcification. The presence of pericardial calcification on a plain film or CT is suggestive of pericardial constriction (Fig. 13) *(8)*. It is important to note that a diagnosis of constrictive pericarditis cannot be established by pericardial calcifications on CT alone unless there is coexisting hemodynamic diastolic constriction on invasive ventricular

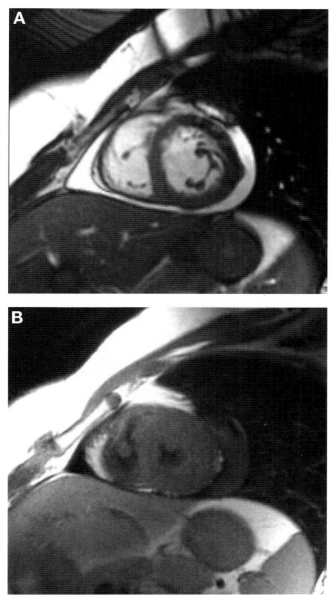

Fig. 8. Patient with systemic lupus erythematosus and pericarditis. A patient with a long history of systemic lupus erythematosus presented with pericarditis. Note the pericardial fluid on cine SSFP imaging (**A**). The fluid has medium signal intensity (adjacent to the lateral wall of the left ventricle) on T_1W fast spin echo imaging, suggestive of an exudative composition (**B**) (*see* figure 8 movie in CD).

pressure tracing or signs and symptoms of constriction. The absence of pericardial calcification cannot be used to rule out constrictive pericarditis because pericardial calcification is absent by X-ray or CT in 50% of surgically confirmed constrictive pericarditis. The pericardium of effusive constrictive pericarditis during the early stage of the disease may be soft and spongy without fibrosis and calcifications.

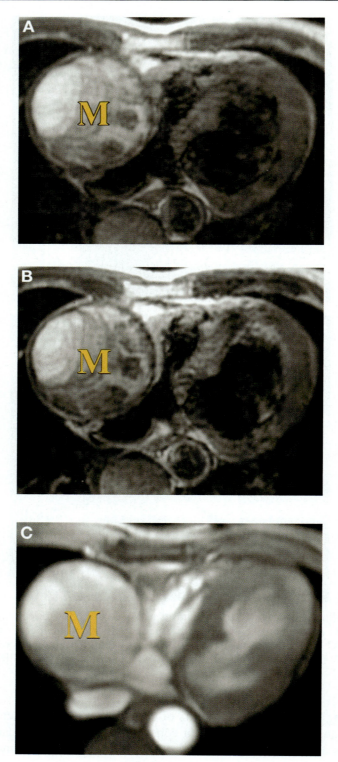

Fig. 9. *(Continued)*

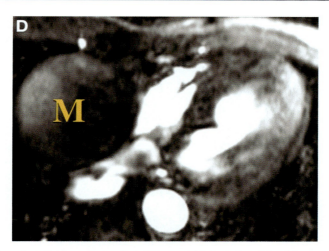

Fig. 9. Organized pericardial hematoma in a 70-year-old woman with a history of coronary artery disease and angioplasty of the right coronary artery (1 of 4) axial ECG-gated T_1W spin echo image shows a mass (M) with heterogeneous signal intensity in the right atrioventricular groove. (Reproduced from ref. 7 with permission from the Radiological Society of North America.)

In addition, the diagnosis of constrictive pericarditis is greatly aided by the excellent pericardial delineation by CMR. Pericardial thickness of 4 mm or more on CMR T_1W spin echo indicates abnormal thickening, and when accompanied by clinical findings of heart failure, it is strongly suggestive of constrictive pericarditis (Fig. 14). MR imaging also has a high reported accuracy (93%) in differentiating constrictive pericarditis from restrictive cardiomyopathy on the basis of depiction of thickened pericardium when accompanied by patient symptoms *(9)*. Pericardial thickening may be limited to the right side of the heart or to a small area, such as the right atrioventricular groove, which would be very difficult for echocardiography to detect.

However, it is important to understand that neither pericardial thickness on either CMR or CT should be interpreted without assessment of radiological findings suggestive of constrictive physiology. Pericardial thickening is non specific and could be seen in conditions like post-pericardiotomy state and acute pericarditis without constriction. Other diagnostic clues to the presence of significant constriction include the presence of dilated inferior vena cava, hepatic veins, and right atrium. These can be clearly displayed on SSFP cine CMR imaging. The right ventricle tends to be small in cavity and often assumes an elongated or conical shape. Tagged cine MRI could show tight adhesion of the thickened pericardium to the myocardium of the right and left ventricles, indicated by the persistent concordance of tagged signals between the pericardium and the myocardium throughout the diastolic and systolic phases (Fig. 15) *(10)*.

It is always important to distinguish restrictive from constrictive pericarditis. Real-time cine MRI can be used to detect ventricular coupling noted in constriction. A sigmoid-shaped ventricular septum or prominent leftward-convex ventricular septum is seen in some cases. The respiratory effects on septal position and configuration during early ventricular filling on breath-hold cine MRI studies can also help differentiate constrictive from restrictive pericarditis. In constriction, there is a leftward inversion or flattening of the septum during early ventricular filling. This pattern is not seen in

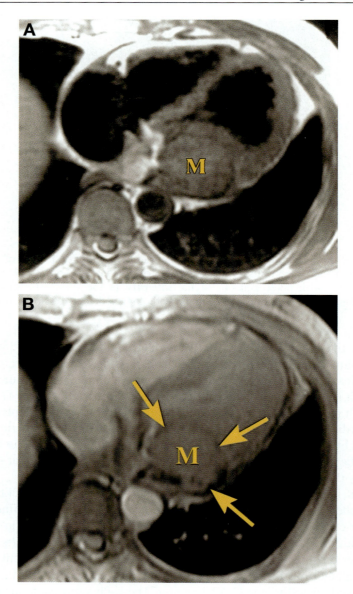

Fig. 10. Chronic organized pericardial hematoma in a 39-year-old man who presented with syncope and chest discomfort and had a history of blunt chest trauma 8 years prior (1 of 2) axial ECG-gated T_1W spin echo image shows a well-circumscribed mass (M) with intermediate signal intensity in the left atrioventricular groove; the mass compresses the left atrium and ventricle. (Reproduced from ref. *7* with permission from the Radiological Society of North America.)

patients with restrictive pericarditis *(11)*. Abnormal septal motion yielded a sensitivity of 81%, specificity of 100%, accuracy of 90%, positive predictive value of 100%, and negative predictive value of 83% in the detection of constrictive pericarditis *(12)*.

The amount of ventricular coupling could be evaluated by quantifying the difference in the maximal septal excursion between inspiration and expiration. This parameter, normalized to the biventricular diameter, was significantly larger in patients with

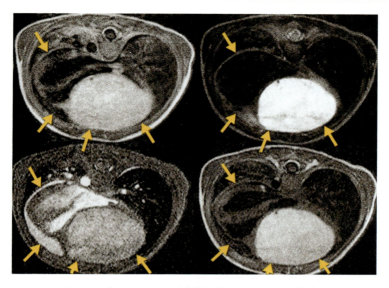

Fig. 11. Transverse midventricular spin echo CMR of a large pericardial cyst demonstrating effect of different MR contrast techniques. Top left: T_1W spin echo image with repetition time (TR) of one R–R. Note the right ventricular compression by the large cyst (yellow arrowheads). There is also a moderate-size transudative (low-intensity) pericardial effusion (yellow arrows). Note the substantially different signal intensities of the pericardial effusion and the pericardial cyst. Top right: Gradient echo CMR at the same level. Note the different signal intensities of the pericardial effusion and pericardial cyst. Bottom left: T_2W spin echo CMR with marked enhancement within the pericardial cyst. The pericardial effusion is less well defined than on the two upper images. Bottom right: T_1W spin echo CMR following gadolinium-DTPA infusion. The pericardial fluid still has a relatively low signal intensity, indicating that it has relatively low protein and cellular content (transudative). In contrast, the cyst has a high signal intensity, consistent with a high protein content. At surgery, the high protein content of the cyst was confirmed. (Reproduced from ref. *16* with permission.)

A   **Causes of Constrictive Pericarditis**

(Western Nations)

Great Majority: Unknown or uncertain etiology/ "Idiopathic pericarditis"

Relatively Common

○ Infectious

  • Viral or probable viral

  • Tuberculous

  • Pyogenic

○ Therapeutic irradiation

○ Cardiopericardial surgery

Fig. 12. *(Continued)*

B **Causes of Constrictive Pericarditis**
(Western Nations)

Relatively Uncommon (increased incidence in special populations)

○ Neoplasia
  • Metastatic
  • Mesothelioma
    • Pericardial
    • Pleural
○ Uremia (on dialysis)
○ Vasculitis/connective tissue disease group
    • Especially rheumatoid arthritis, lupus, scleroderma (including CREST syndrome)
○ Infectious
  • Fungal
  • Parasitic
○ Myocardial infarct-related
    • Post hemopericardium (from thrombolysis)
    • Post-myocardial infarction (Dressler) syndrome
○ Trauma
  • Blunt
  • Penetrating
○ Drugs
  • Procainamide (lupus)
  • Methysergide
  • Practolol
  • Hydralazine (lupus)
○ Hemopericardium/encapsulated hemopericardium in hemorrhagic disorders

C **Causes of Constrictive Pericarditis**
(Western Nations)

Rare

  ○ Cholesterol pericarditis
  ○ Chylopericardium
  ○ Intrapericardial instrumentation
      • Automatic implantable cardioverter-defibrillator
      • Epicardial pacemaker
  ○ Whipple disease
  ○ Wegener granulomatosis
  ○ Hypereosinophilic syndromes
  ○ Cardiac transplant
  ○ Hereditary: mulibrey nanism
  ○ Sarcoidosis
  ○ Asbestosis
  ○ Pericardial amyloidosis
  ○ Dermatomyositis
  ○ Lassa fever
  ○ Chemical trauma: sclerotherapy of esophageal varices

Fig. 12. Causes of constrictive pericarditis. (Reproduced from ref. *6* with permission from Elsevier Science.)

constrictive pericarditis (20.0 ± 4.5%, $p < 0.0001$) than in normals and those with restrictive pericarditis. A cutoff value of 11.8% (mean normals +2 standard deviations [SD]) enabled differentiation of patients with constrictive pericarditis from normals and those with restrictive patients completely (Figs. 16–18) *(13)*. In some cases, pericardial constriction can also be demonstrated by the sudden restricted left ventricular diastolic

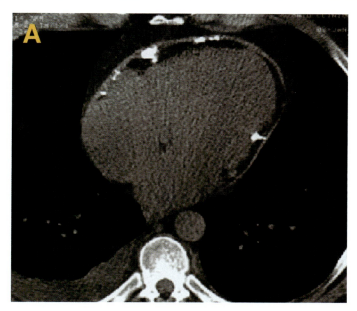

Fig. 13. CT scans of focal pericardial calcifications. Most of the pericardium is mildly or minimally thickened. Despite this, the patient has clinical findings of constriction. The noncontrast examination is sufficient to make the diagnosis. (Reproduced from ref. *8* with permission.)

filling by quantifying ventricular volume vs time (Fig. 19) or by a diminished vena caval forward flow during ventricular systole by phase velocity mapping (Fig. 20). Cine CMR imaging may allow visualization of pericardial adhesions either from the excellent spatial resolution and image contrast of SSFP imaging (Fig. 21) or myocardial labeling of tagged motion imaging (Fig. 15) *(10)*.

OTHER PERICARDIAL CONDITIONS

Other pericardial conditions encountered clinically include pericardial neoplasms, cysts, and congenital absence of the pericardium. CMR and CT better detect these rare conditions because of their better tissue contrast and wider field of imaging than echocardiography.

Metastatic pericardial tumors are much more common than primary pericardial tumors. Up to 10–12% of patients with breast or lung cancer, lymphoma, or melanoma have evidence of pericardial metastasis on autopsy. Tumor may involve the heart and pericardium by one of four pathways: retrograde lymphatic extension, hematogenous spread, direct contiguous extension, or transvenous extension. Impairment of cardiac function occurs in approximately 30% of patients and is usually attributable to pericardial effusion. Hemorrhagic pericardial effusions are common in pericardial metastasis and usually demonstrate high signal intensity on T_1W spin echo images. Most pericardial metastases have low signal intensity on T_1W images and high signal intensity on T_2W images. Metastatic melanoma is an exception because of the short T_1 effect from the paramagnetic metals bound by melanin and as a result will demonstrate high signal pericardial densities on T_1W spin echo imaging.

Primary neoplasms of the pericardium are rare. Benign pericardial tumors include lipoma, fibroma, and hemangioma; malignant tumors include mesothelioma, lymphoma,

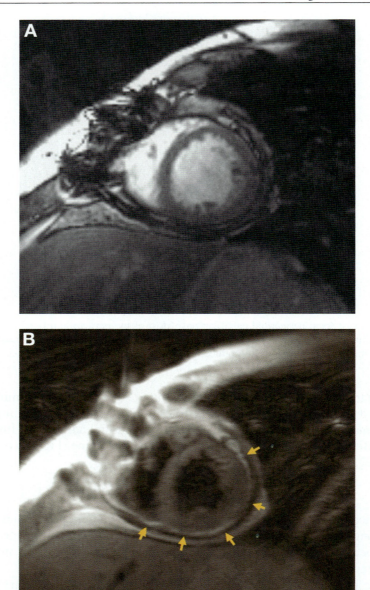

Fig. 14. Markedly thickened pericardium in a case of constrictive pericarditis (*see* figure 14 movie in CD).

sarcoma, and liposarcoma. The short T_1 from the fatty content of lipoma demonstrates high signal intensity on T_1W SE images. Fibroma usually demonstrates low signal intensity because of its fibrous content and does not always enhance from gadolinium-DPTA administration because of its poor vascular supply. Primary malignant tumors usually cannot be definitively diagnosed by imaging techniques and require biopsy and histopathological diagnosis. CMR or CT is helpful in anatomically localizing the tumor for the planning of surgical biopsy in most cases. Pericardial mesothelioma may

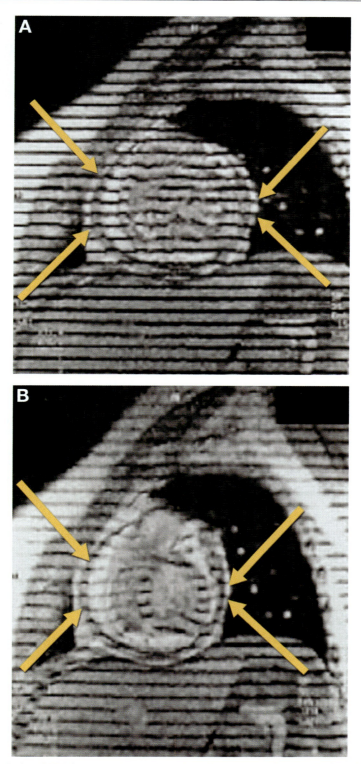

Fig. 15. Tagged cine MRI images at end diastole. (Reproduced from ref. *10* with permission. Copyright 1999, Massachusetts Medical Association. All rights reserved.)

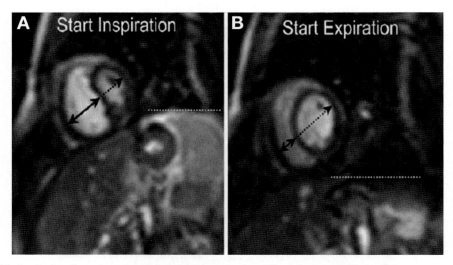

Fig. 16. Analysis of respiratory-related septal excursion. The relative position of the septum can be obtained by dividing the distance between right ventricular free wall and septum (full line) by the biventricular distance (dashed line). If done during inspiration and expiration, at early ventricular filling, then the respiratory-related septal excursion can be quantified. The horizontal dashed white line indicates the position of the left hemidiaphragm, which is used to determine the phase of the respiratory cycle. In this patient with CP, paradoxical septal inversion was visible at the onset of inspiration, with enhanced right-sided excursion during onset of expiration. The relative septal position at end-inspiration is 56.6% and 31.0% at end-expiration, giving a relative septal excursion of 25.6%. (Reproduced from ref. *13*.)

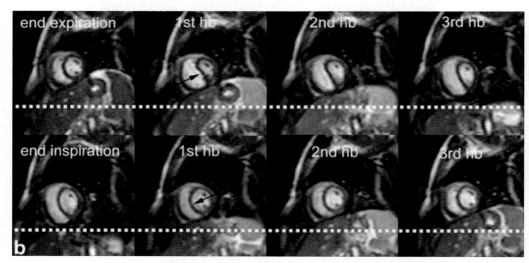

Fig. 17. Constrictive pericarditis in a 28-year-old male patient. (**A**) T_1W axial fast spin echo MRI shows diffuse pericardial thickening (arrows), which is most pronounced over the right ventricle. The pericardium has a hypointense signal and is irregularly defined. (**B**) Short-axis real-time cine MRI during operator-guided breathing shows abnormal septal motion with septal inversion during onset of inspiration (arrow in upper row). The abnormal septal motion rapidly disappears; during expiration, an increased rightward motion is noticed (arrow in lower row). The respiratory-related septal excursion was 25.6%. All images shown were obtained at the moment of early ventricular filling. The dashed white line represents the end-inspiratory position of the diaphragm. (Reproduced from ref. *13*.)

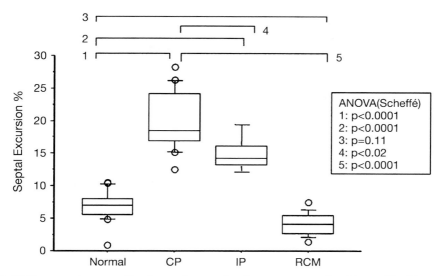

Fig. 18. Differences in normalized septal excursion between normal subjects, IP, CP, and RCM patients (Reproduced from ref. *13.*)

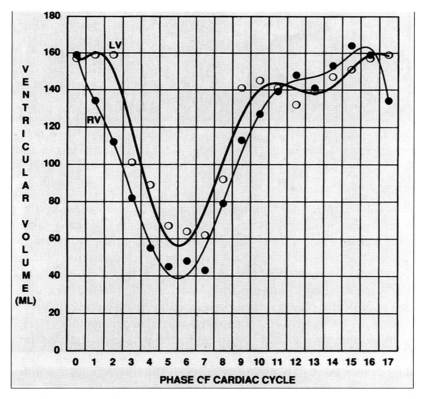

Fig. 19. Pericarditis (cine, gradient echo for time-vs-ventricular volume curve analysis). Rapid early ventricular filling followed by abrupt limitation of late diastolic filling of the ventricles, in the setting of preserved systolic emptying of the left and right ventricles, indicate constrictive pericarditis. (Reproduced from ref. *17* with permission from Blackwell Futura.)

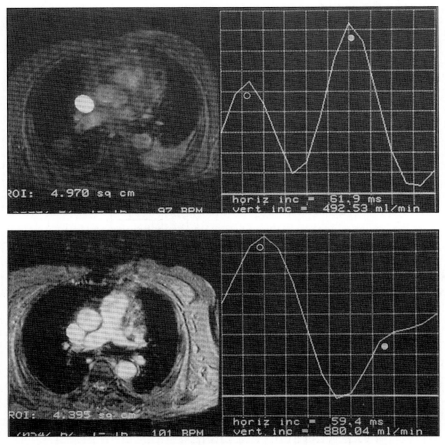

Fig. 20. Pericarditis (phase velocity mapping for systemic venous flow analysis). In the superior vena cava, the decrease in ratio of peak flow in systole (open circle) relative to that in diastole (closed circle) because of the constrictive pericarditis (top) is improved after surgical pericardial stripping (bottom). (Reproduced from ref. *17* with permission from Blackwell Futura.)

contain pericardial effusion and multiple pericardial nodules and may show signs of local invasion. Lymphoma, liposarcoma, and angiosarcoma typically appear as large heterogeneous masses frequently associated with serosanguineous pericardial effusion. In a patient who has received radiation therapy, the pericardium may appear thickened and nodular, mimicking metastatic disease.

Congenital pericardial cysts are congenital malformation of the pericardium that are usually benign clinically. Rarely, large pericardial cysts may result in compression of cardiac chambers. They usually contain transudative fluid and therefore typically appear as a thin-wall structure with fluid low or intermediate signal intensity on T_1W spin echo images and homogeneous high intensity on T_2W spin echo images. Occasionally, pericardial cysts may contain highly proteinaceous fluid, which demonstrates high signal intensity on T_1W spin echo images, and do not enhance with the administration of gadolinium-DTPA. Pericardial cysts are most often found in the right cardiophrenic angle, but they may occur from any region of the pericardium and may be indistinguishable from a bronchogenic cyst or thymic cyst.

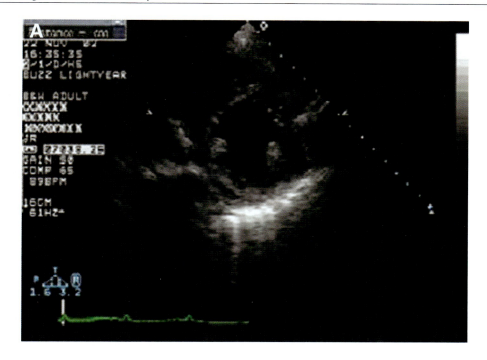

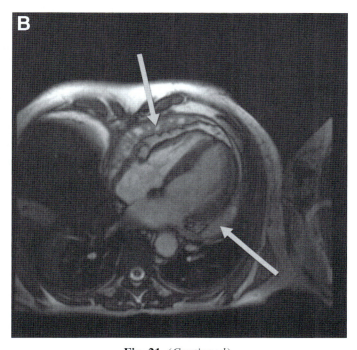

Fig. 21. (*Continued*).

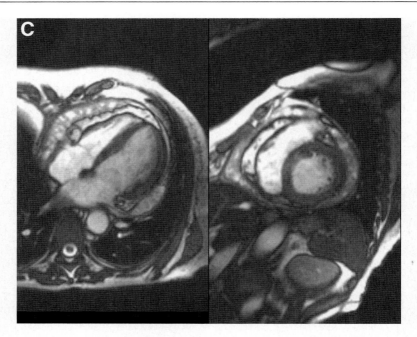

Fig. 21. (*Continued*) Echocardiography of a patient with previous radiation therapy for breast carcinoma who presented with recurrent symptoms of heart failure. Although the pericardium adjacent to the left ventricle appeared thickened, the extent of the pericardial thickening and the content of the pericardial cavity were difficult to characterize. Cine SSFP CMR imaging of this patient showed diffuse pericardial thickening with fibrous adhesions (arrows) in the pericardial cavity (*see* figure 21 movie A and C).

Complete or partial absence of the pericardium is an uncommon congenital pericardial condition. Partial absence of the pericardium on the left heart may cause chest pain from localized herniation and strangulation of the left atrium and the left ventricle. A circumscribed crease in the left atrial or ventricular walls suggests strangulation. Because this may result in sudden cardiac death, elective surgical repair is often indicated in asymptomatic partial absence of the pericardium. Rarely, lung tissue may herniate into the pericardial cavity through the defect. A definitive diagnosis of congenital absence of the pericardium can be obtained with either CMR or CT. Patients with pericardial defects also may have other congenital abnormalities, such as atrial septal defect, patent ductus arteriosus, mitral valve stenosis, or tetralogy of Fallot, which should be part of the CMR assessment.

ACKNOWLEDGMENT

The content of this chapter is reproduced in part from ref. *14*.

REFERENCES

1. Ferrans V IT, Roberts WC. In: editors. Pericardial disease. Anatomy of the pericardium. New York: Raven Press; 1982.
2. Hayashi H, Kawamata H, Machida M, Kumazaki T. Tuberculous pericarditis: MRI features with contrast enhancement. Br J Radiol 1998;71:680–682.

3. Taylor AM, Dymarkowski S, Verbeken EK, Bogaert J. Detection of pericardial inflammation with late-enhancement cardiac magnetic resonance imaging: initial results. Eur Radiol 2006;16:569–574.
4. Watanabe A, Hara Y, Hamada M, et al. A case of effusive-constrictive pericarditis: an efficacy of GD-DTPA enhanced magnetic resonance imaging to detect a pericardial thickening. Magn Reson Imaging 1998;16:347–350.
5. Kovanlikaya A, Burke LP, Nelson MD, Wood J. Characterizing chronic pericarditis using steady-state free-precession cine MR imaging. AJR Am J Roentgenol 2002;179:475–476.
6. Spodick DH. Pericardial diseases. In: Braunwald E, Zipes DP, Libby P, eds. Heart disease. 6th ed. New York: Saunders; 2001:1849.
7. Wang ZJ, Reddy GP, Gotway MB, Yeh BM, Hetts SW, Higgins CB. CT and MR imaging of pericardial disease. Radiographics 2003;23:167S–180S.
8. Breen JF. Imaging of the pericardium. J Thorac Imaging 2001;16:47–54.
9. Masui T, Finck S, Higgins CB. Constrictive pericarditis and restrictive cardiomyopathy: evaluation with MR imaging. Radiology 1992;182:369–373.
10. Kojima S, Yamada N, Goto Y. Diagnosis of constrictive pericarditis by tagged cine magnetic resonance imaging. N Engl J Med 1999;341:373–374.
11. Giorgi B, Mollet NR, Dymarkowski S, Rademakers FE, Bogaert J. Clinically suspected constrictive pericarditis: MR imaging assessment of ventricular septal motion and configuration in patients and healthy subjects. Radiology 2003;228:417–424.
12. Francone M, Dymarkowski S, Kalantzi M, Bogaert J. Real-time cine MRI of ventricular septal motion: a novel approach to assess ventricular coupling. J Magn Reson Imaging 2005;21:305–309.
13. Francone M, Dymarkowski S, Kalantzi M, Rademakers FE, Bogaert J. Assessment of ventricular coupling with real-time cine MRI and its value to differentiate constrictive pericarditis from restrictive cardiomyopathy. Eur Radiol 2006;16:944–951.
14. Cardiovascular magnetic resonance self-assessment program (CMRSAP). Bethesda, MD: American College of Cardiology Foundation; 2004. Cardiovascular Structure and Function: Pericardial Disease. Bethesda, MD: American College of Cardiology Foundation; 2004.
15. White CS, et al. Topics Magn Reson Imaging 1995;7:258–266.
16. Manning WJ, Pennell DJ. Cardiovascular magnetic resonance. London: Churchill Livingstone; 2002.
17. Higgins CB, Ingwall JS, Pohost G, eds. Current and future applications of magnetic resonance in cardiovascular disease. Armonk, NY: Futura, 1998.

23 Valvular Heart Disease

Vignendra Ariyarajah
and Raymond Y. Kwong

CONTENTS

BASIC CONCEPTS OF VALVULAR HEART IMAGING
ASSESSING VALVULAR STENOSIS
ASSESSING VALVULAR REGURGITATION
SPECIAL CONSIDERATIONS
SUMMARY
REFERENCES

Cardiovascular magnetic resonance (CMR) imaging can accurately assess cardiac structure and physiology vital in evaluating regurgitant or stenotic valvular heart disease. Its versatility in providing comprehensive anatomical and functional assessment in valvular heart disease stems from its ability to qualitatively and quantitatively measure flow volumes, velocities, and flow fractions in any oblique cardiac plane.

BASIC CONCEPTS OF VALVULAR HEART IMAGING

Various pulse sequence techniques in CMR highlight different aspects crucial to the assessment of valvular heart disease. The increased tissue contrast of the multislice spin echo sequence compared to that of the gradient echo sequence better delineates the anatomy of the valvular apparatus and the associated changes in cardiac chamber dimensions *(1)*. However, the static fast spin echo technique is susceptible to a longer imaging duration and may not provide adequate detail to optimally assess the functional anomaly of the valve *(2)*. With a fast gradient echo sequence *(3)*, blood has bright signal intensity because of inflowing magnetically unsaturated blood; turbulence in blood flow produces intravoxel spin dephasing that is depicted as a quantifiable signal loss or flow void *(4)*. The severity and the size of the flow jets in valvular conditions, however, depends on window width and level, flip angle, and echo time (TE) and can be highly variable in relation to the severity of the valvular disease (Fig. 1) *(5)*. Velocities of stenotic or regurgitant valvular jets, along with direct cross-sectional planimetry of the dysfunctional valvular orifice, can be comprehensively measured with CMR cine flow-sensitive phase contrast mapping (phase-encoded or velocity-encoded cine imaging) *(6)*.

From: *Current Clinical Practice: Primary Care Sleep Medicine*
Edited by: James F. Pagel, and S.R. Pandi-Perumal

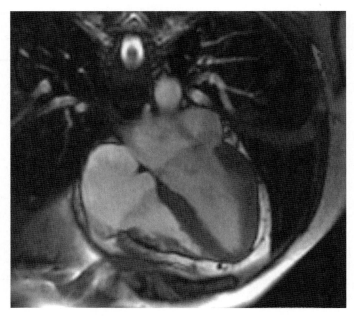

Fig. 1. (movie video included). Cine steady-state free precession gradient echo imaging of a patient with severe mitral regurgitation. Note that the severity of the mitral regurgitation is substantially underestimated by the size and severity of the mitral regurgitation jet demonstrated by this sequence. A short echo time (TE) of 1.2 ms was used.

Awareness of the respective strengths and weaknesses of the different imaging parameters for the assessment of the valvular abnormality is therefore crucial.

Flow and velocity mapping techniques in phase contrast imaging are conceptualized on the theory that, in a magnetic gradient, the phase of the flowing spins relative to the stationary spins changes in direct proportion to flow velocity (7). Blood flow profile of a given region of interests can be expressed as either velocity or flow volume per unit of time (8). Phase contrast CMR techniques can process quantitative information into two sets of images matching in slice location (5). Magnitude images can be reconstructed to provide anatomic data, whereas matching phase images can provide flow velocity data. On the phase images, through-plane flow away from the viewer appears bright; conversely, flow in the opposite direction appears dark (Fig. 2) (5,9). These images can be further enhanced with color coding of the anterograde (red) and retrograde (blue) dynamic flow. Gray values in stationary structures (e.g., skeletal muscles) can be used for background subtraction for noise. A misalignment of 20° between true and measured flow jets in stenosis or regurgitation produces a negligible error (of about 6%) and can be so determined by the equation)

$$V_{measured} = V_{true} \, (\cos \theta)$$

where $V_{measured}$ is the measured velocity, V_{true} is the true velocity, and θ is the angle of misalignment between flow encoding and flow direction (10). Peak velocity (centimeters/second) can be measured for each pixel within a region of interest by tracing all or part of its cross-sectional area or across the valvular orifice annulus (11). The product of cross-sectional area (as determined from the magnitude image) and spatial mean velocity (the average velocity for all pixels in the cross-sectional area on the phase image) yields

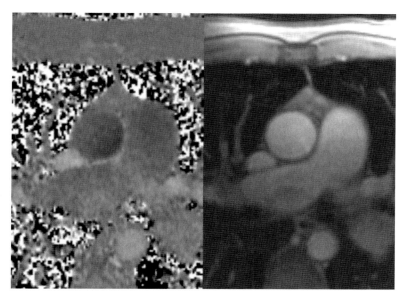

Fig. 2. (movie video included). Phase contrast cine gradient echo imaging: magnitude images (left) and location-matched phase images (right) for the assessment of the systolic forward flow of the ascending aorta.

the instantaneous flow volume (milliliters) for each time frame during the cardiac cycle *(12)*. Integration of all instantaneous flow volumes throughout the cardiac cycle yields the absolute flow volume per heartbeat. The advantages of the phase contrast CMR technique compared to echocardiographic Doppler assessment include a lack of the requirement for assumption of cross-section anatomy of the vessel or valvular orifice and unrestricted scan planes and field of imaging.

ASSESSING VALVULAR STENOSIS

General Assessment

To start a general qualitative assessment of heart valve stenosis, fast gradient echo CMR cine imaging, with cine steady-state free precession currently the more popular technique, is the usual sequence of choice. Thickening or doming, decreased leaflet excursion, calcification and anatomical defects (e.g., bicuspid valves) of the valvular leaflets, and associated valvular apparatus and cardiac chamber involvement can be appreciated *(2,5,12,13)*. However, these markers by no means conclusively diagnose valvular stenoses but could be used in context in supplementing physiological blood flow assessment by phase contrast techniques.

High-velocity blood flow through a stenotic orifice produces a distinguishable anterograde signal void *(4,14)*. There is usually a region of acceleration just distal to the orifice, where the narrowest central flow of parallel streamlines forms the jet core. As it extends into the receiving chamber, the jet may dissipate quickly or, commonly, forms a notable parajet of intense turbulence that is swept to the sides or more distally *(13,14)*. The jet complex is naturally dependant on properties that affect flow, such as orifice size, valve morphology and velocity, and nature of image acquisition as described here. Although the gross appearance of the jet size is relatively commensurate with the pressure gradient across the valve, inherent anatomical anomalies of the valvular apparatus could cause turbulent blood flow and misleadingly depict a signal void *(12,14)*.

Assessment of Transvalvular Pressure Gradient and Valve Area

Increase in flow velocity across a stenotic orifice can be measured using phase contrast cine imaging. The pressure gradient across the stenotic valve can be derived using the modified Bernoulli equation:

$$P_1 - P_2 = 4(V_2 - V_1) \text{ or } \Delta P = 4V^2$$

where ΔP is the pressure drop across the stenosis, and V is the peak velocity (in meters per second) measured in the stenotic jet. The stenotic pressure gradients measured by CMR correlate closely with gradients determined by Doppler echocardiography ($r = 0.96$) and cardiac catheterization ($r = 0.97$) *(14–16)*. Parajet turbulence is believed not to interfere significantly with measurements within the true jet *(13)*.

Proper perpendicular alignment of the phase contrast technique with the signal in the jet core is necessary for obtaining the most accurate assessment of the maximal jet velocity. The encoding velocity (venc) of the phase contrast technique should be set just above the expected peak velocity to obviate aliasing *(13,17)*. Higher velocities require minimization of the TE to lessen signal loss or interference from artifacts *(13)*. In newer CMR scanning software, the parameters for velocity encoding are incorporated as a venc setting, for which high-velocity flow like that across the aortic valve optimally requires higher settings (>350 cm/second), and vice-versa, lower-velocity flow like that across the pulmonic valve requires lower settings (<150 cm/second) unless significant stenosis exists. Although in-plane imaging allows a long-axis visualization of the transvalvular jet, it is often subject to limitation from the jet moving out of the imaging plane throughout the cardiac cycle and partial volume effect *(5,13)*.

It is therefore advisable also to utilize through-plane imaging, by which the selected imaging plane is perpendicular to the flow jet just distal to the stenotic orifice *(5,13)*. This allows for assessment of the cross-sectional area of the flow jet and enables velocity mapping in the slice-select directional gradient. We in general obtain a stack of three to five parallel slices to ensure data acquisition closest to the stenotic orifice, where maximum jet can be accurately assessed.

Aortic Stenosis

Aortic stenosis is characterized by congenital or acquired impedence of blood flow from the left ventricle into the aorta and may manifest as subvalvular, supravalvular, or, most commonly, valvular abnormality. Current guidelines of the American Heart Association/American College of Cardiology (AHA/ACC) *(18)* recommend aortic valve surgery in virtually all symptomatic patients with severe aortic stenosis (class I) and support surgical intervention for asymptomatic patients who demonstrate left ventricular systolic dysfunction or exertional hypotension (class IIa).

A comprehensive evaluation of valvular aortic stenosis should not only include quantification of the degree of stenosis but also extend to assessment of left ventricular function, volume, and mass. In cine CMR imaging, the optimal planes for identifying the signal void corresponding to the abnormal flow jet are the coronal plane centered on the left ventricular outflow tract (LVOT) and the long axis of the left ventricle *(12,13)*.

Importantly, the maximum jet velocity across a stenotic valvular orifice in systole should be quantified via phase contrast imaging perpendicular to the direction of flow (5) and with proper venc to avoid aliasing (14,16). Although the aortic valve area can be obtained by planimetry directly on cross-sectional slices through the plane of the valve at the point of maximal stenosis, it can also be calculated by the use of the continuity equation as in echocardiography. In contrast to echocardiography, the cross-sectional area of the LVOT can be directly measured without making geometric assumption. The continuity equation states that the flow at the LVOT level must equal the flow at the level of the aortic valve.

$$Aortic\ Valve\ Area = \frac{LVOT\ velocity}{Aortic\ Valve\ velocity} \times LVOT\ area$$

Such measurement in CMR has been show to have a high rate of intra- and interobserver reproducibility (16,19). The Gorlin equation (20) states that the aortic valve area is equal to the flow through the aortic valve during ventricular systole divided by the systolic pressure gradient across the valve times a constant and is described as

$$Valve\ Area\ (cm^2) = \frac{Cardiac\ Output\left(\frac{ml}{minute}\right)}{Heart\ rate\left(\frac{beats}{minute}\right) \cdot Systolic\ ejection\ period\ (second) \cdot 44.3 \cdot \sqrt{Gradient\ (mmHg)}}.$$

A simplified version of the Gorlin equation exists in the form of the Hakki equation (21), which relies on the observation that the product of the heart rate, systolic ejection period, and constant is often approximately 1000.

$$Aortic\ Valve\ Area\ (cm^2) \approx \frac{Cardiac\ Output\left(\frac{litre}{minute}\right)}{\sqrt{Gradient\ (mmHg)}}$$

Therefore, the aortic valve area can be estimated by the measured cardiac output and pressure gradient estimated by the peak velocity, both of which can be obtained by phase contrast CMR techniques. Pressure gradient and valvular area measurements obtained with these imaging techniques have been shown to correlate accurately with data from cardiac catheterization and Doppler echocardiography (14,15,19). It may also be useful to acquire delay-enhancement images with gadolinium-diethyltriamine-pentaacetic acid as it has been shown that, among patients with critical stenosis, increased subendocardial enhancement was noted, implying subendocardial wall injury (22). In coarctation of the aorta, increase in flow with phase contrast imaging at the distal aorta (at the level of the diaphragm) compared to that of the proximal aorta (after the level of the stenosis) indicates severity and could be important in planning the operative approach (23).

Mitral Stenosis

Restriction in mitral valve opening during diastole results in mitral stenosis and produces a diastolic pressure gradient between the left atrium and left ventricle. Rheumatic heart disease and endocarditis remain the primary causes of this abnormality. The need for CMR assessment in mitral stenosis most often arises when the preferred Doppler echocardiography is inconclusive or insufficient, such as in cases involving a limited acoustic window or complex flow patterns. In this respect, CMR is able to supplement and also better demonstrate such flow patterns in various tomographic planes (24). The signal void corresponding to the abnormal flow jet is most clearly depicted on the four-chamber view and the coronal oblique view encompassing the left atrium and the left ventricle (12,24). Again, phase contrast imaging can provide data on the maximum velocity within the jet, and the transvalvular pressure gradient can be calculated (5).

ASSESSING VALVULAR REGURGITATION

General Assessment

As in the case of valvular stenosis, general assessment with cine fast-gradient echo imaging should be the first step in evaluating valvular regurgitation. Some of the findings on cine CMR imaging are thickening, abnormal movement, decreased or abnormal coaptation and anatomical defects (e.g., bicuspid valves) of the valvular leaflets, and associated valvular apparatus as well as cardiac chamber involvement (2,5,12,13).

Assessment of Signal Loss

The severity of the valvular insufficiency can be semiquantitatively assessed by manually tracing the area and measuring the greatest length of the depicted signal void in the receiving cavity (25). Although this assessment of jet area ($r = 0.91$) and jet length ($r = 0.85$) is comparable to that of transesophageal echocardiography (26) and provides a crude assessment of the severity of the regurgitant lesion, it cannot be overemphasized that the appearance of the signal void varies depending on the valvular abnormality, volume and pressure in the receiving cavity, and imaging parameters, particularly the degree of dephasing allowed by the predefined TE (4,6).

Assessment of Regurgitant Fraction With Ventricular Volumetrics

When a single valve is affected on either side of the heart, the regurgitant volume can be calculated from the difference of right ventricular and left ventricular stroke volumes using the modified Simpson method, in which the volumes of the ventricles are measured on a stack of parallel short-axis views (27). For regurgitant lesion of the heart valve of either great vessels, regurgitant volume can be directly measured by phase contrast cross-sectional imaging at the level of the heart valve. For regurgitant atrioventricular valves (mitral or tricuspid), regurgitant volumes can be calculated by subtracting the great vessel flow per cardiac cycle (measured by phase contrast mapping) from the ventricular stroke volumes (8,28). A regurgitant fraction can then be calculated by dividing regurgitant volume by the ventricular stroke volume and expressed as a percentage of the ventricular stroke volume.

This method is somewhat similar to that used in cardiac scintigraphy and compares favorably with catheterization and Doppler echocardiography (28–32). The drawback, however, is that such calculation yields more accurate results in the elliptic left ventricle than in the right ventricle, for which it is often more difficult to define its basal segments because of through-plane motion of the right ventricle. Phase contrast imaging may be utilized to calculate right and left ventricular stroke volumes separately by assessing flow in the ascending aorta and pulmonary artery (29). The integration of flow measurements on all systolic images yields the absolute flow in systole and provides stroke volumes.

Assessment of Regurgitant Blood Flow With Phase Contrast Imaging

Regurgitation is detected by phase contrast imaging as black (or blue, if color coded) flow to denote retrograde blood flow after valve closure *(5)*. A magnitude image with the manually traced cross-sectional area of the valvular annulus is transferred to the corresponding phase image for each time frame. This enables measurement of the average velocity and provides the flow volume per heartbeat *(5,8)*. As with stenotic valves, measurements must be obtained proximal to the site of the incompetent valve to avoid artifacts from leaflet motion and jet eccentricity *(29)*. Therefore, when assessing aortic regurgitation, imaging should be performed approximately at the level of the right pulmonary artery, where regurgitant aortic regurgitation jet can be clearly appreciated. Data are then used to plot a flow-vs-time graph to depict regurgitant volume precisely *(8)*.

Aortic Regurgitation

Aortic regurgitation is a congenital or acquired insufficiency of the aortic valve apparatus that results in backflow of blood from the aorta into the LVOT, thereby increasing left ventricular end-diastolic volume *(18)*. Frequent causes that may precipitate an acute or chronic process according to underlying pathology are rheumatic heart disease, aortoannular ectasia, endocarditis, and aortic root dilatation (as with aortitis, arteritis, or Marfan's syndrome) or dissection, among others.

Although severity of symptoms often dictates the need for surgical intervention, CMR can play an important noninvasive role in assessing the degree of regurgitation and compromise of the left ventricular chamber and function. Because color Doppler flow mapping by echocardiography is considered semiquantitative for aortic regurgitation assessment, the AHA/ACC has recommended that quantitation of aortic regurgitation by CMR can be helpful in patient management *(18)*. CMR also enables visualization of the aortic arch and may help determine the etiology. For example, uniform dilatation of the aortic annulus and proximal ascending aorta is a finding that is compatible with aortoannular ectasia.

The AHA/ACC guidelines recommend aortic valve replacement in patients with severe aortic regurgitation in presence of symptoms or any evidence of left ventricular dysfunction (class I). Aortic valve replacement is supported (class IIa) by the guidelines in asymptomatic patients with severe left ventricular dilatation (>75 mm end-diastolic and >55 mm end-systolic echocardiographic diameters) *(18)*. Therefore, a comprehensive cine CMR assessment should always quantify the degree of the aortic regurgitation as well as left ventricular function, volume, and mass and appropriately image the aortic arch. The signal void of the regurgitant flow in diastole is best demonstrated by multiplanar imaging in the coronal plane centered on the LVOT and in the long axis of the left ventricle *(33)*. However, for optimal quantification of the degree of regurgitation, regurgitant fraction and phase contrast imaging of the diastolic retrograde volume should be obtained *(5,31)*. The area bounded by the curve under the baseline on a flow-vs-time graph indicates the amount and significance of the regurgitant volume (Fig. 3) *(8)*.

Mitral Regurgitation

Mitral regurgitation is caused by insufficiency of an abnormal mitral valvular apparatus that results in backward flow of blood from the left ventricle into the left atrium and

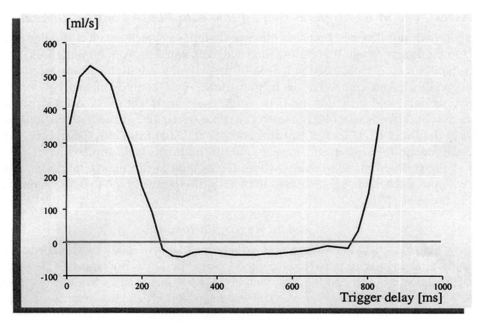

Fig. 3. Flow profile of a patient with mild aortic regurgitation. By dividing the diastolic regurgitant flow (quantified by the area confined by the curve below the base line) by the systolic forward flow (area under the curve above the base line), an aortic regurgitant fraction of 16% was obtained. Note the time shift of the curve during the time delay from gating triggering to data acquisition.

produces an increase in total stroke volume. Rheumatic heart disease and mitral valve prolapse are the most common causes. The AHA/ACC guidelines currently recommend valve replacement in patients with severe mitral regurgitation with symptoms of congestive heart failure or left ventricular systolic dysfunction *(18)*. Echocardiographic assessment, however, is semiquantitative, and as such the role of cine CMR imaging is to provide a more comprehensive noninvasive quantification of the regurgitant volume. This signal void of the regurgitant flow jet in systole is best demonstrated on the four-chamber view and in the coronal oblique view encompassing the left atrium and left ventricle and ideally should be assessed in both planes (Fig. 4).

A good correlation has been found between the ratio of maximum flow void area to left atrial and left ventricular area and the severity of mitral regurgitation as estimated by echocardiography *(32)*. The regurgitant fraction in isolated mitral regurgitation can be calculated by ventricular volumetrics as described elsewhere *(28,33)*. Several phase contrast methods exist for quantifying the severity of mitral regurgitation. The common methods rely on measuring the mitral regurgitant volume by the difference in the systolic flow volume through the ascending aorta and the left ventricular stroke volume from cine imaging (Fig. 5).

Mitral regurgitant volume (and regurgitant volume index) can also be quantified by phase contrast imaging as the difference between the diastolic inflow across the mitral annulus and the systolic outflow through the ascending aorta *(8)*. The difference between the areas of the two superimposed curves corresponds to the volume of mitral regurgitation. Quantitation of the diastolic inflow by this technique can be limited by the mitral annular motion.

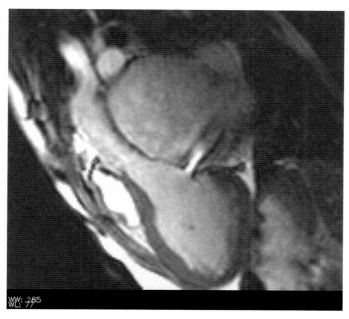

Fig. 4. (movie video included). Cine gradient echo imaging of a patient with severe mitral regurgitation.

Another method is to calculate the difference between the stroke volumes for the left and right ventricles by measuring flow in the ascending aorta and pulmonary artery *(29)*. The difference yields the regurgitant volume.

In general, result consistency should be checked among the different methods. The regurgitant fraction in percentage can then be determined by dividing the regurgitant volume by the left ventricular stroke volume. All these measurements have been shown to have good correlation with those obtained with three-dimensional echocardiography, cardiac catheterization, and angiography *(28,29,34)*.

SPECIAL CONSIDERATIONS

Prosthetic Heart Valves

Mechanical heart valves often produce complex flow patterns that make precise assessment via Doppler echocardiography challenging. In this respect, CMR can be helpful in addition to defining structure, position, flow across the orifice, and associated changes in the valvular apparatus and chambers. However, these valves can induce susceptibility artifacts and often necessitate phase contrast imaging in particular to be acquired outside the magnetic field distortion *(12,35)*. Currently, all mechanical valves are considered safe for imaging in a 1.5-T environment because heating and torque caused by the magnetic field are considerably small *(35,36)* unless clinical valvular dehiscence is suspected; then, CMR imaging may pose additional risk to the patient with an already impaired heart artificial valve.

Pre- and Postsurgical Assessment

The versatility of CMR in postsurgical assessment is encouraging. Not only can CMR provide comprehensive information on valvular function, but also it may

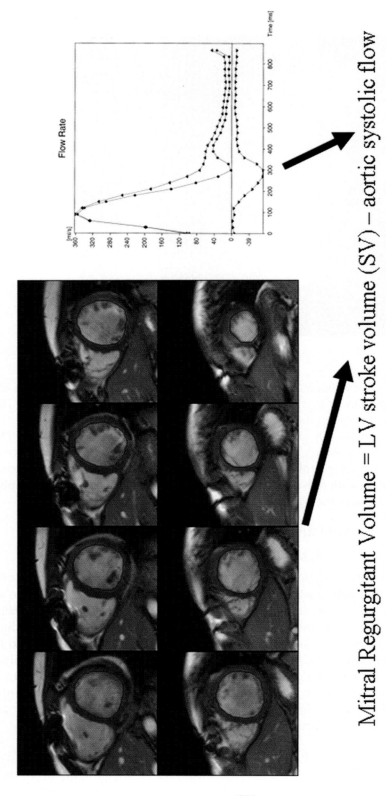

Mitral Regurgitant Volume = LV stroke volume (SV) – aortic systolic flow

Mitral Regurgitant Fraction = Regurgitant Volume / SV x 100%

Fig. 5. Quantitation of mitral regurgitant volume and regurgitant fraction by the differences of the left ventricular stroke volume and the systolic aortic flow volume.

assist in determining the type of surgical procedure and the impact it holds on cardiac hemodynamics during recovery. In patients who had received a mechanical valve compared to those with nonmechanical ones, CMR was able to demonstrate a greater decrease in the absolute value of systolic strain *(37)*.

Effects on left ventricular mass among patients with severe aortic stenosis who had undergone stentless vs stented porcine valve replacement can also be compared with some precision with CMR *(38)*. The extent of left atrial and left ventricular reverse remodeling and impact on absolute left ventricular strain has also been demonstrated by CMR *(39)*.

Tissue tagging is another useful tool in CMR for comparing the type of prosthetic valve used in aortic valve replacement and its impact on incompletely recovered systolic strain in chronic aortic regurgitation *(37,40)*. CMR is also an excellent modality for follow-up after valve-sparing aortic root reconstruction or replacement (David procedure) for which flow mapping of aortic regurgitation has shown good correlation with color Doppler echocardiography $(p < 0.0001)$ *(41)*.

Moreover, CMR is able to assess surgical approaches to valve sparing regarding preservation of the native sinuses of Valsalva, for which it has demonstrated that such aortic vortical blood flow is absent in postoperative patients with Marfan syndrome *(42)*. The determination of regurgitant fraction, ventricular dimensions and functions, and graft diameters allows standardized imaging protocols with high reproducibility, which may lead to favor for this technique for the follow-up of patients after surgery involving the heart valves or the great vessels.

Lesions and Masses Affecting Heart Valves

Atrial fibrillation, which can complicate mitral stenosis, is a harbinger for left atrial electromechanical dysfunction and left atrial thrombus. Frequently, thrombi and other masses such as atrial myxoma or Libmann-Sachs vegetations may cross the plane of the involved valve and distort flow as well as function *(2)*. Although spin echo images may demonstrate the mass, slow-moving blood in the atrium could increase the signal intensity and be falsely interpreted as a mass. Gradient echo with phase contrast imaging should therefore also be done. Addition of gadolinium-diethyltriaminepentaacetic acid during imaging could increase the signal intensity and enable better visualization of the suspected mass *(2,43)*.

SUMMARY

CMR is a good noninvasive tool that provides comprehensive multiplanar quantification of function and volumes in regurgitation and stenosis. However, limitations such as suboptimal electrocardiogram gating in atrial tachyarrhythmias and inability to image those with poor breath holding such as in acutely ill patients exist apart from issues inherent to most magnetic resonance imaging. As such, it is always important to use clinical judgment when determining suitability, imaging sequences and parameters, and indications when imaging stenotic or regurgitant valves. In essence, evaluation of valvular heart disease should ideally be comprehensive and should always include quantification of the severity of the valvular lesion, assessment of the entire valvular apparatus, and assessment of the adaptive mechanisms of the cardiac chambers.

REFERENCES

1. Arai AE, Epstein FH, Bove KE, Wolff SD. Visualization of aortic valve leaflets using black blood MRI. J Magn Reson Imaging 1999;10:771–777.
2. Globits S, Higgins CB. Assessment of valvular heart disease by magnetic resonance imaging. Am Heart J 1995;129:369–381.
3. Krombach GA, Kuhl H, Bucker A, et al. Cine MR imaging of heart valve dysfunction with segmented true fast imaging with steady state free precession. J Magn Reson Imaging 2004;19:59–67.
4. Keegan J, Gatehouse PD, John AS, Mohiaddin RH, Firmin DN. Breath-hold signal-loss sequence for the qualitative assessment of flow disturbances in cardiovascular MR. J Magn Reson Imaging 2003; 18:496–501.
5. Suzuki JI, Caputo GR, Kondo C, Higgins CB. Cine MR imaging of valvular heart disease: display and imaging parameters affect the size of the signal void caused by valvular regurgitation. AJR Am J Roentgenol 1990;155:723–727.
6. Gatehouse PD, Keegan J, Crowe LA, et al. Applications of phase-contrast flow and velocity imaging in cardiovascular MRI. Eur Radiol 2005;15:2172–2184.
7. Firmin DN, Nayler GL, Kilner PJ, Longmore DB. The applications of phase shifts in NMR for flow measurements. Magn Reson Med 1990;14:230–241.
8. Sechtem U, Pflugfelder PW, Cassidy MM, et al. Mitral or aortic regurgitation: quantification of regurgitant volumes with cine MR imaging. Radiology 1988;167:425–430.
9. Kilner PJ, Manzara CC, Mohiaddin RH, et al. Magnetic resonance jet velocity mapping in mitral and aortic valve stenosis. Circulation 1993;87:1239–1248.
10. Stahlberg F, Sondergaard L, Thomsen C, Henriksen O. Quantification of complex flow using MR phase imaging—a study of parameters influencing the phase/velocity relation. Magn Reson Imaging 1992;10:13–23.
11. Debl K, Djavidani B, Seitz J, et al. Planimetry of aortic valve area in aortic stenosis by magnetic resonance imaging. Invest Radiol 2005;40:631–636.
12. Duerinckx AJ, Higgins CB. Valvular heart disease. Radiol Clin North Am 1994;32:613–630.
13. Mohiaddin RH, Kilner PJ: Valvular heart disease. In: Manning WJ, Pennell DJ, eds. Cardiovascular magnetic resonance. Philadelphia: Churchill Livingstone; 2002:387–404.
14. Kilner PJ, Firmin DN, Rees RS, et al. Valve and great vessel stenosis: assessment with MR jet velocity mapping. Radiology 1991;178:229–235.
15. Eichenberger AC, Jenni R, von Schulthess GK. Aortic valve pressure gradients in patients with aortic valve stenosis: quantification with velocity-encoded cine MR imaging. AJR Am J Roentgenol 1993; 160:971–977.
16. Kupfahl C, Honold M, Meinhardt G, et al. Evaluation of aortic stenosis by cardiovascular magnetic resonance imaging: comparison with established routine clinical techniques. Heart 2004;90:893–901.
17. Henk CB, Grampp S, Koller J, et al. Elimination of errors caused by first-order aliasing in velocity encoded cine-MR measurements of postoperative jets after aortic coarctation: in vitro and in vivo validation. Eur Radiol 2002;12:1523–1531.
18. ACC/AHA guidelines for the management of patients with valvular heart disease. A report of the American College of Cardiology/American Heart Association. Task Force on Practice Guidelines (Committee on Management of Patients with Valvular Heart Disease). J Am Coll Cardiol 1998;32: 1486–1588.
19. Sondergaard L, Hildebrandt P, Lindvig K, et al. Valve area and cardiac output in aortic stenosis: quantification by magnetic resonance velocity mapping. Am Heart J 1993;126:1156–1164.
20. Gorlin R, Gorlin SG. Hydraulic formula for calculation of the area of the stenotic mitral valve, other cardiac valves, and central circulatory shunts. I. Am Heart J 1951;41:1–29.
21. Hakki AH, Iskandrian AS, Bemis CE, et al. A simplified valve formula for the calculation of stenotic cardiac valve areas. Circulation 1981;63:1050–1055.
22. Ochiai K, Ishibashi Y, Shimada T, Murakami Y, Inoue S, Sano K. Subendocardial enhancement in gadolinium-diethylene-triamine-pentaacetic acid-enhanced magnetic resonance imaging in aortic stenosis. Am J Cardiol 1999;83:1443–1446.
23. Julsrud PR, Breen JF, Felmlee JP, Warnes CA, Connolly HM, Schaff HV. Coarctation of the aorta: collateral flow assessment with phase-contrast MR angiography. AJR Am J Roentgenol 1997;169: 1735–1742.
24. Casolo GC, Zampa V, Rega L, et al. Evaluation of mitral stenosis by cine magnetic resonance imaging. Am Heart J 1992;123:1252–1260.

25. Wagner S, Auffermann W, Buser P, et al. Diagnostic accuracy and estimation of the severity of valvular regurgitation from the signal void on cine magnetic resonance images. Am Heart J 1989;118:760–767.

26. Nishimura T, Yamada N, Itoh A, Miyatake K. Cine MR imaging in mitral regurgitation: comparison with color Doppler flow imaging. AJR Am J Roentgenol 1989;153:721–724.

27. Baldy C, Douek P, Croisille P, Magnin IE, Revel D, Amiel M. Automated myocardial edge detection from breath-hold cine-MR images: evaluation of left ventricular volumes and mass. Magn Reson Imaging 1994;12:589–598.

28. Hundley WG, Li HF, Willard JE, et al. Magnetic resonance imaging assessment of the severity of mitral regurgitation. Comparison with invasive techniques. Circulation 1995;92:1151–1158.

29. Fujita N, Chazouilleres AF, Hartiala JJ, et al. Quantification of mitral regurgitation by velocity-encoded cine nuclear magnetic resonance imaging. J Am Coll Cardiol 1994;23:951–958.

30. Ohnishi S, Fukui S, Kusuoka H, Kitabatake A, Inoue M, Kamada T. Assessment of valvular regurgitation using cine magnetic resonance imaging coupled with phase compensation technique: comparison with Doppler color flow mapping. Angiology 1992;43:913–924.

31. Pflugfelder PW, Landzberg JS, Cassidy MM, et al. Comparison of cine MR imaging with Doppler echocardiography for the evaluation of aortic regurgitation. AJR Am J Roentgenol 1989;152:729–735.

32. Pflugfelder PW, Sechtem UP, White RD, Cassidy MM, Schiller NB, Higgins CB. Noninvasive evaluation of mitral regurgitation by analysis of left atrial signal loss in cine magnetic resonance. Am Heart J 1989;117:1113–1139.

33. Sechtem U, Pflugfelder PW, Cassidy MM, et al. Mitral or aortic regurgitation: quantification of regurgitant volumes with cine MR imaging. Radiology 1988;167:425–430.

34. Albers J, Nitsche T, Boese J, et al. Regurgitant jet evaluation using three-dimensional echocardiography and magnetic resonance. Ann Thorac Surg 2004;78:96–102.

35. Edwards MB, Taylor KM, Shellock FG. Prosthetic heart valves: evaluation of magnetic field interactions, heating, and artifacts at 1.5 T. J Magn Reson Imaging 2000;12:363–369.

36. Edwards MB, Draper ER, Hand JW, Taylor KM, Young IR. Mechanical testing of human cardiac tissue: some implications for MRI safety. J Cardiovasc Magn Reson 2005;7:835–840.

37. Pomerantz BJ, Krock MD, Wollmuth JR, et al. Aortic valve replacement for aortic insufficiency: valve type as a determinant of systolic strain recovery. J Card Surg 2005;20:524–529.

38. Perez de Arenaza D, Lees B, Flather M, et al. ASSERT (Aortic Stentless vs Stented valve Assessed by Echocardiography Randomized Trial) Investigators. Randomized comparison of stentless vs stented valves for aortic stenosis: effects on left ventricular mass. Circulation 2005;112:2696–2702.

39. Westenberg JJ, van der Geest RJ, Lamb HJ, et al. MRI to evaluate left atrial and ventricular reverse remodeling after restrictive mitral annuloplasty in dilated cardiomyopathy. Circulation 2005;112(9 suppl): I437–I442.

40. Moustakidis P, Cupps BP, Pomerantz BJ, et al. Noninvasive, quantitative assessment of left ventricular function in ischemic cardiomyopathy. J Surg Res 2004;116:187–196.

41. Givehchian M, Kramer U, Miller S, et al. Aortic root remodeling: functional MRI as an accurate tool for complete follow-up. Thorac Cardiovasc Surg 2005;53:267–273.

42. Kvitting JP, Ebbers T, Wigstrom L, Engvall J, Olin CL, Bolger AF. Flow patterns in the aortic root and the aorta studied with time-resolved, three-dimensional, phase-contrast magnetic resonance imaging: implications for aortic valve-sparing surgery. J Thorac Cardiovasc Surg 2004;127:1602–1607.

43. Kaminaga T, Takeshita T, Kimura I. Role of magnetic resonance imaging for evaluation of tumors in the cardiac region. Eur Radiol 2003;13(suppl 6):L1–L10.

24

Magnetic Resonance Imaging Evaluation of Complex Congenital Heart Disease

Adam L. Dorfman and Tal Geva

INTRODUCTION

Congenital heart disease (CHD) occurs in approximately 8 of every 1000 live births, half of whom require surgical or other forms of treatment. Complex CHD has no precise acceptable definition. For the purposes of this chapter, we define complex CHD to include conotruncal anomalies and single-ventricle heart disease. *Conotruncal anomalies* refer to a group of congenital heart defects involving the outflow tracts of the heart and the great vessels. *Single-ventricle heart disease* refers to a heterogeneous group of anomalies in which one of the two ventricular sinuses is absent (anatomical single ventricle) or to hearts with complex anatomy in which biventricular physiology cannot be attained (functional single ventricle).

Cardiovascular magnetic resonance (CMR) imaging plays an important role in the evaluation of patients with complex CHD. It overcomes many of the limitations of echocardiography (e.g., restricted acoustic windows), computed tomography (e.g., exposure to ionizing radiation, limited functional information), and cardiac catheterization (e.g., exposure to ionizing radiation, morbidity, high cost). This chapter discusses the clinical aspects of conotruncal anomalies and single-ventricle heart disease and their evaluation by CMR.

From: *Contemporary Cardiology: Cardiovascular Magnetic Resonance Imaging*
Edited by: Raymond Y. Kwong © Humana Press Inc., Totowa, NJ

TETRALOGY OF FALLOT

Tetralogy of Fallot (TOF) is the most common type of cyanotic CHD, with an incidence of 356 per million live births *(1)*. Although TOF involves several anatomical components, the anomaly is thought to result from a single developmental anomaly: underdevelopment of the subpulmonary infundibulum (conus) *(2,3)*. The anatomy is characterized by infundibular and valvar pulmonary stenosis associated with anterior, superior, and leftward deviation of the infundibular (conal) septum, hypoplasia of the pulmonary valve annulus and thickened leaflets. The degree of right ventricular outflow tract (RVOT) obstruction varies from mild to complete obstruction (i.e., TOF with pulmonary atresia).

The size of the mediastinal pulmonary arteries varies considerably. Although in some patients they can be dilated (e.g., TOF with absent pulmonary valve syndrome), more commonly their diameter ranges from normal to hypoplastic. In some patients, the pulmonary arteries are discontinuous or absent. In patients with pulmonary atresia or diminutive or absent branch pulmonary arteries, pulmonary blood flow may come from a patent ductus arteriosus, from collateral vessels arising from the aorta or its branches, or from both sources.

The ventricular septal defect (VSD) in TOF is usually located between the malaligned conal septum superiorly and the muscular septum inferiorly (termed *conoventricular septal defect; 4)*. The VSD is usually large, but it can rarely be restrictive *(5)*.

The aortic valve is rotated clockwise (as viewed from the apex) and is positioned above the ventricular septal crest, committing to both the left ventricle (LV) and to the right ventricle (RV). In 5–6% of patients with TOF, a major coronary artery crosses the RVOT *(6)*. Most commonly, the left anterior descending coronary artery originates from the right coronary artery and traverses the infundibular free wall before reaching the anterior interventricular groove. Preoperative identification of a major coronary artery crossing the RVOT is important to avoid inadvertent damage to the coronary artery during surgery.

The etiology of TOF is unknown, but data suggest that genetic abnormalities may play an important role, especially chromosome 22q11 deletion *(7–14)*. Additional cardiovascular and noncardiac anomalies can be associated with TOF *(15)*. Although the clinical presentation and course of patients with TOF vary, most develop cyanosis during the first year of life. Some patients with mild or no RVOT obstruction are not cyanotic at birth ("pink TOF") and may exhibit signs and symptoms of pulmonary overcirculation similar to patients with a large VSD. As these patients grow, the subpulmonary infundibulum becomes progressively obstructive and cyanosis ensues *(16)*.

Surgical repair of TOF is usually performed during the first year of life, often during the first 6 months *(17)*. A typical repair includes patch closure of the VSD and relief of the RVOT obstruction using a combination of resection of obstructive muscle bundles and an overlay patch. When the pulmonary valve annulus is moderately or severely hypoplastic, the RVOT patch extends across the pulmonary valve into the main pulmonary artery (MPA), resulting in pulmonary regurgitation. In patients with TOF and pulmonary atresia, or when a major coronary artery crosses the RVOT, a conduit—either a homograft or a prosthetic tube—is placed between the RVOT and the pulmonary arteries.

The results of surgical repair of TOF have improved dramatically since the introduction of open heart surgery. Early mortality is currently less than 2%, and the 20-years survival nears 90% *(18–20)*. The majority of these patients, however, have residual hemodynamic abnormalities, primarily caused by RV volume load from chronic pulmonary regurgitation. Other sequelae include RV hypertension from RVOT or pulmonary arterial obstruction, RV dysfunction, tricuspid regurgitation, LV volume load from a residual shunt or a patch margin VSD, and aortic dilatation. Conduction and rhythm abnormalities are another major source of late morbidity and mortality in this growing patient population *(21–27)*.

CMR Evaluation

TOF is the most frequent diagnosis among patients referred for CMR evaluation at Children's Hospital Boston. Unlike in infants, in whom echocardiography generally provides all the necessary diagnostic information for surgical repair *(6,28)*, CMR assumes an increasing role in adolescents and adults with TOF, in whom the acoustic windows are frequently limited *(29)*. CMR is useful in both pre- and postoperative assessment of TOF, but the focus of the examination is different.

Preoperative CMR

In most patients with unrepaired TOF, the central question for the CMR examination is to delineate all sources of pulmonary blood flow: pulmonary arteries, aorto-pulmonary collaterals, and the ductus arteriosus. Several studies have shown that spin echo and two-dimensional gradient echo cine CMR techniques provide excellent imaging of the central pulmonary arteries and major aorto-pulmonary collaterals *(30–33)*. However, these CMR techniques require relatively long scan times for complete anatomical coverage and small vessels (<2 mm) may not be detected. Furthermore, these two-dimensional techniques are not optimal for imaging long and tortuous blood vessels, some of which arise from the brachiocephalic arteries or from the abdominal aorta.

Gadolinium-enhanced three-dimensional (3D) magnetic resonance angiography (MRA) is ideally suited for imaging these vessels (Figs. 1 and 2). Compared with conventional X-ray angiography, MRA has been shown to be highly accurate in depicting all sources of pulmonary blood supply in patients with complex pulmonary stenosis or atresia, including infants with multiple small aorto-pulmonary collaterals *(34)*.

An electrocardiogram (ECG)-triggered gradient echo cine CMR, preferably steady-state free precession (SSFP), is used to assess ventricular dimensions and function, the RVOT, as well as dynamic flow imaging of valve function. When the origins and proximal course of the left and right coronary arteries are not known from other imaging studies, they should be evaluated by a sequence designed for coronary imaging. Particular attention is paid to the exclusion of a major coronary artery crossing the RVOT.

Postoperative CMR

CMR has been used extensively for assessment of postoperative TOF patients of all ages, but its greatest clinical utility is in adolescents and adults *(29,35)*. Quantitative assessment of RV and LV dimensions and function is a key element of CMR evaluation in patients with repaired TOF. The degree of RV dysfunction is an important determinant of clinical status late after TOF and is also closely associated with LV dysfunction, likely through ventricular-ventricular interaction (Fig. 3) *(36)*. Many studies have

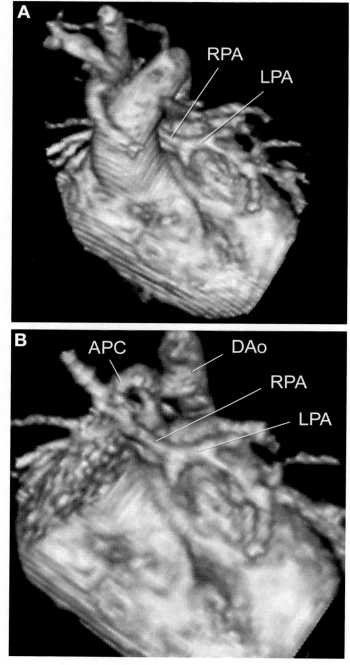

Fig. 1. (Movies in CD) Sources of pulmonary blood supply in a newborn with TOF and pulmonary atresia evaluated by Gd-enhanced 3D magnetic resonance angiography (MRA). **(A)** 3D reconstruction showing hypoplastic central pulmonary arteries. LPA, left pulmonary artery; RPA, right pulmonary artery. **(B)** The aorta was removed to expose the distal RPA. Note an aortopulmonary collateral (APC) vessel from the descending aorta (DAo) connecting to the distal RPA. **(C)** Subvolume maximum intensity projection (MIP) image in the axial plane showing hypoplastic RPA. **(D)** Subvolume MIP image in the axial plane showing hypoplastic LPA. **(E)** Subvolume MIP image in the axial plane showing a large APC arising from the DAo and splitting into two large branches, one to the left lung and one to the right lung.

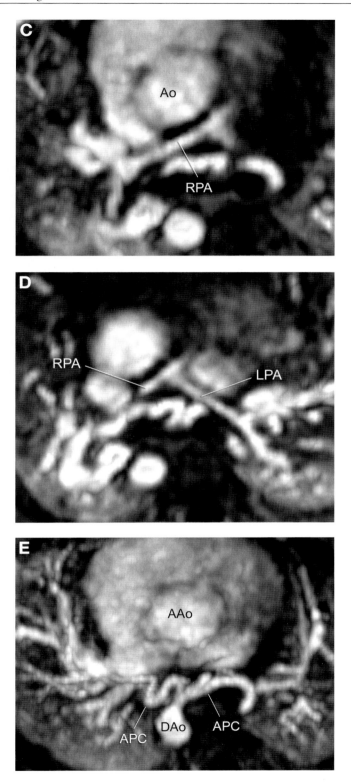

Fig. 1. *(Opposite Page)*

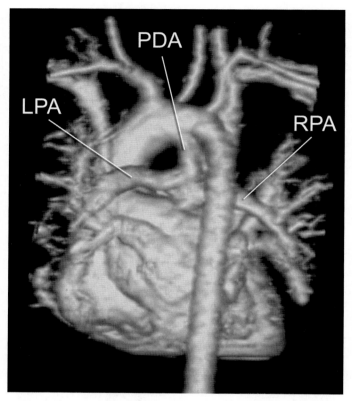

Fig. 2. (Movie in CD) 3D reconstruction of Gd-enhanced MRA in a 1.3-kg newborn with heterotaxy syndrome, dextrocardia, TOF, and pulmonary atresia. Pulmonary blood supply is exclusively through a patent ductus arteriosus (PDA), which supplies good-size confluent left pulmonary artery (LPA) and right pulmonary artery (RPA).

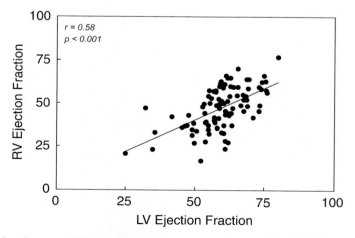

Fig. 3. Correlation between RV and LV ejection fractions in 100 patients evaluated by CMR at a median of 21 years after TOF repair *(36)*. The linear correlation suggests ventricular-ventricular interaction, resulting in a decrease in LV function as RV function decreases.

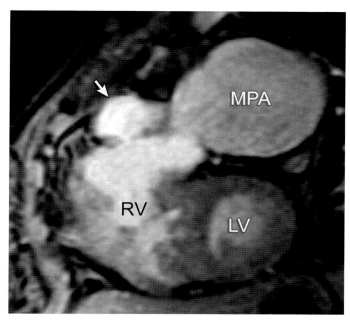

Fig. 4. (Movie in CD) ECG-gated gradient echo cine magnetic resonance (MR) showing an aneurysm of the right ventricular outflow tract (RVOT) (arrow) after TOF repair. LV, left ventricle; MPA, main pulmonary artery; RV, right ventricle.

shown that the degree of pulmonary regurgitation measured by velocity-encoded cine (VEC) CMR is closely associated with the degree of RV dilation *(37–40)*.

Another factor that affects RV function is the presence and extent of an aneurysm in the RVOT (Fig. 4) *(41)*. Taken together with clinical assessment and electrophysiological data, information derived from CMR on pulmonary regurgitation fraction, RV and LV dimensions and function, presence and extent of an RVOT aneurysm, and presence of branch pulmonary artery stenosis is used to direct clinical care in patients with repaired TOF.

Another technique that is increasingly used in patients with repaired CHD is post-gadolinium myocardial delayed enhancement (MDE) for assessment of myocardial fibrosis (Fig. 5) *(42)*. The clinical significance of positive MDE in patients with repaired TOF awaits further study.

The goals of the CMR examination therefore include (1) quantitative assessment of LV and RV volumes, mass, stroke volumes, and ejection fraction; (2) imaging the anatomy of the RVOT, pulmonary arteries, aorta, and aorto-pulmonary collaterals; and (3) quantification of pulmonary regurgitation, tricuspid regurgitation, cardiac output, and pulmonary-to-systemic flow ratio. These objectives can be achieved by the following protocol:

- Three-plane localizing images
- ECG-gated cine SSFP sequences in the two- and four-chamber planes
- ECG-gated cine SSFP sequence in the short-axis plane across the ventricles from base to apex (12 slabs with adjustment of the slice thickness and the interslice space to completely cover both ventricles) for quantitative assessment of ventricular dimensions and function
- ECG-gated cine SSFP sequence parallel to the RVOT and pulmonary arteries

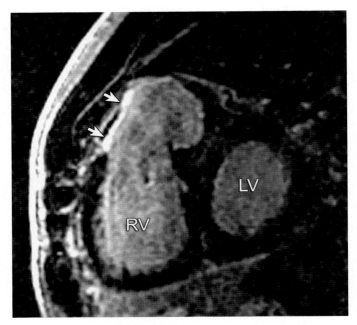

Fig. 5. MDE imaging in postoperative TOF. Images were acquired in the short-axis plane approximately 12 minutes after intravenous administration of gadopentetate dimeglumine (0.2 mmol/kg). Note the enhanced signal in the area of the RVOT patch (arrows).

- ECG-gated VEC CMR sequences perpendicular to the MPA (with or without branch pulmonary arteries), ascending aorta, and atrioventricular (AV) valves
- Gadolinium-enhanced 3D MRA
- Postgadolinium MDE may be used to evaluate the presence of scar tissue

SSFP cine sequences are acquired with breath holding whenever possible. Fast (turbo) spin echo with double inversion recovery sequence may be used to minimize artifacts from metallic implants, when present. Under optimal conditions, the above study protocol requires 60 minutes to complete. The use of sensitivity encoding or other parallel processing imaging techniques can further shorten the examination time.

TRANSPOSITION OF THE GREAT ARTERIES

Transposition of the great arteries (TGA) is defined as discordant connections between the ventricles and the great arteries; the aorta arises from the RV, and the pulmonary artery arises from the LV. There are several anatomical types of TGA, depending on the viscero-atrial situs (solitus or inversus) and the type of ventricular loop (D or L) *(43)*. The most common type of TGA is in viscero-atrial situs solitus (S), ventricular D-loop (D), and dextro malposition of the aortic valve relative to the pulmonary valve (D). This anatomical arrangement can be summarized as {S,D,D} TGA. Note that the term *D-TGA* is nonspecific as the D might relate to the ventricular loop or to the spatial position of the aortic and pulmonary valves. This ambiguity can be avoided by using the term *D-loop TGA*. The incidence of D-loop TGA is estimated at 303 per million live births *(1)*.

The principal physiological abnormality in D-loop TGA is that systemic venous blood returns to the aorta, and oxygenated pulmonary venous blood returns to the lungs, resulting in profound hypoxemia. Consequently, survival is dependent on communications that allow mixing of blood between the systemic and pulmonary circulations. The most common sites of shunting are through the ductus arteriosus, atrial septal defect, or VSD. Associated anomalies include VSD in approximately 45% of patients, coarctation or interrupted aortic arch (IAA) in approximately 12%, pulmonary stenosis in approximately 5%, RV hypoplasia in approximately 4%, juxtaposition of the atrial appendages in approximately 2%, and other anomalies in 1% of patients or less, each *(44)*.

Surgical management of D-loop TGA in the 1960s and 1970s consisted mostly of an atrial switch procedure—the Senning or Mustard operations. In both procedures, the systemic and pulmonary venous blood returns are redirected within the atria so that the pulmonary venous blood reaches the tricuspid valve, RV, and aorta, whereas the systemic venous blood reaches the mitral valve, LV, and pulmonary arteries. The main technical difference between these procedures is that in the Mustard operation the surgeon uses pericardium to redirect the blood flow, and in the Senning operation the surgeon uses native atrial tissue *(45)*. The main drawbacks of the atrial switch operations include RV (systemic ventricle) dysfunction, sinus node dysfunction, atrial arrhythmias, obstruction of the systemic or pulmonary venous pathways, and baffle leaks *(46–48)*.

Beginning in the late 1970s and rapidly gaining popularity in the 1980s, the arterial switch operation (ASO) largely replaced the atrial switch procedures *(49,50)*. The advantages of the ASO over the atrial switch procedures include reestablishment of the LV as the systemic ventricle and avoidance of extensive suture lines in the atria. Recent data on late outcome of the ASO continues to show excellent overall survival with low morbidity *(51–56)*. The Rastelli operation is another surgical option for patients with an associated subvalvular and valvular pulmonary stenosis and a VSD. It consists of patch closure of the VSD to the aortic valve and placement of a conduit between the RV and the pulmonary arteries.

The second most common type of TGA is in viscero-atrial situs solitus (S), L-ventricular loop (L), and levo-malposition of the aortic valve relative to the pulmonary valve (L). This anatomical arrangement can be summarized as {S,L,L} TGA or L-loop TGA *(57–60)*. It is also known as "physiologically corrected" TGA because the systemic venous return reaches the pulmonary circulation through the right-sided LV, and the pulmonary venous return reaches the aorta through the left-sided RV. Associated anomalies include tricuspid valve abnormalities (e.g., Ebstein anomaly), RV hypoplasia, VSD, subvalvar and valvar pulmonary stenosis, as well as conduction abnormalities, including complete heart block. Outcome is determined primarily by the associated lesions and RV (the systemic ventricle) function *(57–60)*.

CMR Evaluation

CMR is seldom requested for preoperative assessment of infants with D-loop TGA because echocardiography usually provides all necessary diagnostic information *(44)*. In postoperative TGA, CMR assumes an increasing role because of its ability to noninvasively evaluate most clinically relevant issues *(61–69)*.

Postoperative Atrial Switch

The goals of CMR evaluation of postoperative atrial switch include (1) quantitative evaluation of the size and function of the systemic RV *(62)*; (2) imaging of the systemic and pulmonary venous pathways for obstruction or baffle leaks; (3) assessment of tricuspid valve regurgitation; (4) evaluation of the left ventricular outflow tract (LVOT) and RVOT for obstruction; and (5) detection of aorto-pulmonary collateral vessels and other associated anomalies. In patients with RV dysfunction, postgadolinium delayed myocardial enhancement can be used to detect myocardial fibrosis *(70)*. The response of the systemic RV to pharmacological stress (dobutamine) or to exercise can be tested by CMR, but the clinical utility of this information awaits further study *(67,69)*. These objectives can be achieved by the following protocol:

- Three-plane localizing images.
- ECG-gated cine SSFP sequence in the four-chamber or axial plane with multiple contiguous slices from the level of the diaphragm to the level of the transverse arch (provides dynamic imaging of the venous pathways, qualitative assessment of ventricular function, AV valve regurgitation, and imaging of the great arteries) (Fig. 6A).
- Based on the previous sequence, ECG-gated cine SSFP sequence in multiple oblique coronal planes parallel to the superior vena cava (SVC) and inferior vena cava (IVC) pathways to image them in their long axis (Fig. 6B).
- ECG-gated cine SSFP sequence in the short-axis plane across the ventricles from base to apex (12 slabs) for quantitative assessment of ventricular dimensions and function (Fig. 6C).
- ECG-gated VEC CMR sequences perpendicular to the AV valves, MPA, and the ascending aorta; additional VEC CMR sequences may be obtained to evaluate specific areas suspected for obstruction (71)
- Gd-enhanced 3D MRA.

SSFP cine sequences are acquired with breath holding whenever possible. Fast (turbo) spin echo with double inversion recovery sequence may be used to minimize artifacts from metallic implants, and postgadolinium delayed myocardial enhancement may be used to evaluate the presence of scar tissue *(42)*.

Postoperative Arterial Switch

The long-term concerns in patients after the ASO relate primarily to the technical challenges of the operation—transfer of the coronary arteries from the native aortic root to the neoaortic root (native pulmonary root) and the transfer of the pulmonary arteries anterior to the neoascending aorta (Fig. 7). Consequently, the goals of CMR evaluation of postoperative arterial switch include (1) evaluation of global and regional LV and RV size and function; (2) evaluation of the LVOT and RVOT for obstruction; (3) qualitative estimation of RV systolic pressure based on the configuration of the interventricular septum; (4) imaging of the great vessels with emphasis on evaluation of the pulmonary arteries for stenosis and the aortic root for dilatation; and (5) detection of aorto-pulmonary collaterals and other associated anomalies. The role of myocardial perfusion and viability imaging in this population deserves further study. These objectives can be achieved by the following protocol:

- Three-plane localizing images.
- ECG-gated cine SSFP sequence in the axial plane with multiple contiguous slices from the midventricular level to the level of the transverse arch (provides axial dynamic imaging of the outflow tracts and the great arteries, qualitative assessment of ventricular function, and AV valve regurgitation)
- ECG-gated cine SSFP sequence in the coronal or oblique sagittal planes parallel to the LVOT and RVOT

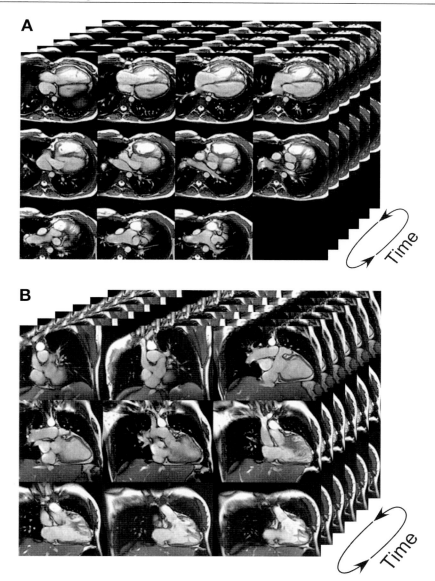

Fig. 6. (Movies in CD) Evaluation of Mustard pathways by ECG-gated steady-state free precession (SSFP) cine MR (magnetic resonance). **(A)** Multiple contiguous slices in the four-chamber plane from the level of the diaphragm to the level of the branch pulmonary arteries. The image data set provides dynamic imaging of the venous pathways, qualitative assessment of ventricular function, AV valve regurgitation, and imaging of the great arteries. **(B)** Based on the previous sequence, ECG-gated SSFP cine MR in multiple oblique coronal planes showing the superior and inferior systemic venous pathways. **(C)** ECG-gated SSFP cine MR in the short-axis plane for assessment of biventricular volumes, mass, and function.

- ECG-gated cine SSFP sequences in the two- and four-chamber planes, followed by a short-axis stack across the ventricles from base to apex (12 slabs) for quantitative assessment of ventricular dimensions and function
- ECG-gated VEC CMR sequences perpendicular to the main and branch pulmonary arteries and the ascending aorta; additional VEC CMR sequences may be obtained to evaluate specific areas suspected for obstruction *(71)*
- Gd-enhanced 3D MRA.

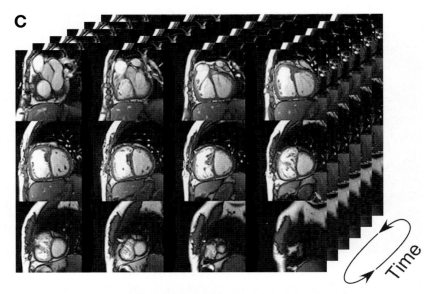

Fig. 6. *(Continued)*

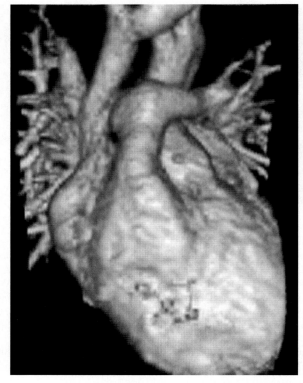

Fig. 7. (Movie in CD) 3D reconstruction of Gd-enhanced MRA in postoperative arterial switch operation.

SSFP cine sequences are acquired with breath-holding whenever possible. Fast (turbo) spin echo with double inversion recovery sequence may be used to minimize artifacts from metallic implants. Pharmacological stress testing—either adenosine or dobutamine—for evaluation of myocardial ischemia and MDE for detection of myocardial fibrosis is increasingly incorporated into the clinical imaging protocol in patients with repaired TGA.

DOUBLE-OUTLET RIGHT VENTRICLE

Double-outlet right ventricle (DORV) is defined as a specific type of ventriculo-arterial alignment in which both great vessels arise from the RV or from the infundibulum. The incidence of DORV is estimated at 127 per million live births *(1)*. It is important to recognize the wide spectrum of anatomical and physiological variations that share this type of ventriculo-arterial alignment. In fact, the clinical course and management of patients with DORV are dictated in large part by the size and location of the VSD in relation to the semilunar valves, the anatomy of the infundibulum and the semilunar valves, the position of the infundibular septum, the size of the LV and RV sinuses, and the anatomy of the AV valves. The LV can be normal in size, hypoplastic, or absent. The RV is usually good size, but in rare circumstances it can be hypoplastic or even absent (double-outlet infundibulum). Both semilunar valves can be patent, but stenosis or atresia is relatively common. The presence of a straddling mitral or tricuspid valve is particularly important for surgical planning. Examples of some of the common anatomical-physiological variations encountered in patients with DORV include

- VSD physiology: DORV with subaortic VSD and no pulmonary stenosis
- TOF physiology: DORV with subaortic VSD and pulmonary stenosis
- TGA physiology: DORV with subpulmonary VSD with or without systemic (aortic) outflow obstruction (Taussig-Bing-type DORV)
- Single-ventricle physiology: DORV with mitral atresia, unbalanced AV canal, or severe hypoplasia of one of the ventricular sinuses (often in association with heterotaxy syndrome)

The ultimate goal of surgical management of DORV is to align the LV with the systemic outflow and the RV with the pulmonary outflow. In DORV with a subaortic VSD, the LV can be aligned with the aorta by placing a patch on the RV aspect of the defect, leaving the aortic valve on the LV side. Resection of RVOT obstruction, with or without an outflow patch, may be necessary in patients with subvalvar or valvar pulmonary stenosis, analogous to TOF repair. In DORV with a subpulmonary VSD (Taussig-Bing variety), the VSD is closed with a patch that directs the blood from the LV to the pulmonary valve accompanied by an arterial switch procedure. Concomitant repair of an aortic arch anomaly (e.g., hypoplasia, interruption, or coarctation) is often required as well. More complex forms of DORV with heterotaxy syndrome, severe hypoplasia or absence of one of the ventricular sinuses, major straddling of an AV valve, or mitral atresia are palliated as a single ventricle with an eventual Fontan procedure.

Late complications in patients with repaired DORV are relatively common and vary with their underlying anatomy, physiology, and surgical repair. Subaortic stenosis can develop after the LV is baffled to the aorta *(72)*. The complications after repair of DORV with pulmonary outflow tract obstruction are similar to those seen after TOF repair, including chronic pulmonary regurgitation, dilation and dysfunction of the

RV, and arrhythmia. Aortic arch obstruction can be found in patients after coarctation or interrupted aortic arch IAA repair. Those who undergo an arterial switch operation may have the same problems described above for this procedure.

Preoperative CMR

Because echocardiography is usually sufficient for diagnosis and surgical planning in most newborns or infants with DORV, CMR is seldom requested for preoperative evaluation in this age group. Exceptions include patients with complex anomalies of the aortic arch, pulmonary arteries, aorto-pulmonary collaterals, and systemic or pulmonary venous anomalies that are not completely delineated by echocardiography. Several investigators demonstrated the use of CMR for the assessment of the relationship between the great vessels and the VSD as well as the position of the great vessels in relation to the conal septum (73–77).

The imaging strategy is tailored to address the specific clinical questions. In general, gadolinium-enhanced 3D MRA is particularly helpful for evaluation of great vessel anatomy (Fig. 8A). Intracardiac anatomy is assessed by SSFP cine CMR and by fast (turbo) spin echo with double inversion recovery (Fig. 8B–D). Sorensen et al. described the use of a free-breathing, ECG triggered, navigator-gated, isotropic 3D SSFP sequence that holds promise for assessment of both intra- and extracardiac anatomy (78). Although the quality of the images obtained in children younger than 7 years was inferior to those in older patients, further refinements may prove this technique helpful for assessment of complex intracardiac anatomy.

Postoperative CMR

The role of CMR after DORV repair increases as patients grow and their acoustic windows become progressively more limited. The examination strategy is tailored based on the underlying anatomy, the operations performed, and the specific clinical and other diagnostic findings. Although no single generic imaging protocol covers all possible scenarios after DORV repair, certain patterns are recognized. Patients with a "TOF-like" DORV repair have similar long-term sequelae as those after TOF repair, and the CMR examination protocol is comparable (*see* section on TOF). Similarly, in those with Taussig-Bing-type DORV, the postoperative issues are similar to those encountered after the arterial switch operation for TGA (*see* section on TGA). The importance of modifying the examination protocol to address anatomical and functional abnormalities specific to the individual patient cannot be overstated. This requires on-line evaluation of the imaging data because previously unsuspected abnormalities may only be detected during the scan.

TRUNCUS ARTERIOSUS

Truncus arteriosus is an uncommon conotruncal anomaly with a reported incidence of 94 per million live births (1). It is defined by the presence of a single artery arising from the heart with a single semilunar valve, giving rise to the coronary arteries, aorta, and at least one branch pulmonary artery. Van Praagh and Van Praagh (79) modified the original classification of Collett and Edwards (80):

- Type I: The branch pulmonary arteries arise from a short MPA.
- Type II: The branch pulmonary arteries arise directly from the arterial trunc through separate orifices.

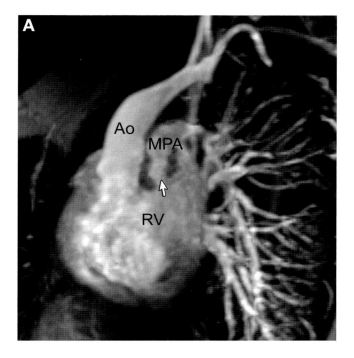

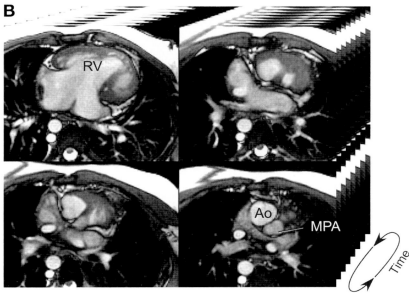

Fig. 8. CMR evaluation of heterotaxy syndrome, common AV canal, and double-outlet right ventricle with pulmonary stenosis. **(A)** Subvolume MIP image of Gd-enhanced 3D MRA showing origin of the aorta (Ao) and main pulmonary artery (MPA) from the right ventricle (RV). Note the subvalvar pulmonary stenosis (arrow). **(B)** (movie in CD) Multislice ECG-gated SSFP cine MR in the axial plane. The left upper slice shows the RV-dominant common AV canal. The right upper slice shows the subaortic and subpulmonary conus. The right lower slice shows the great arteries with the larger Ao to the right and anterior relative to the smaller MPA. **(C)** (movie in CD) Diastolic frame of an ECG-gated SSFP cine MR in an oblique coronal plane showing the narrowed subpulmonary conus (arrow). **(D)** Systolic frame in the same location as **C** showing two jets (arrows); the inferior jet is caused by subvalvar stenosis, and the superior jet caused by pulmonary valve stenosis.

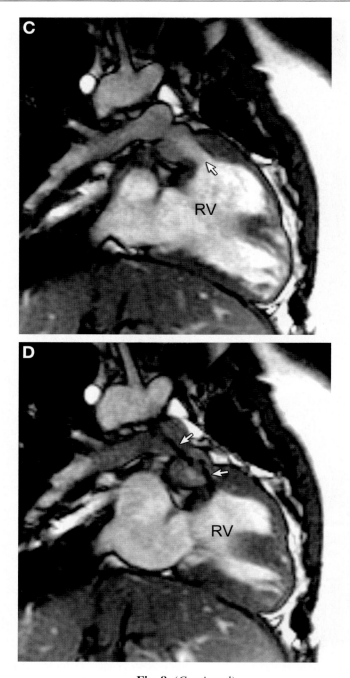

Fig. 8. *(Continued)*

- Type III: Only one branch pulmonary artery arises from the ascending segment of the trunc. Collateral vessels usually supply the contralateral lung.
- Type IV: This truncus arteriosus has aortic arch hypoplasia, coarctation, or interruption (usually type B distal to the left common carotid artery). In this anatomical variation, there is usually a well-formed MPA and a small ascending aorta.

In the majority of cases, there is a subtruncal VSD over which the truncal valve sits, similar to TOF. Rarely, the ventricular septum is intact. The conal septum is usually absent, and the truncal valve is in direct fibrous continuity with the mitral valve. In rare circumstances, the truncal valve may be supported by a complete infundibulum and relate exclusively to the RV. The truncal valve is most commonly tricommissural, followed by bicommissural morphology, and least common is a quadricommissural valve. The valve can be thickened and redundant with stenosis, regurgitation, or both.

Associated cardiovascular and noncardiac anomalies are frequent. Examples of associated cardiovascular anomalies include multiple VSDs, partial and complete AV canal defects, mitral atresia, mitral stenosis, aortic atresia, hypoplastic LV, double-inlet LV, tricuspid atresia, straddling tricuspid valve, Ebstein malformation, heterotaxy syndrome, aberrant origin of the right or left subclavian artery, coarctation of the aorta, secundum atrial septal defect, partially and totally anomalous pulmonary venous connections, left SVC to coronary sinus, retroaortic innominate vein, and left pulmonary artery sling (81). Various noncardiac anomalies have been described in patients with truncus arteriosus. DiGeorge syndrome, velocardiofacial syndrome, and chromosome 22q11 deletion are frequently associated. A large series found the 22q11 deletion in 34.5% of patients with truncus arteriosus (82).

Most patients with truncus arteriosus are diagnosed early in life, and echocardiography is sufficient for diagnosis and surgical planning in almost all. Surgical repair usually follows the diagnosis. Typically, the VSD is closed with a patch so that the truncal valve is aligned with the LV (becoming the neoaortic valve), and the pulmonary arteries are detached from the arterial trunk and connected to the RV with a valved homograft. Surgical repair of the truncal valve for stenosis or regurgitation is uncommon during the initial repair. Surgical mortality is low and has improved with the overall advances in surgical management of infants. The use of a nongrowing homograft in infancy makes additional operations inevitable as patients grow.

Important residual lesions after truncus arteriosus repair include progressive stenosis and regurgitation of the RV-to-pulmonary artery homograft, branch pulmonary artery stenosis, and regurgitation or stenosis of the neoaortic (truncal) valve. Aortic arch obstruction can complicate the course of patients with coarctation or IAA repair.

Preoperative CMR

CMR is rarely requested for preoperative evaluation in an infant with truncus arteriosus because echocardiography is almost always adequate (83). Exceptions include complex aortic arch or pulmonary venous anomalies that require further delineation and the occasional older patient with an unrepaired truncus arteriosus (Fig. 9).

Postoperative CMR

The role of CMR in patients with repaired truncus arteriosus increases with their age. The anatomical and functional issues in these patients are similar to those encountered in patients with repaired TOF, especially in those with TOF and pulmonary atresia. Neoaortic valve dysfunction and aortic arch obstruction are additional issues that may require investigation. Therefore, the goals of the CMR examination after truncus repair include (1) quantitative assessment of LV and RV volumes, function, and mass; (2) measurements of pulmonary and neoaortic valve regurgitation; (3) imaging of the RVOT, the homograft, and the branch pulmonary arteries; (4) assessment of residual shunts; and (5) imaging of the aortic arch and isthmus. These objectives can be

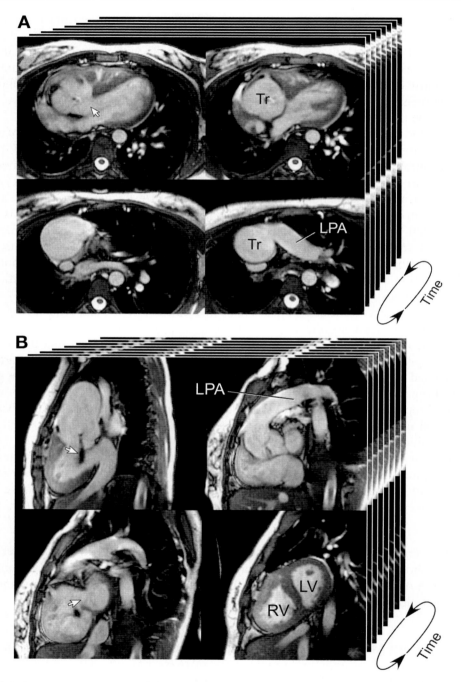

Fig. 9. CMR evaluation of truncus arteriosus with absent right pulmonary artery (truncus arteriosus type III of Van Praagh). **(A)** (movie in CD) Multislice ECG-gated SSFP cine MR in the axial plane. The left upper slice shows the conoventricular septal defect (arrow). The right upper slice shows the large truncal root (Tr). The right lower slice shows the origin of the left pulmonary artery (LPA) from the Tr. **(B)** (movie in CD) Multislice ECG-gated SSFP cine MR in the short-axis plane. The left upper slice shows truncal valve regurgitation (arrow). The right upper slice shows the origin of the LPA above the truncal root. The left lower slice shows the conoventricular septal defect (arrow). The right lower slice shows the ventricles in short axis. **(C)** (movie in CD) 3D reconstruction of Gd-enhanced MRA showing the origin of the left pulmonary artery from the truncal root.

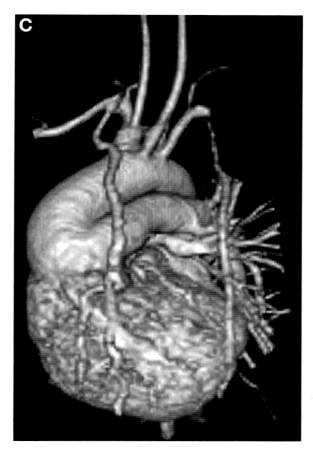

Fig. 9. *(Continued)*

achieved with modifications of the protocol described for TOF and individualized for the patient's anatomical and hemodynamic issues.

INTERRUPTED AORTIC ARCH

IAA is an uncommon congenital cardiovascular malformation characterized by anatomical discontinuity between segments of the aortic arch. The prevalence of IAA is 19 per million live births or 1.3% of infants with CHD in the New England Regional Infant Cardiac Program *(84)*. This condition should be distinguished from aortic arch atresia, for which there is anatomical continuity between the arch segments through a fibrous strand, but the aortic lumen is completely obstructed. Because of their identical hemodynamic consequences, both conditions are discussed together.

The classification proposed by Celoria and Patton in 1959 is widely used to date *(85)*. Type A denotes interruption distal to the left subclavian artery, type B between the left common carotid and the left subclavian arteries, and type C between the common carotid arteries. Type B is the most common anatomical variation, accounting for approximately 62% of IAA cases, type A for 37%, and type C for 1%. Other morphological variations associated with IAA have been described. Aberrant origin of the right subclavian artery from the proximal descending aorta is found in roughly 50% of patients with type B IAA but only in a minority of those with type A interruption. Other rare variations include interruption of a right aortic arch (86) and interruption of a cervical arch (87).

Survival of patients with IAA depends on a patent ductus arteriosus. Intravenous administration of prostaglandin E begins immediately once the diagnosis is suspected and is followed by surgical repair. In most institutions, the preferred surgical approach is direct anastomosis of the interrupted (or atretic) aortic segments. When the distance between the interrupted aortic arch segments is large, homograft augmentation may be added to the arch reconstruction. The use of a tubular conduit to bridge between the arch segments is usually reserved for unusually long segment interruptions or for reoperations. In patients with an associated VSD, the defect is closed at the time of the arch repair. In type B IAA with posterior malalignment of the conal septum and markedly hypoplastic LVOT, the VSD can be baffled to the pulmonary valve, the MPA is transected and anastomosed to the ascending aorta, and a conduit (usually a valved homograft) is placed between the RV and the pulmonary arteries.

CMR Evaluation

Echocardiography is usually adequate for preoperative diagnosis of interrupted aortic arch and associated anomalies (88). CMR is used in selected patients in whom the anatomy is not clearly defined by echocardiography (89,90). CMR assumes a larger role in patients with repaired IAA as they grow and their acoustic windows become restricted.

Preoperative CMR

The goal of the CMR examination is to delineate the anatomy of the aortic arch and the branching pattern of the brachiocephalic arteries (Fig. 10). It is important to fully evaluate the vascular anatomy to exclude any associated anomalies (e.g., systemic and pulmonary venous anomalies). Gadolinium-enhanced 3D MRA is the most robust and time-efficient technique to achieve these goals (Fig. 11) (90). The use of gradient echo cine and black blood imaging is tailored to the clinical and imaging issues of individual patients. Evaluation of intracardiac anatomy is usually not necessary because the information should be available from echocardiography.

Postoperative CMR

The goal of the CMR examination after IAA surgery is to evaluate residual or recurrent anatomical and hemodynamic problems. Often, the focus is on imaging of the aortic arch and the repair site for evaluation of obstruction or aneurysm formation (Fig. 12). However, other abnormalities, such as LVOT obstruction, aortic valve stenosis or regurgitation, residual VSD, left ventricular size and function, and other anomalies should be examined as well. The hemodynamic severity of residual or recurrent aortic arch obstruction can be assessed based on body surface area-adjusted smallest cross-sectional area of the aortic arch or isthmus (from Gd-enhanced 3D MRA) and the heart rate-adjusted mean deceleration rate in the descending aorta (from VEC CMR) as described by Nielsen et al. (91). These objectives can be achieved with the following protocol:

- Three-plane localizing images
- ECG-gated cine SSFP sequences in the two- and four-chamber planes

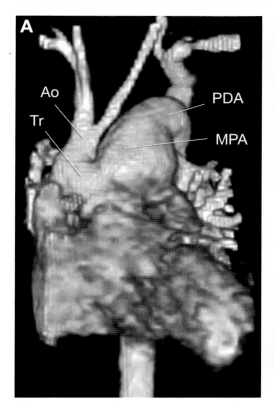 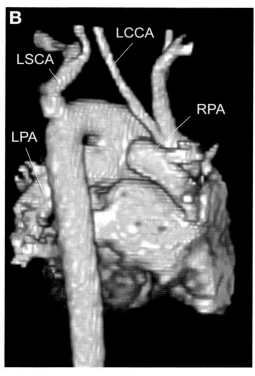

Fig. 10. (Movie in CD) 3D reconstruction of Gd-enhanced MRA in a newborn with truncus arteriosus and type B interrupted aortic arch (truncus type IV of Van Praagh). **(A)** Anterior view showing the ascending aorta (Ao), which gives rise to the right innominate and to the left common carotid arteries (LCCAs). The main pulmonary artery (MPA) continues as a large patent ductus arteriosus (PDA). **(B)** Posterior view showing the interruption between the LCCA and the left subclavian artery (LSCA), which arises from the proximal descending aorta.

- ECG-gated cine SSFP sequence in the short-axis plane across the ventricles from base to apex (12 slabs with adjustment of the slice thickness and the interslice space to completely cover both ventricles) for quantitative assessment of ventricular dimensions and function
- ECG-gated cine SSFP sequence parallel to the LVOT
- ECG-gated cine SSFP sequence in the long axis of the aortic arch
- Optional: ECG-gated fast (turbo) spin echo in the long axis of the aortic arch
- ECG-gated VEC CMR sequences perpendicular to the ascending and descending aorta, with additional flow measurements obtained based on clinical relevance (e.g., assessment of aortic regurgitation)
- Gadolinium-enhanced 3D MRA

SINGLE VENTRICLE

The normal human heart is composed of three chambers at the ventricular level (between the AV valves and the semilunar valves): the LV sinus, the RV sinus, and the infundibulum. From an anatomical standpoint, *single ventricle* is defined as a

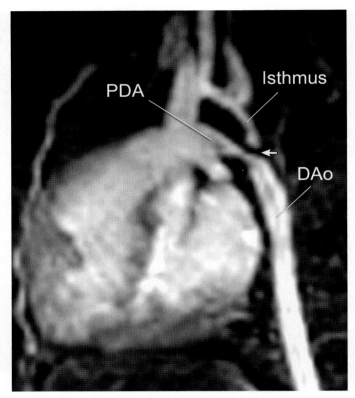

Fig. 11. Subvolume MIP image of Gd-enhanced 3D MRA showing type A interrupted aortic arch distal to the left subclavian artery. Note the short segment of luminal discontinuity (arrow) between the aortic isthmus and the descending aorta (DAo).

circumstance in which one of the two ventricular sinuses is absent. The infundibulum is always present and has been described by various terms, such as infundibular outlet chamber, rudimentary or hypoplastic RV, and rudimentary chamber. As defined, single ventricle accounts for approximately 1% of CHD, with a median incidence of 85 per million live births (1). There are other congenital cardiac anomalies in which the anatomy precludes establishment of biventricular physiology. These conditions, which are often treated with one of the modifications of the Fontan operation, are often grouped under the term *functional single ventricle* or *functional univentricular hearts.* Examples include tricuspid atresia, mitral atresia, unbalanced common AV canal defect, pulmonary atresia with intact ventricular septum and diminutive RV and tricuspid valve, and others.

From an anatomical perspective, there are two types of single ventricle:

1. Single LV: Several anatomical types of single LV are recognized. Common to all is the absence of the RV sinus and the presence of a LV and an infundibulum. The following anatomical features characterize hearts with a single LV:

    a. The different anatomical types of single LV vary according to the type of ventricular loop present and the types of AV and ventriculoarterial alignments.
    b. There is communication between the LV and the infundibulum, termed the *bulboventricular foramen.*

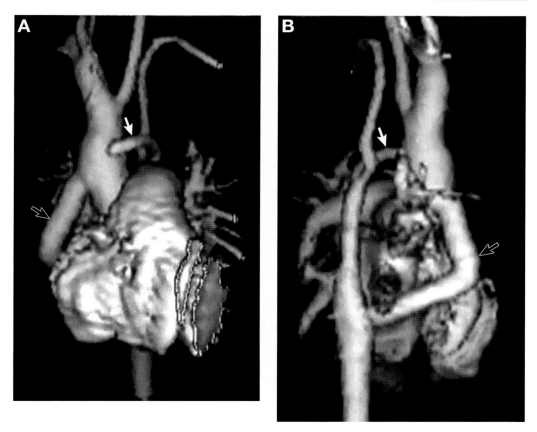

Fig. 12. 3D reconstruction of Gd-enhanced MRA in postoperative type B interrupted aortic arch initially repaired with a left-sided conduit between the distal ascending aorta and the proximal descending aorta (white arrow). When that conduit became obstructive, a second conduit was placed on the patient's right side (black arrow). **(A)** Anterior view. **(B)** Posterior view.

    c. When two AV valves enter the LV (double-inlet LV), their different papillary muscle architectures reflect their identity. The tricuspid valve is typically closer to the septum (septophilic); it may have chordal attachments on the septum, to the inferior VSD margin, or both and sometimes into the infundibulum. By contrast, the mitral valve attaches to the free-wall papillary muscles (septophobic). If the two AV valves share the LV cavity, then usually one, and rarely both, is abnormal. If only the mitral valve enters the LV (i.e., tricuspid atresia), then it is typically structurally normal. Other types of AV alignments in single LV include common inlet, when a common AV valve is present, and mitral atresia with a large LV.

    d. The types of ventriculoarterial connections include (1) normally related great arteries (Holmes heart), in which the aorta arises from the LV and the pulmonary artery from the infundibulum; (2) TGA, in which the pulmonary artery arises from the LV and the aorta from the infundibulum; and (3) double-outlet infundibulum, in which both aorta and pulmonary artery arise from the infundibulum. Pulmonary stenosis or atresia, aortic stenosis or atresia, and aortic arch anomalies (most commonly coarctation) may be associated with single LV.

2. Single RV: In hearts with a single RV, the ventricular mass consists of the RV sinus and the infundibulum, both forming a common chamber. The septal band is present, indicating the location of a ventricular septum, but there is no macroscopically recognizable LV sinus on the other side of the septum. Several anatomical types of single RV are recognized:

   a. Double-inlet RV: Both AV valves open into the RV. The tricuspid valve attaches in the inlet (sinus) portion of the RV, and the mitral valve attaches in the outflow or infundibulum. Both valves exhibit attachments to the septal band.

   b. Common-inlet single RV: A single AV valve connects both atria with the RV. The morphology is often that of a tricuspid valve, but the presence of an ostium primum defect and the alignment of both atria with the single RV indicate that this is a common AV valve mimicking a tricuspid valve. This type of single RV usually occurs in association with visceral heterotaxy and asplenia. Associated malformations include anomalies of the systemic and pulmonary venous connections, absence or marked hypoplasia of the atrial septum, absence of the coronary sinus, and pulmonary outflow tract stenosis or atresia. In both types of single RV, both great arteries originate from the infundibulum, and the resulting ventriculoarterial alignment is that of double-outlet RV.

Single-ventricle physiology is characterized by complete mixing of the systemic and pulmonary venous return flows. The proportion of the ventricular output distributed to the pulmonary or systemic vascular bed is determined by the relative resistance to flow in the two circuits. The clinical presentation and course in patients with single ventricle depends on the hemodynamic profile:

1. Diminished pulmonary blood flow: patients are cyanotic with arterial oxygen saturation typically less than 75%; there are no signs and symptoms of congestive heart failure.
2. Increased pulmonary blood flow: patients may be asymptomatic in the newborn and early neonatal periods; arterial oxygen saturation typically is greater than 85%, and cyanosis may not be evident; signs and symptoms of congestive heart failure develop during the first few weeks of life as pulmonary vascular resistance decreases and pulmonary blood flow increases.
3. Balanced circulation: patients exhibit mild or moderate cyanosis with arterial oxygen saturation of 75–85%; there are no signs and symptoms of congestive heart failure.
4. Closing duct: patients with a duct-dependent pulmonary circulation and a closing duct present with profound cyanosis and acidemia. Patients with a duct-dependent systemic circulation present with a clinical picture of shock, hypoperfusion, poor peripheral pulses, oliguria or anuria, and acidemia.
5. Atypical clinical picture: This is caused by the progressive nature of certain anatomical and hemodynamic factors (e.g., progressive narrowing of a bulboventricular foramen leading to severe subaortic stenosis).

The goals of current surgical therapy in patients with single ventricle are to separate the systemic and pulmonary circulations and to eliminate volume overload on the ventricle. These goals are often achieved with staged palliative procedures, leading to one of the modifications of the Fontan operation (Fig. 13). The principal aim of the procedure is to divert the systemic venous return from the IVC and SVC to the pulmonary arteries, which separates the poorly oxygenated systemic venous return from the oxygenated pulmonary venous return.

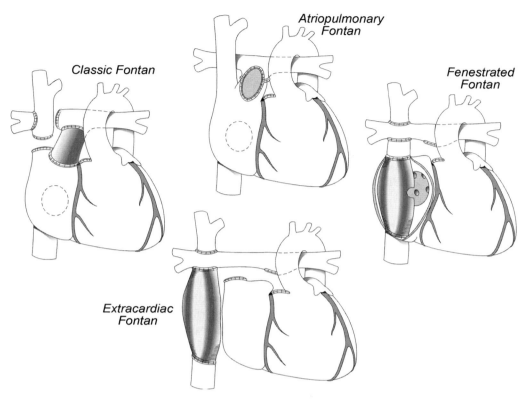

Fig. 13. Diagrams of four variations of the Fontan operation.

Since it was first described in 1971 *(92)*, the Fontan operation has undergone multiple modifications, including direct anastomosis of the right atrial appendage to the MPA (called atriopulmonary anastomosis) *(93)*, RA-to-RV conduit, lateral tunnel between the IVC and the undersurface of the ipsilateral branch pulmonary artery *(94)*, fenestration of the lateral tunnel baffle *(95)*, and an extracardiac conduit between the IVC and the ipsilateral branch pulmonary artery *(96)*. With refinement of the criteria for patient selection, management strategies, and surgical techniques, the short- and medium-term results of the Fontan operation have gradually improved *(97)*. Nevertheless, this growing patient population continues to be at risk for complications, such as systemic ventricular dysfunction, thromboembolism, dilation of the systemic venous atrium, obstruction of the Fontan pathways, pulmonary artery stenosis, compression of the pulmonary veins, AV valve regurgitation, and arrhythmias *(97–103)*. Prompt detection of these complications is therefore an important element of managing these patients.

CMR Evaluations

CMR is particularly well suited for the detailed investigation of the divergent and often complex anatomy of single-ventricle heart disease. Although echocardiography is typically adequate for initial diagnosis in the neonate with a single ventricle, CMR is assuming an increasingly important role in the evaluation of patients before and after later stages of palliation.

CMR Evaluation During Staged Palliation of Single Ventricle

Staged palliation of single-ventricle disease often includes the superior cavo-pulmonary anastomosis (bidirectional Glenn) operation, typically performed at 4–6 months of age. Traditionally, this procedure is preceded by diagnostic cardiac catheterization for anatomical and physiological information. CMR may offer an alternative for cardiac catheterization in selected cases. The goals of CMR in the pre-bidirectional Glenn patient include (1) quantitative assessment of ventricular mass, volume, and function; (2) imaging the anatomy of the pulmonary veins, pulmonary arteries, and aortic arch; (3) imaging the anatomy of any prior surgical intervention (e.g., aortic arch reconstruction); (4) evaluating for the presence of aortopulmonary or veno-venous collateral vessels; and (5) quantification of AV or semilunar valve regurgitation. These objectives can be achieved by the following protocol:

- Three-plane localizing images
- ECG-gated cine SSFP sequence in the axial plane for evaluation of the anatomy, with particular attention to the atrial septum, pulmonary veins, and pulmonary arteries
- ECG-gated cine SSFP sequence of the systemic ventricle in its long axis followed by short-axis cine imaging from the level of the AV valves to the apex (12 slices are prescribed with slice thickness and interslice gap adjusted to cover the desired anatomy)
- ECG-gated cine SSFP sequence in an oblique sagittal plane to image the aortic arch
- ECG-gated fast (turbo) spin echo with double inversion recovery to image the branch pulmonary arteries and aortic arch (optional)
- ECG-gated VEC CMR sequences perpendicular to the AV valves, ascending aorta, descending aorta, and (optional) branch pulmonary arteries
- Gadolinium-enhanced 3D MRA

Postgadolinium late myocardial enhancement may be performed for evaluation of endocardial fibroelastosis or myocardial fibrosis.

Post-Fontan CMR

Several reports have utilized CMR as an investigational tool to study blood flow dynamics within the Fontan pathways and to delineate the distribution of IVC and SVC flow to each lung (104–107). Myocardial tagging has proved an important investigational tool in the evaluation of myocardial mechanics in patients with functional single ventricle and Fontan circulation, demonstrating asynchrony and impaired regional wall motion (108). The clinical utility of CMR in patients with the Fontan circulation increases as these patients grow and their acoustic windows become more restricted (Fig. 14).

The goals of the CMR examination in patients with the Fontan circulation include (1) assessment of the pathways from the systemic veins to the pulmonary arteries for obstruction and for thrombus; (2) detection of Fontan baffle fenestration or leaks; (3) evaluation of the pulmonary veins for compression; (4) systemic ventricular volumes, mass, and function; (5) imaging of the systemic ventricular outflow tract for obstruction; (6) quantitative assessment of the AV and semilunar valves for regurgitation; (7) imaging the aorta for obstruction or an aneurysm; and (8) detection of aortopulmonary, systemic venous, or systemic-to-pulmonary venous collateral vessels. A representative imaging protocol begins with localizing images and continues with the following sequences:

- ECG-gated cine SSFP sequence in the axial plane from the level of the IVC-hepatic veins confluence to the level of the cranial end of the SVC

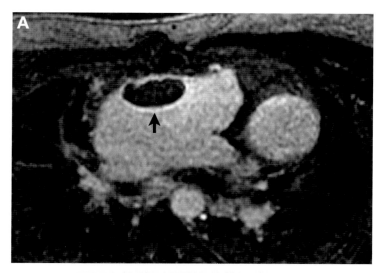

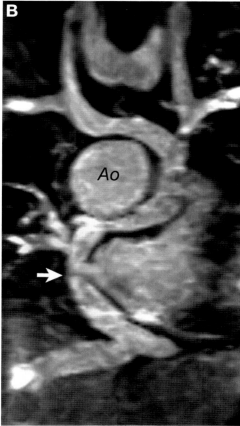

Fig. 14. CMR evaluation of the Fontan operation. **(A)** Post-Gd delayed-enhancement image in the axial plane showing a large thrombus (arrow) in the right atrium. **(B)** Subvolume maximum intensity projection image in the coronal plane showing an extracardiac conduit (arrow) extending from the hepatic veins to the right pulmonary artery in a patient with heterotaxy syndrome and interrupted IVC with azygos extension to the left SVC. Note the connection between the left SVC and the left pulmonary artery and the absence of a right SVC. Ao, aorta.

- Additional cine SSFP sequences may be obtained in coronal or oblique planes to image areas of the Fontan pathways or other areas that are suspected based on the previous sequence to be abnormal
- ECG-gated cine SSFP sequence of the systemic ventricle in its long axis followed by short-axis cine imaging from the level of the AV valves to the apex (12 slices are prescribed with slice thickness and interslice gap adjusted to cover the desired anatomy)
- VEC CMR sequences perpendicular to the AV valves and systemic arterial root for flow quantification; based on clinical relevance, additional flow measurements are obtained in selected areas of the Fontan pathways and the systemic veins to evaluate pulmonary-to-systemic flow ratio and differential pulmonary blood flow
- Gd-enhanced 3D MRA of the Fontan pathways, systemic and pulmonary veins, and the aorta

SSFP cine sequences are acquired with breath holding whenever possible. Fast (turbo) spin echo with double inversion recovery sequence may be used to minimize artifacts from metallic implants, which are common in this patient population *(109)*. Additional sequences such as myocardial perfusion or viability and myocardial tagging can be performed when the information provided by these sequences is clinically desired.

ACKNOWLEDGMENTS

We thank the physicians, technologists, nurses, and support personnel in the Cardiovascular CMR Program at Children's Hospital Boston for their help. Parts of the text and figures of this chapter have been included in other chapters recently written by the authors on CMR evaluation of CHD.

REFERENCES

1. Hoffman JI, Kaplan S. The incidence of congenital heart disease. J Am Coll Cardiol 2002;39: 1890–1900.
2. Van Praagh R, Van Praagh S, Nebesar RA, Muster AJ, Sinha SN, Paul MH. Tetralogy of Fallot: underdevelopment of the pulmonary infundibulum and its sequelae. Am J Cardiol 1970;26:25–33.
3. Van Praagh R. Etienne-Louis Arthur Fallot and his tetralogy: a new translation of Fallot's summary and a modern reassessment of this anomaly. Eur J Cardiothorac Surg 1989;3:381–386.
4. Van Praagh R, Geva T, Kreutzer J. Ventricular septal defects: how shall we describe, name and classify them? J Am Coll Cardiol 1989;14:1298–1299.
5. Flanagan MF, Foran RB, Van Praagh R, Jonas R, Sanders SP. Tetralogy of Fallot with obstruction of the ventricular septal defect: spectrum of echocardiographic findings. J Am Coll Cardiol 1988;11: 386–395.
6. Need LR, Powell AJ, del Nido P, Geva T. Coronary echocardiography in tetralogy of Fallot: diagnostic accuracy, resource utilization and surgical implications over 13 years. J Am Coll Cardiol 2000;36: 1371–1377.
7. Lu JH, Chung MY, Betau H, Chien HP, Lu JK. Molecular characterization of tetralogy of Fallot within Digeorge critical region of the chromosome 22. Pediatr Cardiol 2001;22:279–284.
8. Marino B, Digilio MC, Toscano A, et al. Anatomic patterns of conotruncal defects associated with deletion 22q11. Genet Med 2001;3:45–48.
9. Momma K, Takao A, Matsuoka R, et al. Tetralogy of Fallot associated with chromosome 22q11.2 deletion in adolescents and young adults. Genet Med 2001;3:56–60.
10. Boudjemline Y, Fermont L, Le Bidois J, Lyonnet S, Sidi D, Bonnet D. Prevalence of 22q11 deletion in fetuses with conotruncal cardiac defects: a 6-years prospective study. J Pediatr 2001;138:520–524.
11. Goldmuntz E, Geiger E, Benson DW. NKX2.5 mutations in patients with tetralogy of Fallot. Circulation 2001;104:2565–2568.
12. Hokanson JS, Pierpont E, Hirsch B, Moller JH. 22q11.2 microdeletions in adults with familial tetralogy of Fallot. Genet Med 2001;3:61–64.

13. McElhinney DB, Krantz ID, Bason L, et al. Analysis of cardiovascular phenotype and genotype-phenotype correlation in individuals with a JAG1 mutation and/or Alagille syndrome. Circulation 2002;106:2567–2574.

14. Masuda K, Nomura Y, Yoshinaga M, et al. Inverted duplication/deletion of the short arm of chromosome 8 in two patients with tetralogy of Fallot. Pediatr Int 2002;44:534–536.

15. Marino B, Digilio MC, Grazioli S, et al. Associated cardiac anomalies in isolated and syndromic patients with tetralogy of Fallot. Am J Cardiol 1996;77:505–508.

16. Geva T, Ayres NA, Pac FA, Pignatelli R. Quantitative morphometric analysis of progressive infundibular obstruction in tetralogy of Fallot. A prospective longitudinal echocardiographic study. Circulation 1995;92:886–892.

17. Kaulitz R, Jux C, Bertram H, Paul T, Ziemer G, Hausdorf G. Primary repair of tetralogy of Fallot in infancy—the effect on growth of the pulmonary arteries and the risk for late reinterventions. Cardiol Young 2001;11:391–398.

18. Bacha EA, Scheule AM, Zurakowski D, et al. Long-term results after early primary repair of tetralogy of Fallot. J Thorac Cardiovasc Surg 2001;122:154–161.

19. Murphy JG, Gersh BJ, Mair DD, et al. Long-term outcome in patients undergoing surgical repair of tetralogy of Fallot. N Engl J Med 1993;329:593–599.

20. Nollert G, Fischlein T, Bouterwek S, Bohmer C, Klinner W, Reichart B. Long-term survival in patients with repair of tetralogy of Fallot: 36-year follow-up of 490 survivors of the first year after surgical repair. J Am Coll Cardiol 1997;30:1374–1383.

21. Saul JP, Alexander ME. Preventing sudden death after repair of tetralogy of Fallot: complex therapy for complex patients. J Cardiovasc Electrophysiol 1999;10:1271–1287.

22. Kugler JD. Predicting sudden death in patients who have undergone tetralogy of Fallot repair: is it really as simple as measuring ECG intervals? J Cardiovasc Electrophysiol 1998;9:103–106.

23. Bricker JT. Sudden death and tetralogy of Fallot. Risks, markers, and causes. Circulation 1995;92: 158–159.

24. Gatzoulis MA, Till JA, Somerville J, Redington AN. Mechanoelectrical interaction in tetralogy of Fallot. QRS prolongation relates to right ventricular size and predicts malignant ventricular arrhythmias and sudden death. Circulation 1995;92:231–237.

25. Berul CI, Hill SL, Geggel RL, et al. Electrocardiographic markers of late sudden death risk in postoperative tetralogy of Fallot children. J Cardiovasc Electrophysiol 1997;8:1349–1356.

26. Hokanson JS, Moller JH. Significance of early transient complete heart block as a predictor of sudden death late after operative correction of tetralogy of Fallot. Am J Cardiol 2001;87:1271–1277.

27. Hamada H, Terai M, Jibiki T, Nakamura T, Gatzoulis MA, Niwa K. Influence of early repair of tetralogy of Fallot without an outflow patch on late arrhythmias and sudden death: a 27-years follow-up study following a uniform surgical approach. Cardiol Young 2002;12:345–351.

28. Mackie AS, Gauvreau K, Perry SB, del Nido PJ, Geva T. Echocardiographic predictors of aortopulmonary collaterals in infants with tetralogy of Fallot and pulmonary atresia. J Am Coll Cardiol 2003;41:852–857.

29. Geva T, Sahn, DJ, Powell AJ. Magnetic resonance imaging of congenital heart disease in adults. Prog Pediatr Cardiol 2003;17:21–39.

30. Vick GW 3rd, Wendt RE 3rd, Rokey R. Comparison of gradient echo with spin echo magnetic resonance imaging and echocardiography in the evaluation of major aortopulmonary collateral arteries. Am Heart J 1994;127:1341–1347.

31. Powell AJ, Chung T, Landzberg MJ, Geva T. Accuracy of MRI evaluation of pulmonary blood supply in patients with complex pulmonary stenosis or atresia. Int J Card Imaging 2000;16:169–174.

32. Holmqvist C, Hochbergs P, Bjorkhem G, Brockstedt S, Laurin S. Pre-operative evaluation with MR in tetralogy of Fallot and pulmonary atresia with ventricular septal defect. Acta Radiol 2001;42:63–69.

33. Beekman RP, Beek FJ, Meijboom EJ. Usefulness of MRI for the pre-operative evaluation of the pulmonary arteries in tetralogy of Fallot. Magn Reson Imaging 1997;15:1005–1015.

34. Geva T, Greil GF, Marshall AC, Landzberg M, Powell AJ. Gadolinium-enhanced three-dimensional magnetic resonance angiography of pulmonary blood supply in patients with complex pulmonary stenosis or atresia: comparison with X-ray angiography. Circulation 2002;106:473–478.

35. Helbing WA, de Roos A. Clinical applications of cardiac magnetic resonance imaging after repair of tetralogy of Fallot. Pediatr Cardiol 2000;21:70–79.

36. Geva T, Sandweiss BM, Gauvreau K, Lock JE, Powell AJ. Factors associated with impaired clinical status in long-term survivors of tetralogy of Fallot repair evaluated by magnetic resonance imaging. J Am Coll Cardiol 2004;43:1068–1074.

37. Roest AA, Helbing WA, Kunz P, et al. Exercise MR imaging in the assessment of pulmonary regurgitation and biventricular function in patients after tetralogy of Fallot repair. Radiology 2002;223:204–211.

38. Rebergen SA, Chin JG, Ottenkamp J, van der Wall EE, de Roos A. Pulmonary regurgitation in the late postoperative follow-up of tetralogy of Fallot. Volumetric quantitation by nuclear magnetic resonance velocity mapping. Circulation 1993;88:2257–2266.

39. Niezen RA, Helbing WA, van Der Wall EE, van Der Geest RJ, Vliegen HW, de Roos A. Left ventricular function in adults with mild pulmonary insufficiency late after Fallot repair. Heart 1999;82:697–703.

40. Niezen RA, Helbing WA, van der Wall EE, van der Geest RJ, Rebergen SA, de Roos A. Biventricular systolic function and mass studied with MR imaging in children with pulmonary regurgitation after repair for tetralogy of Fallot. Radiology 1996;201:135–140.

41. Davlouros PA, Kilner PJ, Hornung TS, et al. right ventricular function in adults with repaired tetralogy of Fallot assessed with cardiovascular magnetic resonance imaging: detrimental role of right ventricular outflow aneurysms or akinesia and adverse right-to-left ventricular interaction. J Am Coll Cardiol 2002;40:2044–2052.

42. Prakash A, Powell AJ, Krishnamurthy R, Geva T. Magnetic resonance imaging evaluation of myocardial perfusion and viability in congenital and acquired pediatric heart disease. Am J Cardiol 2004;93: 657–661.

43. Van Praagh R. The importance of segmental situs in the diagnosis of congenital heart disease. Semin Roentgenol 1985;20:254–271.

44. Blume ED, Altmann K, Mayer JE, Colan SD, Gauvreau K, Geva T. Evolution of risk factors influencing early mortality of the arterial switch operation. J Am Coll Cardiol 1999;33:1702–1709.

45. Levinsky L, Srinivasan V, Alvarez-Diaz F, Subramanian S. Reconstruction of the new atrial septum in the Senning operation. New technique. J Thorac Cardiovasc Surg 1981;81:131–134.

46. Myridakis DJ, Ehlers KH, Engle MA. Late follow-up after venous switch operation (Mustard procedure) for simple and complex transposition of the great arteries. Am J Cardiol 1994;74:1030–1036.

47. Redington AN, Rigby ML, Oldershaw P, Gibson DG, Shinebourne EA. Right ventricular function 10 years after the Mustard operation for transposition of the great arteries: analysis of size, shape, and wall motion. Br Heart J 1989;62:455–461.

48. Deanfield J, Camm J, Macartney F, et al. Arrhythmia and late mortality after Mustard and Senning operation for transposition of the great arteries. An eight-year prospective study. J Thorac Cardiovasc Surg 1988;96:569–576.

49. Van Praagh R, Jung WK. The arterial switch operation in transposition of the great arteries: anatomic indications and contraindications. Thorac Cardiovasc Surg 1991;39(suppl 2):138–150.

50. Wernovsky G, Jonas RA, Colan SD, et al. Results of the arterial switch operation in patients with transposition of the great arteries and abnormalities of the mitral valve or left ventricular outflow tract. J Am Coll Cardiol 1990;16:1446–1454.

51. Rehnstrom P, Gilljam T, Sudow G, Berggren H. Excellent survival and low complication rate in medium-term follow-up after arterial switch operation for complete transposition. Scand Cardiovasc J 2003;37:104–106.

52. Kramer HH, Scheewe J, Fischer G, Uebing A, Harding P, Schmiel F, Cremer J. Long term follow-up of left ventricular performance and size of the great arteries before and after one- and two-stage arterial switch operation of simple transposition. Eur J Cardiothorac Surg 2003;24:898–905.

53. Prifti E, Crucean A, Bonacchi M, et al. Early and long term outcome of the arterial switch operation for transposition of the great arteries: predictors and functional evaluation. Eur J Cardiothorac Surg 2002;22:864–873.

54. Dunbar-Masterson C, Wypij D, Bellinger DC, et al. General health status of children with D-transposition of the great arteries after the arterial switch operation. Circulation 2001;104:I138–I142.

55. Losay J, Touchot A, Serraf A, et al. Late outcome after arterial switch operation for transposition of the great arteries. Circulation 2001;104:I121–I126.

56. Mahle WT, McBride MG, Paridon SM. Exercise performance after the arterial switch operation for D-transposition of the great arteries. Am J Cardiol 2001;87:753–758.

57. Van Praagh R, Papagiannis J, Grunenfelder J, Bartram U, Martanovic P. Pathologic anatomy of corrected transposition of the great arteries: medical and surgical implications. Am Heart J 1998;135: 772–785.

58. Beauchesne LM, Warnes CA, Connolly HM, Ammash NM, Tajik AJ, Danielson GK. Outcome of the unoperated adult who presents with congenitally corrected transposition of the great arteries. J Am Coll Cardiol 2002;40:285–290.

59. Colli AM, de Leval M, Somerville J. Anatomically corrected malposition of the great arteries: diagnostic difficulties and surgical repair of associated lesions. Am J Cardiol 1985;55:1367–1372.

60. Van Praagh R. What is congenitally corrected transposition? N Engl J Med 1970;282:1097–1098.

61. Chung KJ, Simpson IA, Glass RF, Sahn DJ, Hesselink JR. Cine magnetic resonance imaging after surgical repair in patients with transposition of the great arteries. Circulation 1988;77:104–109.

62. Lorenz CH, Walker ES, Graham TP Jr, Powers TA. Right ventricular performance and mass by use of cine MRI late after atrial repair of transposition of the great arteries. Circulation 1995;92:II233–II239.

63. Hardy CE, Helton GJ, Kondo C, Higgins SS, Young NJ, Higgins CB. Usefulness of magnetic resonance imaging for evaluating great-vessel anatomy after arterial switch operation for D-transposition of the great arteries. Am Heart J 1994;128:326–332.

64. Beek FJ, Beekman RP, Dillon EH, et al. MRI of the pulmonary artery after arterial switch operation for transposition of the great arteries. Pediatr Radiol 1993;23:335–340.

65. Theissen P, Kaemmerer H, Sechtem U, et al. Magnetic resonance imaging of cardiac function and morphology in patients with transposition of the great arteries following Mustard procedure. Thorac Cardiovasc Surg 1991;39(suppl 3):221–224.

66. Rees S, Somerville J, Warnes C, et al. Comparison of magnetic resonance imaging with echocardiography and radionuclide angiography in assessing cardiac function and anatomy following Mustard's operation for transposition of the great arteries. Am J Cardiol 1988;61:1316–1322.

67. Tulevski II, Lee PL, Groenink M, et al. Dobutamine-induced increase of right ventricular contractility without increased stroke volume in adolescent patients with transposition of the great arteries: evaluation with magnetic resonance imaging. Int J Card Imaging 2000;16:471–478.

68. Tulevski II, van der Wall EE, Groenink M, et al. Usefulness of magnetic resonance imaging dobutamine stress in asymptomatic and minimally symptomatic patients with decreased cardiac reserve from congenital heart disease (complete and corrected transposition of the great arteries and subpulmonic obstruction). Am J Cardiol 2002;89:1077–1081.

69. Roest AA, Lamb HJ, van der Wall EE, et al. Cardiovascular response to physical exercise in adult patients after atrial correction for transposition of the great arteries assessed with magnetic resonance imaging. Heart 2004;90:678–684.

70. Babu-Narayan SV, Goktekin O, Moon JC, et al. Late gadolinium enhancement cardiovascular magnetic resonance of the systemic right ventricle in adults with previous atrial redirection surgery for transposition of the great arteries. Circulation 2005;111:2091–2098.

71. Videlefsky N, Parks WJ, Oshinski J, et al. Magnetic resonance phase-shift velocity mapping in pediatric patients with pulmonary venous obstruction. J Am Coll Cardiol 2001;38:262–267.

72. Belli E, Serraf A, Lacour-Gayet F, et al. Surgical treatment of subaortic stenosis after biventricular repair of double-outlet right ventricle. J Thorac Cardiovasc Surg 1996;112:1570–1578; discussion 1578–1580.

73. Yoo SJ, Kim YM, Choe YH. Magnetic resonance imaging of complex congenital heart disease. Int J Card Imaging 1999;15:151–160.

74. Beekmana RP, Roest AA, Helbing WA, et al. Spin echo MRI in the evaluation of hearts with a double outlet right ventricle: usefulness and limitations. Magn Reson Imaging 2000;18:245–253.

75. Beekman RP, Beek FJ, Meijboom EJ, Wenink AC. MRI appearance of a double inlet and double outlet right ventricle with supero-inferior ventricular relationship. Magn Reson Imaging 1996;14:1107–1112.

76. Igarashi H, Kuramatsu T, Shiraishi H, Yanagisawa M. Criss-cross heart evaluated by colour Doppler echocardiography and magnetic resonance imaging. Eur J Pediatr 1990;149:523–525.

77. Niezen RA, Beekman RP, Helbing WA, van der Wall EE, de Roos A. Double outlet right ventricle assessed with magnetic resonance imaging. Int J Card Imaging 1999;15:323–329.

78. Sorensen TS, Korperich H, Greil GF, et al. Operator-independent isotropic three-dimensional magnetic resonance imaging for morphology in congenital heart disease: a validation study. Circulation 2004;110:163–169.

79. Van Praagh R, Van Praagh S. The anatomy of common aorticopulmonary trunk (truncus arteriosus communis) and its embryologic implications. A study of 57 necropsy cases. Am J Cardiol 1965;16:406–425.

80. Collett RW, Edwards JE. Persistent truncus arteriosus: a classification according to anatomic types. Surg Clin North Am 1949;29:1245–1270.

81. Litovsky SH, Ostfeld I, Bjornstad PG, Van Praagh R, Geva T. Truncus arteriosus with anomalous pulmonary venous connection. Am J Cardiol 1999;83:801–804, A10.

82. Goldmuntz E, Clark BJ, Mitchell LE, et al. Frequency of 22q11 deletions in patients with conotruncal defects. J Am Coll Cardiol 1998;32:492–498.

83. Tworetzky W, McElhinney DB, Brook MM, Reddy VM, Hanley FL, Silverman NH. Echocardiographic diagnosis alone for the complete repair of major congenital heart defects. J Am Coll Cardiol 1999;33: 228–233.

84. Fyler DC, Buckley LP, Hellenbrand WE, Cohn HE. Report of the New England Regional Infant Cardiac Program. Pediatrics 1980;65:377–461.

85. Celoria GC, Patton RB. Congenital absence of the aortic arch. Am Heart J 1959;58:407–413.

86. Geva T, Gajarski RJ. Echocardiographic diagnosis of type B interruption of a right aortic arch. Am Heart J 1995;129:1042–1045.

87. Kutsche LM, Van Mierop LH. Cervical origin of the right subclavian artery in aortic arch interruption: pathogenesis and significance. Am J Cardiol 1984;53:892–895.

88. Kaulitz R, Jonas RA, van der Velde ME. Echocardiographic assessment of interrupted aortic arch. Cardiol Young 1999;9:562–571.

89. Varghese A, Gatzoulis M, Mohiaddin RH. Images in cardiovascular medicine: Magnetic resonance angiography of a congenitally interrupted aortic arch. Circulation 2002;106:E9–E10.

90. Tsai-Goodman B, Geva T, Odegard KC, Sena LM, Powell AJ. Clinical role, accuracy, and technical aspects of cardiovascular magnetic resonance imaging in infants. Am J Cardiol 2004;94:69–74.

91. Nielsen J, Powell AJ, Gauvreau K, Marcus E, Geva T. Magnetic resonance imaging predictors of the hemodynamic severity of aortic coarctation. J Am Coll Cardiol 2004;43:24A.

92. Fontan F, Baudet E. Surgical repair of tricuspid atresia. Thorax 1971;26:240–248.

93. Kreutzer GO, Vargas FJ, Schlichter AJ, et al. Atriopulmonary anastomosis. J Thorac Cardiovasc Surg 1982;83:427–436.

94. Jonas RA, Castaneda AR. Modified Fontan procedure: atrial baffle and systemic venous to pulmonary artery anastomotic techniques. J Card Surg 1988;3:91–96.

95. Bridges ND, Mayer JE Jr, Lock JE, et al. Effect of baffle fenestration on outcome of the modified Fontan operation. Circulation 1992;86:1762–1769.

96. Tireli E. Extracardiac Fontan operation without cardiopulmonary bypass: how to perform the anastomosis between inferior vena cava and conduit. Cardiovasc Surg 2003;11:225–227.

97. Gentles TL, Mayer JE Jr, Gauvreau K, et al. Fontan operation in 500 consecutive patients: factors influencing early and late outcome. J Thorac Cardiovasc Surg 1997;114:376–391.

98. Wilson WR, Greer GE, Tobias JD. Cerebral venous thrombosis after the Fontan procedure. J Thorac Cardiovasc Surg 1998;116:661–663.

99. Day RW, Boyer RS, Tait VF, Ruttenberg HD. Factors associated with stroke following the Fontan procedure. Pediatr Cardiol 1995;16:270–275.

100. Jacobs ML. Complications associated with heterotaxy syndrome in Fontan patients. Semin Thorac Cardiovasc Surg Pediatr Card Surg Annu 2002;5:25–35.

101. Lam J, Neirotti R, Becker AE, Planche C. Thrombosis after the Fontan procedure: transesophageal echocardiography may replace angiocardiography. J Thorac Cardiovasc Surg 1994;108:194–195.

102. Deal BJ, Mavroudis C, Backer CL. Beyond Fontan conversion: surgical therapy of arrhythmias including patients with associated complex congenital heart disease. Ann Thorac Surg 2003;76: 542–553; discussion 553–554.

103. Kreutzer J, Keane JF, Lock JE, et al. Conversion of modified Fontan procedure to lateral atrial tunnel cavopulmonary anastomosis. J Thorac Cardiovasc Surg 1996;111:1169–1176.

104. Hjortdal VE, Emmertsen K, Stenbog E, et al. Effects of exercise and respiration on blood flow in total cavopulmonary connection: a real-time magnetic resonance flow study. Circulation 2003;108: 1227–1231.

105. Be'eri E, Maier SE, Landzberg MJ, Chung T, Geva T. In vivo evaluation of Fontan pathway flow dynamics by multidimensional phase-velocity magnetic resonance imaging. Circulation 1998;98: 2873–2882.

106. Fogel MA, Weinberg PM, Rychik J, et al. Caval contribution to flow in the branch pulmonary arteries of Fontan patients with a novel application of magnetic resonance presaturation pulse. Circulation 1999;99:1215–1221.

107. Fratz S, Hess J, Schwaiger M, Martinoff S, Stern HC. More accurate quantification of pulmonary blood flow by magnetic resonance imaging than by lung perfusion scintigraphy in patients with fontan circulation. Circulation 2002;106:1510–1513.

108. Fogel MA, Gupta KB, Weinberg PM, Hoffman EA. Regional wall motion and strain analysis across stages of Fontan reconstruction by magnetic resonance tagging. Am J Physiol 1995;269:H1132–H1152.

109. Garg R, Powell AJ, Sena L, Marshall AC, Geva T. Effects of metallic implants on magnetic resonance imaging evaluation of Fontan palliation. Am J Cardiol 2005;95:688–691.

25 Congenital Heart Disease
Indications, Patient Preparation, and Simple Lesions

Rachel M. Wald and Andrew J. Powell

CONTENTS

INTRODUCTION

Technical advances over the past two decades have greatly expanded the diagnostic role of cardiac magnetic resonance (CMR) imaging in patients with congenital heart disease. In addition to high-resolution anatomical information, CMR provides physiological information about the cardiovascular system, such as ventricular function and blood flow. Along with these improved capabilities, the speed and efficiency of imaging have increased, thereby allowing a comprehensive examination to be obtained within a time frame acceptable to both patient and operator.

The first part of this chapter reviews the indications, patient preparation and monitoring, and sedation strategies for CMR in patients with congenital heart disease. The second part details the CMR evaluation of several "simple" congenital heart lesions: atrial septal defect (ASD) and other interatrial communications, ventricular septal defect (VSD), patent ductus arteriosus (PDA), partially anomalous pulmonary venous connection (PAPVC), and coarctation of the aorta. More "complex" lesions are discussed in Chapter 26. Despite classification as simple, many of the conditions in this chapter have important anatomical subtypes and variable physiology. Thus, summaries of the anatomical considerations and clinical management are provided for each lesion.

From: *Contemporary Cardiology: Cardiovascular Magnetic Resonance Imaging*
Edited by: Raymond Y. Kwong © Humana Press Inc., Totowa, NJ

Table 1
Primary Referral Diagnoses in 1119 Consecutive Patients With Congenital and Acquired Pediatric Heart Disease at Children's Hospital Boston

Referral diagnosis	n
Tetralogy of Fallot	256 (22.9%)
Aorta	182 (16.3%)
Coarctation	112
Other	70
Complex two ventricle	144 (12.9%)
TGA status-post arterial switch operation	47
TGA status-post atrial switch operation	28
Other	69
Single ventricle	110 (9.8%)
Ventricular function	81 (7.2%)
Possible ARVC	52 (4.6%)
Pulmonary veins	49 (4.4%)
Valve regurgitation	47 (4.2%)
Septal defects	39 (3.5%)
ASD	32
VSD	7
Vascular ring	29 (2.6%)
Pulmonary atresia with intact ventricular septum	21 (1.9%)
Congenital coronary anomaly	21 (1.9%)
Vascular anomalies	17 (1.5%)
Cardiac tumor	11 (1%)
Other	60 (5.4%)

ARVC, arrhythmogenic right ventricular cardiomyopathy; TGA, transposition of the great arteries.

INDICATIONS FOR MAGNETIC RESONANCE IMAGING EVALUATION OF CONGENITAL HEART DISEASE

The indications for CMR in patients with congenital heart disease continue to expand with time. Table 1 summarizes the primary reasons for CMR in 1119 consecutive patients evaluated at Children's Hospital Boston, illustrating the wide range of cardiovascular anomalies evaluated. Given that CMR has been shown to provide helpful diagnostic information in most types of congenital heart disease, it is not practical to list individual anomalies in which the test is recommended. More generally, the clinical indications for a CMR examination involve one or more of the following situations:

1. When transthoracic echocardiography is incapable of providing the required diagnostic information.
2. When clinical assessment and other diagnostic tests are inconsistent.
3. As an alternative to diagnostic cardiac catheterization with its associated risks and higher cost.
4. To obtain diagnostic information for which CMR offers unique advantages.

It is worth noting that the role of CMR in infants and toddlers is more limited than that in older patients. Because young children typically have excellent acoustic windows, echocardiography can provide the necessary diagnostic information in nearly all patients. CMR, which requires sedation or anesthesia, is reserved for the relatively rare case when additional information is required. A review of 99 consecutive CMR examinations in patients under 1 year of age during a 4-years period at Children's Hospital Boston found that delineation of the thoracic vasculature was the most common indication (55%), followed by assessment of airway compression (25%), and evaluation of cardiac tumors (6%) *(1)*.

In the future, CMR will likely assume a greater role in this age group, primarily as an alternative to diagnostic cardiac catheterization. Such scenarios include delineation of sources of pulmonary blood supply in tetralogy of Fallot with pulmonary atresia and preoperative assessment of candidates for a bidirectional Glenn shunt or Fontan procedure.

PATIENT PREPARATION, SEDATION, AND MONITORING

Patients undergoing CMR examinations must remain still in the scanner bore for up to 60 minutes to minimize motion artifact during image acquisition and allow planning of successive imaging sequences. Accordingly, the need for performing the examination under sedation or anesthesia and an assessment of the risk/benefit ratio for proceeding under these circumstances should be determined well before the examination date. Multiple factors are taken into account when deciding whether a patient should have an examination without sedation, including the length of the anticipated examination protocol, the child's developmental age and maturity, the child's experience with prior procedures, and the parents' opinion of their child's capability to cooperate with the examination.

True claustrophobia in the pediatric age group is rare. In general, most children 7 years of age and older can cooperate sufficiently for a good-quality CMR study. Parents should be provided with a detailed description of the examination and asked to discuss it with their child in an age-appropriate manner in advance to increase the likelihood of a successful study. After proper screening, parents can be allowed into the scanner room to help their child complete the examination.

Strategies for sedation and anesthesia in CMR vary and often depend on institutional preference and resources, such as availability of qualified pediatric anesthesiologists. Although it is possible to wait for young children to fall into a natural sleep, this approach may be time consuming and complicated by early awakening. Sedation can be achieved with a variety of medications (e.g., pentobarbital, propofol, fentanyl, midazolam, chloral hydrate) and is a reasonable approach *(2–7)*. Its principal drawbacks are an unprotected airway and reliance on spontaneous respiratory effort with the associated risks of aspiration, airway obstruction, and hypoventilation. In addition, because images are often acquired over several seconds, respiratory motion will degrade image quality. This motion artifact can be reduced by synchronizing image data acquisition to the respiratory cycle, tracked by either a bellows device around the abdomen or by navigator echoes that concurrently image the position of the diaphragm or heart. An alternative strategy to reduce respiratory motion artifact is to acquire multiple images at the same location and average them, thereby minimizing variations from respiration. The principal limitations of both of these strategies are prolonged scan times and incomplete elimination of respiratory motion, which can lead to reduced image quality.

Because of these safety and image quality concerns, we and others frequently prefer to perform CMR examinations under general anesthesia in children who cannot undergo an awake examination *(8,9)*. This approach, described in detail elsewhere *(1,10)*, is safe, consistently achieves adequate sedation, protects the airway, and offers control of ventilation. Respiratory motion artifact can be completely eliminated by suspending ventilation in conjunction with neuromuscular blockade. Breath-hold periods of 30–60 seconds are typically well tolerated and allow multiple locations to be scanned efficiently.

When utilizing either sedation or anesthesia, is it important that both the nurses and physicians have sufficient experience with these procedures in children with cardiovascular disorders. Continuous monitoring of the electrocardiogram (ECG), pulse oximetry, end-tidal carbon dioxide, anesthetic gases, temperature, and blood pressure with a magnetic resonance imaging (MRI)-compatible physiological monitoring system is required. MRI-compatible anesthesia machines are available that can be located in the scanner room and connected to the patient's endotracheal tube by an extended breathing circuit. To maximize patient safety and examination quality, it is recommended that different health care providers be responsible for supervising the imaging and sedation/anesthesia aspects of the study, and that both communicate closely with each other.

Prior to bringing the patient into the scanner room, the physician and technologists should review the patient's history, safety screening form, and the most recent chest radiograph to identify implanted devices that may be hazardous in the MRI environment or produce image artifact. Previously, pacemakers and defibrillators were considered to be absolute contraindications to undergoing MRI examinations (11,12); however, reports have challenged this position and proposed specific safety protocols for scanning patients with these devices (13–15). Sternal wires; prosthetic heart valves; and stents, occluders, and vascular coils in place for greater than 6 weeks have been deemed safe (11,16–18). The recommendation to defer MRI for 6 weeks after device implantation, however, is not supported by conclusive published data. A decision to perform a MRI examination shortly after cardiac surgery or implantation of a biomedical device must weigh the risk/benefit ratio for the individual patient. More detailed safety information regarding specific devices can be obtained by consulting comprehensive databases (e.g., www.mrisafety.com).

Following safety screening, physiological monitoring devices and hearing protection (for both awake and anesthetized patients) are put in place. A high-quality ECG signal is essential for optimum image quality in cardiac-gated sequences. The signal should be checked both when the patient is outside and then inside the scanner bore. In patients with dextrocardia, ECG leads are best placed on the right chest. Because young children dissipate body heat faster than adults, the scanner room temperature should be adjusted and prewarmed blankets applied to minimize heat loss.

The imaging coil should be chosen to maximize the signal-to-noise ratio over the entire body region to be examined. Because congenital heart disease often involves abnormalities of the thoracic vasculature, the coil will usually need to be large enough to cover the entire thorax rather than just the heart. Adult head or knee coils are often appropriate for infants weighing less than 10 kg, and adult cardiac coils can be used for medium-size children weighing between 10 and 40 kg. Adequate coil coverage and placement should be confirmed early in the examination by reviewing the localizing images.

PRINCIPLES OF MAGNETIC RESONANCE IMAGING EVALUATION OF CONGENITAL HEART DISEASE

Detailed preexamination planning is crucial given the wide array of imaging sequences available and the often-complex nature of the clinical, anatomical, and functional issues in patients with congenital heart disease. The importance of a careful review of the patient's medical history, including details of all cardiovascular surgical procedures,

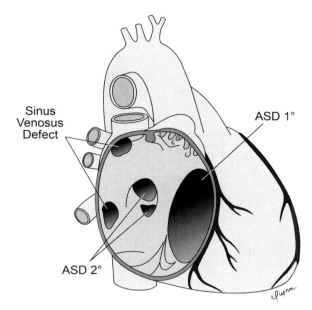

Fig. 1. Anatomical types of atrial communications (*see* text for details). ASD 1° denotes primum ASD; ASD 2° denotes secundum atrial septal defect.

interventional catheterizations, findings of previous diagnostic tests, and current clinical status, cannot be overemphasized.

As with echocardiography and cardiac catheterization, CMR examination of congenital heart disease is a dynamic diagnostic procedure that requires on-line review and interpretation of the data by the supervising physician. The unpredictable nature of the anatomy and hemodynamics often requires adjustment of the examination protocol, imaging planes, pulse sequences, and imaging parameters. Reliance on standardized protocols and postexamination review alone in these patients may result in incomplete or even erroneous interpretation.

SIMPLE CONGENITAL HEART LESIONS

Atrial Septal Defects and Other Interatrial Communications

ANATOMY

Anatomically, five different defects can lead to an interatrial shunt (Fig. 1).

1) A patent foramen ovale is bordered on the left by septum primum and by the superior limbic band of the fossa ovalis (septum secundum) on the right. It is an important and nearly universally present communication during fetal life. Following the transition to postnatal circulation, septum primum opposes the superior limbic band of the fossa ovalis, and the foramen ovale narrows. A patent foramen ovale is seen in almost all newborns and with decreasing frequency throughout life *(19)*.

2) A secundum ASD is the most common cause of an atrial-level shunt after patent foramen ovale. Usually, the defect is caused by deficiency of septum primum (the valve of the fossa ovalis), but rarely it results from a deficiency of septum secundum (the muscular limb of the fossa ovalis). The defect may be single or multiple with several fenestrations of septum primum.

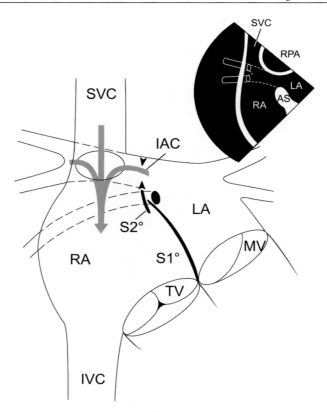

Fig. 2. Diagrammatic representation of a sinus venosus septal defect. Absence of the common wall between the right superior vena cava (SVC) and the right upper pulmonary vein allows drainage of blood from the right upper pulmonary vein into the SVC and right atrium (RA). The interatrial communication (IAC) is not a defect; rather, it is the anatomical orifice of the right upper pulmonary vein (arrowheads), which allows blood to flow from the left atrium (LA) into the RA. The inset shows the normal course of the right upper pulmonary vein posterior to the SVC. AS, atrial septum; IVC, inferior vena cava; MV, mitral valve; RPA, right pulmonary artery; S1°, septum primum; S2°, septum secundum; TV, tricuspid valve.

3) A primum ASD is a variant of incomplete common atrioventricular canal, and is the third most common interatrial communication. This defect involves the septum of the atrioventricular canal and is almost always associated with a cleft anterior mitral valve leaflet. Any associated defect within the fossa ovale (secundum ASD) is regarded as a separate abnormality.

4) A sinus venosus septal defect results from deficiency of the sinus venosus septum, which separates the pulmonary veins from the systemic veins and the sinus venosus component of the right atrium (Fig. 2). Most commonly, a sinus venosus defect is between the right upper pulmonary vein and the cardiac end of the superior vena cava. Rarely, the defect involves the right lower and or middle pulmonary veins and the inferior aspect of the right atrium at its junction with the inferior vena cava. From an anatomical standpoint, a sinus venosus defect is not an ASD because it does not allow direct communication between the left and right atria. Instead, the interatrial flow travels between the left atrium, one or more of the pulmonary veins, the sinus venosus septal defect, the superior (or inferior) vena cava, and the right atrium. The defect usually

allows pulmonary vein flow to drain to the right atrium through the defect as well. Patients with sinus venosus defects commonly have additional accessory right upper pulmonary veins that connect to the superior vena cava or azygous vein.

5) A coronary sinus septal defect is a rare type of interatrial communication in which the septum between the coronary sinus and the left atrium is either partially or completely unroofed, allowing the right and left atria to communicate through the defect and the coronary sinus orifice. Sometimes, there is also a persistent left superior vena cava draining to the coronary sinus. If the coronary sinus is completely unroofed, then the left superior vena cava will appear to be connected to the left atrium. The association of a coronary sinus septal defect and persistent left superior vena cava is termed *Raghib syndrome* and may result in cyanosis *(20)*.

CLINICAL COURSE AND MANAGEMENT

Regardless of the specific anatomical type, the amount of shunting through an interatrial communication is determined by the defect size and relative compliance of the right and left ventricles. Over the first few months of life, right ventricular compliance typically rises, leading to an increasing left-to-right shunt. During adulthood, left ventricular compliance normally decreases further, augmenting the left-to-right flow. Shunt flow through the right heart and lungs leads to dilation of the right atrium, right ventricle, pulmonary arteries, and pulmonary veins. Most young children tolerate this increased pulmonary blood flow well and are asymptomatic; a few develop dyspnea or growth failure. Defects in this age group are typically detected after auscultation of a heart murmur or incidentally when an echocardiogram is obtained for other indications. Up to 5–10% of patients with significant left-to-right shunts may develop pulmonary vascular disease by adulthood, leading to pulmonary hypertension. Adults with unrepaired ASDs are also at risk for exercise intolerance, atrial arrhythmias, and paradoxical emboli.

In general, current practice is to refer patients for ASD closure if the patient is symptomatic or the defect results a significant left-to-right shunt. Evidence for the latter includes a defect diameter greater than 5 mm, right ventricular dilation, flattening of the ventricular septum in diastole (caused by elevated right ventricular diastolic pressure from the volume load), and a pulmonary-to-systemic flow ratio larger than 1.5–2.0. One must also be aware that smaller secundum ASDs may close spontaneously or become smaller in the first few years of life; thereafter, defects tend to become larger with time *(21)*. Primum ASDs, sinus venosus septal defects, and coronary sinus septal defects almost never become smaller with time. Although a patent foramen ovale typically produces only a small shunt, closure may be indicated when there is a history consistent with a paradoxical embolus.

All of these defect types can be closed surgically with low mortality and morbidity in centers with expertise. The timing of surgery depends on multiple factors, including the size of the defect, associated cardiac abnormalities, symptoms, and local experience, but there is rarely a reason to delay surgical closure beyond 3 years of age. Transcatheter treatment for secundum ASDs and patent foramen ovales by occluding them with various devices has become available at specialized centers. Although device closure is generally favored over surgical closure for patent foramen ovale *(22)*, there is yet no consensus on the specific circumstances under which device closure is superior in secundum ASD.

Regarding surgical technique, secundum ASDs are closed either primarily or with a patch. For primum ASDs, the defect is closed with a patch, and in some cases, the associated mitral valve cleft is partially sutured. Sinus venosus septal defects can often be closed by simply placing a patch to reconstruct the missing portion of the sinus venosus septum, thereby eliminating interatrial and right pulmonary vein to right atrial flow. In some cases, especially when a right upper pulmonary vein drains relatively high to the superior vena cava, the superior vena cava is transected superior to the anomalous veins and the distal caval end anastomosed to the right atrial appendage. The sinus venosus septal defect is then closed in such a way that the proximal superior vena cava and anomalous veins drain to the left atrium. For a coronary sinus septal defect, the os of the coronary sinus is usually patched closed. If a left superior vena cava is present, then it is redirected to the right atrial side either through ligation, when an adequate left innominate vein is present, or via a baffle to the right atrium.

Much less commonly, interatrial flow through the various types of defects is bidirectional or right to left. This typically occurs when right ventricular compliance is low as the result of right ventricular outflow tract obstruction or pulmonary hypertension (i.e., increased pulmonary vascular resistance). Right-to-left shunt flow causes cyanosis and its sequelae, including exercise intolerance, paradoxical emboli, and polycythemia. Closure of defects in this clinical setting is often contraindicated as it would exacerbate pulmonary hypertension and right heart failure.

MRI EVALUATION

Transthoracic echocardiography is the primary imaging technique for the evaluation of ASDs and is usually sufficient for clinical decision making in the pediatric age range. However, CMR can often be helpful in patients, usually adolescents and adults, with a known or suspected ASD and inconclusive clinical or transthoracic echocardiographic findings. For example, CMR provides a noninvasive alternative to transesophageal echocardiography and to diagnostic catheterization in patients with evidence of right ventricular volume overload in whom transthoracic echocardiography cannot demonstrate the source of the left-to-right shunt. The advent of transcatheter occlusion of ASDs has also increased the need for accurate anatomical information to help determine whether a patient is an appropriate candidate for this intervention vs surgery.

In the preintervention situation, the specific goals of the CMR examination include delineation of the location, size, rims, and number of ASDs; evaluation of pulmonary venous return; determination of suitability for transcatheter closure; estimation of right ventricular pressure; and assessment of the hemodynamic burden by quantifying the pulmonary-to-systemic flow (Qp/Qs) ratio and right ventricular size and systolic function. In patients who have undergone transcatheter device closure of an ASD, additional goals include excluding device malposition, interference with the atrioventricular valves and venous blood flow, thrombus formation, and a residual shunt. Patients who have undergone a repair of a sinus venosus defect are at risk for superior vena cava and right pulmonary vein obstruction. Mitral regurgitation from a residual cleft is often present after primum ASD repair and should be assessed quantitatively with velocity-encoded cine (VEC) MRI.

The anatomical issues should be addressed by acquiring high-resolution images of the atrial septum and adjacent structures, including the vena cavae, the pulmonary veins, and the atrioventricular valves. Our preference is to image in at least two planes by acquiring a contiguous stack of locations in the axial or four-chamber plane and a stack in an oblique sagittal plane (Fig. 3). The most useful commonly available techniques for this

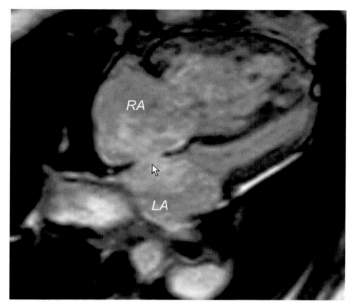

Fig. 3. (Movie in CD) ECG-triggered steady-state free precession cine MRI in the four-chamber plane showing a secundum ASD (arrow). Note the dilated right atrium (RA) and right ventricle. LA, left atrium.

work are fast (turbo) spin echo and segmented k-space cine steady-state free precession pulse sequences, both performed with breath holding and ECG gating.

Unless image quality is optimal, thin structures such as septum primum may not be clearly demonstrated, leading to an overestimation of the defect's size or to a false-positive diagnosis. Moreover, it may be difficult to appreciate the precise anatomy of a secundum ASD with multiple fenestrations. For these reasons, it is also useful to image the atrial septum using VEC MRI both in the plane of the septum to yield an *en face* view as well as in orthogonal planes planned from the *en face* view. A non-ECG-gated gadolinium-enhanced three-dimensional magnetic resonance angiogram (3D MRA) sequence is not ideally suited for evaluation of ASDs because of blurring of intracardiac structures from heart motion. However, this technique is helpful in the anatomical evaluation of the pulmonary veins, especially in patients with sinus venosus septal defects, which invariably involve the pulmonary veins (Fig. 4).

In patients with known or suspected ASDs, left and right ventricular size and systolic function should be quantified by acquiring a stack of cine steady-state free precession images in a ventricular short-axis plane. This image series also allows one to make a qualitative estimate of right ventricular systolic pressure based on the configuration of the ventricular septum. The septal geometry is concave toward the right ventricle when the right ventricle-to-left ventricle pressure ratio is low and assumes a flat configuration or even a concave shape toward the left ventricle as the right ventricle-to-left ventricle pressure ratio increases. Interpretation of the septal configuration may be confounded by factors such as dysynchronous contraction of the right ventricle, intraventricular conduction delay (e.g., right or left bundle branch block, preexcitation), and a high left ventricular pressure.

Measurement of the Qp/Qs ratio is clinically useful in patients with ASDs. Multiple studies have shown that VEC MRI calculation of the Qp/Qs ratio by measuring flow in the

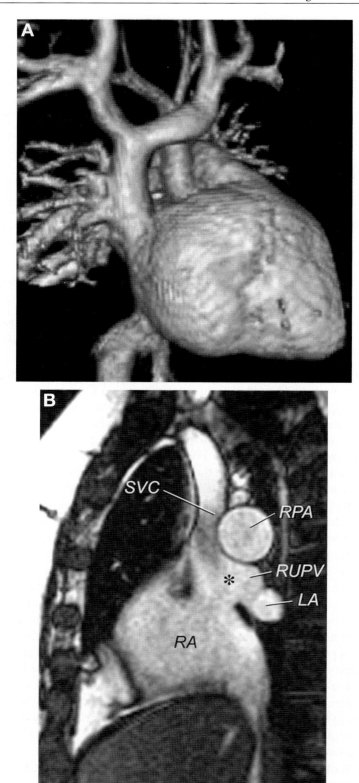

Fig. 4. *(Continued)*

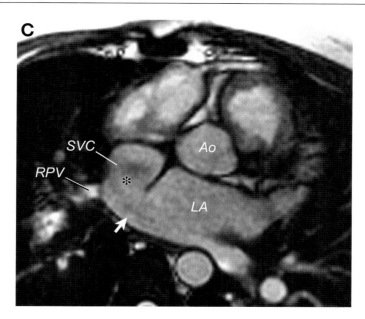

Fig. 4. (Movie in CD) Sinus venosus defect. **(A)** 3D reconstruction of gadolinium-enhanced 3D MRA showing several pulmonary veins from the right upper lobe draining into the superior vena cava. **(B)** ECG-triggered steady-state free precession cine MR in the sagittal plane showing the defect (*) between the right upper pulmonary vein (RUPV) and the superior vena cava (SVC). **(C)** ECG-triggered steady-state free precession cine MRI in the axial plane showing the defect between the RUPV and the SVC (*). The arrow points to the left atrial orifice of the RUPV. Left-to-right shunt results from drainage of the RUPV to the SVC and from left atrial blood entering the right atrium (RA) through the orifice of the RUPV (arrow) and the unroofed wall between the RUPV and the SVC (*). Ao, ascending aorta; LA, left atrium.

main pulmonary artery (Qp) and ascending aorta (Qs) agrees closely with catheterization-based oximetry measurements of *Qp/Qs (23–26)*. In the absence of significant valve regurgitation or an additional shunt, *Qp/Qs* can also be derived from the right (Qp) and left (Qs) ventricular stroke volumes calculated from the short-axis cine stack of the ventricles. In clinical practice, it is recommended to measure the *Qp/Qs* ratio by both of these methods and check the data for consistency.

In addition to case reports, several studies have assessed the role of CMR in evaluating ASDs. Early reports utilized conventional spin echo imaging to compare the apparent defect size with measurements made at surgery and yielded generally good agreement *(27–29)*. Subsequently, Holmvang et al. evaluated defect size by performing VEC MRI carefully positioned in the plane of the ASD to visualize the defect *en face (30)*. These measurements agreed closely with those made at surgery or with balloon sizing at catheterization in 30 patients, mostly adults. However, measurements from conventional spin echo imaging in planes perpendicular to the ASD overestimated the defect size; the discrepancy was attributed to "signal dropout" in the thin portion of the septum.

Beerbaum et al. studied 65 children with clinically suspected ASDs and inconclusive transthoracic echocardiogram results *(31)*. Defect size and rim measurements were assessed using VEC MRI oriented in the ASD plane for *en face* visualization and in orthogonal planes for the distance to adjacent structures. Time-of-flight angiography was also performed to assess systemic and pulmonary venous return. Based on the CMR examination findings, 30 patients underwent transcatheter device closure and accompanying transesophageal echocardiography. Five of these patients were subsequently referred for surgery because stretched-balloon sizing revealed an unexpectedly large defect. The other 35 children were referred directly to surgery because the defect was deemed unsuitable for device closure or there was associated partial anomalous pulmonary venous return. The accuracy of this determination was confirmed in all cases at surgery. Defect size measurements by CMR agreed well with those by transesophageal echocardiography and at surgery. Rim distances to adjacent structures agreed less well but were usually within 5 mm. The CMR measurement of septal length was larger than that by transesophageal echocardiography but agreed with surgical results. Rim distance to the coronary sinus and minor septal fenestrations less than 1 mm were difficult to identify by CMR. All 9 patients with multiple hemodynamically relevant ASDs were correctly diagnosed by *en face* phase contrast imaging, and all 4 patients with partially anomalous pulmonary venous return were accurately identified by time-of-flight angiography. The authors concluded that in children with suspected ASDs and inconclusive transthoracic echocardiograms, CMR is useful for the determination of ASD size, rim distances, and venous connections.

In another study, Durongpisitkul et al. reported on 66 children and adults with secundum ASDs who underwent transthoracic echocardiography, transesophageal echocardiography, and CMR to evaluate their suitability for Amplatzer device closure *(32)*. Compared with transesophageal echocardiography, the major axis ASD diameter was significantly larger by CMR (30 ± 3.9 mm vs 24.4 ± 3 mm, $p = 0.021$) and correlated better with ASD balloon-stretched diameter measured at catheterization. The authors also noted that the posterior inferior ASD rim was not seen adequately in 10 patients by transesophageal echocardiography but could be visualized well in all patients by CMR. Based on these two advantages, the authors suggested that CMR may be more useful than transesophageal echocardiography to assess suitability for Amplatzer device closure.

The application of CMR to diagnose patent foramen ovale in adults suspected of having a paradoxical embolism is now under evaluation by several CMR laboratories. In the most common technique, the atria and pulmonary veins are imaged rapidly (gradient echo with echo planar imaging) during the infusion of gadolinium contrast while the patient performs a Valsalva maneuver. The appearance of contrast in the left atrium after the right atrium but prior to the pulmonary veins indicates a patent foramen ovale. A pilot study using this approach correctly categorized all 15 patients with and all 5 without a patent foramen ovale *(33)*. The 3 patients with atrial septal aneurysms were also appropriately diagnosed; however, the study did not evaluate the accuracy of CMR to identify left atrial thrombus, often a pertinent question in patients suspected of having embolic events.

Ventricular Septal Defect

ANATOMY

A VSD is a communication between the right and left ventricles through an opening in the ventricular septum. It is one of the most common forms of congenital heart disease and is found frequently in association with complex heart disease. This section focuses on isolated or multiple VSDs in the absence of complex congenital heart disease.

Several VSD anatomical classification systems are in use. Figure 5 shows the anatomical location of VSDs modified from Van Praagh et al., which includes the following: (1) defects at the junction between the conal septum and the muscular septum

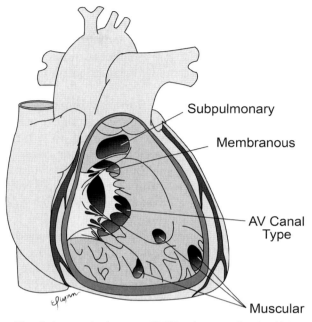

Fig. 5. Anatomical types of VSDs (*see* text for details).

that may be confined to the membranous portion (referred to as membranous or perimembranous defects) or be associated with malalignment of the conal septum (conoventricular defects); (2) defects in the muscular septum (called muscular or trabecular defects); (3) defects in the inlet septum (known as atrioventricular canal-type or inlet defects); and (4) defects in the outlet septum (variably called outlet, doubly committed subarterial, subpulmonary, conal septal, or supracristal defects) *(34)*.

CLINICAL COURSE AND MANAGEMENT

The natural history of a VSD is related to the size and location of the defect. Defects in the membranous or muscular septum often become smaller over time and may spontaneously close. In contrast, malalignment conoventricular defects, outlet septum defects, and atrioventricular canal-type defects are usually large and remain so. Consequently, such patients often undergo surgical closure in infancy. Venturi effects associated with VSDs in the membranous or outlet septum may cause aortic valve leaflets (usually the right coronary cusp) to prolapse through the defect. Although the leaflet prolapse typically reduces the effective orifice size of the defect, it may also lead to aortic insufficiency. VSDs, particularly those associated with turbulent flow jets, also predispose patients to the development of endocarditis.

Symptoms are predominantly determined by the size of the shunt through the VSD, which in turn is related to the defect size and the relative resistances of the pulmonary vascular and the systemic vascular beds. In most situations, pulmonary resistance is lower than systemic resistance, and there is a left-to-right shunt. The resulting increased blood flow to the lungs and left heart may lead to dilation of the pulmonary arteries, pulmonary veins, left atrium, and left ventricle. Because most of the shunt flow passes through the VSD into the right ventricle in systole, right ventricular dilation is usually not present.

If the shunt is small, then the patient is asymptomatic, and intervention to close the defect is not warranted. When the shunt is large, symptoms from pulmonary overcirculation (e.g., tachypnea, diaphoresis, poor feeding, and slow weight gain) may develop in the first few months of life. If the defect is unlikely to become small over time or if these symptoms cannot be managed medically, then surgical closure in infancy is recommended.

Untreated, patients with VSDs and large left-to-right shunts may develop irreversible pulmonary hypertension from elevated pulmonary vascular resistance. In such cases, the flow through the defect will become increasingly right-to-left, resulting in cyanosis (Eisenmenger syndrome). Occasionally, one may encounter older patients with VSDs of intermediate size who are minimally symptomatic and have normal pulmonary artery pressure yet have a large enough shunt to result in left ventricular dilation. VSD closure is probably warranted under these circumstances given its low risk and the potential beneficial impact on ventricular function long-term.

A surgical approach is by far the most common technique used to close VSDs and carries a low mortality even when performed in the first few months of life (35). Typically, the surgeon works through the tricuspid valve and applies a patch to cover the defect. Experience with transcatheter delivery of occlusion devices is growing, and this approach may be appropriate in selected circumstances (36,37).

MRI EVALUATION

Transthoracic echocardiography is the primary diagnostic imaging modality in patients with suspected or known VSDs and is usually adequate. Occasionally in larger patients, acoustic windows may be insufficient, and CMR is indicated to define the defect size and location as well as identify associated conditions such as aortic valve prolapse. CMR may also be of use when the hemodynamic burden of a defect is uncertain by providing reliable quantitative data on the *Qp/Qs* ratio and ventricular dimensions and function.

VSD location and size can be demonstrated by cine gradient echo (preferably steady-state free precession) or spin echo sequences (38–40). Very small defects may be difficult to resolve; however, the associated turbulent flow can be made quite conspicuous on gradient echo sequences provided the echo time is long enough to allow for sufficient spin dephasing (Fig. 6). It is useful to assess the ventricular septum using stacks of images oriented in at least two planes. The four-chamber plane provides base-to-apex localization, whereas the short-axis plane shows the location in the anterior-to-posterior axis (Fig. 7).

Additional imaging in other planes can be used as needed to demonstrate defect position relative to key adjacent structures (e.g., atrioventricular or semilunar valves). Bremerich and colleagues reported that CMR is an important noninvasive test in the diagnosis and management of defects in the outlet septum as echocardiography was felt to image this region of the ventricular septum inadequately (41). Yoo and colleagues demonstrated how CMR can provide an *en face* view of a VSD, which is particularly advantageous in complex anatomy, such as double-inlet ventricle with transposed great arteries, in which systemic blood flow is dependent on passage through the defect (42,43).

An ECG- and navigator-gated isotropic 3D steady-state free precession sequence was developed to assess intracardiac anatomy in patients with congenital heart disease. The resulting high-resolution block of anatomical data can be reformatted in multiple

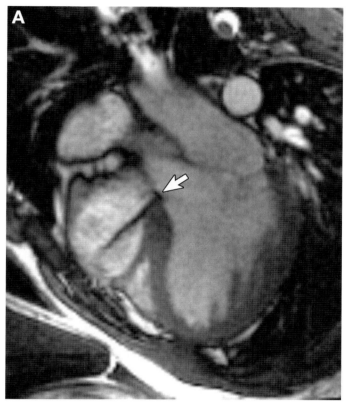

Fig. 6. (Movie in CD) Membranous VSD (arrow). **(A)** ECG-triggered steady-state free precession cine MRI in a four-chamber plane showing the defect and associated flow jet into the right ventricle. **(B)** ECG-gated fast spin echo image in a four-chamber plane.

planes to characterize VSDs and other abnormalities *(44)*. Image quality with this approach, however, was significantly worse in younger patients (approximately <7 years).

Measurement of ventricular dimensions and function is also a key element of the CMR evaluation in a patient with a VSD. This can be done from the ventricular short-axis cine MRI image stack. Larger left-to-right shunts will result in left ventricular dilation but not right ventricular dilation. Ventricular systolic function is usually normal. As described in the section on ASDs, ventricular septal configuration can be used to estimate right ventricular pressure. Finally, quantification of the VSD shunt should be performed by calculating the *Qp/Qs* ratio. This can be accomplished by measuring the net blood flow in the main pulmonary artery (Qp) and the ascending aorta (Qs) using VEC MRI *(24,26,45)*. Alternatively, in the absence of significant valve regurgitation or other shunts, the ventricular volumetric data can be used. The *Qp/Qs* ratio is equal to left ventricular stroke volume divided by right ventricular stroke volume. In practice, both approaches are recommended, and the two results should be compared for consistency.

Patent Ductus Arteriosus

ANATOMY, CLINICAL COURSE, AND MANAGEMENT

The ductus arteriosus is a vascular channel that usually connects the aortic isthmus with the origin of either the left or the right pulmonary artery. During fetal life, the ductus

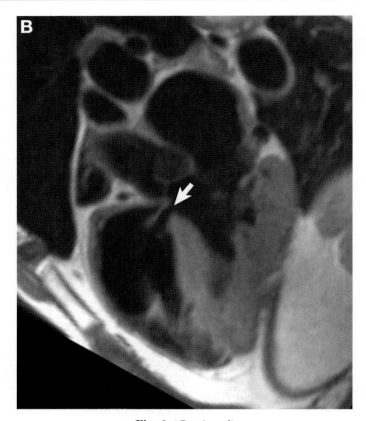

Fig. 6. *(Continued)*

arteriosus allows the majority of the right ventricular output to bypass the lungs by carrying blood flow to the descending aorta. Normally, the ductus arteriosus closes shortly after birth. It may persist in patients with congenital heart disease, allowing communication between the systemic and pulmonary circulations. A persistent PDA is common in premature infants and is associated with increased morbidity.

In full-term infants and children, the clinical course and sequelae of an isolated PDA are usually related to the ductus size and the direction of flow. In the absence of elevated pulmonary vascular resistance, isolated PDAs have left-to-right flow, leading to increased pulmonary flow and a volume load to the left heart. Larger PDAs cause a significant left-to-right shunt and, if untreated, lead to pulmonary overcirculation, respiratory distress, growth failure, and eventually pulmonary vascular disease. Smaller ducts place the patient at risk for infective endarteritis. Thus, in the absence of elevated pulmonary vascular resistance, most isolated persistent PDAs should be closed. This can be accomplished either surgically or in the catheterization laboratory using occluding devices.

MRI Evaluation

CMR is seldom requested primarily for assessment of an isolated PDA as this usually presents in childhood and is a straightforward echocardiographic diagnosis. In several types of complex congenital heart disease, evaluation of the ductus arteriosus is an important

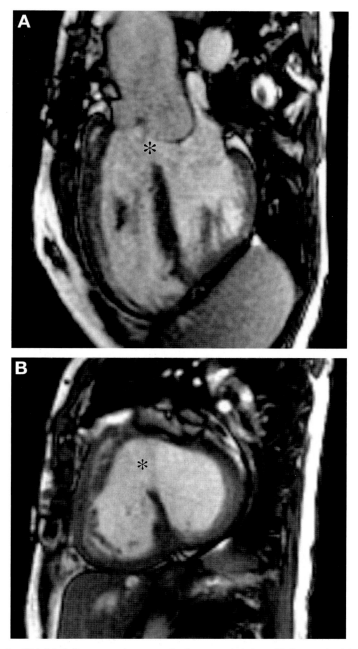

Fig. 7. (Movies in CD) Malalignment conoventricular septal defect (*) imaged with ECG-triggered steady-state free precession cine MRI in ventricular long axis (**A**) and short axis (**B**).

element of the examination. For example, in patients with tetralogy of Fallot and pulmonary atresia, the ductus arteriosus may persist and can be an important source of pulmonary blood supply. Gadolinium-enhanced 3D MRA is a particularly helpful imaging technique in these patients because it allows accurate delineation of all sources of pulmonary blood supply, including a PDA, aortopulmonary collaterals, and the central

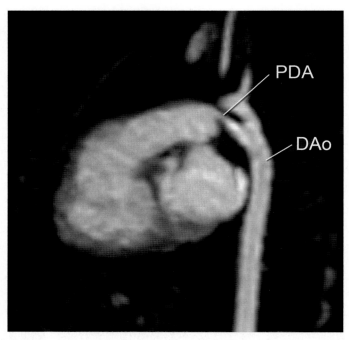

Fig. 8. (Movie in CD) Gadolinium-enhanced 3D MRA (oblique sagittal subvolume maximal intensity projection) in an infant illustrating a patent ductus arteriosus (PDA). DAo, descending aorta.

pulmonary arteries (Fig. 8) (movie in CD) *(46)*. Cine MRI is also useful in detecting PDAs, particularly those that are small with turbulent flow. As with VSD jets, a longer echo time will allow more time for spin dephasing and make the turbulent flow more conspicuous.

When a PDA is detected, VEC MRI is useful to evaluate the direction of flow across the ductus and quantify the *Qp/Qs* ratio. Note that with a PDA and no other shunting lesions, systemic flow (Qs) is equal to the main pulmonary artery flow, and pulmonary flow (Qp) is equal to ascending aorta flow. In patients with a PDA, it is also helpful to measure ventricular volumes and function and assess right ventricular pressure by evaluating ventricular septal position in systole.

Partially Anomalous Pulmonary Venous Connection

ANATOMY

In PAPVC, one or more, but not all, of the pulmonary veins connect to a systemic vein. PAPVC may be seen in isolation or as a component in complex congenital heart lesions, particularly heterotaxy syndrome with polysplenia. There is wide variability in the number of abnormal veins, the site of their termination, and the caliber of the associated connecting vessels. A detailed description of the variety of lesions captured by this diagnosis may be found elsewhere *(47)*.

Common PAPVC types include anomalous connection to the left innominate vein, to the right superior vena cava, to the azygous vein, or to the inferior vena cava. Anomalous connection of some or all of the right pulmonary veins to the inferior vena cava is termed *scimitar syndrome* (movie in CD). The name is derived from the curvilinear shadow in the right lung on chest radiography; this is caused by the anomalous vein as it descends toward the right hemidiaphragm, which resembles a scimitar or Turkish sword. Other abnormalities commonly seen in scimitar syndrome include hypoplasia of the right lung and pulmonary artery, secondary dextrocardia, and anomalous systemic arterial supply, usually from the descending aorta to the right lung *(48)*.

CLINICAL COURSE AND MANAGEMENT

PAPVC results in a left-to-right shunt: blood draining from the lungs returns to the lungs via the systemic veins and right heart without passing through the systemic arterial circulation. This physiology leads to increased pulmonary blood flow and resembles that of an ASD. The magnitude of the shunt is determined by the number of involved veins, the site of their connections, the pulmonary vascular resistance, and the presence of associated defects. Dilation is commonly seen in the systemic veins downstream of the anomalous pulmonary vein insertion site, the right atrium and ventricle, and the pulmonary arteries.

Young patients are usually asymptomatic; dyspnea on exertion becomes increasingly common in the third and fourth decades of life. Development of pulmonary hypertension is rare. Patients may come to attention after auscultation of a pulmonary flow murmur or when diagnostic imaging is performed for another indication. Evidence of right ventricular volume overload with no apparent intracardiac shunt should prompt a search for PAPVC.

The presentation of scimitar syndrome varies widely, depending on the severity of the associated abnormalities. Infants may be critically ill with respiratory compromise; adults may have minimal symptoms. Pulmonary hypertension may develop from a combination of stenosis of the pulmonary veins, arterial blood supply from the descending aorta, pulmonary hypoplasia and parenchymal pulmonary abnormalities.

For the most part, anomalous veins can be surgically corrected, but the likelihood of success and probable benefits must be weighed carefully. A single, small, anomalous pulmonary vein is associated with a modest left-to-right shunt and does not require intervention. In those with most or all of the left pulmonary veins returning to the left innominate vein, the connecting vertical vein is usually large and long enough to detach from the innominate vein and anastomose to the left atrium. For veins connecting to the superior vena cava, a baffle within the superior vena cava and across the atrial septum can be constructed to channel the pulmonary venous return to the left atrium. Alternatively, the superior vena cava can be transected superior to the anomalous veins and the caval end anastomosed to the right atrial appendage. A baffle across the atrial septum is then created to direct the pulmonary venous flow in the cardiac end of the superior vena cava to the left atrium. Pulmonary veins entering the inferior vena cava can be baffled successfully to the left atrium.

The most common postoperative complications seen in patients with PAPVC correction are obstruction and residual leaks in the created channels.

MRI EVALUATION

If a clinical concern for PAPVC cannot be resolved by echocardiography with confidence, then MRI is the most appropriate additional diagnostic imaging test. The acoustic properties of lung tissue may make it difficult by echocardiography to trace

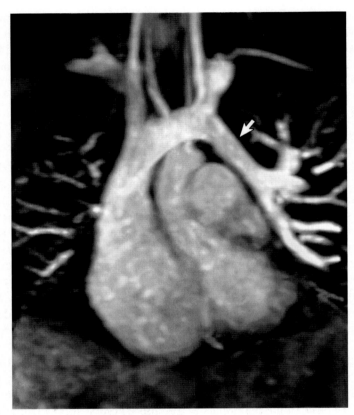

Fig. 9. Gadolinium-enhanced 3D MRA (oblique coronal subvolume maximal intensity projection) illustrating PAPVC of the left upper pulmonary vein (arrow) to the left innominate vein (movie in CD).

possible anomalous veins back into the lungs to confirm that they are pulmonary rather than systemic veins. This limitation it not encountered with CMR.

The goals of CMR evaluation of PAPVC include precise delineation of the anatomy and quantification of the imposed hemodynamic burden. Gadolinium-enhanced 3D MRA is an effective and efficient technique to define the thoracic vasculature anatomy, including the pulmonary veins, pulmonary arteries, and aortopulmonary collateral vessels (Figs. 9 and 10). The image data set can be reformatted in any plane to illustrate spatial relationships and has sufficient resolution to detect vessels smaller than 1 mm. For added confidence, additional imaging of the vascular anatomy can be obtained using cine gradient echo or fast spin echo with blood signal nulling sequences.

Several studies assessing the accuracy and utility of gadolinium-enhanced 3D MRA have shown similar results *(49–51)*. There was a high level of agreement between findings on MRA compared with surgical inspection and X-ray angiography. MRA was uniformly more accurate than transthoracic and transesophageal echocardiography. CMR studies often diagnosed previously unknown PAPVC or added new clinically important information regarding PAPVC anatomy.

Patients with PAPVC should also have their ventricular dimensions and function measured using a stack of cine MRI oriented in the ventricular short-axis plane.

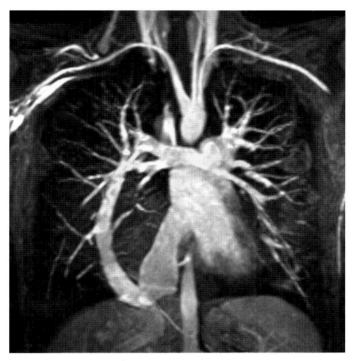

Fig. 10. (Movie in CD) Gadolinium-enhanced 3D MRA (oblique coronal subvolume maximal intensity projection) in an adult with scimitar syndrome.

Particular attention should be devoted to quantifying right ventricular end-diastolic volume as this should be related to the size of the left-to-right shunt. The shunt should also be measured directly by obtaining VEC MRI flow measurements in the main pulmonary artery (Qp) and the ascending aorta (Qs). In some cases, it may also be possible to measure the flow in the anomalously draining vein itself. In the absence of significant valvular insufficiency, the ventricular stoke volume differential should also be equal to the shunt size, thus serving as a useful check.

It is worth noting that, in patients with PAPVC, Qp/Qs ratio measurements by oximetry in the catheterization laboratory are inherently inaccurate because of the difficulty in obtaining a reliable, representative mixed systemic venous saturation. Because blood flow is measured directly, these concerns do not apply to the MRI measurements. When there is a hypoplastic pulmonary artery or pulmonary venous pathway obstruction, it is also useful to calculate differential pulmonary blood flow using VEC MRI measurements in the branch pulmonary arteries.

Coarctation of the Aorta

ANATOMY

Coarctation of the aorta is a discrete narrowing most commonly located just distal to the left subclavian artery at the site of insertion of the ductus arteriosus. It is thought to arise either from an abnormal flow pattern through the arch during development or from extension of ductal tissue into the aortic wall. Hypoplasia and elongation of the distal transverse arch are frequent associations. Coarctation may be present alone or in combination with other heart lesions, including bicuspid aortic valve (the most frequent intracardiac defect), aortic stenosis (valvular or subvalvular), mitral valve abnormalities, ASD, VSD, persistent PDA, and conotruncal anomalies *(52,53)*.

CLINICAL COURSE AND MANAGEMENT

Infants tend to present with symptoms of heart failure and systemic hypoperfusion as the ductus arteriosus closes and, if untreated, may progress to shock or death. Older children and adults typically have isolated coarctation and are usually relatively asymptomatic. A heart murmur, systemic hypertension, or rib notching on a chest X-ray from collateral vessels often lead to the diagnosis. Even in asymptomatic patients, relief of the aortic obstruction is indicated for hemodynamically significant lesions because of the high rate of late complications, including congestive heart failure, systemic hypertension, premature coronary artery disease, ruptured aortic or cerebral aneurysms, stroke, aortic dissection, infective endarteritis, and premature death *(54)*.

Therapeutic options for coarctation include surgical repair and percutaneous balloon angioplasty, sometimes with stent placement. Currently, resection of the coarctation with an end-to-end anastomosis and augmentation of the transverse arch if needed is the most widely practiced surgical repair and has the lowest incidence of recurrent obstruction. Other approaches have included subclavian flap aortoplasty, patch augmentation, and conduit interposition. These techniques have fallen out of favor as postoperative complications, such as aneurysm formation at the site of the prosthetic patch and recurrent arch obstruction, have become increasingly recognized *(55,56)*.

Coarctation in infants is treated surgically in the majority of centers because of the lower risk of residual obstruction, recurrence, and technique-related complications compared with percutaneous interventions *(57)*. For isolated coarctation, the surgical mortality approaches zero *(58)*. In the event of recurrent coarctation following surgical repair, balloon angioplasty with or without stent placement is often the first line of therapy. Coarctation in older children or adults is increasingly treated primarily by percutaneous interventions, which thus far have shown a low risk of recoarctation and aneurysm formation *(59,60)*.

MRI EVALUATION

Transthoracic echocardiography is usually the only diagnostic imaging needed for evaluation of young children with suspected coarctation or following intervention for coarctation. With increasing age, acoustic windows typically deteriorate, leading to an incomplete anatomical assessment by echocardiography. In these circumstances, CMR is able to provide high-quality anatomical imaging of the aortic arch in its entirety, an assessment of the hemodynamic severity of the obstruction, and evaluation of left ventricular mass and function.

In a retrospective study of 84 adult patients following intervention for coarctation of the aorta, Therrien and colleagues showed that the combination of clinical assessment and CMR on every patient was more "cost-effective" for detecting complications than combinations that relied on echocardiography or chest radiography as imaging modalities *(61)*. Other studies have shown the utility of CMR in infants and children with coarctation and other anomalies of the aortic arch *(62–64)*. Computed tomography can also provide excellent anatomical imaging of the aorta but little functional information regarding the left ventricle or pressure gradient across any obstruction. It has the additional disadvantage of ionizing radiation exposure, making it a less-attractive modality for serial follow-up.

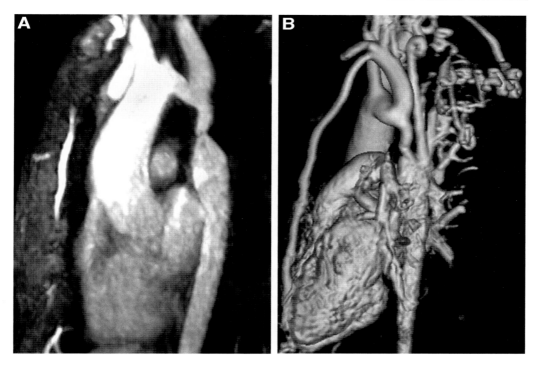

Fig. 11. (Movies in CD) Gadolinium-enhanced 3D MRA. **(A)** Oblique sagittal subvolume maximal intensity projection showing elongation of the distal transverse arch, hypoplastic aortic isthmus with severe discrete coarctation at the junction between the isthmus and descending thoracic aorta. **(B)** Volume reconstruction shows the coarctation as well as several large tortuous collateral vessels and a dilated left internal mammary artery.

A comprehensive CMR evaluation of patients with suspected coarctation or following intervention for coarctation includes assessment of aortic anatomy; cine MRI sequences to measure ventricular size, function, and mass; and VEC MRI sequences to evaluate the severity of obstruction. Regarding aortic anatomy, attention should be given to transverse aortic arch and isthmus, the brachiocephalic vessels, collateral vessels that may bypass obstruction, and possible aneurysms or dissections at the repair sites. Abnormal vessels should ideally be measured in cross section as elliptical segments are common. If a coarctation is present, its diameter, length, and distance to neighboring vessels should be reported as this may influence decisions regarding percutaneous intervention. Given the association of bicuspid aortic valve with coarctation, the aortic valve morphology should be noted as well as the dimensions of the aortic root and ascending aorta.

Gadolinium-enhanced 3D MRA is an efficient technique to assess aortic anatomy (Fig. 11). Using subvolume maximal intensity projections and reformatting, most of the relevant issues can be addressed and measurements performed *(3,65–67)*. Cine gradient echo imaging of the aortic arch in long axis is useful to identify the sites of obstruction because the associated high-velocity turbulent jets produce systolic signal voids. Cine MRI is also helpful for assessment of the aortic valve morphology and aortic root dimensions. Finally, turbo spin echo sequences with nulling of the blood signal can be used to produce high-resolution, high-contrast images of the aorta. They are particularly valuable following endovascular stent placement because there is less metallic susceptibility artifact than with gradient echo sequences. For anatomical definition of the coarctation site, multiple investigators have demonstrated good correlation between these various CMR imaging techniques and X-ray angiography *(68–74)*.

MRI evaluation of coarctation should also include calculation of left ventricular dimensions, systolic function, mass, and mass-to-volume ratio by acquiring a stack of cine steady-state free precession images in a ventricular short-axis plane. These data are clinically relevant because hypertension is often present and may lead to ventricular hypertrophy and dysfunction. Upper body hypertension may be caused by aortic arch obstruction, but systemic hypertension is also prevalent following coarctation repair even without residual coarctation, particularly in patients who had surgery later in life. It is good practice to measure upper and lower extremity cuff blood pressures at the time of the CMR examination to help identify patients with hypertension and estimate the pressure gradient across any aortic obstruction. Note that there may be little upper-to-lower extremity blood pressure differential even with important aortic obstruction when there is a significant collateral circulation bypassing the obstruction.

VEC MRI measurements have been used to gain insight into the functional significance of an obstruction. One approach has been to assess the flow pattern in the descending aorta distal to the coarctation. Flow characteristics suggestive of a hemodynamically significant coarctation include decreased peak flow, decreased time-averaged flow, delayed onset of descending aorta flow compared with the onset of flow in the ascending aorta, decreased acceleration rate, and prolonged deceleration with increased antegrade diastolic flow *(70,75,76)*.

A model to predict the probability of a hemodynamically significant coarctation pressure gradient (defined as $\geq$ 20 mmHg measured during cardiac catheterization) was developed at our institution *(77)*. A combination of the smallest cross-sectional area of the aorta (measured from the gadolinium-enhanced 3D MRA) and the heart rate-adjusted mean deceleration of flow in the descending aorta (measured by VEC MRI distal to the coarctation) predicted a gradient of 20 mm Hg or more with 95% sensitivity and 82% specificity, 90% positive and negative predictive values, and an area under the receiver-operator characteristics curve of 0.94.

Another approach to assessing severity is to measure the peak coarctation jet velocity and estimate a pressure gradient using the modified Bernoulli equation. Mohiaddin et al. compared peak coarctation jet velocity measured by VEC MRI with that obtained by continuous-wave Doppler and found a high correlation ($r = 0.95$) as well as close agreement (mean difference = 0.12 ± 0.23 m/second) *(75)*. Nevertheless, they noted that such measurements are technically difficult in a long, tortuous coarctation segment, and that such pressure estimates may not be indicative of anatomical severity because of collateral flow. In support of the latter notion, they found a poor inverse correlation between peak coarctation jet velocity and coarctation diameter ($r = -0.48$). Consequently, they performed additional VEC MRI flow measurements in the ascending and descending aorta distal to the coarctation. Compared to controls, coarctation patients had a significantly lower descending-to-ascending aorta flow ratio as well as a smaller, more blunted descending aortic flow profile.

Similarly, Steffens et al. found that, although there was close correlation between gradients obtained by VEC MRI and Doppler echocardiography ($r = 0.95$), both methods showed poorer correlation with cuff blood pressure gradients ($r = 0.63$ for Doppler echocardiography and $r = 0.54$ for VEC MRI) *(76)*. In an effort to improve accuracy,

Oshinski et al. proposed that the Bernoulli equation be adapted to take into account hemodynamic variables associated with stenosis severity *(78)*.

Finally, VEC MRI has been used to quantify collateral flow entering the descending aorta distal to the obstruction via retrograde flow from the intercostal arteries or vessels arising off the aortic arch and arch branches in patients with coarctation *(76,79–81)*. Increased collateral flow suggests more severe obstruction. Moreover, higher collateral flow would be expected to decrease the likelihood of spinal cord ischemic injury during surgical correction that involves interruption of aortic flow. If little collateral flow is suspected, then the surgeon may elect to perform left heart bypass to the descending aorta during the repair.

Steffens et al. attempted to directly quantify collateral flow entering the descending aorta via retrograde flow from the intercostal arteries by performing flow measurements slightly distal to the coarctation site and at the level of the diaphragm *(76)*. Total flow from proximal to distal descending aorta decreased by $7 \pm 6\%$ in normal volunteers compared to an increase of $83 \pm 50\%$ in patients with moderate-to-severe coarctation ($p < 0.01$). The amount of flow increase in the distal aorta correlated directly with the severity of anatomical narrowing ($r = 0.94$) and the extremity cuff blood pressure gradient ($r = 0.84$). Nevertheless, the added clinical benefit of this approach is unclear because the extent of collateral flow necessitating left heart bypass to prevent spinal cord ischemic injury during surgical correction has not been defined.

SUMMARY

CMR is a valuable tool for the diagnosis and management of children and adults with congenital heart disease. Although transthoracic echocardiography remains the primary imaging modality for this group, deterioration of acoustic windows as patients grow or undergo surgery often limits its utility. In such circumstances, CMR provides a noninvasive alternative to transesophageal echocardiography and cardiac catheterization. Moreover, the superior ability of CMR to depict anatomy in three dimensions, evaluate ventricular size and function, and measure vessel-specific blood flow make it the preferred imaging modality in a variety of clinical circumstances involving simple congenital heart lesions. To ensure a high-quality, complete CMR evaluation in these situations, the supervising physician should have a thorough understanding of the relevant anatomical and physiological issues as well as CMR techniques. One must also be mindful that CMR strategies for evaluating congenital heart disease will continue to evolve as experience grows and new imaging techniques are developed.

ACKNOWLEDGMENT

We thank the physicians, technologists, nurses, and support personnel in the Cardiovascular MRI Program at Children's Hospital Boston for their help. Parts of the text and figures of this chapter have been included in other chapters recently written by the authors on MRI evaluation of congenital heart disease.

REFERENCES

1. Tsai-Goodman B, Geva T, Odegard KC, Sena LM, Powell AJ. Clinical role, accuracy, and technical aspects of cardiovascular magnetic resonance imaging in infants. Am J Cardiol 2004;94:69–74.
2. Gutierrez FR. Magnetic resonance imaging of congenital heart disease. Top Magn Reson Imaging 1995;7:246–257.

3. Masui T, Katayama M, Kobayashi S, et al. Gadolinium-enhanced MR angiography in the evaluation of congenital cardiovascular disease pre- and postoperative states in infants and children. J Magn Reson Imaging 2000;12:1034–1042.

4. Schlesinger AE, Hernandez RJ. Magnetic resonance imaging in congenital heart disease in children. Tex Heart Inst J 1996;23:128–143.

5. Fogel MA, Donofrio MT, Ramaciotti C, Hubbard AM, Weinberg PM. Magnetic resonance and echocardiographic imaging of pulmonary artery size throughout stages of Fontan reconstruction. Circulation 1994;90:2927–2936.

6. Beekman RP, Hoorntje TM, Beek FJ, Kuijten RH. Sedation for children undergoing magnetic resonance imaging: efficacy and safety of rectal thiopental. Eur J Pediatr 1996;155:820–822.

7. Didier D, Ratib O, Beghetti M, Oberhaensli I, Friedli B. Morphologic and functional evaluation of congenital heart disease by magnetic resonance imaging. J Magn Reson Imaging 1999;10:639–655.

8. Baker E. What's new in magnetic resonance imaging? Cardiol Young 2001;11:445–452.

9. Holmqvist C, Larsson E-M, Stahlberg F, Laurin S. Contrast-enhanced thoracic 3D-MR angiography in infants and children. Acta Radiol 2001;42:50–58.

10. Odegard KC, DiNardo JA, Tsai-Goodman B, Powell AJ, Geva T, Laussen PC. Anaesthesia considerations for cardiac MRI in infants and small children. Paediatr Anaesth 2004;14:471–476.

11. Ahmed S, Shellock FG. Magnetic resonance imaging safety: implications for cardiovascular patients. J Cardiovasc Magn Reson 2001;3:171–182.

12. Shellock FG, O'Neil M, Ivans V, et al. Cardiac pacemakers and implantable cardioverter defibrillators are unaffected by operation of an extremity MR imaging system. AJR Am J Roentgenol 1999;172:165–170.

13. Martin ET, Coman JA, Shellock FG, Pulling CC, Fair R, Jenkins K. Magnetic resonance imaging and cardiac pacemaker safety at 1.5-T. J Am Coll Cardiol 2004;43:1315–1324.

14. Loewy J, Loewy A, Kendall EJ. Reconsideration of pacemakers and MR imaging. Radiographics 2004;24:1257–1267.

15. Roguin A, Zviman MM, Meininger GR, et al. Modern pacemaker and implantable cardioverter/defibrillator systems can be magnetic resonance imaging safe: in vitro and in vivo assessment of safety and function at 1.5 T. Circulation 2004;110:475–482.

16. Shellock FG. Prosthetic heart valves and annuloplasty rings: assessment of magnetic field interactions, heating, and artifacts at 1.5 T. J Cardiovasc Magn Reson 2001;3:317–324.

17. Shellock FG, Shellock VJ. Cardiovascular catheters and accessories: ex vivo testing of ferromagnetism, heating, and artifacts associated with MRI. J Magn Reson Imaging 1998;8:1338–1342.

18. Shellock FG, Morisoli SM. Ex vivo evaluation of ferromagnetism and artifacts of cardiac occluders exposed to a 1.5-T MR system. J Magn Reson Imaging 1994;4:213–215.

19. Hagen PT, Scholz DG, Edwards WD. Incidence and size of patent foramen ovale during the first 10 decades of life: an autopsy study of 965 normal hearts. Mayo Clin Proc 1984;59:17–20.

20. Raghib G, Ruttenberg HD, Anderson RC, Amplatz K, Adams P Jr, Edwards JE. Termination of the left superior vena cava in left atrium, atrial septal defect, and absence of coronary sinus; a developmental complex. Circulation 1965;31:906–918.

21. Radzik D, Davignon A, van Doesburg N, Fournier A, Marchand T, Ducharme G. Predictive factors for spontaneous closure of atrial septal defects diagnosed in the first 3 months of life. J Am Coll Cardiol 1993;22:851–853.

22. Homma S, Sacco RL. Patent foramen ovale and stroke. Circulation 2005;112:1063–1072.

23. Powell AJ, Tsai-Goodman B, Prakash A, Greil GF, Geva T. Comparison between phase-velocity cine magnetic resonance imaging and invasive oximetry for quantification of atrial shunts. Am J Cardiol 2003;91:1523–1525, A9.

24. Beerbaum P, Korperich H, Barth P, Esdorn H, Gieseke J, Meyer H. Noninvasive quantification of left-to-right shunt in pediatric patients: phase-contrast cine magnetic resonance imaging compared with invasive oximetry. Circulation 2001;103:2476–2482.

25. Hundley WG, Li HF, Lange RA, et al. Assessment of left-to-right intracardiac shunting by velocity-encoded, phase-difference magnetic resonance imaging. A comparison with oximetric and indicator dilution techniques. Circulation 1995;91:2955–2960.

26. Arheden H, Holmqvist C, Thilen U, et al. Left-to-right cardiac shunts: comparison of measurements obtained with MR velocity mapping and with radionuclide angiography. Radiology 1999;211:453–458.

27. Diethelm L, Dery R, Lipton MJ, Higgins CB. Atrial-level shunts: sensitivity and specificity of MR in diagnosis. Radiology 1987;162:181–186.

28. Dinsmore RE, Wismer GL, Guyer D, et al. Magnetic resonance imaging of the interatrial septum and atrial septal defects. AJR Am J Roentgenol 1985;145:697–703.

29. Sakakibara M, Kobayashi S, Imai H, Watanabe S, Masuda Y, Inagaki Y. [Diagnosis of atrial septal defect using magnetic resonance imaging]. J Cardiol 1987;17:817–829.

30. Holmvang G, Palacios IF, Vlahakes GJ, et al. Imaging and sizing of atrial septal defects by magnetic resonance. Circulation 1995;92:3473–3480.

31. Beerbaum P, Korperich H, Esdorn H, et al. Atrial septal defects in pediatric patients: noninvasive sizing with cardiovascular MR imaging. Radiology 2003;228:361–369.

32. Durongpisitkul K, Tang NL, Soongswang J, Laohaprasitiporn D, Nanal A. Predictors of successful transcatheter closure of atrial septal defect by cardiac magnetic resonance imaging. Pediatr Cardiol 2004;25:124–130.

33. Mohrs OK, Petersen SE, Erkapic D, et al. Diagnosis of patent foramen ovale using contrast-enhanced dynamic MRI: a pilot study. AJR Am J Roentgenol 2005;184:234–240.

34. Van Praagh R, Geva T, Kreutzer J. Ventricular septal defects: how shall we describe, name and classify them? J Am Coll Cardiol 1989;14:1298–1299.

35. Bol-Raap G, Weerheim J, Kappetein AP, Witsenburg M, Bogers AJ. Follow-up after surgical closure of congenital ventricular septal defect. Eur J Cardiothorac Surg 2003;24:511–515.

36. Kumar K, Lock JE, Geva T. Apical muscular ventricular septal defects between the left ventricle and the right ventricular infundibulum. Diagnostic and interventional considerations. Circulation 1997;95:1207–1213.

37. Knauth AL, Lock JE, Perry SB, et al. Transcatheter device closure of congenital and postoperative residual ventricular septal defects. Circulation 2004;110:501–507.

38. Didier D, Higgins CB, Fisher MR, Osaki L, Silverman NH, Cheitlin MD. Congenital heart disease: gated MR imaging in 72 patients. Radiology 1986;158:227–235.

39. Lowell DG, Turner DA, Smith SM, et al. The detection of atrial and ventricular septal defects with electrocardiographically synchronized magnetic resonance imaging. Circulation 1986;73: 89–94.

40. Baker EJ, Ayton V, Smith MA, et al. Magnetic resonance imaging at a high field strength of ventricular septal defects in infants. Br Heart J 1989;62:305–310.

41. Bremerich J, Reddy GP, Higgins CB. MRI of supracristal ventricular septal defects. J Comput Assist Tomogr 1999;23:13–15.

42. Yoo SJ, Lim TH, Park IS, Hong CY, Song MG, Kim SH. Defects of the interventricular septum of the heart: *en face* MR imaging in the oblique coronal plane. AJR Am J Roentgenol 1991;157:943–946.

43. Yoo SJ, Kim YM, Choe YH. Magnetic resonance imaging of complex congenital heart disease. Int J Card Imaging 1999;15:151–160.

44. Sorensen TS, Korperich H, Greil GF, et al. Operator-independent isotropic three-dimensional magnetic resonance imaging for morphology in congenital heart disease: a validation study. Circulation 2004;110:163–169.

45. Mohiaddin RH, Underwood R, Romeira L, et al. Comparison between cine magnetic resonance velocity mapping and first-pass radionuclide angiocardiography for quantitating intracardiac shunts. American Journal of Cardiology 1995;75:529–532.

46. Geva T, Greil GF, Marshall AC, Landzberg M, Powell AJ. Gadolinium-enhanced three-dimensional magnetic resonance angiography of pulmonary blood supply in patients with complex pulmonary stenosis or atresia: comparison with X-ray angiography. Circulation 2002;106:473–478.

47. Geva T, Van Praagh S. Anomalies of the pulmonary veins. In: Allen HD, Gutgessel HP, Clark EB, Driscoll DJ, eds. Moss and Adams' heart disease in infants, children, and adolescents. Philadelphia: Lippincott Williams and Wilkins; 2001:736–772.

48. Neill CA, Ferencz C, Sabiston DC, Sheldon H. The familial occurrence of hypoplastic right lung with systemic arterial supply and venous drainage "scimitar syndrome." Bull Johns Hopkins Hosp 1960;107:1–21.

49. Greil GF, Powell AJ, Gildein HP, Geva T. Gadolinium-enhanced three-dimensional magnetic resonance angiography of pulmonary and systemic venous anomalies. J Am Coll Cardiol 2002;39:335–341.

50. Prasad SK, Soukias N, Hornung T, et al. Role of magnetic resonance angiography in the diagnosis of major aortopulmonary collateral arteries and partial anomalous pulmonary venous drainage. Circulation 2004;109:207–214.

51. Ferrari VA, Scott CH, Holland GA, Axel L, Sutton MS. Ultrafast three-dimensional contrast-enhanced magnetic resonance angiography and imaging in the diagnosis of partial anomalous pulmonary venous drainage. J Am Coll Cardiol 2001;37:1120–1128.

52. Roos-Hesselink JW, Scholzel BE, Heijdra RJ, et al. Aortic valve and aortic arch pathology after coarctation repair. Heart 2003;89:1074–1077.

53. Konen E, Merchant N, Provost Y, McLaughlin PR, Crossin J, Paul NS. Coarctation of the aorta before and after correction: the role of cardiovascular MRI. AJR Am J Roentgenol 2004;182:1333–1339.
54. Campbell M. Natural history of coarctation of the aorta. Br Heart J 1970;32:633–640.
55. Bogaert J, Gewillig M, Rademakers F, et al. Transverse arch hypoplasia predisposes to aneurysm formation at the repair site after patch angioplasty for coarctation of the aorta. J Am Coll Cardiol 1995;26:521–527.
56. Parks WJ, Ngo TD, Plauth WH, et al. Incidence of aneurysm formation after Dacron patch aortoplasty repair for coarctation of the aorta: long-term results and assessment utilizing magnetic resonance angiography with three-dimensional surface rendering. J Am Coll Cardiol 1995;26:266–271.
57. Rao PS, Jureidini SB, Balfour IC, Singh GK, Chen SC. Severe aortic coarctation in infants less than 3 months: successful palliation by balloon angioplasty. J Invasive Cardiol 2003;15:202–208.
58. Corno AF, Botta U, Hurni M, et al. Surgery for aortic coarctation: a 30 years experience. Eur J Cardiothorac Surg 2001;20:1202–1206.
59. Walhout RJ, Lekkerkerker JC, Ernst SM, Hutter PA, Plokker TH, Meijboom EJ. Angioplasty for coarctation in different aged patients. Am Heart J 2002;144:180–186.
60. Fawzy ME, Awad M, Hassan W, Al Kadhi Y, Shoukri M, Fadley F. Long-term outcome (up to 15 years) of balloon angioplasty of discrete native coarctation of the aorta in adolescents and adults. J Am Coll Cardiol 2004;43:1062–1067.
61. Therrien J, Thorne SA, Wright A, Kilner PJ, Somerville J. Repaired coarctation: a "cost-effective" approach to identify complications in adults. J Am Coll Cardiol 2000;35:997–1002.
62. Simpson IA, Chung KJ, Glass RF, Sahn DJ, Sherman FS, Hesselink J. Cine magnetic resonance imaging for evaluation of anatomy and flow relations in infants and children with coarctation of the aorta. Circulation 1988;78:142–148.
63. Mendelsohn AM, Banerjee A, Donnelly LF, Schwartz DC. Is echocardiography or magnetic resonance imaging superior for precoarctation angioplasty evaluation? Cathet Cardiovasc Diagn 1997;42:26–30.
64. Rupprecht T, Nitz W, Wagner M, Kreissler P, Rascher W, Hofbeck M. Determination of the pressure gradient in children with coarctation of the aorta by low-field magnetic resonance imaging. Pediatr Cardiol 2002;23:127–131.
65. Prince MR, Narasimham DL, Jacoby WT, et al. Three-dimensional gadolinium-enhanced MR angiography of the thoracic aorta. AJR Am J Roentgenol 1996;166:1387–1397.
66. Krinsky GA, Rofsky NM, DeCorato DR, et al. Thoracic aorta: comparison of gadolinium-enhanced three-dimensional MR angiography with conventional MR imaging. Radiology 1997;202:183–193.
67. Bogaert J, Kuzo R, Dymarkowski S, et al. Follow-up of patients with previous treatment for coarctation of the thoracic aorta: comparison between contrast-enhanced MR angiography and fast spin-echo MR imaging. Eur Radiol 2000;10:1847–1854.
68. Simpson IA, Chung KJ, Glass RF, Sahn DJ, Sherman FS, Hesselink J. Cine magnetic resonance imaging for evaluation of anatomy and flow relations in infants and children with coarctation of the aorta. Circulation 1988;78:142–148.
69. Fawzy ME, von Sinner W, Rifai A, et al. Magnetic resonance imaging compared with angiography in the evaluation of intermediate-term result of coarctation balloon angioplasty. Am Heart J 1993;126:1380–1384.
70. Muhler EG, Neuerburg JM, Ruben A, et al. Evaluation of aortic coarctation after surgical repair: role of magnetic resonance imaging and Doppler ultrasound. Br Heart J 1993;70:285–290.
71. Riquelme C, Laissy JP, Menegazzo D, et al. MR imaging of coarctation of the aorta and its postoperative complications in adults: assessment with spin-echo and cine-MR imaging. Magn Reson Imaging 1999;17:37–46.
72. Godart F, Labrot G, Devos P, McFadden E, Rey C, Beregi JP. Coarctation of the aorta: comparison of aortic dimensions between conventional MR imaging, 3D MR angiography, and conventional angiography. Eur Radiol 2002;12:2034–2039.
73. Stern HC, Locher D, Wallnofer K, et al. Noninvasive assessment of coarctation of the aorta: comparative measurements by two-dimensional echocardiography, magnetic resonance, and angiography. Pediatr Cardiol 1991;12:1–5.
74. Gutberlet M, Hosten N, Vogel M, et al. Quantification of morphologic and hemodynamic severity of coarctation of the aorta by magnetic resonance imaging. Cardiol Young 2001;11:512–520.
75. Mohiaddin RH, Kilner PJ, Rees S, Longmore DB. Magnetic resonance volume flow and jet velocity mapping in aortic coarctation. J Am Coll Cardiol 1993;22:1515–1521.
76. Steffens JC, Bourne MW, Sakuma H, O'Sullivan M, Higgins CB. Quantification of collateral blood flow in coarctation of the aorta by velocity encoded cine magnetic resonance imaging. Circulation 1994;90:937–943.

77. Nielsen JC, Powell AJ, Gauvreau K, Marcus EN, Prakash A, Geva T. Magnetic resonance imaging predictors of coarctation severity. Circulation 2005;111:622–628.
78. Oshinski JN, Parks WJ, Markou CP, et al. Improved measurement of pressure gradients in aortic coarctation by magnetic resonance imaging. J Am Coll Cardiol 1996;28:1818–1826.
79. Holmqvist C, Stahlberg F, Hanseus K, et al. Collateral flow in coarctation of the aorta with magnetic resonance velocity mapping: correlation to morphological imaging of collateral vessels. J Magn Reson Imaging 2002;15:39–46.
80. Araoz PA, Reddy GP, Tarnoff H, Roge CL, Higgins CB. MR findings of collateral circulation are more accurate measures of hemodynamic significance than arm-leg blood pressure gradient after repair of coarctation of the aorta. J Magn Reson Imaging 2003;17:177–183.
81. Julsrud PR, Breen JF, Felmlee JP, Warnes CA, Connolly HM, Schaff HV. Coarctation of the aorta: collateral flow assessment with phase-contrast MR angiography. AJR Am J Roentgenol 1997; 169:1735–1742.

26 Magnetic Resonance Angiography of the Aorta and Peripheral Arteries

Servet Tatli

INTRODUCTION

Magnetic resonance angiography (MRA) has virtually replaced diagnostic conventional X-ray angiography and has become the primary imaging tool for the evaluation of the diseases of the aorta and branches for many indications *(1–13)*. Development of faster magnetic resonance imaging (MRI) scanners with shorter TR (relaxation time) and TE (echo time) and powerful gradients, allowing completion of principal MRA sequences within single breath hold, has led this revolution *(2)*. Improvements in coil, computer hardware/software technology, and postprocessing techniques have also contributed to this transition and made MRA a rapid and robust technique.

MRA has many advantages over conventional X-ray angiography; it is noninvasive and requires no direct arterial access. MRA uses no ionizing radiation or potentially nephrotoxic iodine-based contrast material as in conventional X-ray angiography or computed tomography (CT). The paramagnetic contrast material used for contrast-enhanced (CE) MRA have much more favorable safety profiles in recommended doses compared to iodine-based contrast material, which makes MRA an ideal tool to evaluate patients with aortic and peripheral vascular disease (PVD), who also frequently have concomitant poor renal function *(14–17)*. MRA also has advantages compared to color Doppler ultrasound because of less dependence on the operator and lack of difficulties with acoustic window limitations *(3)*.

From: *Contemporary Cardiology: Cardiovascular Magnetic Resonance Imaging*
Edited by: Raymond Y. Kwong © Humana Press Inc., Totowa, NJ

MRA is such a versatile imaging tool because of its inherent nature. Multiplanar capability of the technique allows obtaining an image in any direction depending on the course of the vessel to be imaged. The use of various MRA sequences permits evaluation not only of the lumen of a vessel, as in conventional angiography, but also of the wall of the vessel and the adjacent soft tissue and organs *(9)*. This important advantage of MRA has improved the detection, characterization, and understanding of many aortic diseases, such as in intramural hematoma (IMH) *(9)*. In addition, physiological properties of blood flow can be accurately calculated by specific MRA techniques, namely, phase contrast (PC) MRA, in the same examination session.

PRINCIPAL MAGNETIC RESONANCE ANGIOGRAPHIC TECHNIQUES

Currently, there are several MRA techniques used in daily clinical practice. MRA techniques are briefly divided into two major categories according to the mechanism of depiction of the blood vessel. Flow-dependent MRA techniques rely on the direction of the blood flow to demonstrate a vessel, such as time-of-flight (TOF) MRA, and PC MRA; however, flow-independent MRA techniques, such as contrast-enhanced MRA, employ the T_1-shortening effect of circulating gadolinium-containing contrast material (Gd-DTPA, gadolinium-**diethyltriaminepentaacetic acid**) and not effected by inherent blood flow characteristics *(13)*. Comprehensive evaluation of the aorta and branches requires a combination of these techniques, depending on the clinical question. Understanding the basic principles of these techniques is essential to acquire consistently diagnostic MRA images and evaluate these images accurately.

In this chapter, first the main MRA techniques are reviewed briefly, and then applications of these techniques are discussed with some illustrated examples.

TIME-OF-FLIGHT MAGNETIC RESONANCE ANGIOGRAPHY

As the oldest MRA technique, TOF MRA has limited value today because of inherent limitations, and it is not used in routine clinical imaging of the aorta *(18)*. However, some important and well-validated applications remain, primarily in the distal runoff vessels *(19–23)*. TOF MRA relies on flow-related enhancement of the spins in the flowing blood. The saturation of the signal from background tissue is achieved by applying multiple radio-frequency pulses into the imaging section. The vessel in this imaging section appears much brighter compared to stationary background tissue because of continuous inflow of fresh unsaturated blood (Fig. 1A). The technique uses a two-dimensional (2D) flow-compensated gradient echo sequence to acquire multiple, thin, sequential sections, which can be either viewed individually or reformatted with maximum intensity projection (MIP) technique to obtain a three-dimensional (3D) projectional image (Fig. 1B). Selective arterial imaging can be obtained by using presaturation pulse placed inferior to the imaging sections to eliminate the signal from the veins.

In addition to being extremely time consuming (imaging of the lower extremity can take more than 60 minutes), TOF MRA has important limitations, explaining its rapid replacement by CE MRA. These limitations include (1) complex flow producing loss of signal because intravoxel dephasing may simulate disease; (2) vessels not truly perpendicular to the acquired section plane are more likely to show saturation effect, which causes low signal and simulates disease (Fig. 2); (3) triphasic

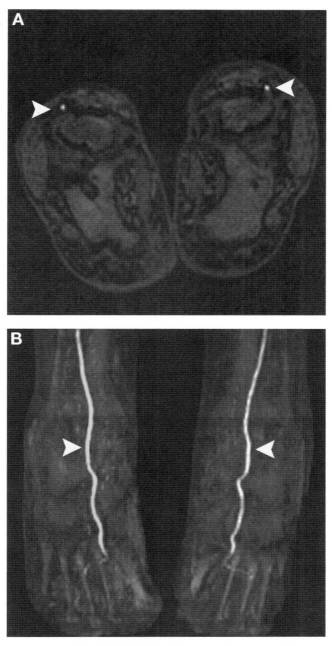

Fig. 1. Axial **(A)** and coronal MIP **(B)** TOF MRA image of both feet. The dorsalis pedis arteries (arrowheads) are widely patent on both sides, but the planter arteries show no flow bilaterally, consistent with total occlusion.

pulsatile flow in vessels with relatively preserved inflow produces ghost artifact unless cardiac gating is used, which further prolongs imaging time; and (4) retrograde flow in collateral and reconstituted vessels may also be saturated, obscuring the true level of obstruction and simulating an occluded segment that is longer than the actual length *(21,24,25)*.

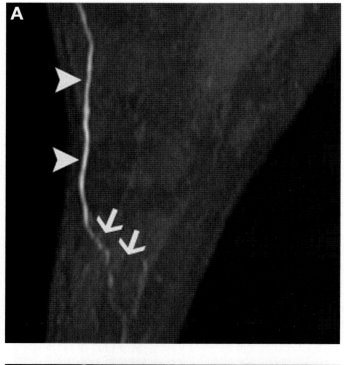

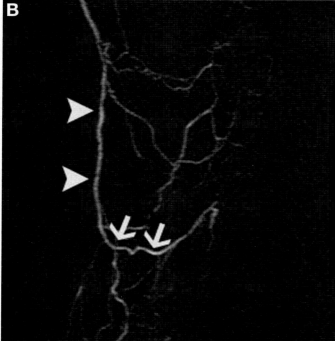

Fig. 2. MIP reformations of TOF (**A**) and CE MRA (**B**) of a foot. The dorsalis pedis artery (arrowheads) is patent on both images. The plantar arch (arrows) is patent on CE MRA, whereas it shows no flow on TOF MRA because of in-plane saturation caused by the course of the vessel, which is parallel to the imaging slice.

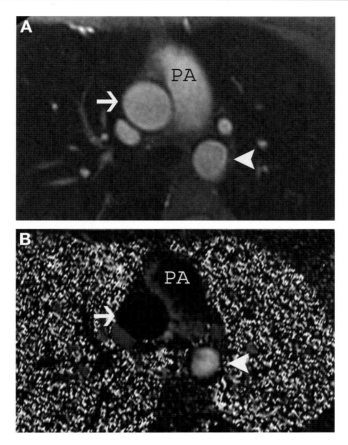

Fig. 3. Axial magnitude **(A)** and phase image **(B)** of PC MRA from the level of the main pulmonary artery (PA). The ascending thoracic aorta (arrow) appears black, and the descending thoracic aorta (arrowhead) is white because the flow-encoded gradient is chosen as superior to inferior. Using special software, the velocity and volume of the blood flow can be calculated.

PHASE CONTRAST MAGNETIC RESONANCE ANGIOGRAPHY

PC MRA is a unique MRA technique because of its ability to evaluate physiological properties of blood flow *(26,27)*. Currently, it is used as an adjunct to CE MRA to evaluate the hemodynamic significance of a detected stenosis *(11)*. Appropriately performed PC MRA can calculate blood flow accurately with a 5% deviation from the true flow *(28,29)*. PC MRA has been shown to be superior to Doppler sonography for measurement of mean flow because Doppler sonography assumes a constant velocity over the whole vessel area; however, PC MRA can take into account the variation of flow in the vessel *(30,31)*.

PC MRA is a 2D sequence usually acquired during a breath hold, and cardiac gating is used to synchronize the measurement of PC MRA to the cardiac cycle. Like moving along a magnetic field gradient, a spin within flowing blood acquires a shift in its rotation in comparison to stationary spins. This phase shift of a moving spin is proportional to the velocity of this spin and can be detected through bipolar gradients. The system performs both flow-sensitive and flow-compensated reference acquisitions, which are automatically subtracted and processed into two sets: magnitude and phase images (Fig. 3).

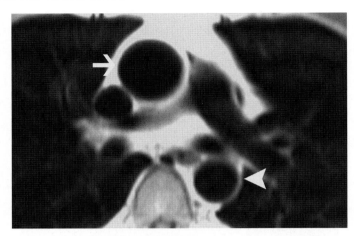

Fig. 4. Axial DIR MRA image obtained with cardiac gating and breath holding shows excellent suppression of the intraluminal signal in the ascending (arrow) and descending (arrowhead) thoracic aorta.

The magnitude images resemble a normal bright blood image and are used for anatomical orientation *(30)*. The phase images are constituted by tones of gray for each pixel that represents velocity information, with higher signal intensities demonstrating higher flow velocities. Blood flowing in the direction opposite to the flow-encoded gradient will return no signal and thus appear dark. Although the PC MRA sequence is available in most clinical MRI units, special software is necessary for postprocessing to calculate flow velocity and volume.

There are several drawbacks of PC MRA, including (1) the velocity-encoding factor needs to be actively chosen before the acquisition according to the expected velocity of the vessel to be imaged (which is typically 150–200 cm/second in the aorta), with larger velocity-encoding values increasing noise, and smaller velocity-encoding values causing aliasing artifacts; (2) the imaging plane needs to be perpendicular to the vessel of interest for more accurate flow measurement; and (3) low temporal and spatial resolution may cause underestimation of the flow and peak velocity *(30)*.

BLACK-BLOOD MAGNETIC RESONANCE ANGIOGRAPHY

Traditionally, T_1-weighted spin echo images have been obtained prior to CE MRA to overview of gross anatomy and for a good road map for subsequent MRA prescriptions *(32)*. These images are called black blood MRA because of the color of the blood on the images, and they typically are obtained in axial orientation with or without fat suppression or intravenous Gd-DTPA and are valuable for evaluation of vessel wall, adjacent soft tissue, and organs. Flowing blood appears dark in signal intensity in conventional spin echo or fast spin echo images because of the washout phenomenon that results from moving the magnetized spins out from the imaging slice before the sampling of the echo. If the blood flow is too slow, turbulent, or the TE is not long enough, then the lumen of the vessel may appear incompletely dark, obscuring proper visualization of intraluminal and mural detail, and may simulate a disease *(4)*.

To overcome this problem, the dedicated double-inversion recovery (DIR) sequence has been developed, eliminating any signal from flowing blood *(32–34)* (Fig. 4).

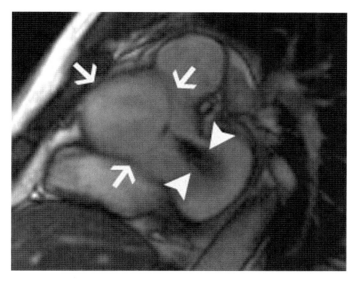

Fig. 5. Oblique sagittal image from cine steady-state free precession (SSFP) acquisition obtained with cardiac gating and breath holding at the level of the aortic root (arrows) shows retrograde flow during diastole (arrowheads).

The technique applies two 180° inversion pulses; one is non-slice selective, suppressing the signal in the imaging volume, and the second is slice selective, restoring the signal in the slice. A time delay (time of inversion) is allowed before obtaining the imaging sequence (generally fast spin echo) to the suppressed blood from the imaging volume flow into the imaging slice. Although this imaging sequence is typically fast spin echo, it can be any sequence depending on availability *(33)*. The technique obtains sequential sections using cardiac gating and breath holding, with TR time equal to one R–R interval and a TE of 20–30 ms, producing T_1-weighted images, or proton density images depending on the length of TR. To maximize the black blood effect, the imaging plane should be chosen as perpendicular to the vessel of interest.

STEADY-STATE FREE PRECESSION

Steady-state free precession (SSFP) or true FISP **(fast imaging with steady-state precession)** is a T_2-weighted, gradient echo technique that widely used in cine imaging of the heart and produces high signal from the blood without need for a contrast agent *(35,36)* (Fig. 5). SSFP has a short imaging time (6–8 seconds for each section) and can be implemented as either a single-shot or cine technique for imaging of the aorta, especially for the aortic root and ascending aorta *(37)* (Movie 1).

CONTRAST-ENHANCED MAGNETIC RESONANCE ANGIOGRAPHY

Basic Principles of CE MRA

CE MRA is the backbone of MRA. It is fast, robust, and accurate without the limitations of flow-dependent MRA techniques mentioned in this chapter *(2,24)*. CE MRA has become possible with the advent of faster MRI scanners, allowing acquisition times within a single breath hold (20–30 seconds), which permits imaging of the arterial first pass of a rapidly injected bolus of paramagnetic contrast material (Gd-DTPA). Gd-DTPA shortens the T_1 of spins, providing bright signal intensity in the lumen of the vessel regardless of flow pattern, direction, or velocity (Fig. 6A–C). Signal intensity of the blood and the overall image quality depend on the intra-arterial contrast material concentration; therefore, synchronization of image acquisition and the intra-arterial Gd-DTPA concentration are crucial.

k-*Space Filling*

Contrast of an MRI depends mainly on the central k-space data, whereas the peripheral lines of k-space contain data primarily for spatial resolution (38). For this reason, filling the central portion of the k-space is necessary during the peak arterial transit of the contrast bolus to obtain selective arterial enhancement. Several contrast timing methods have been developed to estimate contrast travel time accurately; these are discussed in a separate section.

The type of k-space filling (sequential, centric, elliptical centric) can be selected manually by the MRI operator depending on the vessel of interest; the type is typically centric k-space filling for the aorta, but elliptical centric when there is a high risk for venous contamination (such as the aortic arch, thigh and calf stations of peripheral runoff). In centric k-space filling, phase-encoding data begin to be collected from the central lines. Filling the central lines of k-space before the contrast arrival results in suboptimal images with very low signal and ringing artifacts, whereas filling the central lines of k-space too long after the peak arterial contrast produces images with not only arterial enhancement but also enhancement of veins and soft tissue, which limits use of 3D reformats (39–41) (Fig. 7).

Imaging Parameters

CE MRA technique uses a 3D T_1-weighted gradient echo sequence with minimum TR and TE. Flip angle is chosen in the range between 30 and 40° to obtain better background suppression, and bandwidth is generally narrow (31.25 kHz) to achieve images with less noise and high signal-to-noise ratio. Use of a rectangular field of view (FOV) is one way of decreasing imaging time. Parallel imaging techniques such as SENSE can be implemented to decrease imaging time or to increase resolution or signal-to-noise ratio if available (40). The imaging plane can be optimized, depending on the vessel studied (sagittal oblique for thoracic aorta; coronal for aortic arch, abdominal aorta, and renal arteries; sagittal for mesenteric arteries).

Contrast Dose, Rate, and Timing

In CE MRA, signal intensity of an artery is directly related to the intraluminal concentration of the Gd-DTPA at the time of acquisition, especially during the filling of central k-space. Typically, 40 cc intravenous Gd-DTPA is used for CE MRA of the aorta at the infusion rate of 2.5 cc/second. Contrast injection should be followed by saline solution (typically 20 cc at the same rate as Gd-DTPA) to ensure that the contrast material is delivered into the central venous system and does not pool within the tubing or peripheral veins (4).

There are several methods used to determine the optimal delay between the start of intravenous contrast material injection and the start of image acquisition (39). Empirical timing with delay times of 25 seconds for thoracic aorta and 30 seconds for

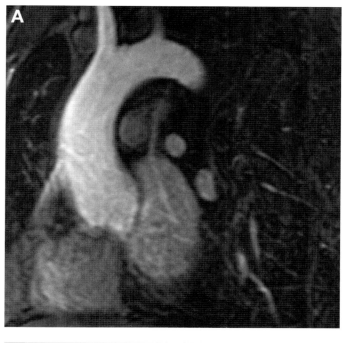

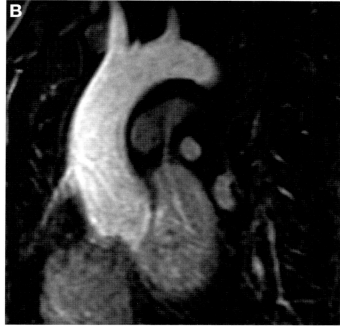

Fig. 6. *(Continued)*

abdominal aorta are generally reliable *(42)*; however, occasionally timing errors can occur. More precise methods to estimate contrast material travel time include a timing bolus scan, automatic detection of contrast bolus passage, or magnetic resonance (MR) fluoroscopic triggering *(39,43–45)*. One of these methods should be used routinely depending on the availability and preference of the operator.

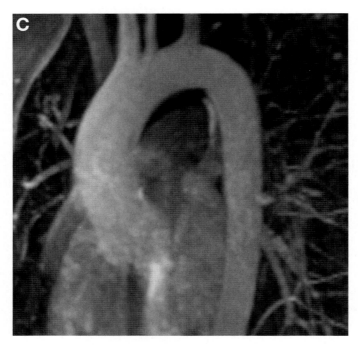

Fig. 6. Sagittal oblique source **(A)**, masked **(B)**, MIP **(C)** image from a CE MRA of the thoracic aorta. Note better background suppression on the masked image compared to the source image, resulting in good quality of MIP reconstruction.

Breath Holding

Image acquisition should be obtained with breath holding, which significantly improves image quality, especially in thoracic aortic imaging. Breath-holding capacity can be improved by supplemental oxygen and hyperventilation *(46)*. In patients with limited breath-holding capacity, normal shallow breathing often results in adequate diagnostic images. Both mask and actual CE MRA acquisitions should be obtained with breath holding for better matching of images.

Image Optimization

Phased array coils significantly increase signal-to-noise ratio compared to body coil and should be preferred whenever possible. Obtaining a mask image prior to CE MRA sequence optimizes background suppression (Fig. 6B). Image reconstructions are obtained following subtraction of the mask image from the CE MRA. A second scan should be routinely obtained and can be helpful in recovering diagnostic information in cases of early scan or to evaluate late-enhancing vascular structures.

Postprocessing

The subtracted images are reconstructed to obtain final MRA images used for the evaluation. Generally, postprocessing is performed on the scanners using available software or can be performed on a commercially available workstation. The obtained images can be interpreted individually or can be placed in a cine loop for demonstration (Movie 2).

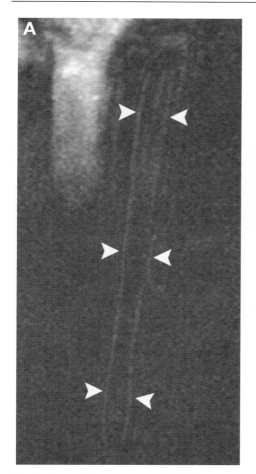
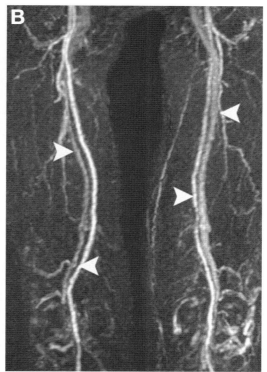

Fig. 7. Coronal image from a CE MRA of the abdominal aorta **(A)** shows very low intraluminal signal with ringing artifacts (arrowhead) because of filling the central lines of *k*-space before the contrast arrival. Coronal MIP reformation of CE MRA **(B)** from thigh station of another patient shows not only arterial enhancement, but also enhancement of veins (arrowheads), which is superimposing on the arteries and limiting use of 3D reformat.

MIP is the most commonly used postprocessing technique and produces projection images as in conventional angiography (Fig. 6C). These images allow overall evaluation of the anatomy interested and are much preferred by referring physicians and surgeons in comparison to viewing the source images. The technique extracts the brightest pixel along the user-defined direction, incorporating 3D data into a 2D image *(47–49)*. The areas with poor flow, such as edges of blood vessels or small vessels with slow flow, can be obscured by overlapping with brighter stationary tissues *(49)*. The filling defects in the center of the vessel may not be demonstrated with this technique. It is well known that MIP reconstructions tend to overestimate the degree of stenosis *(2)*. To overcome these drawbacks, any abnormality seen on MIP images should be correlated with source CE MRA images.

In addition to MIP, axial reformations should be obtained routinely from the subtracted images; these reformations are necessary to evaluate the third dimension of blood vessels because the anterior-posterior dimension of a blood vessel cannot be optimally evaluated

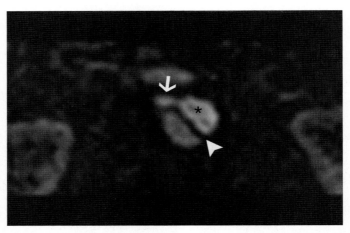

Fig. 8. Axial reformation of CE MRA of a patient with aortic dissection clearly shows intimal flap (arrowhead). Note the right renal artery (arrow) is arising from the true lumen (asterisk).

on coronal MIP images. Axial reformations are also helpful for evaluation of the presence of intraluminal filling defects, such as thrombus, intimal flaps, or atheromas, which cannot be seen well on MIP images (Fig. 8).

Many image postprocessing systems support reformation of a 3D volume into the three main orientations (transverse, sagittal, and coronal) at the same time, so-called multiplanar reformation, and allow viewing the anatomy on one of the orientation and changing the other two orientations interactively as needed according to the course of the vessel of interest. Multiplanar reformation is most effective if the process that needs to be evaluated is limited in spatial extent, such as in the evaluation of the extent and degree of focal stenosis *(47)*.

Volume rendering (VR) is an advanced postprocessing method used to generate a 3D image *(47,50)*. This technique renders images using a ray-casting algorithm that selects visible voxels within the data set from a viewing point positioned outside the vessel, maps these voxels for the degree of signal intensity, and assigns a color to this signal intensity value. A VR image retains all the information from source image regarding the surface of the vessel lumen, which can be identified by thresholding according to the intensity of the vessel of interest. Although VR is excellent in 3D appreciation of the outer surface of the lumen, allowing comprehensive viewing of complex vascular anatomy, it provides no information from within the lumen of the vessel (Fig. 9).

Time-Resolved CE MRA

Time-resolved CE MRA techniques such as time-resolved imaging of contrast kinetics (TRICKS) have been developed and have found widespread use in clinical practice, especially in peripheral runoff *(51–58)*. In this technique, multiple sets of 3D image data are collected so rapidly (in several seconds), eliminating a need for a bolus timing technique, triggering method, or separate acquisition for precontrast mask image (Fig. 10). The TRICKS technique not only simplifies contrast timing but also provides temporal information about relative rates of enhancement of various structures

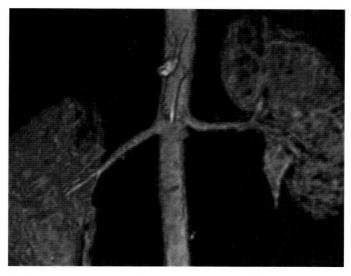

Fig. 9. Coronal CE MRA reconstructed with volume rendering (VR) technique, allowing comprehensive evaluation of outer surface of the vessel lumen but providing no information within the lumen.

within the FOV as in conventional angiography (Movie 3). This multiphase feature of TRICKS could help to assess hemodynamic significance of any vascular disease visualized. However, there is some reduction in spatial resolution when compared with the standard CE MRA technique.

CE MRA of Peripheral Arteries

To evaluate the arterial system of the lower extremity, demonstration of a long segment of vascular tree from the abdomen to the ankle is needed, which requires at least three stations (aortoiliac, thigh, and calf) because of limited length (z-axis) of the magnet. In patients with limb-threatening ischemia, dedicated evaluation of the symptomatic foot is also required. Although a technique of multiple, separate injections for each station has been described, it has not been practical in routine clinical use *(59)*.

Introduction of moving-table technology has allowed "chasing" the contrast bolus distally and imaging all three stations following a single contrast injection *(60,61)*. Table translation from one station to another can be achieved either manually or with help from dedicated software, which can be found in most of today's modern scanners. Although imaging of all three stations with a single contrast injection using the moving-table and bolus-chasing technique produces excellent diagnostic images at the first two stations (aortoiliac and thigh), nondiagnostic calf images are a problem because the current technology is not fast enough to catch contrast material from the aorta to the calf in all cases before venous contamination occurs. This problem especially is seen in higher frequency in patients with limb-threatening ischemia, in whom the demonstration of the status of tibial vessel is crucial for proper surgical planning. Although obtaining high-resolution TOF images of the symptomatic calf and ankle in addition to CE MRA can be helpful, hybrid methods with dual injections have been implemented to overcome this problem.

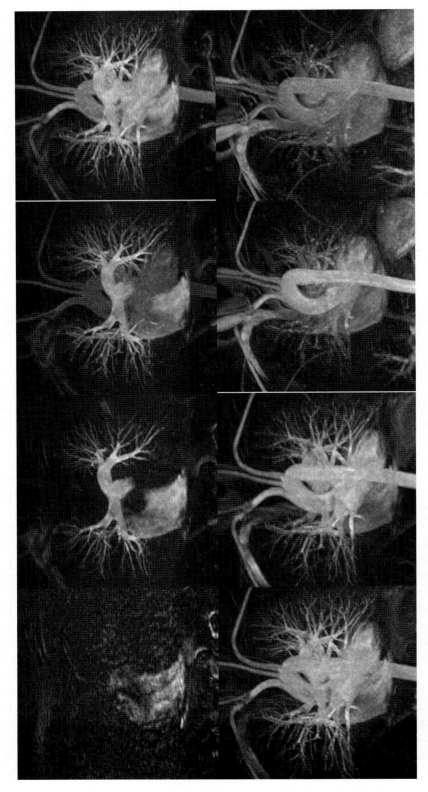

Fig. 10. Series of coronal images from CE MRA of chest obtained with TRICKS shows relative enhancement order of the cardiovascular structures as contrast bolus reach these structures. Note enhancement of the right atrium (the first image in the upper row), the pulmonary artery (the second image in the upper row), the left ventricle and aorta (the third image in the upper row), and then superior vena cava and branches (the images in the lower row) (*see* movie in CD).

In the hybrid method, two sets of CE MRA are performed with separate contrast material injections; first is CE MRA of the calf, followed by two-station CE MRA of aortoiliac and thigh stations *(62–64)* (Fig. 11). Mask images obtained before each injection prevent contrast material contamination from the earlier injection *(60)*. Use of time-resolved techniques for calf station and foot has been useful *(58)* (Movies 4, 5).

CLINICAL APPLICATIONS

Aorta

IMAGING PROTOCOL

The typical imaging protocol of the aorta includes a combination of CE MRA with axial, T_1-weighted, black blood images to visualize both the lumen and the wall of the aorta. Coronal MIP and axial reformation should be obtained to review CE MRA. Postcontrast 2D or 3D gradient echo T_1-weighted images (SPGR) with fat suppression can also be obtained following the CE MRA and are helpful for some pathological conditions of the aorta, such as infectious inflammatory diseases, and for evaluation of surrounding soft tissue and organs.

CONGENITAL AORTIC DISEASE IN ADULT

MRA is a valuable tool in the postoperative evaluation of congenital aortic diseases in adults, such as aortic coarctation. In addition to CE MRA, which is capable of demonstrating postoperative changes or residual stenosis of the coarctation (Fig. 12), the cross-sectional flow through the aorta can be measured using PC MRA to evaluate the hemodynamic significance of the coarctation *(65)*. The flow measurement is performed at two levels: just distal to the coarctation and at the level of diaphragm. In the case of hemodynamically significant coarctation, the distal flow exceeds the proximal flow (ratio greater than 1) because of reverse flow through the intercostal arteries.

The aortic arch anomalies may cause compression on the esophagus or the trachea and may be silent until adulthood. The right arch with aberrant left subclavian artery is the most common right arch variant seen in adults, and aneurysmal dilation of the origin of the aberrant left subclavian artery is called the diverticulum of Kommerell *(66)* (Fig. 13). The right aortic arch with mirror image branching may be associated with congenital heart diseases.

AORTIC ANEURYSM

An *aneurysm* is defined as increased outer diameter of the aorta at least 50% greater than normal, which is approximately 3.5 cm at the aortic root, 3.0 cm at the ascending thoracic, 2.5 cm at the descending thoracic, and 2.0 cm at the abdominal aorta levels *(67)*. The smaller degree of dilation is referred to as ectasia. Atherosclerosis is the underlying cause for most aortic aneurysms, affecting elderly individuals and most commonly involving the infrarenal abdominal aorta (Fig. 14). The atherosclerotic aneurysms are typically fusiform in shape and true aneurysms (all three layers of the wall are involved), in contrast to a false aneurysm, in which the aortic wall layers are disrupted and the aortic lumen is surrounded by periarterial soft tissue. If an aneurysmal dilation of the proximal portion of the ascending aorta including the aortic root and sinotubular junction is seen in a young person, then a possibility of Marfan's syndrome should be sought *(68)* (Fig. 15). An aortic valvular disease, such as aortic stenosis, can

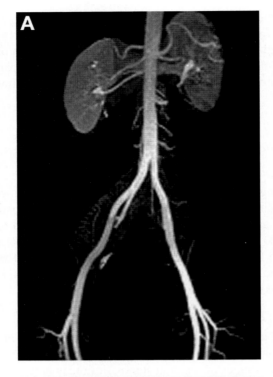

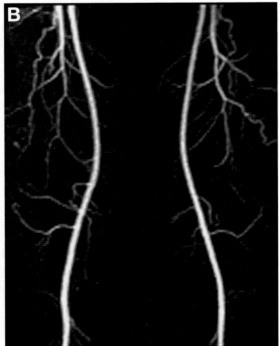

Fig. 11. *(Continued)*

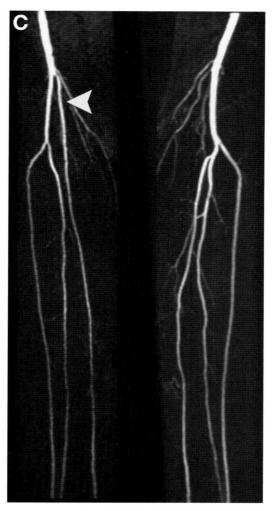

Fig. 11. Coronal MIP reformations of pelvis (**A**), thigh (**B**), and calf (**C**) stations of CE MRA of the lower extremity obtained with a hybrid technique using a separate injection for the calf but a single injection for the pelvis and thigh stations. Only arterial structures enhance, and there is excellent background suppression. Note anomalous high origin of the right posterior tibial artery (arrowhead on image **C**).

also cause aneurysmal dilation of the proximal ascending aorta, but the sinotubular junction remains uninvolved.

Saccular aneurysms are relatively rare compared to fusiform aneurysms and can be secondary to atherosclerosis, traumatic injury, or infection. Mycotic aneurysms result from weakening of the vessel wall by bacterial infection, causing saccular aneurysms and most commonly involving the abdominal aorta, especially at the suprarenal portion (Fig. 16).

If it reaches a diameter of 6 cm or more, then an aneurysm carries a high risk for rupture and should be treated with either surgery or endoluminal stent placement *(69)*.

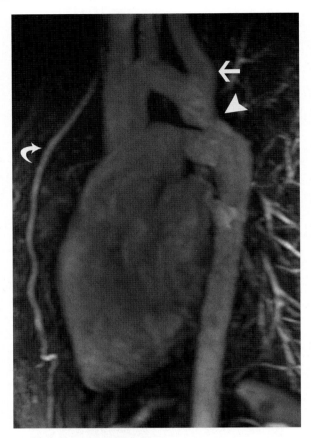

Fig. 12. Oblique sagittal MIP reformation of CE MRA of thoracic aorta of 27-years-old woman with a history of repaired aortic coarctation and now complaining of weakness and claudication in her lower extremities. The image shows focal narrowing in the descending thoracic aorta (arrowhead) just distal to the left subclavian artery (arrow), consistent with aortic coarctation. Note a large internal mammary artery (curved arrow), indicating hemodynamic significance of coarctation.

Imaging surveillance of an asymptomatic aneurysm is recommended to prevent this life-threatening complication. An aneurysm may become quite large and compress adjacent structures. Although the resolution still remains lower than that of multidetector CTA, coronal 3D and axial reformatted images of CE MRA are highly accurate and allow a comprehensive evaluation, including the proximal and distal extent of the aneurysm and relationship to branch vessels (involvement or concomitant occlusion) *(70)*.

CE MRA is especially valuable in patients with contraindications to iodinated contrast material and renal failure who require imaging surveillance. Because CE MRA demonstrates only the lumen and contains little information about the morphology of the aortic wall and adjacent soft tissue, it should be complemented by axial, black blood, T_1-weighted and postcontrast, fat-suppressed, T_1-weighted images *(34)*. The diameter of an aneurysm should always be measured on these T_1-weighted images through a line perpendicular to the course of the vessel and running from outer to outer contour because CE MRA is a luminogram and fails to show mural thromboses, which must be included in the measurement (Fig. 17).

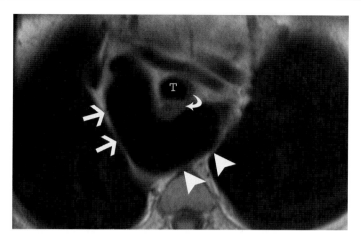

Fig. 13. Axial T_1-weighted DIR image at the level of aortic arch shows a right-sided aortic arch (arrows) on this 76-years-old man. There is also a large vessel (arrowheads) arising from the arch and crossing the midline posterior to the esophagus (curved arrow) and trachea (T), consistent with aneurysmal dilation of the origin of the aberrant left subclavian artery, which is also called the diverticulum of Kommerell. The patient had no complaint related to these anomalies.

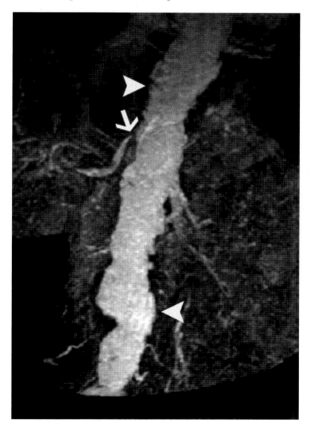

Fig. 14. Coronal MIP reformation of CE MRA shows diffuse fusiform aneurysmal dilation of the abdominal aorta (arrowheads) involving supra- as well as infrarenal segments of the aorta. The contour irregularities are caused by severe atherosclerosis. Note also a focal high-grade stenosis (arrow) at the origin of the right renal artery.

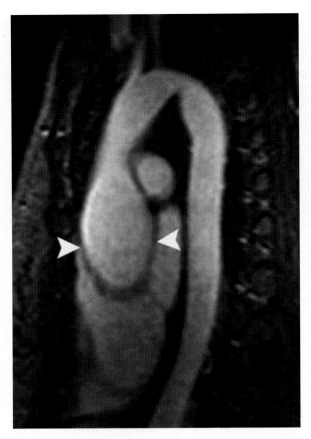

Fig. 15. Oblique sagittal MIP reconstruction of CE MRA of a 33-years-old man with a history of Marfan syndrome shows aneurysmal dilation of the proximal ascending aorta, including the aortic root and sinotubular junction (arrowheads), which is classic for this syndrome.

AORTIC DISSECTION

Aortic dissection occurs when blood enters into the media of the aortic wall because of an intimal interruption, resulting in two lumens: the normal anatomical true lumen, which is surrounded by an intimal flap, and a false lumen, which is an artificial lumen between the intimal flap and the remaining layers of the aortic wall. Initial interruption of the intima frequently starts at two sites, including the proximal ascending aorta and the proximal descending aorta just distal to the origin of the left subclavian artery.

Aortic dissections are divided into two groups according to the segment involved: Stanford type A when the ascending aorta is involved and Stanford type B if the descending aorta is dissected with sparing of the ascending aorta (Fig. 18). The abdominal aorta may or may not be involved. Stanford type A dissection is a surgical emergency with high mortality and may be complicated by contained rupture into the pericardium, which may cause cardiac tamponade; involvement of coronary arteries, causing acute myocardial ischemia; and extension to the arch arteries, compromising brain perfusion *(71–75)*. In some cases, the aortic valve may be disrupted, resulting in aortic regurgitation, which may lead to congestive heart failure.

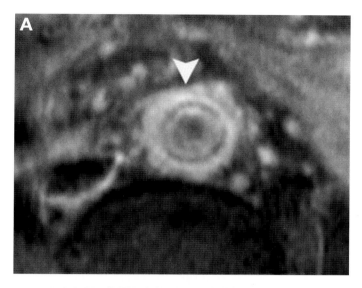

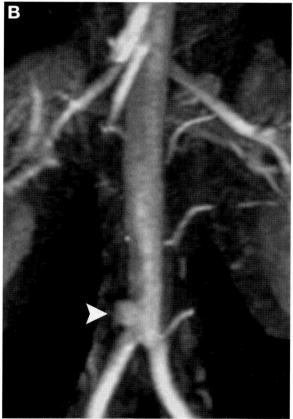

Fig. 16. For a 56-years-old immunosuppressed woman with disseminated fungal infection in the setting of lung transplantation, the axial, fat-suppressed, postcontrast T_1-weighted image (**A**) shows marked circumferential wall thickening of the abdominal aorta (arrowhead), which also shows significant enhancement consistent with infectious aortitis. Coronal MIP reformation of CE MRA (**B**) obtained 3 months later shows interval development of a saccular aneurysm (so-called mycotic aneurysm) at the same level.

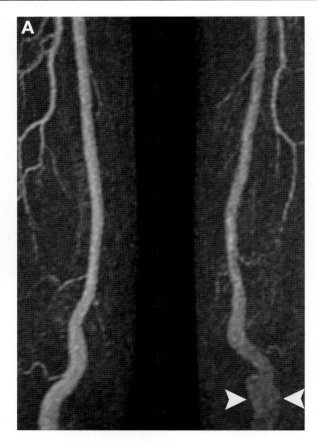

Fig. 17. *(Continued)*

Stanford type B dissections are treated medically unless there is evidence of significant aortic expansion or persistent clinical symptoms. Paraplegia caused by spinal cord ischemia because of disruption of the Adamkiewicz artery is a frequent complication of surgery of the descending thoracic aorta and is observed in up to 30% of individuals after such surgery *(72)*.

CT with multidetector technology is the first-line imaging modality for patients with suspected aortic dissection. It is fast, well tolerated by patients, and widely available. It is highly accurate, especially when cardiac gating is used. MRA is considered the most sensitive method and has the same specificity as CT in the diagnosis of aortic dissection *(73)*, but its use is limited in the emergency setting and reserved only for patients with allergy to iodine and renal failure; however, it is the preferred imaging tool for chronic dissections and postsurgical follow-up *(8,9)*. The extent of the dissection, true and false lumen size, false lumen patency, and branch vessel involvement are important imaging features and can be adequately evaluated by MRA.

In the diagnosis of aortic dissection, the demonstration of an intimal flap is the key finding. Artifacts such as those caused by pulsation may sometimes mimic an intimal flap. These artifacts typically do not persist on all sequences and are seen as a linear signal intensity through the lumen of the aorta, extending beyond the contour of the

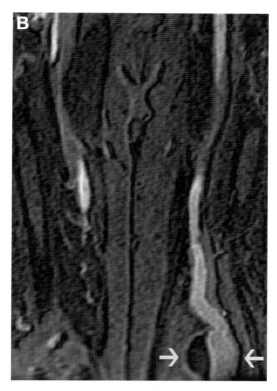

Fig. 17. Coronal MIP reformation (**A**) and source image (**B**) from a CE MRA of thigh shows an aneurysm of the left popliteal artery (arrowheads). Note the maximal diameter of the aneurysm (arrows) is significantly underestimated if the measurement is performed on MIP reformation.

vessel (Fig. 19). Although use of cardiac gating and better breath holding can help to eliminate these artifacts, obtaining axial reformations of CE MRA or postcontrast T_1-weighted images is also helpful in recognizing these artifacts. The false lumen has greater cross-sectional area and slower flow and is usually crescent shaped surrounding the true lumen.

The amount of thrombus in the false lumen is an indirect indicator of the degree of communication between the true and false lumens. In cases with absent or inadequate reentry site (distal intimal tear), the thrombus in the false lumen may progress and threaten to compromise the branches originating from it, or sometimes the size of the false lumen may enlarge over time because of intraluminal high pressure and wall stress, resulting in either significant external compression to the true lumen or an aneurysm with a risk of rupture (Fig. 20). Cine SSFP images can be added to the imaging protocol in cases of ascending aortic dissection to evaluate the presence of aortic valve involvement or sometimes to identify entry and reentry sites.

Aortic dissections have been further classified *(76)*, considering classical dissection (class 1) as a spectrum of more comprehensive pathological process involving the aorta and including IMH (class 2), intimal tear without hematoma (class 3), penetrating atherosclerotic ulcer (PAU) (class 4), and iatrogenic/traumatic dissection (class 5).

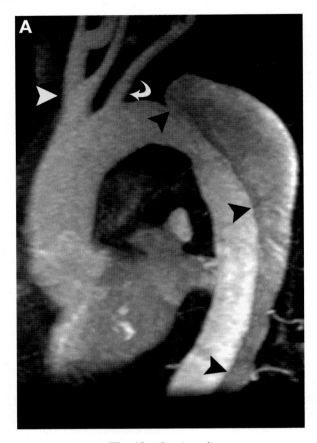

Fig. 18. *(Continued)*

INTRAMURAL HEMATOMA

Intramural hematoma (IMH) is characterized by aortic wall hematoma without visible intimal flap *(77)* and is considered an atypical form of classical aortic dissection. With widespread clinical use of high-resolution cross-sectional imaging techniques, it has been increasingly diagnosed, accounting for 12–22% of patients with acute aortic syndromes in published series *(72,78,79)*. Arterial hypertension has been the most frequent predisposing factor *(79)*. Spontaneous rupture of the vasovasorum of the aortic wall or PAU has been suggested as an initiating factor *(80,81)*.

IMH most frequently involves the ascending aorta and proximal segment of the descending thoracic aorta, as in those with classical dissection *(8)*. IMH is generally considered to be a precursor of classical dissection instead of a separate entity *(79)*. Therefore, the clinical symptoms, prognostic impact of the location, and its standard treatment have been considered similar to those of classic aortic dissection; however, there have been published studies reporting favorable responses to medical treatment with complete absorption of type A IMH without surgical intervention *(77,82–85)*.

On MRA, IMH is diagnosed as a localized wall thickening of the aorta, which is generally crescent shape but could also be circumferential (Fig. 21). The signal intensity of IMH is variable, depending on the age of the blood, and is usually

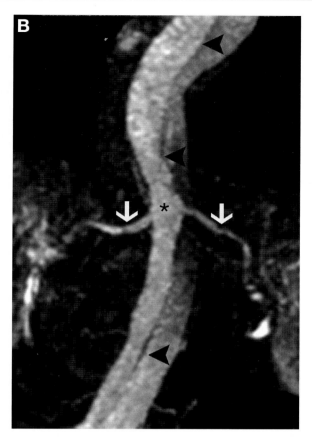

Fig. 18. MIP reformation of CE MRA for thoracic **(A)** and abdominal **(B)** aorta on a patient with type B dissection. There is an intimal flap (black arrowheads) starting just distal to the origin of the left subclavian artery (curved arrow) and extending distally to the abdominal aorta. Both renal arteries (arrows) are arising from the true lumen (asterisk). Note a common origin of right brachocephalic and left common carotid arteries (white arrowhead), a so-called bovine type arch.

bright on T_1-weighted images. Fat-saturated images may be helpful for demonstration of this signal intensity difference and separation of the wall of the aorta from the mediastinal fat. When the signal intensity of the IMH is not high, it may be difficult to differentiate IMH from mural thrombus of atherosclerosis, especially in elderly individuals. In these cases, nonenhanced CT might be useful for confirming the diagnosis.

Penetrating Atherosclerotic Ulcer

A PAU occurs when an atherosclerotic plaque penetrates through the intima into the media of the aortic wall, causing an outpouching of the lumen beyond its expected contour. It is usually seen in elderly individuals with hypertension and severe atherosclerotic disease *(86)* and typically involves the descending thoracic aorta. PAU can be associated with a variable amount of hematoma within the aortic wall in the acute stage, or IMH may develop a focal outpouching resembling PAU *(86–89)*. The majority of PAUs are diagnosed in asymptomatic patients undergoing imaging for other reasons and

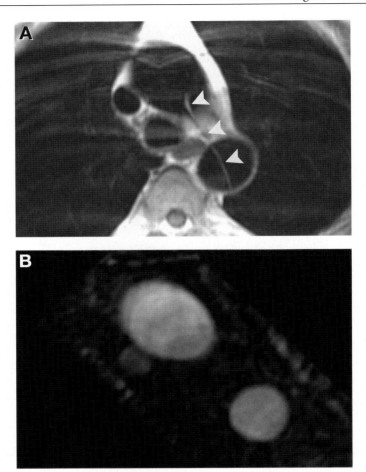

Fig. 19. Axial T_1-weighted DIR **(A)** and axial reformation of CE MRA **(B)** at the level of aortic arch on this study performed to rule out an aortic dissection for a patient presenting with chest pain. On T_1-weighted image **(A)**, there is linear signal intensity (arrowheads) within the lumen of the descending aorta, which could be misinterpreted as an intimal flap. Note the linear signal intensity extends beyond the contour of the aorta, suggestive of an artifact, which likely arose from the aortic arch because of pulsation. No intimal flap is seen on the postcontrast image **(B)**.

remain stable over time *(90)*. However, a PAU can be complicated by saccular aneurysm (caused by a tear through the adventitia), fusiform aneurysm, classical dissection, or aortic rupture *(86,88–90)*. A PAU located in the ascending aorta is treated surgically as in classical dissection, whereas a more distal PAU without clinical signs of instability is managed medically and followed by sequential imaging *(91)*. Unstable descending aorta PAU is considered for more aggressive treatment such as stent-graft placement, which is becoming a popular method to treat this entity given that the disease tends to occur in elderly patients who carry a high risk for surgery because of other comorbidities *(88)*.

On MRA, a PAU is seen as a focal outpouching extending beyond the expected contour of the lumen (Fig. 22). Axial reformations of the CE MRA are especially useful for demonstrating this focal outpouching, which is connected to the lumen of the aorta and fills with contrast material. Sometimes it may be difficult to differentiate a PAU

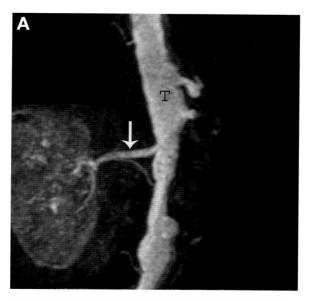

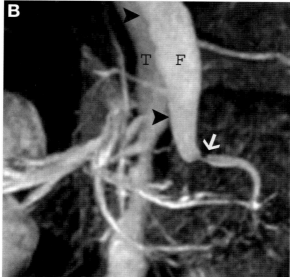

Fig. 20. *(Continued)*

from focal saccular aneurysms, which tend to contain a significant amount of mural thrombus compared to a PAU. In fact, this differentiation may not be clinically relevant if the patient is asymptomatic because both entities are treated medically with imaging surveillance to ensure stability.

INFECTIOUS AND INFLAMMATORY DISEASE OF THE AORTA

Takayasu's arteritis is inflammation of the aorta and major branches (thoracic aorta and arch branches are involved the most), resulting in stenoses and occlusions; therefore, it is also called pulselessness syndrome *(92)*. The disease most frequently

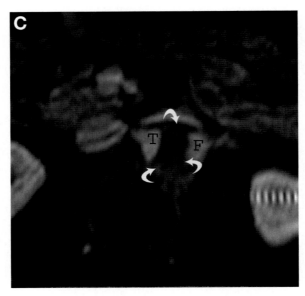

Fig. 20. Coronal first phase **(A)** and second phase **(B)** MIP and axial reformation **(C)** of CE MRA show enhancement of the true lumen (T) on the first phase from which the right renal artery (long arrow) is arising. The false lumen (F) is filled only on the second phase because of slow flow and gives rise to the left renal artery, which shows a focal narrowing at the origin (arrow). Note extensive thrombus (curved arrows) in the false lumen, likely because of lack of a reentry tear, preventing unrestricted blood flow through the false lumen.

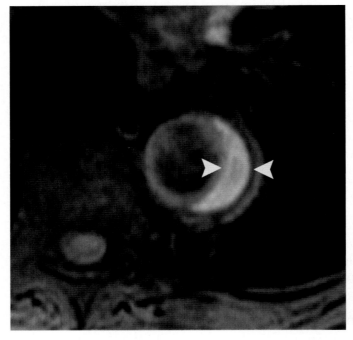

Fig. 21. Axial, fat-suppressed DIR, T_1-weighted image shows crescent shape high signal intensity (arrowheads) in the wall of the descending aorta suggestive of IMH.

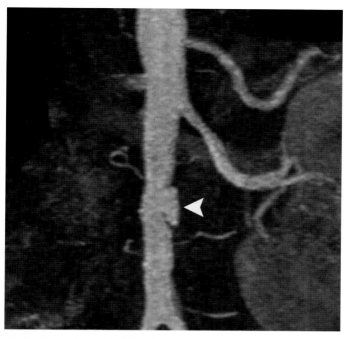

Fig. 22. Coronal MIP reformation of CE MRA shows a focal outpouching (arrowhead) that extends beyond the expected contour of the lumen and likely represents a PAU.

affects young Asian women and is characterized by systemic signs and symptoms initially. The significant imaging feature of this early phase is aorta wall thickening. The occlusive complications of the late phase usually take years to develop. Axial, black blood, T_1-weighted images are highly sensitive for demonstrating the wall thickening of the early phase *(8,92,93)*. Fat-suppressed, T_1-weighted, postcontrast images are used to reveal the enhancement of the thickened wall, which is suggestive of active inflammation *(93)*. MIP reformations of the CE MRA are helpful in determining the degree and extent of occlusive disease of the aorta and arch branches during the late phase *(8)* (Fig. 23).

Giant cell arteritis is the most common form of vasculitis seen in whites, occurring most commonly in elderly women and involving the primary and secondary branches of the aorta and rarely the aorta itself *(94)*.

AORTA AFTER SURGICAL REPAIR

As discussed, many symptomatic aortic diseases, especially the ones involving the ascending thoracic aorta, are treated by surgical repair. In surgery, the diseased aortic segment can either be completely replaced by a synthetic graft (most commonly a Dacron graft) or left in vivo but wrapped around the inserted graft *(95)*. After the surgery, follow-up imaging is routinely recommended to identify graft stability and possible complications, such as graft dehiscence and pseudoaneurysm, or to ensure the stability of the remaining unrepaired segments of the aorta.

On MRA, the graft is recognized as a segment showing an abrupt caliber change relative to the native aorta, which commonly shows atherosclerotic change (Fig. 24).

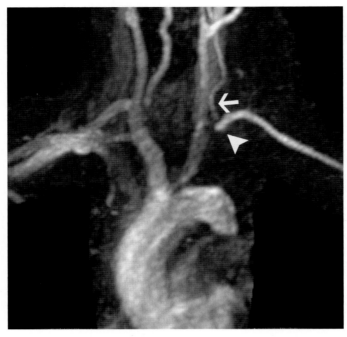

Fig. 23. For a 55-years-old female with a known history of Takayasu disease, the coronal MIP reformation of CE MRA shows total occlusion of the proximal segment of the left subclavian artery (arrowhead), which is patent distally likely because of a retrograde flow through the left vertebral artery (arrow) (so-called subclavian steal syndrome).

A replaced aortic valve is seen as a signal void area in the expected location of the aortic valve because of magnetic susceptibility artifact from the metallic prosthetic valve. Fluid or soft tissue signal intensity material surrounding or adjacent to the aortic graft likely represent an old hematoma and may remain long after the surgery. Metallic stents, which are used for endovascular repair of the descending aorta, create metallic artifact on MRA, and CT should be preferred for evaluating such patients in the absence of contraindications.

Renal Arteries

IMAGING PROTOCOL

CE MRA is the principal MRA technique for evaluation of renal arteries. Patients should be imaged in the supine position, lying on a torso phased array coil to maximize signal-to-noise ratio, and coronal FOV should be placed to start below the heart and cover the iliac arteries inferiorly because accessory renal arteries, rarely, may arise from these arteries. The image volume should include the entire aorta anteriorly and the majority of the renal parenchyma posteriorly, excluding the most posterior portion of the renal parenchyma to decrease the number of slices and the acquisition time. Coronal MIP as well as thin axial reformations should be obtained. Axial or coronal T_2-weighted sequence and postcontrast fat-suppressed T_1-weighted gradient echo (2D or 3D) sequence can be obtained to evaluate renal parenchyma and adrenal glands.

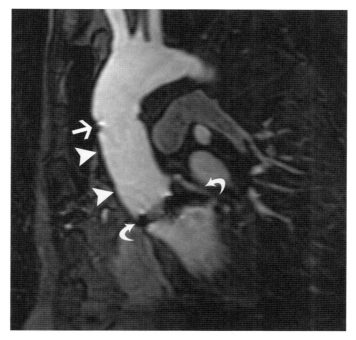

Fig. 24. Oblique sagittal CE MRA image of a patient with a history of ascending aorta repair with a Dacron graft (arrowheads). Note the distal anastomosis (arrow) and metallic susceptibility artifact from the prosthetic aortic valve (curved arrows).

Sagittal 2D cine PC images obtained perpendicular to each renal artery for flow measurements *(96)* or 3D PC images, on which hemodynamically significant stenosis is associated with turbulance-related signal void *(97)*, could be added to the imaging protocol as a complementary sequence.

ATHEROSCLEROTIC DISEASES OF THE RENAL ARTERIES

Renal artery stenosis is a well-known cause of high blood pressure, accounting for approximately 5% of patients with hypertension. These patients are frequently elderly men, and the majority (90–95%) of renovascular hypertension is caused by atherosclerosis.

With recent developments, CE MRA of renal arteries has become a practical screening method for renovascular disease. It is easy to perform and is capable of providing reliable depiction of renal artery morphology with high spatial resolution and with fewer artifacts. The technique has high diagnostic accuracy, with sensitivity and specificity over 90% for lesions greater than 50% of lumen narrowing *(98–101)*. On MRA, atherosclerotic lesions characteristically involve the origin and proximal segment of the renal arteries and commonly are seen as eccentric and irregular lumen narrowing, frequently with a poststenotic dilatation (Fig. 25). Reviewing thin axial reformations from the source images in addition to coronal MIP images is important and helps to prevent overlooking the plaques involving only the anteroposterior dimension of the vessel, which cannot be evaluated properly on coronal MIP images. Every abnormality seen on MIP reformations should be confirmed on source images, and a reader should keep in mind that the degree of stenosis tends to be overestimated on MIP reformations (Fig. 25).

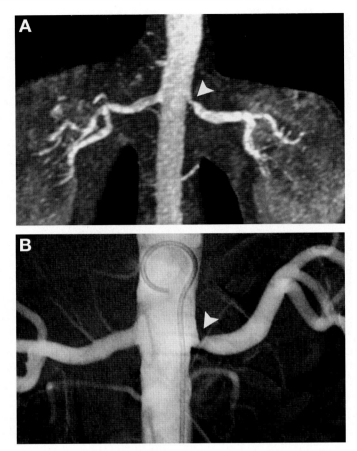

Fig. 25. Coronal MIP reformation of CE MRA **(A)** and digital subtraction contrast angiography **(B)** show focal stenosis (arrowhead) at the origin of the left renal artery. Note the overestimation of the degree of stenosis on the MIP image.

FIBROMUSCULAR DYSPLASIA

Fibromuscular dysplasia (FMD) is a much less frequent cause of renovascular hypertension. It occurs mainly in young women and commonly affects both renal arteries, most frequently mid and distal segments of the arteries. On imaging, FMD is seen as alternating areas of short segmental narrowings and aneurysmal dilations, a so-called string-of-beads appearance (Fig. 26). The resolution of MRA may not be adequate for identifying the disease involving the distal segment, and any patient who is suspected of having FMD should be further evaluated with conventional angiography.

OTHERS

CE MRA is a safe, noninvasive method to evaluate the artery of a transplant kidney. Arterial inflow stenosis, is a treatable cause of graft failure, of a transplant kidney *(102)* (Fig. 27). CE MRA can be used for comprehensive evaluation of potential renal donors prior to harvesting, including number, length, and location of renal arteries, noting any anatomical variant of renal arteries as well as veins *(103)* (Fig. 28). In this indication, a delayed coronal 3D gradient echo sequence can be added to

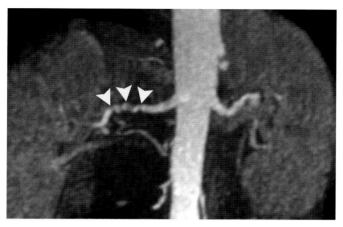

Fig. 26. Coronal MIP of CE MRA of a 47-years-old woman presenting with high blood pressure shows beading appearance (arrowhead) in the midsegment of the right renal artery, which could be caused by fibromuscular dysplasia. Confirmation of the disease with conventional angiography is necessary because artifacts sometimes may mimic this appearance.

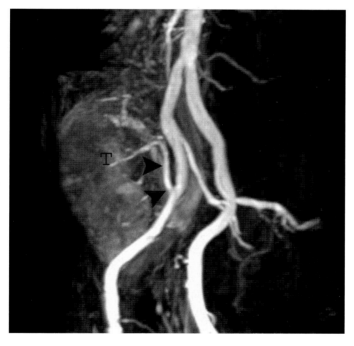

Fig. 27. Oblique coronal MIP of CE MRA shows patent artery (arrowheads) of a transplanted kidney (T) originating from the right external iliac artery.

the imaging protocol to demonstrate the collecting system. For better delineating the collecting system, a small amount of diuretic can be administered intravenously to increase the amount of gadolinium excretion.

Saccular aneurysms of the renal artery can be secondary to atherosclerosis; a high incidence of renal artery aneurysms has been also reported in presence of FMD,

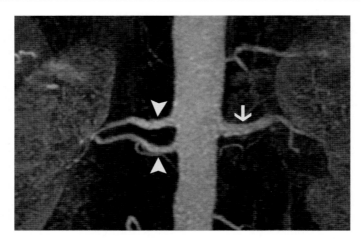

Fig. 28. Oblique coronal MIP of CE MRA of a health renal donor shows two renal arteries on the right side (arrowheads), which is important for surgeon to know prior to surgery. Note a single left renal artery (arrow).

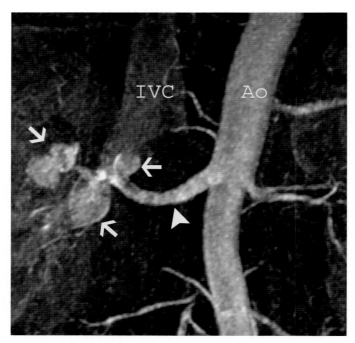

Fig. 29. Coronal MIP reformation of CE MRA of a 47-years-old woman presenting with hematuria shows a large right renal artery (arrowhead) and multiple contrast-filled vascular structures in the renal hilum (arrows) and early filling of the renal vein and inferior vena cava (IVC) consistent with renal arteriovenous malformation.

neurofibromatosis, and polyarteritis nodosa *(104)* (Movie 6). Although CE MRA can demonstrate well the aneurysms of main renal arteries, smaller intraparenchymal aneurysms such as those seen in polyarteritis nodosa are beyond the resolution of CE MRA. Rarely, arteriovenous malformations may involve the kidneys (Fig. 29).

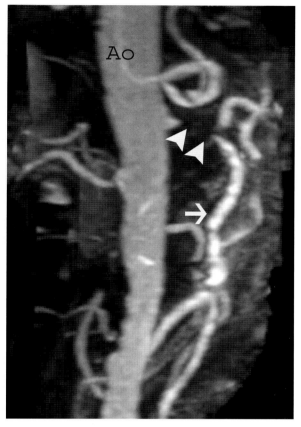

Fig. 30. Oblique sagittal MIP of CE MRA of a patient with a history of significant PVD and multiple episodes of mesenteric ischemia shows occlusion of the proximal segment of the superior mesenteric artery (SMA) (arrowheads) with diffuse distal aneurymastic dilatation (arrow). Note the visualized segment of the SMA shows significant contour irregularities caused by atherosclerosis.

Mesenteric Arteries

IMAGING PROTOCOL

CE MRA with a sagittal imaging plane is used. Flow measurements with PC MRA of superior mesenteric artery and veins *(105,106)* can be added as a complementary sequence.

ATHEROSCLEROTIC DISEASES OF MESENTERIC ARTERIES

Mesenteric ischemia occurs when the blood supply to the intestine is insufficient. The majority of mesenteric ischemia is secondary to atherosclerotic disease and seen in elderly individuals. Because of a rich splanchnic collateral network, mesenteric arterial disease may be clinically silent unless at least two of three mesenteric arteries are severely narrowed or occluded. Atherosclerotic disease typically involves the proximal segments of the mesenteric arteries, which CE MRA has the capability to display with excellent diagnostic accuracy (Fig. 30). The distal mesenteric branches, however, may not be demonstrated well on CE MRA.

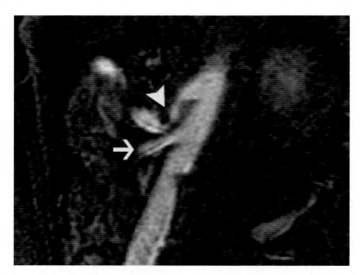

Fig. 31. Sagittal CE MRA of a 50-years-old woman presenting with postprandial epigastric pain and epigastric bruit on clinical exam shows inferiorly displaced proximal segment of the celiac artery with a suggestion of superior external compression (arrowhead). This appearance is typical for median arcuate ligament compression in an appropriate clinical setting. Note patent superior mesenteric artery (arrow).

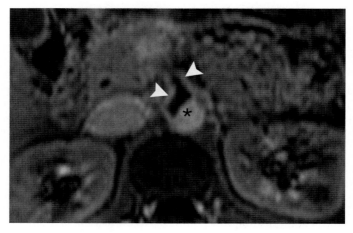

Fig. 32. Axial, T_1-weighted postcontrast image of a 36-years-old otherwise healthy woman presenting with abdominal pain and diarrhea. The image at the level of SMA shows hypointense filling defects in the SMA (arrowhead) and the right renal artery (not shown here), consistent with thrombus. Note patent abdominal aorta (asterisk).

OTHERS

The celiac artery can sometimes be compressed by the adjacent median arcuate ligament, which joins both diaphragmatic crus. On MRA, this extrinsic compression has a characteristic appearance; the celiac axis is displayed inferiorly rather than its normal perpendicular course relative to the aorta (Fig. 31). In rare cases, spontaneous

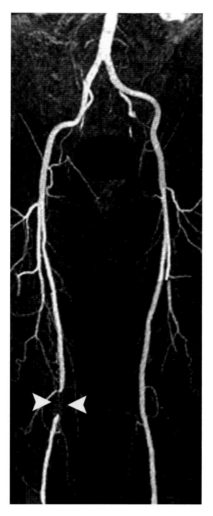

Fig. 33. Coronal MIP reformation of CE MRA of pelvis and thigh using moving-table technique shows occlusion of the right superior femoral artery (arrowheads) at the level of the adductor canal with reconstitution after a short segment.

dissection of the superior mesenteric artery can be seen. An embolic event can be identified by CE MRA if the embolus lodges in the proximal segment of the artery (Fig. 32). Not infrequently, a small saccular aneurysm arising from the mesenteric arteries may be seen on MRA obtained for other purposes.

Arteries of the Lower Extremity

IMAGING PROTOCOL

Although CE MRA with moving-table and bolus-chasing technique after a single injection of contrast material complemented by TOF MRA may be sufficient, hybrid techniques with dual injections as described in the MRA techniques section is more reliable. The TRICKS technique should be used if available for the calf and foot.

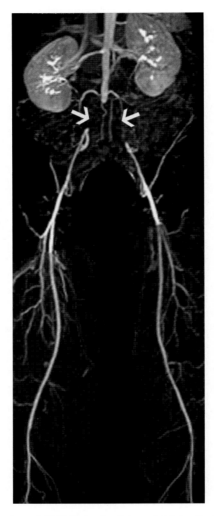

Fig. 34. Coronal MIP reformation of CE MRA of pelvis and thigh of a 48-years-old woman presenting with severe buttock and thigh claudication shows occlusion of the distal abdominal aorta and both iliac arteries (arrows). The patient had hypertension and tobacco use as risk factors.

ATHEROSCLEROTIC DISEASE OF PERIPHERAL ARTERIES

PVD is a common problem, especially in developed countries, affecting 8–12 million Americans *(107)*. Patients may present with claudication, chronically threatened limb, or acute limb-threatening event, resulting in nonhealing wound, gangrene, and even amputations. Although abnormal pressure measurements may indicate the presence of disease, the planning of surgical or percutaneous transluminal revascularization requires precise anatomical mapping. CE MRA is an ideal noninvasive technique for this purpose and has replaced conventional angiography in many centers. CE MRA can demonstrate the location, severity, and extent of the disease with reliable identification of reconstituted vessels. Many investigators have demonstrated the superiority

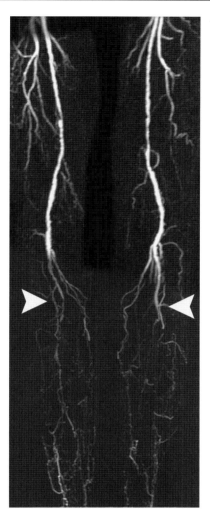

Fig. 35. Coronal MIP reformation of CE MRA of thigh and calf of a 65-years-old woman with diabetes and renal failure presenting with progressive bilateral claudication. The image shows occlusion of both popliteal arteries (arrowheads) at the trifucation with no significant distal reconstitution.

of CE MRA over conventional digital subtraction angiography for the identification of patent arterial segments in infrapopliteal runoff vessels (arteries of the calf and foot) suitable for bypass grafting, especially in patients with limb-threatening ischemia *(108–111)*.

Branching sites and mechanical stress points such as aortic and iliac bifurcations, the origin and distal segment (the segment through the adductor canal) of the superior femoral artery, and popliteal bifurcations are frequent sites of atherosclerotic disease (Fig. 33). The distribution of vascular disease can be specific to underlying systemic diseases, such as isolated aortoiliac disease in middle-aged smokers (Fig. 34) and distal peripheral disease in patients with adult onset diabetes and end-stage renal disease (Fig. 35).

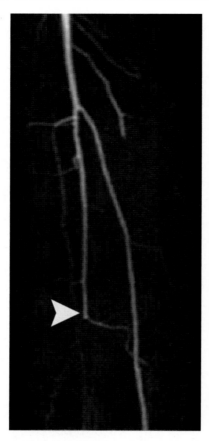

Fig. 36. Coronal MIP of calf CE MRA of 33-years-old woman presenting with right lower extremity claudication following a cesarean section for preeclampsia shows abrupt occlusion of the right peroneal artery (arrowhead), likely caused by an embolic event.

In addition to occlusive disease, atherosclerosis may result in aneurysms. The popliteal artery is the most common site of lower extremity aneurysms and can be complicated by occlusion of the artery because of thrombosis or ischemic symptoms caused by peripheral embolism (Fig. 17). Atherosclerosis is not the only cause for arterial stenosis/occlusions, and asymmetric isolated disease should raise the possibility of other causes, such as embolic event, vasculitis, or external compression (Fig. 36). Popliteal entrapment syndrome is seen in young athletes because of compression of the popliteal artery by the gastrocnemius muscle tendon *(112)*. CE MRA is increasingly utilized for evaluating bypass graft *(113)*. It is important for a reader to know the details of prior vascular surgery or percutaneous intervention as well as the classical appearance of grafts, stents, clips, or other postoperative changes for accurate interpretation (Fig. 37).

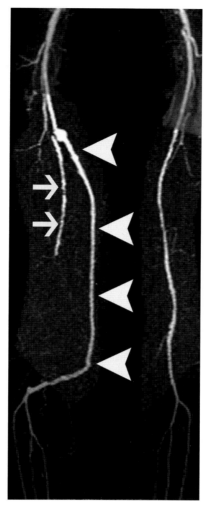

Fig. 37. Coronal MIP reformation of CE MRA of thigh and calf of a patient with prior history of right femoropopliteal bypass grafting shows widely patent graft (arrowheads) with no evidence of disease. Note occluded native right superficial femoral artery (arrows).

REFERENCES

1. Koelemay MJ, Lijmer JG, Stoker J, Legemate DA, Bossuyt PM. Magnetic resonance angiography for the evaluation of lower extremity arterial disease: a meta-analysis. JAMA 2001;285: 1338–1345.
2. Yucel EK, Anderson CM, Edelman RR, et al. AHA scientific statement. Magnetic resonance angiography: update on applications for extracranial arteries. Circulation 1999;100(22):2284–2301.
3. Grist TM. MRA of the abdominal aorta and lower extremities. J Magn Reson Imaging 2000;11:32–43.
4. Ho VB, Corse WR, Hood MN, Rowedder AM. MRA of the thoracic vessels. Semin Ultrasound CT MR 2003;24:192–216.

5. Green D, Parker D. CTA and MRA: visualization without catheterization. Semin Ultrasound CT MR 2003;24:185–191.
6. Czum JM, Corse WR, Ho VB. MR angiography of the thoracic aorta. Magn Reson Imaging Clin N Am 2005;13:41–64.
7. McGuigan EA, Sears ST, Corse WR, Ho VB. MR angiography of the abdominal aorta. Magn Reson Imaging Clin N Am 2005;13:65–89.
8. Tatli S, Lipton MJ, Davison BD, Skorstad RB, Yucel EK. From the RSNA refresher courses: MR imaging of aortic and peripheral vascular disease. Radiographics 2003;23(spec no):S59–S78.
9. Tatli S, Yucel EK, Lipton MJ. CT and MR imaging of the thoracic aorta: current techniques and clinical applications. Radiol Clin North Am 2004;42:565–585.
10. Carroll TJ, Grist TM. Technical developments in MR angiography. Radiol Clin North Am 2002;40:921–951.
11. Carr JC, Finn JP. MR imaging of the thoracic aorta. Magn Reson Imaging Clin N Am 2003;11:135–148.
12. Rajagopalan S, Prince M. Magnetic resonance angiographic techniques for the diagnosis of arterial disease. Cardiol Clin 2002;20:501–512.
13. Neimatallah MA, Ho VB, Dong Q, et al. Gadolinium-enhanced 3D magnetic resonance angiography of the thoracic vessels. J Magn Reson Imaging 1999;10:758–770.
14. Sam AD 2nd, Morasch MD, Collins J, Song G, Chen R, Pereles FS. Safety of gadolinium contrast angiography in patients with chronic renal insufficiency. J Vasc Surg 2003;38:313–318.
15. Rofsky NM, Weinreb JC, Bosniak MA, Libes RB, Birnbaum BA. Renal lesion characterization with gadolinium-enhanced MR imaging: efficacy and safety in patients with renal insufficiency. Radiology 1991;180:85–89.
16. Nelson KL, Gifford LM, Lauber-Huber C, Gross CA, Lasser TA. Clinical safety of gadopentetate dimeglumine. Radiology 1995;196:439–443.
17. Prince MR, Arnoldus C, Frisoli JK. Nephrotoxicity of high-dose gadolinium compared with iodinated contrast. J Magn Reson Imaging 1996;6:162–166.
18. Snidow JJ, Harris VJ, Johnson MS, et al. Iliac artery evaluation with two-dimensional time-of-flight MR angiography: update. J Vasc Interv Radiol 1996;7:213–220.
19. Owen RS, Carpenter JP, Baum RA, Perloff LJ, Cope C. Magnetic resonance imaging of angiographically occult runoff vessels in peripheral arterial occlusive disease. N Engl J Med 1992;326:1577–1581.
20. Carpenter JP, Owen RS, Baum RA, et al. Magnetic resonance angiography of peripheral runoff vessels. J Vasc Surg 1992;16:807–813; discussion 813–815.
21. McCauley TR, Monib A, Dickey KW, et al. Peripheral vascular occlusive disease: accuracy and reliability of time-of-flight MR angiography. Radiology 1994;192:351–357.
22. Huber TS, Back MR, Ballinger RJ, et al. Utility of magnetic resonance arteriography for distal lower extremity revascularization. J Vasc Surg 1997;26:415–423; discussion 423–424.
23. Baum RA, Rutter CM, Sunshine JH, et al. Multicenter trial to evaluate vascular magnetic resonance angiography of the lower extremity. American College of Radiology Rapid Technology Assessment Group. JAMA 1995;274:875–880.
24. Prince MR, Yucel EK, Kaufman JA, Harrison DC, Geller SC. Dynamic gadolinium-enhanced three-dimensional abdominal MR arteriography. J Magn Reson Imaging 1993;3:877–881.
25. Kaufman JA, McCarter D, Geller SC, Waltman AC. Two-dimensional time-of-flight MR angiography of the lower extremities: artifacts and pitfalls. AJR Am J Roentgenol 1998;171:129–135.
26. Walker MF, Souza SP, Dumoulin CL. Quantitative flow measurement in phase contrast MR angiography. J Comput Assist Tomogr 1988;12:304–313.
27. Dumoulin CL. Phase contrast MR angiography techniques. Magn Reson Imaging Clin N Am 1995;3:399–411.
28. Evans AJ, Iwai F, Grist TA, et al. Magnetic resonance imaging of blood flow with a phase subtraction technique. In vitro and in vivo validation. Invest Radiol 1993;28:109–115.
29. Kondo C, Caputo GR, Semelka R, Foster E, Shimakawa A, Higgins CB. Right and left ventricular stroke volume measurements with velocity-encoded cine MR imaging: in vitro and in vivo validation. AJR Am J Roentgenol 1991;157:9–16.
30. Lotz J, Meier C, Leppert A, Galanski M. Cardiovascular flow measurement with phase-contrast MR imaging: basic facts and implementation. Radiographics 2002;22(3):651–671.
31. Lee VS, Spritzer CE, Carroll BA, et al. Flow quantification using fast cine phase-contrast MR imaging, conventional cine phase-contrast MR imaging, and Doppler sonography: in vitro and in vivo validation. AJR Am J Roentgenol 1997;169:1125–1131.

32. Edelman RR, Chien D, Kim D. Fast selective black blood MR imaging. Radiology 1991;181:655–660.
33. Stehling MK, Holzknecht NG, Laub G, Bohm D, von Smekal A, Reiser M. Single-shot T_1- and T_2-weighted magnetic resonance imaging of the heart with black blood: preliminary experience. MAGMA 1996;4:231–240.
34. Jara H, Barish MA. Black-blood MR angiography. Techniques, and clinical applications. Magn Reson Imaging Clin N Am 1999;7:303–317.
35. Carr JC, Simonetti O, Bundy J, Li D, Pereles S, Finn JP. Cine MR angiography of the heart with segmented true fast imaging with steady-state precession. Radiology 2001;219:828–834.
36. Barkhausen J, Ruehm SG, Goyen M, Buck T, Laub G, Debatin JF. MR evaluation of ventricular function: true fast imaging with steady-state precession vs fast low-angle shot cine MR imaging: feasibility study. Radiology 2001;219:264–269.
37. Pereles FS, McCarthy RM, Baskaran V, et al. Thoracic aortic dissection and aneurysm: evaluation with nonenhanced true FISP MR angiography in less than 4 minutes. Radiology 2002;223:270–274.
38. Mezrich R. A perspective on k-space. Radiology 1995;195:297–315.
39. Earls JP, Rofsky NM, DeCorato DR, Krinsky GA, Weinreb JC. Breath-hold single-dose gadolinium-enhanced three-dimensional MR aortography: usefulness of a timing examination and MR power injector. Radiology 1996;201:705–710.
40. Maki JH, Wilson GJ, Eubank WB, Hoogeveen RM. Utilizing SENSE to achieve lower station sub-millimeter isotropic resolution and minimal venous enhancement in peripheral MR angiography. J Magn Reson Imaging 2002;15:484–491.
41. Svensson J, Petersson JS, Stahlberg F, Larsson EM, Leander P, Olsson LE. Image artifacts due to a time-varying contrast medium concentration in 3D contrast-enhanced MRA. J Magn Reson Imaging 1999;10:919–928.
42. Prince MR, Chabra SG, Watts R, et al. Contrast material travel times in patients undergoing peripheral MR angiography. Radiology 2002;224:55–61.
43. Hany TF, McKinnon GC, Leung DA, Pfammatter T, Debatin JF. Optimization of contrast timing for breath-hold three-dimensional MR angiography. J Magn Reson Imaging 1997;7:551–556.
44. Foo TK, Saranathan M, Prince MR, Chenevert TL. Automated detection of bolus arrival and initiation of data acquisition in fast, three-dimensional, gadolinium-enhanced MR angiography. Radiology 1997;203:275–280.
45. Wilman AH, Riederer SJ, King BF, Debbins JP, Rossman PJ, Ehman RL. Fluoroscopically triggered contrast-enhanced three-dimensional MR angiography with elliptical centric view order: application to the renal arteries. Radiology 1997;205(1):137–146.
46. Marks B, Mitchell DG, Simelaro JP. Breath-holding in healthy and pulmonary-compromised populations: effects of hyperventilation and oxygen inspiration. J Magn Reson Imaging 1997;7:595–597.
47. Davis CP, Hany TF, Wildermuth S, Schmidt M, Debatin JF. Postprocessing techniques for gadolinium-enhanced three-dimensional MR angiography. Radiographics 1997;17:1061–1077.
48. Laub G. Displays for MR angiography. Magn Reson Med 1990;14:222–229.
49. Anderson CM, Saloner D, Tsuruda JS, Shapeero LG, Lee RE. Artifacts in maximum-intensity-projection display of MR angiograms. AJR Am J Roentgenol 1990;154:623–629.
50. Cline HE, Dumoulin CL, Lorensen WE, Souza SP, Adams WJ. Volume rendering and connectivity algorithms for MR angiography. Magn Reson Med 1991;18:384–394.
51. Korosec FR, Frayne R, Grist TM, Mistretta CA. Time-resolved contrast-enhanced 3D MR angiography. Magn Reson Med 1996;36:345–351.
52. Barger AV, Block WF, Toropov Y, Grist TM, Mistretta CA. Time-resolved contrast-enhanced imaging with isotropic resolution and broad coverage using an undersampled 3D projection trajectory. Magn Reson Med 2002;48:297–305.
53. Kvitting JP, Ebbers T, Wigstrom L, Engvall J, Olin CL, Bolger AF. Flow patterns in the aortic root and the aorta studied with time-resolved, three-dimensional, phase-contrast magnetic resonance imaging: implications for aortic valve-sparing surgery. J Thorac Cardiovasc Surg 2004;127:1602–1607.
54. Zhang HL, Khilnani NM, Prince MR, et al. Diagnostic accuracy of time-resolved 2D projection MR angiography for symptomatic infrapopliteal arterial occlusive disease. AJR Am J Roentgenol 2005;184:938–947.
55. Du J, Carroll TJ, Brodsky E, et al. Contrast-enhanced peripheral magnetic resonance angiography using time-resolved vastly undersampled isotropic projection reconstruction. J Magn Reson Imaging 2004;20:894–900.

56. Wieben O, Grist TM, Hany TF, et al. Time-resolved 3D MR angiography of the abdomen with a real-time system. Magn Reson Med 2004;52:921–926.

57. Johnson KR, Patel SJ, Whigham A, Hakim A, Pettigrew RI, Oshinski JN. Three-dimensional, time-resolved motion of the coronary arteries. J Cardiovasc Magn Reson 2004;6:663–673.

58. Swan JS, Carroll TJ, Kennell TW, et al. Time-resolved three-dimensional contrast-enhanced MR angiography of the peripheral vessels. Radiology 2002;225:43–52.

59. Rofsky NM, Johnson G, Adelman MA, Rosen RJ, Krinsky GA, Weinreb JC. Peripheral vascular disease evaluated with reduced-dose gadolinium-enhanced MR angiography. Radiology 1997;205:163–169.

60. Ho KY, Leiner T, de Haan MW, Kessels AG, Kitslaar PJ, van Engelshoven JM. Peripheral vascular tree stenoses: evaluation with moving-bed infusion-tracking MR angiography. Radiology 1998;206: 683–692.

61. Meaney JF, Ridgway JP, Chakraverty S, et al. Stepping-table gadolinium-enhanced digital subtraction MR angiography of the aorta and lower extremity arteries: preliminary experience. Radiology 1999;211:59–67.

62. Janka R, Fellner FA, Fellner C, et al. A hybrid technique for the automatic floating table MRA of peripheral arteries using a dedicated phased-array coil combination. Rofo 2000;172:477–481.

63. von Kalle T, Gerlach A, Hatopp A, Klinger S, Prodehl P, Arlart IP. Contrast-enhanced MR angiography (CEMRA) in peripheral arterial occlusive disease (PAOD): conventional moving table technique vs hybrid technique. Rofo 2004;176:62–69.

64. Schmitt R, Coblenz G, Cherevatyy O, et al. Comprehensive MR angiography of the lower limbs: a hybrid dual-bolus approach including the pedal arteries. Eur Radiol 2005;15:2513–2524.

65. Julsrud PR, Breen JF, Felmlee JP, Warnes CA, Connolly HM, Schaff HV. Coarctation of the aorta: collateral flow assessment with phase-contrast MR angiography. AJR Am J Roentgenol 1997;169: 1735–1742.

66. VanDyke CW, White RD. Congenital abnormalities of the thoracic aorta presenting in the adult. J Thorac Imaging 1994;9(4):230–245.

67. Hager A, Kaemmerer H, Rapp-Bernhardt U, et al. Diameters of the thoracic aorta throughout life as measured with helical computed tomography. J Thorac Cardiovasc Surg 2002;123:1060–1066.

68. Nollen GJ, van Schijndel KE, Timmermans J, et al. Magnetic resonance imaging of the main pulmonary artery: reliable assessment of dimensions in Marfan patients on a simple axial spin echo image. Int J Cardiovasc Imaging 2003;19:141–147; discussion 149–150.

69. Elefteriades JA. Natural history of thoracic aortic aneurysms: indications for surgery, and surgical vs nonsurgical risks. Ann Thorac Surg 2002;5:S1877–S1880; discussion S1892–S1898.

70. Prince MR, Narasimham DL, Stanley JC, et al. Gadolinium-enhanced magnetic resonance angiography of abdominal aortic aneurysms. J Vasc Surg 1995;21:656–669.

71. Meszaros I, Morocz J, Szlavi J, et al. Epidemiology and clinicopathology of aortic dissection. Chest 2000;5:1271–1278.

72. Hagan PG, Nienaber CA, Isselbacher EM, et al. The International Registry of Acute Aortic Dissection (IRAD): new insights into an old disease. JAMA 2000;7:897–903.

73. Nienaber CA, von Kodolitsch Y, Nicolas V, et al. The diagnosis of thoracic aortic dissection by noninvasive imaging procedures. N Engl J Med 1993;1:1–9.

74. Nienaber CA, Eagle KA. Aortic dissection: new frontiers in diagnosis and management: Part II: therapeutic management and follow-up. Circulation 2003;6:772–778.

75. Nienaber CA, Eagle KA. Aortic dissection: new frontiers in diagnosis and management: Part I: from etiology to diagnostic strategies. Circulation 2003;5:628–635.

76. Svensson LG, Labib SB, Eisenhauer AC, Butterly JR. Intimal tear without hematoma: an important variant of aortic dissection that can elude current imaging techniques. Circulation 1999;99: 1331–1336.

77. Kaji S, Akasaka T, Horibata Y, et al. Long-term prognosis of patients with type a aortic intramural hematoma. Circulation 2002;106(12 suppl 1):I248–I1252.

78. Evangelista A, Dominguez R, Sebastia C, et al. Long-term follow-up of aortic intramural hematoma: predictors of outcome. Circulation 2003;108:583–589.

79. Nienaber CA, von Kodolitsch Y, Petersen B, et al. Intramural hemorrhage of the thoracic aorta. Diagnostic and therapeutic implications. Circulation 1995;6:1465–1472.

80. Stanson AW, Kazmier FJ, Hollier LH, et al. Penetrating atherosclerotic ulcers of the thoracic aorta: natural history and clinicopathologic correlations. Ann Vasc Surg 1986;1:15–23.

81. Gore I. Pathogenesis of dissecting aneurysm of the aorta. AMA Arch Pathol 1952;53:142–145.

82. Sawhney NS, DeMaria AN, Blanchard DG. Aortic intramural hematoma: an increasingly recognized and potentially fatal entity. Chest 2001;4:1340–1346.

83. Shimizu H, Yoshino H, Udagawa H, et al. Prognosis of aortic intramural hemorrhage compared with classic aortic dissection. Am J Cardiol 2000;6:792–795.

84. Song JK, Kim HS, Kang DH, et al. Different clinical features of aortic intramural hematoma vs dissection involving the ascending aorta. J Am Coll Cardiol 2001;6:1604–1610.

85. Song JK, Kim HS, Song JM, et al. Outcomes of medically treated patients with aortic intramural hematoma. Am J Med 2002;3:181–187.

86. Harris JA, Bis KG, Glover JL, Bendick PJ, Shetty A, Brown OW. Penetrating atherosclerotic ulcers of the aorta. J Vasc Surg 1994;1:90–98; discussion 98–99.

87. Wann S, Jaff M, Dorros G, Sampson C. Intramural hematoma of the aorta caused by a penetrating atheromatous ulcer. Clin Cardiol 1996;19:438–439.

88. Ganaha F, Miller DC, Sugimoto K, et al. Prognosis of aortic intramural hematoma with and without penetrating atherosclerotic ulcer: a clinical and radiological analysis. Circulation 2002;3:342–348.

89. Rubinowitz AN, Krinsky GA, Lee VS. Intramural hematoma of the ascending aorta secondary to descending thoracic aortic penetrating ulcer: findings in two patients. J Comput Assist Tomogr 2002;26:613–616.

90. Quint LE, Williams DM, Francis IR, et al. Ulcerlike lesions of the aorta: imaging features and natural history. Radiology 2001;3:719–723.

91. von Kodolitsch Y, Nienaber CA. Ulcer of the thoracic aorta: diagnosis, therapy and prognosis. Z Kardiol 1998;87:917–927.

92. Choe YH, Kim DK, Koh EM, Do YS, Lee WR. Takayasu arteritis: diagnosis with MR imaging and MR angiography in acute and chronic active stages. J Magn Reson Imaging 1999;10:751–757.

93. Yamada I, Nakagawa T, Himeno Y, Kobayashi Y, Numano F, Shibuya H. Takayasu arteritis: diagnosis with breath-hold contrast-enhanced three-dimensional MR angiography. J Magn Reson Imaging 2000;11:481–487.

94. Hunder G. Vasculitis: diagnosis and therapy. Am J Med 1996;100:37S–45S.

95. Riley P, Rooney S, Bonser R, Guest P. Imaging the post-operative thoracic aorta: normal anatomy and pitfalls. Br J Radiol 2001;74:1150–1158.

96. Schoenberg SO, Knopp MV, Bock M, et al. Renal artery stenosis: grading of hemodynamic changes with cine phase-contrast MR blood flow measurements. Radiology 1997;203:45–53.

97. De Cobelli F, Mellone R, Salvioni M, et al. Renal artery stenosis: value of screening with three-dimensional phase-contrast MR angiography with a phased-array multicoil. Radiology 1996;201: 697–703.

98. Hany TF, Debatin JF, Leung DA, Pfammatter T. Evaluation of the aortoiliac and renal arteries: comparison of breath-hold, contrast-enhanced, three-dimensional MR angiography with conventional catheter angiography. Radiology 1997;204:357–362.

99. Holland GA, Dougherty L, Carpenter JP, et al. Breath-hold ultrafast three-dimensional gadolinium-enhanced MR angiography of the aorta and the renal and other visceral abdominal arteries. AJR Am J Roentgenol 1996;166:971–981.

100. Snidow JJ, Johnson MS, Harris VJ, et al. Three-dimensional gadolinium-enhanced MR angiography for aortoiliac inflow assessment plus renal artery screening in a single breath hold. Radiology 1996;198:725–732.

101. Steffens JC, Link J, Grassner J, et al. Contrast-enhanced, k-space-centered, breath-hold MR angiography of the renal arteries and the abdominal aorta. J Magn Reson Imaging 1997;7:617–622.

102. Ferreiros J, Mendez R, Jorquera M, et al. Using gadolinium-enhanced three-dimensional MR angiography to assess arterial inflow stenosis after kidney transplantation. AJR Am J Roentgenol 1999;172: 751–757.

103. Jha RC, Korangy SJ, Ascher SM, Takahama J, Kuo PC, Johnson LB. MR angiography and preoperative evaluation for laparoscopic donor nephrectomy. AJR Am J Roentgenol 2002;178:1489–1495.

104. Schoenberg SO, Prince MR, Knopp MV, Allenberg JR. Renal MR angiography. Magn Reson Imaging Clin N Am 1998;6:351–370.

105. Li KC, Whitney WS, McDonnell CH, et al. Chronic mesenteric ischemia: evaluation with phase-contrast cine MR imaging. Radiology 1994;190:175–179.

106. Wasser MN, Geelkerken RH, Kouwenhoven M, et al. Systolically gated 3D phase contrast MRA of mesenteric arteries in suspected mesenteric ischemia. J Comput Assist Tomogr 1996;20:262–268.

107. Hirsch AT, Criqui MH, Treat-Jacobson D, et al. Peripheral arterial disease detection, awareness, and treatment in primary care. JAMA 2001;286:1317–1324.

108. Kreitner KF, Kalden P, Neufang A, et al. Diabetes and peripheral arterial occlusive disease: prospective comparison of contrast-enhanced three-dimensional MR angiography with conventional digital subtraction angiography. AJR Am J Roentgenol 2000;174:171–179.

109. Loewe C, Schoder M, Rand T, et al. Peripheral vascular occlusive disease: evaluation with contrast-enhanced moving-bed MR angiography vs digital subtraction angiography in 106 patients. AJR Am J Roentgenol 2002;179:1013–1021.

110. Dorweiler B, Neufang A, Kreitner KF, Schmiedt W, Oelert H. Magnetic resonance angiography unmasks reliable target vessels for pedal bypass grafting in patients with diabetes mellitus. J Vasc Surg 2002;35:766–772.

111. Morasch MD, Collins J, Pereles FS, et al. Lower extremity stepping-table magnetic resonance angiography with multilevel contrast timing and segmented contrast infusion. J Vasc Surg 2003;37:62–71.

112. Atilla S, Ilgit ET, Akpek S, Yucel C, Tali ET, Isik S. MR imaging and MR angiography in popliteal artery entrapment syndrome. Eur Radiol 1998;8:1025–1029.

113. Loewe C, Cejna M, Schoder M, et al. Contrast material-enhanced, moving-table MR angiography vs digital subtraction angiography for surveillance of peripheral arterial bypass grafts. J Vasc Interv Radiol 2003;14(9 pt 1):1129–1137.

27 Assessment of Pulmonary Venous Anatomy

Thomas H. Hauser and Dana C. Peters

The development of radio-frequency ablation for the treatment of atrial fibrillation has led to increased interest in the accurate determination of pulmonary vein anatomy to help plan the procedure and to monitor for postablation stenosis. Contrast-enhanced magnetic resonance angiography readily demonstrates the pulmonary veins and is the method of choice for these required serial imaging studies. In this chapter, we review the techniques for pulmonary vein imaging, normal and variant pulmonary vein anatomy, the utility of imaging prior to and after atrial fibrillation ablation, and congenital pulmonary vein anomalies.

IMAGING TECHNIQUE

The pulmonary veins can be identified using standard anatomical and functional cardiovascular magnetic resonance (CMR) imaging sequences. Although these methods are often able to identify the anatomical relationship of the pulmonary veins to the heart and the other major vascular structures, the pulmonary veins are frequently imaged using contrast-enhanced magnetic resonance angiography.

A three-dimensional (3D) spoiled gradient echo sequence is acquired during the first pass of gadolinium contrast (1). Clinical protocols vary but have many common

From: *Contemporary Cardiology: Cardiovascular Magnetic Resonance Imaging*
Edited by: Raymond Y. Kwong © Humana Press Inc., Totowa, NJ

elements *(2–10)*. This method uses short repetition times (3–6 ms), a high flip angle (30–60°), and fractional echoes to provide T_1-weighting and to minimize flow artifacts. The spatial resolution varies from 1 to 2 × 1 to 2 mm in-plane with 2- to 4-mm slices before interpolation.

A single 3D volume requires an approximately 10-seconds breath hold to suppress ventilatory motion, but scan time can be shortened using smaller fields of view, shorter repetition times, partial Fourier, lower spatial resolution, or parallel imaging. Electrocardiographic (ECG) triggering is not generally used, but it is recognized that the position and shape of the pulmonary veins change throughout the cardiac cycle *(7,11)*. Images obtained with this method appear to reflect the pulmonary veins at their maximal size *(12)*. Slabs are usually acquired in the axial plane using either sequential or centric *k*-space filling. For the pulmonary vasculature, the arterial-venous transit time is short (4–7 seconds) *(13)*, so that artery-vein separation is highly challenging and generally not needed.

Gadolinium contrast is injected with a dose of 0.1–0.3 mmol/kg at a rate of 1–2 mL/second, followed by a saline flush. A precontrast mask can be acquired, but mask subtraction is not needed for pulmonary venography because the background signal in the lungs is low. Often, a second dynamic is acquired immediately after the first-pass image to ensure acquisition during peak contrast. Timing of the acquisition is critical to capture the first pass of contrast through the pulmonary veins and is achieved using either a bolus timing scan *(14)* or fluoroscopic triggering *(15)*. Imaging is timed to begin with the appearance of contrast in the left atrium with either method.

IMAGE DISPLAY

Once obtained, the 3D magnetic resonance angiography data set can be transferred to a workstation for further manipulation and analysis (Fig. 1). The simplest and often most informative method to display the images is to dynamically view two-dimensional (2D) slices within the 3D data set in the axial, coronal, and sagittal planes. The axial images generally provide a good review of the pulmonary veins and their relationship to the left atrium, but the coronal and sagittal images are usually required to determine specific anatomical findings and variant or anomalous pulmonary veins.

Although 2D slices are useful for viewing the individual pulmonary veins, it is difficult to produce a single summary image of the entire anatomy. Maximal intensity projection images and 3D reconstructions displayed as shaded surface or volume-rendered images take full advantage of the 3D data set and provide good summary images. These are most useful when the displayed volume is limited to the left atrium and pulmonary veins. Because the aorta is directly posterior to the left-sided pulmonary vein, it frequently obscures them from a view in the maximal intensity projection images. 3D reconstructed images are often preferred because the aorta can be excluded from the displayed volume. Cine images can also be generated to better display the anatomy. The left atrium and pulmonary veins are viewed in the posterior-anterior orientation by convention. Direct anatomical measurements should be obtained from the 2D slices, not from these postprocessed images.

EMBRYOLOGY OF THE PULMONARY VEINS

An understanding of pulmonary vein embryology is important for the understanding of normal pulmonary vein anatomy, nonpathological variations from the normal anatomy, and congenital anomalies. The pulmonary veins and left atrium are derived from the primitive common pulmonary vein. The primitive pulmonary venous system

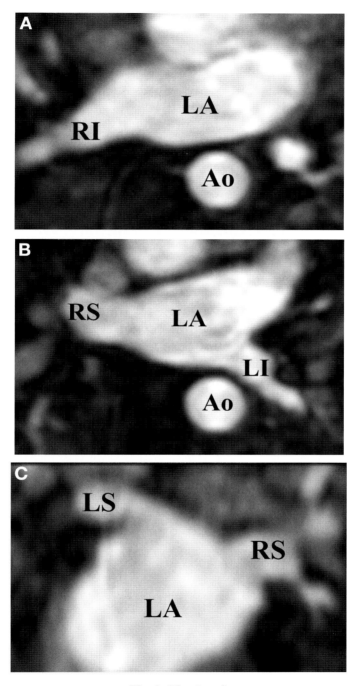

Fig. 1. *(Continued)*

originally has no connection with the heart and drains into the cardinal veins and the umbilicovitelline system.

At approximately the fourth week of gestation, the pulmonary venous drainage merges into a single vessel *(16)*. An outgrowth of the primitive left atrium extends toward the pulmonary venous system to meet this vessel at the same time to form the primitive

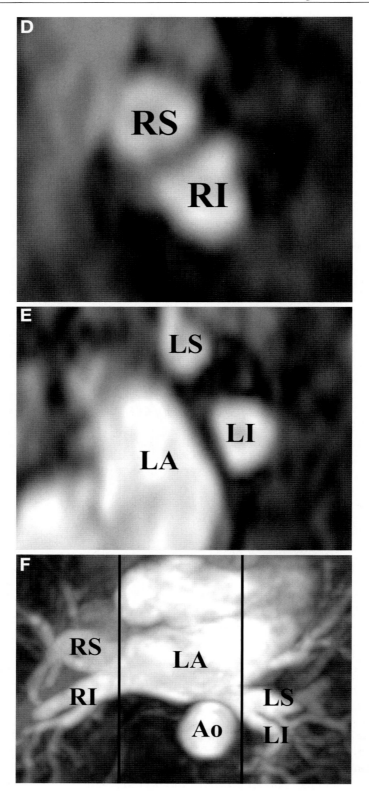

Fig. 1. *(Continued)*

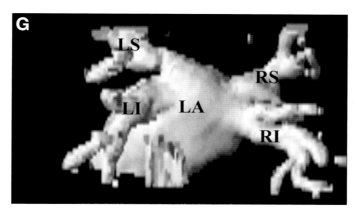

Fig. 1. Normal anatomy and quantification of pulmonary vein size. These images show the four pulmonary veins along with the left atrium (LA) and descending aorta (Ao). The right inferior (RI), right superior (RS), and left inferior (LI) pulmonary veins are shown in the axial plane **(A)** and **(B)**. The left superior (LS) and right superior pulmonary veins are shown in the coronal plane (posterior-anterior orientation) **(C)**. The right-sided **(D)** and left-sided **(E)** pulmonary veins are shown in the sagittal plane (anterior to the left). All of the veins are shown in the axial maximal intensity projection **(F)** and posterior-anterior shaded surface **(G)** images. The aorta has been removed from the shaded surface image to show all of the pulmonary veins. The lines in the maximal intensity projection image **(F)** correspond to the location in the sagittal plane in which the pulmonary veins separate from the left atrium and from each other **(D)** and **(E)**. The maximal diameter, perimeter, and cross-sectional area can be readily measured in the sagittal images.

common pulmonary vein. The venous connections to the cardinal veins and the umbilicovitelline system degenerate. The common pulmonary vein then expands to form the body of the left atrium; the primitive left atrium forms the trabeculated left atrial appendage *(17)*.

The branches of the primitive common pulmonary vein eventually form the adult pulmonary veins. There is asymmetrical development of the left atrium and pulmonary veins, with the two right-sided pulmonary veins developing first; the left-sided pulmonary venous drainage enters the left atrium through a single trunk that eventually bifurcates to form two veins *(18)*.

NORMAL ANATOMY AND COMMON VARIATIONS

There are typically four pulmonary veins that enter the left atrium: left superior, left inferior, right superior, and right inferior (Fig. 1). Each of these veins is directed laterally. The inferior veins are directed posteriorly, and the superior veins are directed anteriorly. The left superior pulmonary vein often has a cranial angulation and may appear to come from the superior portion of the left atrium.

Nonpathological variant pulmonary vein anatomy is common, occurring in approximately 40% of patients *(2,19)*. Although many variations have been described, the most frequent variations in the usual anatomy are the presence of a left common pulmonary vein or a right middle pulmonary vein (Fig. 2) *(3)*. These variations occur because of more or less integration of the primitive common pulmonary vein into the left atrium. Less integration leads to apparent fusion of pulmonary veins prior to entering the left atrium; more integration results in additional pulmonary veins (Fig. 3). It is more common to have additional pulmonary veins on the right because the right-sided veins form first and have more developmental time to be integrated into the left

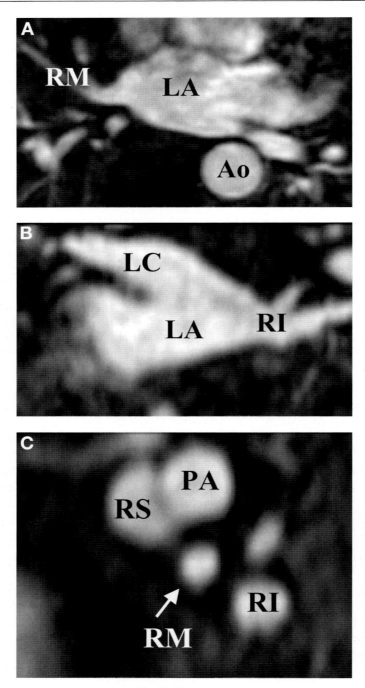

Fig. 2. *(Continued)*

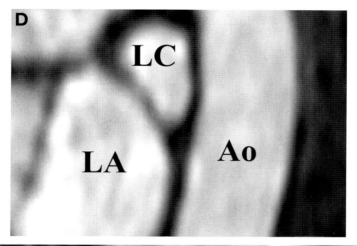

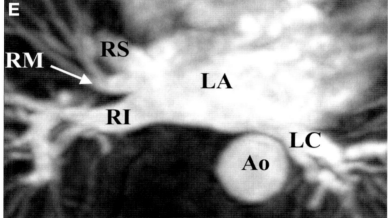

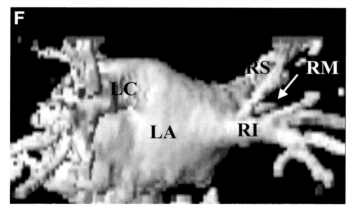

Fig. 2. *(Continued)*

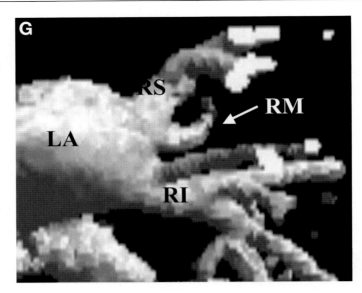

Fig. 2. Variant anatomy. Imaging was performed in a patient with right middle and left common pulmonary veins. The right middle (RM) pulmonary vein is shown in the axial plane (**A**). The left common (LC) pulmonary vein is shown in the coronal plane (posterior-anterior orientation) (**B**). All three right (**C**) and the left common pulmonary veins (**D**) are shown in the sagittal plane (anterior to the left) with the pulmonary artery (PA) adjacent to the right superior pulmonary vein. All of the veins are shown in the axial maximal intensity projection (**E**) and posterior-anterior shaded surface (**F**) images. The aorta has been removed from the shaded surface image. The right middle pulmonary vein is obscured by the right inferior pulmonary vein and is best seen with cranial angulation (**G**). It is often necessary to manipulate the point of view to see all of the pulmonary veins.

atrium. The left-sided pulmonary veins form later and are more likely to have a common trunk. No pathology has been identified as a result of these variations in pulmonary venous anatomy.

PATHOPHYSIOLOGY OF ATRIAL FIBRILLATION
AND THE PULMONARY VEINS

Atrial fibrillation is the most common sustained cardiac arrhythmia, affecting more than 2 million people in the United States *(20)*. It is a major cause of morbidity and mortality, accounting for more than 400,000 hospitalizations each year *(21)* and increasing the risk of death by 50% *(22)*. Atrial fibrillation quintuples the risk of stroke *(23)* and is the attributed cause for 15% of all strokes, more than 100,000 per year *(21)*. The costs for treatment of atrial fibrillation are estimated at over $1 billion *(21)*. Although several antiarrhythmic drugs are available for the treatment of atrial fibrillation, maintenance of sinus rhythm is frequently suboptimal *(24–26)*, and all have significant side effects or associated adverse events *(27)*.

Evidence suggests that the pulmonary veins play a critical role in the pathophysiology of atrial fibrillation. The pulmonary veins and left atrium are each derived from the primitive common pulmonary vein *(17)* and thus have many anatomical similarities. Both are smooth-walled structures that have electrically active myocardium, with atrial myocardium in approximately 90% *(28)*. Although the myocardium in the atrium is uniform, myocardium in the pulmonary veins is often discontinuous and fibrotic.

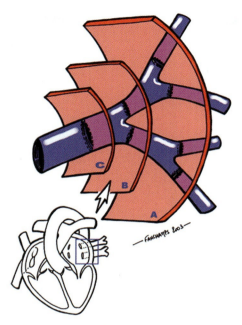

Fig. 3. Integration of the primitive common pulmonary vein into the left atrium. The integration of the primitive common pulmonary vein is variable and results in nonpathological variations in the normal anatomy. This figure shows the results of variable integration of the left-sided pulmonary veins. The most common pattern is two left-sided pulmonary veins (plane B). With less integration of the common pulmonary vein into the left atrium, there is only a single left common pulmonary vein (plane C). With more integration, there are additional pulmonary veins (plane A). (From ref. *74*.)

Patients with a history of atrial fibrillation uniformly have myocardium in the pulmonary veins and an increased rate of structural abnormalities. These structural abnormalities result in abnormal electrical activation with slow and anisotropic conduction *(29)*.

A pivotal study demonstrated that the proarrhythmic electrical activity in pulmonary veins is responsible for the generation of atrial fibrillation in many patients *(30)*. Among those with paroxysmal atrial fibrillation, 94% were found to have ectopic foci in the pulmonary veins that were responsible for the induction of atrial fibrillation. Ablation of these foci resulted in complete suppression of atrial fibrillation in a majority of patients.

Several related procedures were developed for the treatment of atrial fibrillation after the report of these findings *(30–34)*. These procedures use radio-frequency ablation to electrically isolate the pulmonary veins from the left atrium. Short-term success rates range from 65 to 85% in patients with paroxysmal atrial fibrillation, with a reduction in morbidity and improved quality of life *(35)*.

IMAGING AND ATRIAL FIBRILLATION ABLATION

Imaging the pulmonary veins is usually performed before atrial fibrillation ablation to determine the number and position of pulmonary veins and after the procedure to screen for stenosis.

The planning and performance of atrial fibrillation ablation requires accurate determination of pulmonary vein anatomy. The operator must place a series of radio-frequency

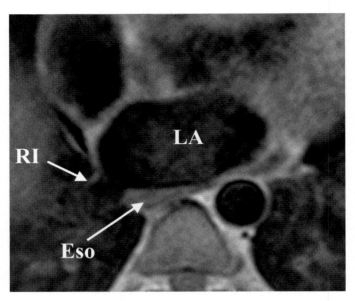

Fig. 4. Relationship of the esophagus to the pulmonary veins and left atrium. This spin echo T_1-weighted image shows the esophagus (Eso) posterior to the left atrium and adjacent to the right inferior pulmonary vein.

lesions that encircle the pulmonary veins and electrically isolate them from the left atrium to achieve success *(36)*. Thus, the pulmonary vein anatomy must be determined prior to the procedure. During initial development of the procedure, the pulmonary veins were identified using invasive contrast venography *(37)*. Although this can be done successfully, it greatly increases the procedure time and only provides projection images of the pulmonary veins. Most centers now use magnetic resonance angiography or computed tomography to determine the pulmonary vein anatomy prior to the procedure. Both techniques provide high-resolution 3D tomographic images of the pulmonary veins and other mediastinal structures. These images can be imported into the 3D electrophysiological mapping systems that are an important part of the procedure to combine anatomical and functional information during the procedure *(38)*.

Excessive heating of the left atrial wall and the adjacent esophagus can rarely lead to the formation of an atrial-esophageal fistula, a catastrophic complication *(39–42)*. Standard anatomical CMR sequences can easily identify the esophagus and its relationship to the left atrium (Fig. 4). The esophagus nearly always directly abuts the left atrium and is frequently closer to the left-sided pulmonary veins, but the location is highly variable *(43–45)*. The esophagus is often within 5 mm of the pulmonary veins *(46,47)*. The risk of an atrial-esophageal fistula may be reduced by avoiding ablation in the region of the left atrium closest to the esophagus. This may be difficult because the esophagus is mobile and may move during the course of the procedure *(48)*.

Pulmonary vein imaging is performed after the procedure to screen for pulmonary vein stenosis. Stenosis is an uncommon, severe complication of atrial fibrillation ablation (Fig. 5) *(2,19,37,49–55)*. Radio-frequency energy application to the pulmonary veins causes intimal proliferation and myocardial necrosis, which can result in stenosis or occlusion *(56)*. Severe stenosis occurs in up to 5% of patients and causes pulmonary hypertension and decreased perfusion of the affected lung segments

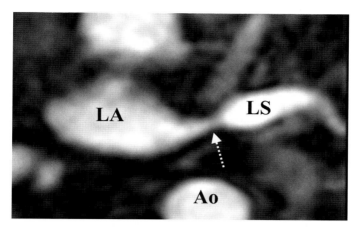

Fig. 5. Pulmonary vein stenosis. There is severe stenosis of the left superior pulmonary vein with prestenotic dilation.

(57,58). Patients frequently present with cough or dyspnea, but a significant percentage are asymptomatic *(51)*.

Stenosis is most likely to occur in smaller pulmonary veins in which the ablation lesions were placed more proximally into the pulmonary vein trunk and with greater extent of ablation *(54,55)*. If stenosis does occur, then pulmonary vein angioplasty is generally successful in restoring normal flow and alleviating symptoms *(59)*. Newer techniques that have emphasized placing ablation lesions closer to the left atrium under intracardiac echocardiographic guidance have reduced the rate of pulmonary vein stenosis *(50)*, but screening is still recommended for all patients.

PULMONARY VEIN SIZE QUANTIFICATION

Accurate measurement of pulmonary vein size is important for serial assessment of pulmonary vein stenosis and to further investigate the role of the pulmonary veins in the generation and maintenance of atrial fibrillation. Most investigators have measured pulmonary vein diameters in a specified plane, usually at the ostia *(2,37,55)*. These measurements tend to have poor reproducibility (Fig. 6). Identification of the true ostia is difficult because the pulmonary veins and left atrium are embryologically related with no clear anatomical border between them. The pulmonary vein ostia are oblong, such that measurements taken at the same location vary significantly with the plane of measurement *(2,3)*.

Most measurements are derived from nongated images while the pulmonary vein size varies significantly over the cardiac cycle *(7,60)*. These difficulties were shown in a study comparing pulmonary vein diameter measurements performed using computed tomography, intracardiac echocardiography, transesophageal echocardiography, and venography in the same patients *(61)*. Each of these methods identified different numbers and positions of pulmonary veins. There was a poor correlation between diameter measurements obtained with each imaging modality.

Tomographic pulmonary vein imaging using CMR has several advantages. All of the anatomical information is obtained in a 3D data set that can be manipulated as needed. This allows for anatomical measurements in any plane, including determination of the perimeter and cross-sectional area that may be more meaningful measures of pulmonary vein size.

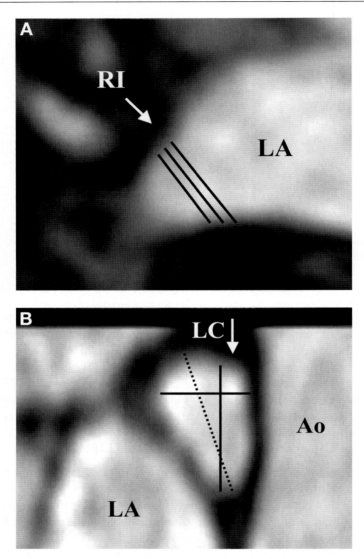

Fig. 6. Difficulty in measurement of pulmonary vein diameters. These images show a right inferior pulmonary vein in the axial plane **(A)** and a left common pulmonary vein in the sagittal plane **(B)**. There is no clear anatomical border between the right inferior pulmonary vein and the left atrium **(A)** such that several potential diameter measurements are possible (solid lines). The left common pulmonary vein is oval **(B)**. The diameters measured in the axial plane (horizontal line) and coronal plane (vertical line) differ from each other and from the true maximal diameter (dashed line).

A simple method for determining pulmonary vein size in the sagittal plane has been described that is highly reproducible and provides these additional measures *(3)*. The maximal diameter, perimeter, and cross-sectional area are measured at the location in the sagittal plane at which the pulmonary veins separate from the left atrium and from each other (Fig. 1). This is determined by scrolling through a reconstruction of the 3D data set in the sagittal plane. Because the measurements are made in a standard plane and location, reproducibility is improved compared to standard diameter

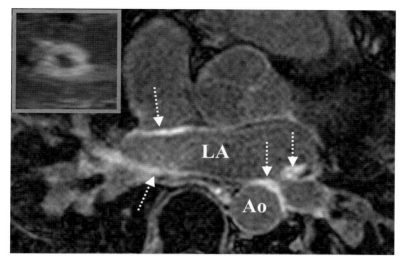

Fig. 7. Delayed-enhancement imaging. This delayed-enhancement image was obtained 6 weeks after atrial fibrillation ablation. There is evidence of scar around the pulmonary veins (dashed arrows). The increased signal in the lumen of the right-sided pulmonary veins is caused by artifact from the ventilatory compensation technique. The inset shows a reformatted image of the left inferior pulmonary vein that demonstrates circumferential scar.

measurements *(3)*. This allows for more accurate determination of interstudy differences in pulmonary vein size and increased statistical power in research studies. Even in the absence of severe stenosis, this method can identify small changes in pulmonary vein size after atrial fibrillation ablation that may be caused by hemodynamic changes related to the restoration of sinus rhythm *(4)*.

It is also advantageous to measure the perimeter and cross-sectional area. Patients with larger summed total pulmonary vein cross-sectional area are more likely to have recurrent atrial fibrillation after ablation independent of the type of atrial fibrillation or left atrial size *(62)*. Diameter measurements do not have predictive value *(35)*.

DELAYED-ENHANCEMENT IMAGING

Radio-frequency ablation results in scarring of the pulmonary vein and left atrium *(56)*. Imaging scar has the potential to noninvasively assess the completeness of ablation by providing a precise anatomical map of the ablation lines. This may be useful after the procedure to assess patient outcomes or as a real-time tool to guide ablation during interventional CMR. Scar can be detected using delayed enhancement *(63)*, in which a strongly T_1-weighted magnetic resonance image is acquired late after the injection of gadolinium contrast *(64)*. Contrast remains concentrated in the regions of scar, compared to muscle or blood, because of reduced clearance and the large contrast distribution volume in fibrotic regions *(65)*. To detect scar in the left atrium, the standard method is modified to achieve higher spatial resolution ($1.3 \times 1.3 \times 5$ mm) by acquiring a 3D volume during free breathing with ventilatory motion-compensated imaging (Fig. 7) *(66)*. The clinical utility of this technique is currently under assessment.

CONGENITAL ANOMALIES

Congenital anomalies of the pulmonary veins account for approximately 3% of all congenital heart disease and up to 2% of all deaths from congenital heart disease in the first year of life (67). The congenital anomalies that may affect the pulmonary veins are atresia, stenosis, and totally or partially anomalous connections. These occur when the normal connections of the primitive pulmonary venous system form abnormally or if embryologic connections to the cardinal vein or umbilicovitelline systems persist. Other major congenital cardiac anomalies are frequently associated with abnormalities of the pulmonary veins (68).

Anomalous connections are the most common congenital pulmonary venous anomaly (67). In total anomalous pulmonary venous connection, there is no connection of the pulmonary veins to the left atrium. All of the pulmonary venous drainage enters the right atrium directly or via a systemic vein. This anomaly is inevitably associated with an atrial right-to-left shunt. Pulmonary venous hypertension is frequent because of bends in the artery or compression from adjacent vascular structures (69). Small atrial septal defects restrict systemic blood flow (70). Either of these conditions may result in cyanosis and congestive heart failure. Although the mortality rate for symptomatic infants is 80% at 1 year (67), surgical repair is often feasible and reduces the mortality rate to less than 25% (71).

In partial anomalous pulmonary venous return, one or more pulmonary veins but not all enter the right atrium or a systemic vein. There is usually an associated atrial septal defect, frequently of the sinus venosus type, with the right superior or right middle pulmonary veins draining into the superior vena cava (67). The physiology of this anomaly is similar to that of an atrial septal defect, depending on the magnitude of the left-to-right shunt and the presence of increased pulmonary vascular resistance (68). If the shunt is relatively small and the pulmonary vascular resistance is normal, then patients are often asymptomatic, and the diagnosis may not be made until adulthood. Named after a characteristic chest radiographic finding, the scimitar syndrome is a specific form of partial anomalous pulmonary venous connection in which all of the venous drainage from the right lung enters the inferior vena cava (Fig. 8). This syndrome is rare and associated with anomalous arterial supply of the right lower lobe from the aorta, dextroposition of the heart, and hypoplasia of the right lung (72).

Congenital pulmonary vein atresia is the absence of any connection of the pulmonary veins to either the left atrium or any other vascular structure. This is a rare condition that is not compatible with life. Infants may survive for a short period of time because of small connections between the pulmonary veins and esophageal or brachial veins (68).

Congenital pulmonary vein stenosis is rare. It can involve a focal segment of one or more pulmonary veins or more diffusely involve an entire pulmonary vein and is usually associated with other congenital cardiac malformations. Severe stenosis often results in cyanosis, congestive heart failure, and death. Surgical repair is possible if only focal stenosis is present (68).

Imaging patients with congenital anomalies using contrast-enhanced magnetic resonance angiography is a helpful method for determining the pulmonary venous anatomy. It is usually able to identify all pulmonary venous anomalies, providing new information in 75% and identifying previously unsuspected anomalies in 30% (73).

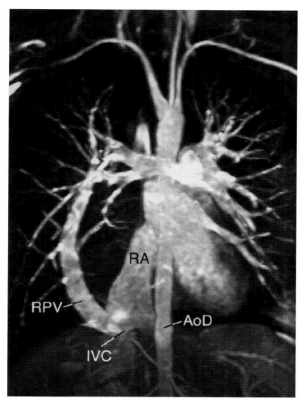

Fig. 8. Scimitar syndrome. This coronal maximal intensity projection image (anterior-posterior orientation) shows the typical findings of the scimitar syndrome. The single right pulmonary vein (RPV) enters the inferior vena cava (IVC). The right atrium (RA) and descending aorta (AoD) are also shown. (Courtesy of Andrew Powell, MD, Children's Hospital, Boston).

SUMMARY

Contrast-enhanced magnetic resonance angiography images the pulmonary veins and is useful for defining normal and anomalous anatomy. Imaging is usually performed before atrial fibrillation ablation to plan for the procedure and after to screen for pulmonary vein stenosis. Pulmonary vein size quantification is important for the comparison of serial studies and is easily accomplished by examining images in the sagittal plane. Delayed-enhancement imaging of the pulmonary veins is a new technique that may be useful to define the extent of ablation.

REFERENCES

1. Prince MR, Narasimham DL, Stanley JC, et al. Breath-hold gadolinium-enhanced MR angiography of the abdominal aorta and its major branches. Radiology 1995;197:785–792.
2. Wittkampf FH, Vonken EJ, Derksen R, et al. Pulmonary vein ostium geometry: analysis by magnetic resonance angiography. Circulation 2003;107:21–23.
3. Hauser TH, Yeon SB, McClennen S, et al. A method for the determination of proximal pulmonary vein size using contrast-enhanced magnetic resonance angiography. J Cardiovasc Magn Reson 2004;6:927–936.

4. Hauser TH, Yeon SB, McClennen S, et al. Subclinical pulmonary vein narrowing after ablation for atrial fibrillation. Heart 2005;91:672–673.

5. Mansour M, Holmvang G, Sosnovik D, et al. Assessment of pulmonary vein anatomic variability by magnetic resonance imaging: implications for catheter ablation techniques for atrial fibrillation. J Cardiovasc Electrophysiol 2004;15:387–393.

6. Mlcochova H, Tintera J, Porod V, Peichl P, Cihak R, Kautzner J. Magnetic resonance angiography of pulmonary veins: implications for catheter ablation of atrial fibrillation. Pacing Clin Electrophysiol 2005;28:1073–1080.

7. Syed MA, Peters DC, Rashid H, Arai AE. Pulmonary vein imaging: comparison of 3D magnetic resonance angiography with 2D cine MRI for characterizing anatomy and size. J Cardiovasc Magn Reson 2005;7:355–360.

8. Tamborero D, Mont L, Nava S, et al. Incidence of pulmonary vein stenosis in patients submitted to atrial fibrillation ablation: a comparison of the selective segmental ostial ablation vs the circumferential pulmonary veins ablation. J Interv Card Electrophysiol 2005;14:21–25.

9. Tsao HM, Wu MH, Huang BH, et al. Morphologic remodeling of pulmonary veins and left atrium after catheter ablation of atrial fibrillation: insight from long-term follow-up of three-dimensional magnetic resonance imaging. J Cardiovasc Electrophysiol 2005;16:7–12.

10. Vonken EP, Velthuis BK, Wittkampf FH, Rensing BJ, Derksen R, Cramer MJ. Contrast-enhanced MRA and 3D visualization of pulmonary venous anatomy to assist radiofrequency catheter ablation. J Cardiovasc Magn Reson 2003;5:545–551.

11. Lickfett L, Dickfeld T, Kato R, et al. Changes of pulmonary vein orifice size and location throughout the cardiac cycle: dynamic analysis using magnetic resonance cine imaging. J Cardiovasc Electrophysiol 2005;16:582–588.

12. Hauser TH, Yeon SB, McClennen S, et al. Variability in pulmonary vein anatomy during the cardiac cycle. Society for Cardiovascular Magnetic Resonance; 2005.

13. Schoenberg SO, Bock M, Floemer F, et al. High-resolution pulmonary arterio- and venography using multiple-bolus multiphase 3D-Gd-mRA. J Magn Reson Imaging 1999;10:339–346.

14. Earls JP, Rofsky NM, DeCorato DR, Krinsky GA, Weinreb JC. Breath-hold single-dose gadolinium-enhanced three-dimensional MR aortography: usefulness of a timing examination and MR power injector. Radiology 1996;201:705–710.

15. Wilman AH, Riederer SJ, King BF, Debbins JP, Rossman PJ, Ehman RL. Fluoroscopically triggered contrast-enhanced three-dimensional MR angiography with elliptical centric view order: application to the renal arteries. Radiology 1997;205:137–146.

16. Blom NA, Gittenberger-de Groot AC, Jongeneel TH, DeRuiter MC, Poelmann RE, Ottenkamp J. Normal development of the pulmonary veins in human embryos and formulation of a morphogenetic concept for sinus venosus defects. Am J Cardiol 2001;87:305–309.

17. Moore KL. The developing human. Philadelphia: Saunders; 1988.

18. Webb S, Kanani M, Anderson RH, Richardson MK, Brown NA. Development of the human pulmonary vein and its incorporation in the morphologically left atrium. Cardiol Young 2001;11:632–642.

19. Kato R, Lickfett L, Meininger G, et al. Pulmonary vein anatomy in patients undergoing catheter ablation of atrial fibrillation: lessons learned by use of magnetic resonance imaging. Circulation 2003;107: 2004–2010.

20. Feinberg WM, Blackshear JL, Laupacis A, Kronmal R, Hart RG. Prevalence, age distribution, and gender of patients with atrial fibrillation. Analysis and implications. Arch Intern Med 1995;155: 469–473.

21. Heart disease and stroke statistics—2004 Update. Dallas, TX: American Heart Association.

22. Benjamin EJ, Wolf PA, D'Agostino RB, Silbershatz H, Kannel WB, Levy D. Impact of atrial fibrillation on the risk of death: the Framingham Heart Study. Circulation 1998;98:946–952.

23. Wolf PA, Abbott RD, Kannel WB. Atrial fibrillation as an independent risk factor for stroke: the Framingham Study. Stroke 1991;22:983–988.

24. Hauser TH, Pinto DS, Josephson ME, Zimetbaum P. Early recurrence of arrhythmia in patients taking amiodarone or class 1C agents for treatment of atrial fibrillation or atrial flutter. Am J Cardiol 2004;93:1173–1176.

25. Singh BN, Singh SN, Reda DJ, et al. Amiodarone vs sotalol for atrial fibrillation. N Engl J Med 2005;352:1861–1872.

26. Roy D, Talajic M, Dorian P, et al. Amiodarone to prevent recurrence of atrial fibrillation. Canadian Trial of Atrial Fibrillation Investigators. N Engl J Med 2000;342:913–920.

27. Hauser TH, Pinto DS, Josephson ME, Zimetbaum P. Safety and feasibility of a clinical pathway for the outpatient initiation of antiarrhythmic medications in patients with atrial fibrillation or atrial flutter. Am J Cardiol 2003;91:1437–1441.

28. Hassink RJ, Aretz HT, Ruskin J, Keane D. Morphology of atrial myocardium in human pulmonary veins: a postmortem analysis in patients with and without atrial fibrillation. J Am Coll Cardiol 2003;42:1108–1114.

29. Arora R, Verheule S, Scott L, et al. Arrhythmogenic substrate of the pulmonary veins assessed by high-resolution optical mapping. Circulation 2003;107:1816–1821.

30. Haissaguerre M, Jais P, Shah DC, et al. Spontaneous initiation of atrial fibrillation by ectopic beats originating in the pulmonary veins. N Engl J Med 1998;339:659–666.

31. Pappone C, Rosanio S, Oreto G, et al. Circumferential radiofrequency ablation of pulmonary vein ostia. A new anatomic approach for curing atrial fibrillation. Circulation 2000;102: 2619–2628.

32. Arentz T, von Rosenthal J, Blum T, et al. Feasibility and safety of pulmonary vein isolation using a new mapping and navigation system in patients with refractory atrial fibrillation. Circulation 2003;108:2484–2490.

33. Haissaguerre M, Jais P, Shah DC, et al. Electrophysiological end point for catheter ablation of atrial fibrillation initiated from multiple pulmonary venous foci. Circulation 2000;101:1409–1417.

34. Oral H, Knight BP, Ozaydin M, et al. Segmental ostial ablation to isolate the pulmonary veins during atrial fibrillation: feasibility and mechanistic insights. Circulation 2002;106:1256–1262.

35. Pappone C, Rosanio S, Augello G, et al. Mortality, morbidity, and quality of life after circumferential pulmonary vein ablation for atrial fibrillation: outcomes from a controlled nonrandomized long-term study. J Am Coll Cardiol 2003;42:185–197.

36. Marine JE, Dong J, Calkins H. Catheter ablation therapy for atrial fibrillation. Prog Cardiovasc Dis 2005;48:178–192.

37. Lin WS, Prakash VS, Tai CT, et al. Pulmonary vein morphology in patients with paroxysmal atrial fibrillation initiated by ectopic beats originating from the pulmonary veins: implications for catheter ablation. Circulation 2000;101:1274–1281.

38. Calkins H. Three dimensional mapping of atrial fibrillation: techniques and necessity. J Interv Card Electrophysiol 2005;13(suppl 1):53–59.

39. Scanavacca MI, D'Avila A, Parga J, Sosa E. Left atrial-esophageal fistula following radiofrequency catheter ablation of atrial fibrillation. J Cardiovasc Electrophysiol 2004;15:960–962.

40. Pappone C, Oral H, Santinelli V, et al. Atrio-esophageal fistula as a complication of percutaneous transcatheter ablation of atrial fibrillation. Circulation 2004;109:2724–2726.

41. Cummings JE, Schweikert RA, Saliba WI, et al. Assessment of temperature, proximity, and course of the esophagus during radiofrequency ablation within the left atrium. Circulation 2005;112: 459–464.

42. Redfearn DP, Trim GM, Skanes AC, et al. Esophageal temperature monitoring during radiofrequency ablation of atrial fibrillation. J Cardiovasc Electrophysiol 2005;16:589–593.

43. Lemola K, Sneider M, Desjardins B, et al. Computed tomographic analysis of the anatomy of the left atrium and the esophagus: implications for left atrial catheter ablation. Circulation 2004;110: 3655–3660.

44. Tsao HM, Wu MH, Higa S, et al. Anatomic relationship of the esophagus and left atrium: implication for catheter ablation of atrial fibrillation. Chest 2005;128:2581–2587.

45. Cury RC, Abbara S, Schmidt S, et al. Relationship of the esophagus and aorta to the left atrium and pulmonary veins: Implications for catheter ablation of atrial fibrillation. Heart Rhythm 2005;2: 1317–1323.

46. Sanchez-Quintana D, Cabrera JA, Climent V, Farre J, Mendonca MC, Ho SY. Anatomic relations between the esophagus and left atrium and relevance for ablation of atrial fibrillation. Circulation 2005;112:1400–1405.

47. Monnig G, Wessling J, Juergens KU, et al. Further evidence of a close anatomical relation between the oesophagus and pulmonary veins. Europace 2005;7:540–545.

48. Good E, Oral H, Lemola K, et al. Movement of the esophagus during left atrial catheter ablation for atrial fibrillation. J Am Coll Cardiol 2005;46:2107–2110.

49. Moak J, Moore H, Lee S, et al. Case report: pulmonary vein stenosis following RF ablation of paroxysmal atrial fibrillation: successful treatment with balloon dilation. J Interv Card Electrophysiol 2000;4:621–631.

50. Saad EB, Rossillo A, Saad CP, et al. Pulmonary vein stenosis after radiofrequency ablation of atrial fibrillation: functional characterization, evolution, and influence of the ablation strategy. Circulation 2003;108:3102–3107.
51. Saad EB, Marrouche NF, Saad CP, et al. Pulmonary vein stenosis after catheter ablation of atrial fibrillation: emergence of a new clinical syndrome. Ann Intern Med 2003;138:634–638.
52. Scanvacca M, Kajita L, Vieira M, Sosa E. Pulmonary vein stenosis complicating catheter ablation of focal atrial fibrillation. J Cardiovasc Electrophysiol 2000;1:677–681.
53. Yang M, Akbari H, Reddy GP, Higgins CB. Identification of pulmonary vein stenosis after radiofrequency ablation for atrial fibrillation using MRI. J Comput Assist Tomogr 2001;25:34–35.
54. Arentz T, Jander N, von Rosenthal J, et al. Incidence of pulmonary vein stenosis 2 years after radiofrequency catheter ablation of refractory atrial fibrillation. Eur Heart J 2003;24:963–969.
55. Dill T, Neumann T, Ekinci O, et al. Pulmonary vein diameter reduction after radiofrequency catheter ablation for paroxysmal atrial fibrillation evaluated by contrast-enhanced three-dimensional magnetic resonance imaging. Circulation 2003;107:845–850.
56. Taylor GW, Kay GN, Zheng X, Bishop S, Ideker RE. Pathological effects of extensive radiofrequency energy applications in the pulmonary veins in dogs. Circulation 2000;101:1736–1742.
57. Kluge A, Dill T, Ekinci O, et al. Decreased pulmonary perfusion in pulmonary vein stenosis after radiofrequency ablation: assessment with dynamic magnetic resonance perfusion imaging. Chest 2004;126:428–437.
58. Arentz T, Weber R, Jander N, et al. Pulmonary haemodynamics at rest and during exercise in patients with significant pulmonary vein stenosis after radiofrequency catheter ablation for drug resistant atrial fibrillation. Eur Heart J 2005;26:1410–1414.
59. Qureshi AM, Prieto LR, Latson LA, et al. Transcatheter angioplasty for acquired pulmonary vein stenosis after radiofrequency ablation. Circulation 2003;108:1336–1342.
60. Bowman AW, Kovacs SJ. Prediction and assessment of the time-varying effective pulmonary vein area via cardiac MRI and Doppler echocardiography. Am J Physiol Heart Circ Physiol 2005;288: H280–H286.
61. Wood MA, Wittkamp M, Henry D, et al. A comparison of pulmonary vein ostial anatomy by computerized tomography, echocardiography, and venography in patients with atrial fibrillation having radiofrequency catheter ablation. Am J Cardiol 2004;93:49–53.
62. Hauser TH, Essebag V, Baldessin F, et al. Larger pulmonary vein cross-sectional area is associated with recurrent atrial fibrillation after pulmonary vein isolation. Circulation 2005;112(S):II-555.
63. Kim RJ, Wu E, Rafael A, et al. The use of contrast-enhanced magnetic resonance imaging to identify reversible myocardial dysfunction. N Engl J Med 2000;343:1445–1453.
64. Simonetti OP, Kim RJ, Fieno DS, et al. An improved MR imaging technique for the visualization of myocardial infarction. Radiology 2001;218:215–223.
65. Judd RM, Lugo-Olivieri CH, Arai M, et al. Physiological basis of myocardial contrast enhancement in fast magnetic resonance images of 2-days-old reperfused canine infarcts. Circulation 1995;92:1902–1910.
66. Peters DC, Wylie JV, Kissinger KV, et al. Detection of pulmonary vein ablation with high resolution MRI. Society for Cardiovascular Magnetic Resonance; 2006.
67. Krabill KA, Lucas RV. Abnormal pulmonary venous connections. In: Emmanouilides GC, Riemenschneider TA, Allen HD, et al., eds. Moss and Adams' heart disease in infants, children and adolescents. Baltimore, MD: Williams and Wilkins; 1995:838.
68. Friedman WF, Silverman N. Congenital heart disease in infancy and childhood. In: Braunwald E, Zipes DP, Libby P, eds. Heart disease. Philadelphia: Saunders; 2001:1552.
69. Wang JK, Lue HC, Wu MH, Young ML, Wu FF, Wu JM. Obstructed total anomalous pulmonary venous connection. Pediatr Cardiol 1993;14:28–32.
70. Ward KE, Mullins CE, Huhta JC, Nihill MR, McNamara DG, Cooley DA. Restrictive interatrial communication in total anomalous pulmonary venous connection. Am J Cardiol 1986;57:1131–1136.
71. Lamb RK, Qureshi SA, Wilkinson JL, Arnold R, West CR, Hamilton DI. Total anomalous pulmonary venous drainage. Seventeen-year surgical experience. J Thorac Cardiovasc Surg 1988;96:368–375.
72. Gao YA, Burrows PE, Benson LN, Rabinovitch M, Freedom RM. Scimitar syndrome in infancy. J Am Coll Cardiol 1993;22:873–882.
73. Greil G, Powell A, Gildein H, Geva T. Gadolinium-enhanced three-dimensional magnetic resonance aniography of pulmonary and systemic venous anomalies. J Am Coll Cardiol 2002;39:335–341.
74. Ghaye B, Szapiro D, Dacher J, Rodriguez L, Timmermans C, Devillers D, Dondelinger R. Percutaneous ablation for arrial fibrillation: the role of cross-sectional imaging. Radiographics 2003;23:19S.

28 Cardiovascular Magnetic Resonance Imaging of Atherothrombosis

W. Yong Kim, Samuel Alberg Kock,
Warren J. Manning, and René M. Botnar

Contents

INTRODUCTION

Atherothrombotic cardiovascular disease remains the leading cause of morbidity and mortality in the Western world and is rapidly becoming the number one killer in the developing countries *(1)*. Atherosclerosis is a systemic and progressive disease involving the intima of large- and medium-size arteries, including the aorta and the carotid, coronary, and peripheral arteries. *Atherothrombosis*, defined as atherosclerotic plaque disruption with superimposed thrombosis, can progress to potential life-threatening conditions, such as myocardial infarction or ischemic stroke. The concept of *vulnerable plaque* has

From: *Contemporary Cardiology: Cardiovascular Magnetic Resonance Imaging*
Edited by: Raymond Y. Kwong © Humana Press Inc., Totowa, NJ

Table 1
Criteria for Defining Vulnerable Plaque

Major criteria
    Active inflammation (monocyte/macrophage ± T-cell infiltration)
    Thin fibrous cap with large lipid core
    Endothelial denudation with superficial platelet aggregation
    Fissured plaque
    Diameter stenosis greater than 90%
Minor criteria
    Superficial calcified nodule
    Glistening yellow
    Intraplaque hemorrhage
    Endothelial dysfunction
    Outward (positive) remodeling (Glagov effect)

Based on the study of culprit plaques. Modified from ref. 2.

been introduced to distinguish thrombosis-prone plaques and plaques with a high probability of undergoing rapid progression. More recently, the term *vulnerable patient* has been proposed in recognition of contributing culprit factors, including vulnerable blood (prone to thrombosis) and vulnerable myocardium (prone to fatal arrhythmia), that identify high-risk patients with high likelihood of developing cardiovascular events in the near future (2).

Integration of vascular biology with noninvasive imaging techniques in the intact human circulation should enhance our current understanding of the natural history and of the pathophysiological mechanisms of atherothrombosis. Currently, the most used noninvasive imaging techniques for atherothrombosis include cardiovascular magnetic resonance (CMR), multidetector computed tomography, and ultrasound. Among these modalities, CMR is emerging as the most comprehensive noninvasive in vivo imaging modality for atherothrombosis (3–5).

With further development, CMR imaging of atherothrombosis in the diseased vessel (carotid, thoracic, and abdominal aorta; coronary) wall may prove to be clinically beneficial in identifying vulnerable patients.

NONINVASIVE DIAGNOSIS OF VULNERABLE PLAQUES

Based on autopsy studies, a number of major and minor criteria for defining vulnerable plaques have been proposed (2). These criteria of vulnerability include morphological features (e.g., size of lipid core and thickness of fibrous cap) (Table 1) as well as markers of plaque activity (e.g., plaque inflammation, superficial platelet aggregation, and fibrin deposition) (Table 2). Most of the proposed features of plaque vulnerability are based on cross-sectional and retrospective studies of culprit lesions. Noninvasive surrogate markers such as coronary vessel wall thickness and plaque burden together with markers of plaque activity could supplement or improve cardiovascular risk stratification, especially in patients with intermediate cardiovascular risk. Noninvasive imaging techniques provide a mechanism for prospective outcome studies to determine if identifying asymptomatic vulnerable patients may allow for primary interventions to reduce clinical cardiovascular events.

Table 2
Markers of Vulnerability at the Plaque Level

Morphology/structure
  Plaque cap thickness
  Plaque lipid core size
  Plaque stenosis (luminal narrowing)
  Remodeling (expansive vs constrictive remodeling)
  Color (yellow, glistening yellow, red, etc.)
  Collagen content vs lipid content, mechanical stability (stiffness and elasticity)
  Calcification burden and pattern (nodule vs scattered, superficial vs deep, etc.)
  Shear stress (flow pattern throughout the coronary artery)
Activity/function
  Plaque inflammation (macrophage density, rate of monocyte infiltration and density of
    activated T cell)
  Endothelial denudation or dysfunction (local NO production, anti- and procoagulation
    properties of the endothelium)
  Plaque oxidative stress
  Superficial platelet aggregation and fibrin deposition (residual mural thrombus)
  Rate of apoptosis (apoptosis protein markers, coronary microsatellite, etc.)
  Angiogenesis, leaking vasa vasorum, and intraplaque hemorrhage
  Matrix-digesting enzyme activity in the cap (MMPs 2, 3, 9, etc.)
  Certain microbial antigens (e.g., heat shock protein 60, *Chlamydia pneumoniae*)
Panarterial
  Transcoronary gradient of serum markers of vulnerability
  Total coronary calcium burden
  Total coronary vasoreactivity (endothelial function)
  Total arterial burden of plaque, including peripheral (e.g., carotid IMT)

Modified from ref. *2*.
MMP, matrix metalloproteinase; NO, nitric oxide; IMT, intima medial thickness.

CARDIOVASCULAR MAGNETIC RESONANCE CORONARY ARTERY IMAGING

The accuracy of coronary magnetic resonance imaging (MRI) was investigated among patients with suspected coronary artery disease (CAD) in a prospective, multicenter study *(6)*. Overall, coronary MRI had an accuracy of 72% (95% confidence interval, 63–81%) in diagnosing CAD (defined as ≥50% diameter reduction on quantitative X-ray angiography) *(6)*. At the current stage of development, coronary MRI was particularly helpful for excluding left main coronary artery or three-vessel disease, with a negative predictive value of 100% *(6)*.

However, coronary MRI remains technically demanding as respiratory and cardiac motion limit the useful data acquisition window. Coronary vessel wall imaging is particularly challenging because of the small vessel size (coronary vessel wall thickness ~0.5–2 mm), tortuous three-dimensional (3D) course of the coronary vessels, and the close proximity to epicardial fat, coronary blood, and myocardium. Advanced motion compensation strategies to meet the challenges of coronary vessel wall imaging have been developed, allowing more consistent visualization of the proximal and mid portions of the native coronary vessel walls.

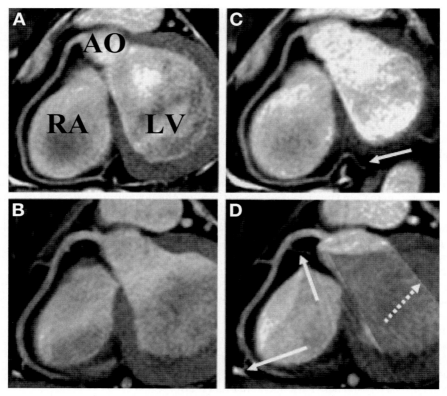

Fig. 1. (A) and **(B)** Reformatted coronary MRI images of the right coronary artery (RCA) obtained with a conventional protocol and **(C)** and **(D)** with the novel sequence comprising high scan efficiency and intra-R–R motion correction. Higher SNR and contrast-to-noise ratio (CNR) are evident in the motion-corrected images. Also, more details, such as small distal branches, could be reconstructed using motion-corrected scanning (solid arrows). Some artifacts resulting from the retrospective correction occurred as regions may comprise image data from a subset of the acquired segments only (dashed arrow). However, these effects do not occur within the region of interest, such as the coronary vessel. AO, aorta; LV, left ventricle; RV, right ventricle. (Reproduced from ref. *9* with permission.)

CARDIAC MOTION

Because of the rapid intrinsic cardiac motion during the cardiac cycle, synchronization of data acquisition to the R-wave of the electrocardiogram is mandatory. Data acquisition is performed only during a relatively short interval comprising less than 10% of the entire cardiac cycle in either end-systole or middiastole (periods of relative myocardial diastasis) *(7,8)*. Subject-specific middiastolic acquisition usually provides the most optimal imaging in subjects with a heart rate below 80 beats per minute. For subjects with heart rates above 80 beats per minute, minimal motion is usually during end-systole.

The timing of the subject-specific image acquisition can be assessed from a cine data set in the four-chamber view by visual inspection or automated analysis. These measures are essential to avoid cardiac motion-induced artifacts but reduce the scan efficiency by a large scale. To overcome this drawback, one could use a longer cardiac acquisition window with intra-R–R motion correction *(9)*. Combining the motion-corrected segments produced a high-resolution image (Fig. 1) *(9)*. The length of the

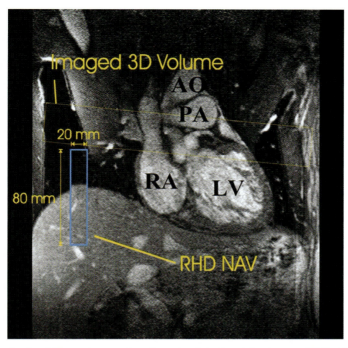

Fig. 2. The 2D selective MR navigator placed on the right hemidiaphragm (RHD NAV) in a coronal view together with a 3D imaging volume intended for imaging the left coronary artery. RHD, right hemidiaphragm; LV, left ventricle; RA, right atrium; AO, aorta; PA, pulmonary artery.

middiastolic or end-systolic rest period (which typically varies from 50 to 350 ms) is inversely related to heart rate *(8)*. Therefore, subjects with heart rates above 60 beats per minute may benefit from β-blockers to slow their heart rates and to increase their rest period duration.

RESPIRATORY MOTION COMPENSATION

During normal breathing, diaphragmatic excursion (10–20 mm), which translates to cardiac motion, will exceed a multiple of the coronary vessel wall thickness (0.5–2 mm) *(10)*. Therefore, either breath-hold techniques or respiratory motion compensation during free breathing are required for coronary vessel wall imaging.

Initial approaches for visualizing cross sections of the proximal coronary vessel wall used two-dimensional (2D) breath-hold techniques with middiastolic image acquisition *(11)*. This approach produces variable image quality because some patients cannot tolerate breath holding for the required 15- to 20-seconds time period. Furthermore, the inadequate spatial coverage of 2D techniques limits the clinical potential because evaluation of the entire proximal coronary vessel wall is likely to be important.

To compensate for respiratory motion during a free-breathing examination, a 2D-selective pencil beam navigator placed on the right hemidiaphragm can be used to monitor respiration and to perform real-time gating and slice tracking (Fig. 2) *(6)*. The use of navigator echoes that record and correct for diaphragmatic motion *(12)* allows for free breathing and eliminates the time constraints of the breath-hold approach, thereby allowing for submillimeter spatial resolution *(13,14)*. Similar to coronary MRI, coronary vessel wall imaging can be combined with the navigator technique and extended to 3D acquisitions, providing higher signal-to-noise ratio (SNR) and improved vessel coverage *(15)*.

The current implementation of respiratory navigators enables slice tracking only in the foot-head direction and accepts data only within a narrow and fixed gating window, typically 5 mm. Therefore, free-breathing coronary MRI with respiratory navigator gating is hampered by prolonged scan time because of irregular breathing patterns that result in low navigator efficiency. A more advanced respiratory motion compensation technique has been proposed that enables the calibration of a 3D affine respiratory motion model to the individual motion pattern of the patient *(16)*. Preliminary results indicate that this approach increases the scan efficiency without sacrificing image quality and therefore has the potential to be more robust for routine clinical usage *(16)*.

CORONARY PLAQUE BURDEN

Early in vivo coronary vessel wall-imaging studies used a 2D fat-suppressed fast spin echo technique *(11,17)*. Coronary blood signal was suppressed using a double-inversion prepulse *(17)*, leading to optimal contrast between lumen and vessel wall. This black blood approach has been implemented in both a 2D breath-hold *(11)* and a free-breathing mode *(17)* and allows for visualization of cross-sectional images of the left anterior descending (LAD) and right coronary artery (RCA) vessel wall in both healthy subjects and patients with CAD. In-plane spatial resolution of these first implementations varied from 0.46*0.46 mm to 0.5*1 mm, with a typical slice thickness of 3–5 mm. Coronary wall thickness was higher in patients with CAD when compared to normal healthy subjects *(11,17)*.

Because of the highly tortuous path of the coronary artery system, cross-sectional vessel wall imaging of the coronary arteries is time inefficient, making a vessel-targeted 3D approach more desirable. Such an approach was implemented using a three-point plan scan method *(18)* and combined with a modified black blood prepulse (local inversion) *(15)*, which allows acquisition of 3D stacks along the major axis of the coronary artery system. This approach allowed for visualization of the proximal and mid portions of the RCA and LAD coronary artery wall with good contrast between coronary blood and the vessel wall *(15)*. Free-breathing 3D black blood coronary CMR identified an increased coronary vessel wall thickness with preservation of lumen size in patients with nonsignificant CAD, consistent with a Glagov-type outward arterial remodeling (Fig. 3) *(19)*.

CORONARY ATHEROTHROMBOSIS IMAGING BY CARDIOVASCULAR MAGNETIC RESONANCE

CMR has shown great promise as a comprehensive imaging modality for in vivo imaging and characterization of atherothrombosis. Multispectral MRI relies on the fact that the MR signal emitted by water protons (^{1}H) varies according to their molecular environment. In principle, each plaque component has an MR-specific "zip code" that is composed of the T_1 and T_2 relaxation times, proton density, molecular diffusion, magnetization transfer, and so on. Because there is an overlap of signal intensities between the different sequences and the different plaque components, unique identification of plaque components can be difficult. Nevertheless, multispectral MRI has been successfully

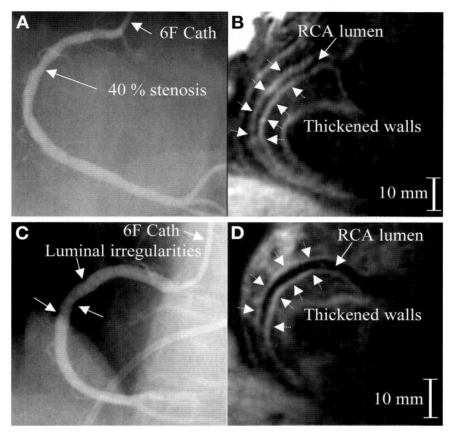

Fig. 3. X-ray angiography in two patients with **(A)** a focal 40% diameter stenosis (white arrow) and **(C)** minor (~10% stenoses) luminal irregularities (white arrows) of the proximal RCA. The corresponding black blood 3D CMR vessel wall scans **(B)** and **(D)** demonstrate an irregularly thickened RCA wall (>2 mm), indicative of an increased atherosclerotic plaque burden. The inner and outer walls are indicated by the black dotted arrows. (Reproduced from ref. *19* with permission.)

demonstrated for plaque characterization in ex vivo vessel specimens *(20–22)*, experimental animals *(4,23,24)*, and human carotid artery *(25)* and aorta *(26,27)* in vivo.

Currently, spatial resolution remains the limiting factor for detailed coronary plaque characterization. Based on simulations and phantom studies, it was demonstrated that at least one pixel is needed across the different tissue layers of the vessel wall (fibrous cap, lipid pool, smooth muscle) to characterize different vessel wall components reliably *(28)*. Furthermore, respiratory motion correction needs to be as accurate as three times the thickness of the tissue layer *(28)*. In principle, these boundaries could be met with the current navigator-based 3D coronary vessel wall sequences *(15,19)*. However, from a practical perspective, high-resolution imaging causes a reduction in SNR. Therefore, the use of exogenous targeted contrast agents *(29,30)*, intravascular coils *(31)*, and higher magnetic field strengths *(32,33)* may be required for detailed vessel wall imaging. Different magnetic resonance (MR) probes have been developed to study various biological processes (e.g., thrombosis, angiogenesis, inflammation, neoplasia) and diseases (e.g., cancer, cardiovascular disease, stroke, diabetes) by targeting a spectrum of molecular markers such as fibrin, selectins, and integrins. Many such agents are in the preclinical stage.

Noninvasive visualization of evolving arterial thrombus would facilitate detection of unstable plaques and thrombosis burden in vulnerable patients. Advances have been made with in vivo imaging of arterial thrombus by fibrin-binding molecular MR contrast agents (29,30). Direct imaging of arterial thrombus by targeted or "molecular" contrast agents (which are engineered to bind to specific target molecules) is advantageous to classical noncontrast multispectral MRI because the demand for high spatial resolution and motion compensation strategies are less stringent. Furthermore, even though several studies have shown high sensitivity of MRI to the detection of carotid and aortic thrombi (34–36), differentiation between complex atherosclerotic plaques and mural thrombosis remains difficult because of the complex composition (e.g., platelets, fibrin, and red blood cells) of thrombus and resultant complex MR signal characteristics on T_1-, T_2-, and proton density-weighted images of arterial thrombi.

The concept of target-specific imaging or molecular imaging was first introduced over a decade ago and has since been further developed by Weissleder (37,38) and others (39) for MRI and optical imaging in recent years. The advantage of CMR molecular plaque imaging is the potential for relatively high spatial resolution. The limitation is the inherently low sensitivity of MR contrast enhancement technology, requiring a relatively high target molecule concentration (>50–100 μM gadolinium [Gd] at target site) for sufficient signal amplification. Initial attempts were made with targeting fibrin (39–41), which is abundant in arterial clots and plays an important role in acute coronary syndromes and stroke.

In vivo MRI of acute and subacute thrombosis following plaque rupture in an animal model of aortic atherosclerosis has been implemented using a small-molecule fibrin-binding peptide derivative, EP-1873 (EPIX Pharmaceuticals, Cambridge, MA) (Fig. 4) (29). This molecular agent allowed for imaging of large-lumen encroaching thrombi as well as submillimeter mural thrombi with signal enhancement of the entire thrombus and excellent differentiation from the vessel wall.

Combining the advent of fibrin-binding molecular MR contrast agents and advances in coronary MRI techniques offers the potential for direct imaging of coronary thrombosis. The feasibility of this approach was demonstrated using a Gd-based fibrin-binding contrast agent, EP-2104R (EPIX Pharmaceuticals), in a swine model of native coronary thrombus (Fig. 5) and in-stent thrombosis using MR-lucent stents (30). Potential applications for direct thrombus imaging include detection and evaluation of acute coronary syndromes and ischemic strokes.

Integrins, such as $\alpha v \beta 3$ are associated with angiogenesis, which is a critical feature of plaque development in atherosclerosis and likely play a key role in plaque rupture leading to myocardial infarction or stroke. Increased angiogenesis was detected as signal enhancement in the MR signal averaged throughout the abdominal aortic wall among hyperlipidemic rabbits that receive $\alpha v \beta 3$-targeted paramagnetic nanoparticles (42). Histology and immunohistochemistry confirmed marked proliferation of angiogenic vessels within the aortic adventitia among cholesterol-fed atherosclerotic rabbits in comparison with sparse incidence of neovasculature in control animals.

Vascular inflammation and associated endothelial activation is believed to play an integral role in initiation and progression of atherosclerosis. Endothelial cells express adhesion molecules such as E- and P-selectin, which facilitate adhesion and migration of monocytes. Differentiation of monocytes into macrophages and subsequent digestion of lipoproteins by macrophages occur in a later stage and eventually lead to the

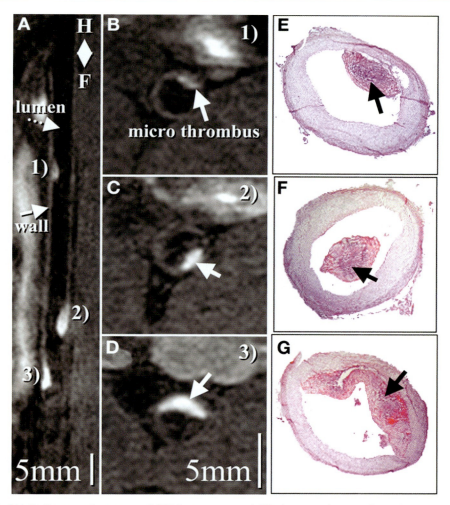

Fig. 4. (A) Reformatted coronary MRI from a coronal 3D data set shows subrenal aorta approximately 20 hours after EP-1873 administration (EPIX Pharmaceuticals) in a rabbit model of atherosclerosis and plaque rupture. Three well-delineated mural thrombi (arrows) can be observed, with good contrast between thrombus (numbered), arterial blood (dotted arrow), and vessel wall (dashed arrow). The in-plane view of the aorta allows simultaneous display of all thrombi, showing head, tail, length, and relative location. **(B)–(D)** Corresponding cross-sectional views show good agreement with histopathology **(E)–(G)**. (Reproduced from ref. *34* with permission.)

accumulation of lipid-filled macrophages, which are believed to be a precursor of rupture-prone vulnerable plaque.

Early endothelial activation has been detected using a novel MR contrast agent in rats with brain inflammation (after interleukin 1β and tumor necrosis factor-α induced E- and P-selectin upregulation) *(43)* and in focal ischemia in mice brains *(44)*. This Gd-labeled contrast agent, Gd-DTPA-B(sLe^x)A *(45)*, consists of the sialyl Lewis^x (sLe^x) carbohydrate, which interacts with both E- and P-selectin. These promising results encourage further studies, including assessment of E- and P-selectin upregulation in early atherosclerotic lesions in the coronary arteries.

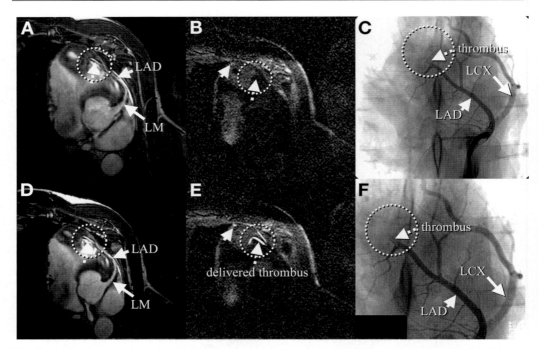

Fig. 5. In vivo MRI of Gd-labeled fibrinogen clots in a swine model of coronary thrombosis. **(A)** and **(D)** Coronary MRI before **(A)** and after **(D)** thrombus delivery. On both scans, no apparent thrombus is visible (circle). **(B)** and **(E)**, Black blood inversion recovery. Turbo Field Echo (TFE) scans before **(B)** and after **(E)** clot delivery (same view as **A** and **D**). After thrombus delivery **(E)**, three bright areas are readily visible (arrows and circle), consistent with location of thrombus. No apparent thrombus was visible on prethrombus **(B)** images (arrow and circle). **(C)** X-ray angiogram confirming MR finding of thrombus in mid-LAD (circle). **(F)** Magnified view of **C**. LM indicates left main. (Reproduced from ref. *30* with permission.)

IMAGING OF CAROTID ARTERIES

Transient ischemic attack and ischemic stroke are the major clinical cerebrovascular complications of atherothrombosis. Among the arteries that carry blood to the brain and eye, atherothrombosis mainly affects large- (ascending aorta) and medium-size arteries at places of branching (e.g., carotid bifurcation), tortuosity (e.g., carotid siphon), and convergence (e.g., basilar artery). Local fluid dynamics, including oscillating and low wall shear stress, in these regions appear to influence the location of atheroma *(46)*.

Several large randomized studies have shown that surgical removal of high-grade carotid plaques significantly reduces the incidence of recurring stroke compared to nonoperatively treated individuals with similar degrees of carotid stenoses *(47,48)*. However, instead of assessing disease severity based on the degree of carotid luminal stenosis, it may prove beneficial to base risk assessment on morphological and functional markers of plaque vulnerability.

Carotid atherothrombosis has been the subject of intense investigation by CMR and other noninvasive imaging modalities. Imaging of the carotid bifurcation is facilitated by the superficial location, relatively large size, and relative immobility. In addition, the carotid bifurcation shows the full spectrum of atherosclerotic lesion types according to the classification of the American Heart Association *(25)*. The carotid artery is also the only vascular bed where intact surgical specimens are readily available for histological examination and comparison to in vivo imaging.

CMR has a unique potential for imaging carotid atherothrombosis achieving high spatial resolution and image quality with excellent soft tissue contrast and sensitivity to flow. Thereby, virtually all of the markers of plaque vulnerability listed in Table 2 can be imaged using CMR. Furthermore, MRI offers the benefit of noninvasively monitoring the atherosclerotic lesions at multiple time points, allowing for enhanced research into the etiology of atherosclerosis as well as monitoring the effect of therapeutic drugs such as statins.

HARDWARE CONSIDERATIONS

As the carotid arteries are superficial structures with a length that is greater than their distance from the surface, their configuration is well suited for the use of phased array surface coils *(49)*. SNR using phased array coils is sufficient to allow for spatial resolutions of $0.25 \times 0.25 \times 2$ mm *(50)*. Furthermore, most dedicated carotid coils employ two sets of coil sections, allowing simultaneous imaging of both the left and right carotid arteries. Head holders are recommended to improve patient comfort as well as minimize patient movement during the scans, thereby allowing repeatable scan positioning.

MULTIPLE CONTRAST WEIGHTINGS

MRI-based tissue quantification is a promising application for prospective longitudinal studies to examine atherosclerotic plaque progression/regression and composition. Early carotid MRI was based solely on T_2-weighted images *(3,51)*. However, sensitivity and specificity improved when multispectral imaging was employed *(25,52)*. Based on previous ex vivo *(20)* and experimental work *(4)*, a standardized carotid plaque imaging protocol has been developed *(50)* utilizing four different contrast weighted images: T_1 weighted (T1W), T_2 weighted (T2W), proton density weighted (PDW), and time of flight (TOF). By comparing the signal intensities obtained with each contrast weighting to the adjacent sternocleidomastoid muscle, the plaque can be divided into distinct tissue types (Table 3): lipid-rich necrotic core, with or without hemorrhagic areas, calcification, loose matrix, and dense fibrous tissue *(53)*. Using multiple contrast-weighted imaging CMR, classification of atherosclerotic plaques can be obtained (Fig. 6) *(25)* with good-to-excellent intra- and interreader reproducibility *(53)*.

Cai et al. *(25)* employed a slightly modified classification optimized for MRI by which American Heart Association plaque types I and II were combined as MRI does not allow discrimination between discrete and multiple foam cell layers. Plaque types IV and V were also combined because MRI does not allow distinguishing between the proteoglycan compositions of type IV vs the dense collagen of type V.

MORPHOLOGY/STRUCTURE

The main criterion in clinical risk assessment of carotid atherosclerosis is the degree of luminal stenosis. Two major randomized clinical studies, the North American Symptomatic Carotid Endarterectomy Trial Collaborators (NASCET) *(47)* and the European Carotid Surgery Trial (ECST) *(48)*, have demonstrated that symptomatic patients with luminal diameter stenosis above 70% could benefit from carotid

Table 3
Tissue Classification Criteria

	TOF	T1W	PDW	T2W
Lipid-rich necrotic core with				
No or little hemorrhage	0	0/+	0/+	–/0
Fresh hemorrhage	+	+	– /0	–/0
Recent hemorrhage	+	+	+	+
Calcification	–	–	–	–
Loose matrix	0	–/0	+	+
Dense (fibrous) tissue	–	0	0	0

Modified from ref. *53*.
TOF, time of flight; T1W, T_1 weighted; PDW, proton density weighted; T2W, T_2 weighted; +, hyperintense; 0, isointense; –, hypointense. All intensities are compared to the adjacent sternocleidomastoid muscle.

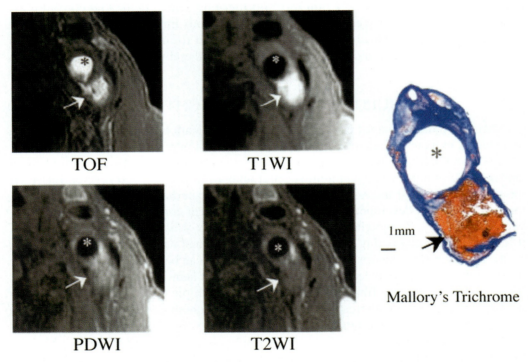

Fig. 6. Example of type VI lesion just distal to carotid bifurcation (acute to subacute mixed hemorrhages were detected by histology). On multicontrast-weighted MR images, acute and subacute mixed hemorrhage had high SI (signal intensity) on both TOF and T1W images, iso-SI to slightly high SI on PDW and T2W images (arrow). The asterisk * indicates lumen. (Reproduced from ref. *25* with permission.)

endarterectomy to remove the carotid plaque. The technique used to define the degree of stenosis was digital subtraction angiography (DSA); the method of choice today is Doppler ultrasound. Studies comparing the sensitivity and specificity of Doppler ultrasound vs MR angiography using DSA as the gold standard concluded that MR angiography has significantly superior discriminatory power to detect stenosis above

70% *(54)*. Conventional DSA techniques are limited to visualization of luminal stenosis; MRI enables quantification of atherosclerotic plaque burden and detects positive arterial remodeling.

The status of the fibrous cap is of decisive importance when determining plaque vulnerability. Rupture of the fibrous cap exposes thrombogenic plaque constituents to the bloodstream and is believed to be the critical event leading to stroke and transient ischemic attacks *(55)*. MRI has the ability to distinguish between intact and ruptured caps as well as determine the thickness of the fibrous cap *(52,56)*, enabling serial prospective studies of the fibrous cap in high-risk patients. Presence of plaque rupture detected using the multiple contrast-weighted technique as outlined has been correlated with recent history of stroke or transient ischemic attack *(57)*.

MRI can accurately determine the size of the lipid-rich necrotic core, another important factor when plaque vulnerability is assessed *(5)*. Stable plaques tend to contain larger amounts of collagen and smaller lipid pools, conferring mechanical stability *(58)*; both collagen and lipid-rich tissue types can reliably be classified using MRI *(53)*.

Calcifications will appear dark on all MRI contrast weightings *(53)* and can be correctly identified using MRI. However, calcium is removed during standard histological preparation, requiring another nonhistological technique, such as Micro-Computed Tomography (μCT), to be used as the gold standard. Clarke and colleagues found an excellent agreement between MRI and μCT classifications *(59)*. In vivo MRI techniques have been developed for determining wall shear stresses (WSSs), the forces acting on the vessel walls caused by the friction of circulating blood *(60,61)*. These techniques have the potential to test the current hypotheses associating low and oscillating wall shear stress with the development of atherosclerosis.

ACTIVITY/FUNCTION

Iron oxide particles, which are used as MRI contrast agents, have differential effects on $1/T_1$ and $1/T_2$ depending on their molecular size *(37)*. Superparamagnetic iron oxide (SPIO) particles produce much larger increases in $1/T_2$ than in $1/T_1$, so they are preferably imaged with T_2-weighted scans, which reveal signal decrease *(62)*. SPIO particles produce a marked disturbance in surrounding magnetic field homogeneity, especially apparent when a nonhomogeneous distribution produces a T_2^* susceptibility effect. Ultrasmall superparamagnetic particles of iron oxide (USPIOs) have a greater effect on $1/T_1$ than SPIO particles, so these agents can also be used for T_1-weighted imaging.

The USPIO contrast agent Sinerem has been used in the evaluation of human carotid atheroma *(63,64)*, in which areas of focal signal loss on in vivo MR images corresponded to accumulation of iron particles in ex vivo specimens. Histological and electron microscopical analyses of the plaques showed USPIOs primarily in macrophages. Trivedi and colleagues examined the time-course for macrophage visualization by USPIO-enhanced MRI of carotid atherothrombosis, showing a signal intensity reduction between pre- and postcontrast images, with an optimal time window after injection of 24–36 hours *(65)*.

Virmani and colleagues *(66)* hypothesized that neovasculature could be the source of intraplaque hemorrhage, which has recently been linked to progression of carotid atherosclerotic plaques by Takaya et al. *(67)*. Kerwin and colleagues *(68)* developed a dynamic contrast technique for quantifying the amount of neovasculature surrounding atherosclerotic plaques providing a means for research into the link between neovasculature and plaque vulnerability.

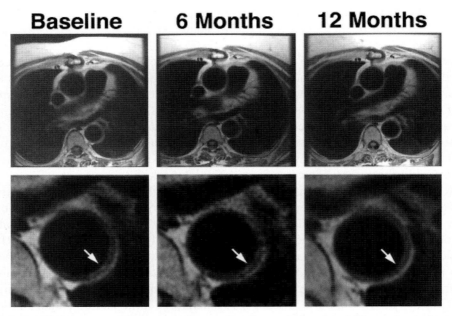

Fig. 7. Serial T2W images of the same patient at baseline and after 6 and 12 months statin therapy. Note the adequate matching of the images with a similar pattern of the coronary vessels (top). In detail of the descending aorta (bottom), arrows indicate maximal atherosclerotic plaque size, showing regression after 12 months statin therapy. (Reproduced from ref. *72* with permission.)

COMPUTATIONAL FLUID DYNAMICS

Using data acquired from MRI scans of an individual subject, velocity profiles and WSS distributions were quantified in an anatomically true model of the human carotid bifurcation. A numerical simulation approach combining the image-processing and computational fluid dynamics (CFD) techniques was developed *(69)*. Combining vessel wall geometries, including the morphological plaque features, with CFD simulations of the blood flow allows for mechanical analysis of human atherosclerotic plaques and could identify critical flow and stress/strain conditions, which are believed to be related to plaque rupture *(70)*. In vivo MRI and CFD techniques could bring new insights into the mechanical properties of plaque rupture, the pathogenesis of atherosclerosis, and estimations of patient-specific WSS levels as part of risk assessments of carotid plaques.

AORTA

Subclinical aortic atherosclerosis is correlated to the Framingham Coronary Risk Score *(26)*, suggesting that CMR imaging of subclinical aortic plaque burden will enhance risk stratification in asymptomatic individuals at intermediate-to-high risk. The principal challenges associated with CMR of the aorta are to obtain sufficient SNR allowing for submillimeter imaging and exclusion of artifacts caused by respiratory motion and blood flow. CMR imaging of plaque size, extent, and composition of thoracic aortic plaques was performed using T1W, T2W, and PDW imaging, showing good correlation to transesophageal echocardiography imaging *(27)*. Furthermore, CMR permits highly reproducible measures of aortic anatomy and atherosclerosis *(71)*, enabling serial studies to investigate the effect of, for example, statin therapy on regression of aortic plaque burden (Fig. 7) *(72)*.

CONCLUSION

Atherothrombosis, defined as atherosclerotic plaque disruption with superimposed thrombus formation, is the major cause of acute coronary syndromes and cardiovascular death. CMR is emerging as the most comprehensive noninvasive imaging technique for imaging of atherothrombosis in large- and medium-size arteries, including the aorta and the carotid, coronary, and peripheral arteries. Carotid atherothrombosis has been the subject of intense investigation by CMR, facilitated by the superficial location, relatively large size, and immobility. In addition, the carotid bifurcation shows the full spectrum of atherosclerotic lesion types, and it is also the only vascular bed where intact surgical specimens are readily available for histological examination and direct comparison to in vivo imaging.

CMR imaging of coronary wall atherothrombosis is particularly challenging because of the small caliber of the vessels combined with respiratory and cardiac motion. Free-breathing 3D CMR coronary vessel wall imaging has enabled in vivo quantification of coronary plaque burden and remodeling as a marker of subclinical CAD. Molecular imaging utilizing target-specific contrast agents such as fibrin-binding agents to detect arterial thrombus shows great promise as the new frontier in noninvasive imaging. Advances in molecular imaging and CMR techniques offer the potential for direct imaging of coronary thrombosis and in-stent thrombosis using fibrin-binding molecular MR contrast agents. Although the current role of noninvasive CMR imaging of atherothrombosis remains investigational, integration of vascular biology with CMR should enhance our understanding of the natural history of acute coronary syndromes and thereby facilitate strategies to prevent acute coronary syndromes and cardiovascular death in vulnerable patients.

REFERENCES

1. Yusuf S, Reddy S, Ounpuu S, Anand S. Global burden of cardiovascular diseases: part I: general considerations, the epidemiologic transition, risk factors, and impact of urbanization. Circulation 2001;104:2746–2753.
2. Naghavi M, Libby P, Falk E, et al. From vulnerable plaque to vulnerable patient: a call for new definitions and risk assessment strategies: part I. Circulation 2003;108:1664–1672.
3. Toussaint JF, LaMuraglia GM, Southern JF, Fuster V, Kantor HL. Magnetic resonance images lipid, fibrous, calcified, hemorrhagic, and thrombotic components of human atherosclerosis in vivo. Circulation 1996;94:932–938.
4. Fayad ZA, Fallon JT, Shinnar M, et al. Noninvasive in vivo high-resolution magnetic resonance imaging of atherosclerotic lesions in genetically engineered mice. Circulation 1998;98:1541–1547.
5. Yuan C, Mitsumori LM, Ferguson MS, et al. In vivo accuracy of multispectral magnetic resonance imaging for identifying lipid-rich necrotic cores and intraplaque hemorrhage in advanced human carotid plaques. Circulation 2001;104:2051–2056.
6. Kim WY, Danias PG, Stuber M, et al. Coronary magnetic resonance angiography for the detection of coronary stenoses. N Engl J Med 2001;345:1863–1869.
7. Wang Y, Vidan E, Bergman GW. Cardiac motion of coronary arteries: variability in the rest period and implications for coronary MR angiography. Radiology 1999;213:751–758.
8. Kim WY, Stuber M, Kissinger KV, Andersen NT, Manning WJ, Botnar RM. Impact of bulk cardiac motion on right coronary MR angiography and vessel wall imaging. J Magn Reson Imaging 2001;14:383–390.
9. Stehning C, Bornert P, Nehrke K, Dossel O. Free breathing 3D balanced FFE coronary magnetic resonance angiography with prolonged cardiac acquisition windows and intra-RR motion correction. Magn Reson Med 2005;53:719–723.
10. Taylor AM, Jhooti P, Wiesmann F, Keegan J, Firmin DN, Pennell DJ. MR navigator-echo monitoring of temporal changes in diaphragm position: implications for MR coronary angiography. J Magn Reson Imaging 1997;7:629–636.

11. Fayad ZA, Fuster V, Fallon JT, et al. Noninvasive in vivo human coronary artery lumen and wall imaging using black-blood magnetic resonance imaging. Circulation 2000;102:506–510.

12. Ehman RL, Felmlee JP. Adaptive technique for high-definition MR imaging of moving structures. Radiology 1989;173:255–263.

13. Li D, Kaushikkar S, Haacke EM, et al. Coronary arteries: three-dimensional MR imaging with retrospective respiratory gating. Radiology 201:857–863.

14. Stuber M, Botnar RM, Danias PG, Kissinger KV, Manning WJ. Submillimeter three-dimensional coronary MR angiography with real-time navigator correction: comparison of navigator locations. Radiology 1999;212:579–587.

15. Botnar RM, Kim WY, Bornert P, Stuber M, Spuentrup E, Manning WJ. 3D coronary vessel wall imaging utilizing a local inversion technique with spiral image acquisition. Magn Reson Med 2001;46:848–854.

16. Manke D, Nehrke K, Bornert P. Novel prospective respiratory motion correction approach for free-breathing coronary MR angiography using a patient-adapted affine motion model. Magn Reson Med 2003;50:122–131.

17. Botnar RM, Stuber M, Kissinger KV, Kim WY, Spuentrup E, Manning WJ. Noninvasive coronary vessel wall and plaque imaging with magnetic resonance imaging. Circulation 2000;102:2582–2587.

18. Stuber M, Botnar RM, Danias PG, et al. Double-oblique free-breathing high resolution three-dimensional coronary magnetic resonance angiography. J Am Coll Cardiol 1999;34:524–531.

19. Kim WY, Stuber M, Bornert P, et al. Three-dimensional black-blood cardiac magnetic resonance coronary vessel wall imaging detects positive arterial remodeling in patients with nonsignificant coronary artery disease. Circulation 2002;106:296–299.

20. Shinnar M, Fallon JT, Wehrli S, et al. The diagnostic accuracy of ex vivo MRI for human atherosclerotic plaque characterization. Arterioscler Thromb Vasc Biol 1999;19:2756–2761.

21. Yuan C, Petty C, O'Brien KD, Hatsukami TS, Eary JF, Brown BG. In vitro and in situ magnetic resonance imaging signal features of atherosclerotic plaque-associated lipids. Arterioscler Thromb Vasc Biol 1997;17:1496–1503.

22. Rogers WJ, Prichard JW, Hu YL, et al. Characterization of signal properties in atherosclerotic plaque components by intravascular MRI. Arterioscler Thromb Vasc Biol 2000;20:1824–1830.

23. Yuan C, Skinner MP, Kaneko E, et al. Magnetic resonance imaging to study lesions of atherosclerosis in the hyperlipidemic rabbit aorta. Magn Reson Imaging 1996;14:93–102.

24. Worthley SG, Helft G, Fuster V, et al. Noninvasive in vivo magnetic resonance imaging of experimental coronary artery lesions in a porcine model. Circulation 2000;101:2956–2961.

25. Cai JM, Hatsukami TS, Ferguson MS, Small R, Polissar NL, Yuan C. Classification of human carotid atherosclerotic lesions with in vivo multicontrast magnetic resonance imaging. Circulation 2002;106:1368–1373.

26. Jaffer FA, O'Donnell CJ, Larson MG, et al. Age and sex distribution of subclinical aortic atherosclerosis: a magnetic resonance imaging examination of the Framingham Heart Study. Arterioscler Thromb Vasc Biol 2002;22:849–854.

27. Fayad ZA, Nahar T, Fallon JT, et al. In vivo magnetic resonance evaluation of atherosclerotic plaques in the human thoracic aorta: a comparison with transesophageal echocardiography. Circulation 2000;101:2503–2509.

28. Schar M, Kim WY, Stuber M, Boesiger P, Manning WJ, Botnar RM. The impact of spatial resolution and respiratory motion on MR imaging of atherosclerotic plaque. J Magn Reson Imaging 2003;17:538–544.

29. Botnar RM, Perez AS, Witte S, et al. In vivo molecular imaging of acute and subacute thrombosis using a fibrin-binding magnetic resonance imaging contrast agent. Circulation 2004;109:2023–2029.

30. Botnar RM, Buecker A, Wiethoff AJ, et al. In vivo magnetic resonance imaging of coronary thrombosis using a fibrin-binding molecular magnetic resonance contrast agent. Circulation 2004;110:1463–1466.

31. Botnar RM, Bucker A, Kim WY, Viohl I, Gunther RW, Spuentrup E. Initial experiences with in vivo intravascular coronary vessel wall imaging. J Magn Reson Imaging 2003;17:615–619.

32. Botnar RM, Stuber M, Lamerichs R, et al. Initial experiences with in vivo right coronary artery human MR vessel wall imaging at 3 T. J Cardiovasc Magn Reson 2003;5:589–594.

33. Koktzoglou I, Simonetti O, Li D. Coronary artery wall imaging: initial experience at 3 T. J Magn Reson Imaging 2005;21:128–132.

34. Johnstone MT, Botnar RM, Perez AS, et al. In vivo magnetic resonance imaging of experimental thrombosis in a rabbit model. Arterioscler Thromb Vasc Biol 2001;21:1556–1560.

35. Corti R, Osende JI, Fayad ZA, et al. In vivo noninvasive detection and age definition of arterial thrombus by MRI. J Am Coll Cardiol 2002;39:1366–1373.
36. Moody AR, Murphy RE, Morgan PS, et al. Characterization of complicated carotid plaque with magnetic resonance direct thrombus imaging in patients with cerebral ischemia. Circulation 2003;107:3047–3052.
37. Weissleder R, Elizondo G, Wittenberg J, Rabito CA, Bengele HH, Josephson L. Ultrasmall superparamagnetic iron oxide: characterization of a new class of contrast agents for MR imaging. Radiology 1990;175:489–493.
38. Weissleder R. Molecular imaging: exploring the next frontier. Radiology 1999;212:609–614.
39. Flacke S, Fischer S, Scott MJ, et al. Novel MRI contrast agent for molecular imaging of fibrin: implications for detecting vulnerable plaques. Circulation 2001;104:1280–1285.
40. Johansson LO, Bjornerud A, Ahlstrom HK, Ladd DL, Fujii DK. A targeted contrast agent for magnetic resonance imaging of thrombus: implications of spatial resolution. J Magn Reson Imaging 2001;13:615–618.
41. Yu X, Song SK, Chen J, et al. High-resolution MRI characterization of human thrombus using a novel fibrin-targeted paramagnetic nanoparticle contrast agent. Magn Reson Med 2000;44:867–872.
42. Winter PM, Morawski AM, Caruthers SD, et al. Molecular imaging of angiogenesis in early-stage atherosclerosis with alpha(v)beta3-integrin-targeted nanoparticles. Circulation 2003;108:2270–2274.
43. Sibson NR, Blamire AM, Bernades-Silva M, et al. MRI detection of early endothelial activation in brain inflammation. Magn Reson Med 2004;51:248–252.
44. Barber PA, Foniok T, Kirk D, et al. MR molecular imaging of early endothelial activation in focal ischemia. Ann Neurol 2004;56:116–120.
45. Laurent S, Vander Elst L, Fu Y, Muller RN. Synthesis and physicochemical characterization of Gd-DTPA-B(sLex)A, a new MRI contrast agent targeted to inflammation. Bioconjug Chem 2004; 15:99–103.
46. Glagov S, Zarins C, Giddens DP, Ku DN. Hemodynamics and atherosclerosis. Insights and perspectives gained from studies of human arteries. Arch Pathol Lab Med 1988;112:1018–1031.
47. Beneficial effect of carotid endarterectomy in symptomatic patients with high-grade carotid stenosis. North American Symptomatic Carotid Endarterectomy Trial Collaborators. N Engl J Med 1991; 325:445–453.
48. MRC European Carotid Surgery Trial: interim results for symptomatic patients with severe (70–99%) or with mild (0–29%) carotid stenosis. European Carotid Surgery Trialists' Collaborative Group. Lancet 1991;337:1235–1243.
49. Hayes CE, Mathis CM, Yuan C. Surface coil phased arrays for high-resolution imaging of the carotid arteries. J Magn Reson Imaging 6:109–112.
50. Yuan C, Kerwin WS. MRI of atherosclerosis. J Magn Reson Imaging 2004;19:710–719.
51. Raynaud JS, Bridal SL, Toussaint JF, et al. Characterization of atherosclerotic plaque components by high resolution quantitative MR and US imaging. J Magn Reson Imaging 1998;8:622–629.
52. Mitsumori LM, Hatsukami TS, Ferguson MS, Kerwin WS, Cai J, Yuan C. In vivo accuracy of multi-sequence MR imaging for identifying unstable fibrous caps in advanced human carotid plaques. J Magn Reson Imaging 2003;17:410–420.
53. Saam T, Ferguson MS, Yarnykh VL, et al. Quantitative evaluation of carotid plaque composition by in vivo MRI. Arterioscler Thromb Vasc Biol 2005;25:234–239.
54. Nederkoorn PJ, van der GY, Hunink MG. Duplex ultrasound and magnetic resonance angiography compared with digital subtraction angiography in carotid artery stenosis: a systematic review. Stroke 2003;34:1324–1332.
55. Falk E. Coronary thrombosis: pathogenesis and clinical manifestations. Am J Cardiol 1991; 68:28B–35B.
56. Hatsukami TS, Ross R, Polissar NL, Yuan C. Visualization of fibrous cap thickness and rupture in human atherosclerotic carotid plaque in vivo with high-resolution magnetic resonance imaging. Circulation 2000;102:959–964.
57. Yuan C, Zhang SX, Polissar NL, et al. Identification of fibrous cap rupture with magnetic resonance imaging is highly associated with recent transient ischemic attack or stroke. Circulation 2002; 105:181–185.
58. Falk E. Why do plaques rupture? Circulation 1992;86:III30–III42.
59. Clarke SE, Hammond RR, Mitchell JR, Rutt BK. Quantitative assessment of carotid plaque composition using multicontrast MRI and registered histology. Magn Reson Med 2003;50:1199–1208.

60. Oyre S, Paaske WP, Ringgaard S, et al. Automatic accurate non-invasive quantitation of blood flow, cross-sectional vessel area, and wall shear stress by modelling of magnetic resonance velocity data. Eur J Vasc Endovasc Surg 1998;16:517–524.

61. Stokholm R, Oyre S, Ringgaard S, Flaagoy H, Paaske WP, Pedersen EM. Determination of wall shear rate in the human carotid artery by magnetic resonance techniques. Eur J Vasc Endovasc Surg 2000;20:427–433.

62. Ferrucci JT, Stark DD. Iron oxide-enhanced MR imaging of the liver and spleen: review of the first 5 years. AJR Am J Roentgenol 1990;155:943–950.

63. Schmitz SA, Taupitz M, Wagner S, Wolf KJ, Beyersdorff D, Hamm B. Magnetic resonance imaging of atherosclerotic plaques using superparamagnetic iron oxide particles. J Magn Reson Imaging 2001;14:355–361.

64. Kooi ME, Cappendijk VC, Cleutjens KB, et al. Accumulation of ultrasmall superparamagnetic particles of iron oxide in human atherosclerotic plaques can be detected by in vivo magnetic resonance imaging. Circulation 2003;107:2453–2458.

65. Trivedi RA, King-Im JM, Graves MJ, et al. In vivo detection of macrophages in human carotid atheroma: temporal dependence of ultrasmall superparamagnetic particles of iron oxide-enhanced MRI. Stroke 2004;35:1631–1635.

66. Virmani R, Narula J, Farb A. When neoangiogenesis ricochets. Am Heart J 1998;136:937–939.

67. Takaya N, Yuan C, Chu B, et al. Presence of intraplaque hemorrhage stimulates progression of carotid atherosclerotic plaques: a high-resolution magnetic resonance imaging study. Circulation 2005; 111:2768–2775.

68. Kerwin W, Hooker A, Spilker M, et al. Quantitative magnetic resonance imaging analysis of neovasculature volume in carotid atherosclerotic plaque. Circulation 2003;107:851–856.

69. Long Q, Xu XY, Ariff B, Thom SA, Hughes AD, Stanton AV. Reconstruction of blood flow patterns in a human carotid bifurcation: a combined CFD and MRI study. J Magn Reson Imaging 2000;11: 299–311.

70. Tang D, Yang C, Zheng J, et al. 3D MRI-based multicomponent FSI models for atherosclerotic plaques. Ann Biomed Eng 2004;32:947–960.

71. Chan SK, Jaffer FA, Botnar RM, et al. Scan reproducibility of magnetic resonance imaging assessment of aortic atherosclerosis burden. J Cardiovasc Magn Reson 2001;3:331–338.

72. Corti R, Fayad ZA, Fuster V, et al. Effects of lipid-lowering by simvastatin on human atherosclerotic lesions: a longitudinal study by high-resolution, noninvasive magnetic resonance imaging. Circulation 2001;104:249–252.

29 Magnetic Resonance Molecular Imaging and Targeted Therapeutics

Anne Morawski Neubauer, Patrick Winter,
Shelton Caruthers, Gregory Lanza,
and Samuel A. Wickline

CONTENTS

INTRODUCTION

Advances in cellular and molecular biology are extending the horizons of medical imaging from gross anatomical description toward delineation of cellular and biochemical signaling processes. The emerging fields of cellular and molecular imaging aim to noninvasively diagnose disease based on the in vivo detection and characterization of complex pathological processes, such as induction of inflammation or angiogenesis. Techniques have been developed to achieve molecular and cellular imaging with most imaging modalities, including nuclear *(1,2)*, optical *(2,3)*, ultrasound *(4,5)*, and magnetic resonance imaging (MRI) *(6,7)*. This chapter focuses on methods under development for detection of atherosclerosis and cardiovascular pathology by MRI molecular imaging. In particular, we focus on the growing role of nanotechnology in the development of new diagnostic and therapeutic constructs that can be used with MRI *(6,8)*.

From: *Contemporary Cardiology: Cardiovascular Magnetic Resonance Imaging*
Edited by: Raymond Y. Kwong © Humana Press Inc., Totowa, NJ

MRI is emerging as a particularly advantageous modality for molecular and cellular imaging given its high spatial resolution and the opportunity to extract both anatomical and physiological information simultaneously (7,9). Molecularly targeted MRI contrast agents consist of carrier molecules or particles that can bring a sufficient amount of paramagnetic or superparamagnetic materials to a selected site to permit in vivo visualization (10). In cardiovascular disease, novel targeted MRI contrast agents are under development to detect unstable lesions through identification of fibrin deposited within plaque microfissures (11–14), adhesion or thrombogenic molecules expressed on endothelium of vulnerable plaques (15–18), or angiogenesis (i.e., expanding vasa vasorum) supporting plaque development (19).

Atherosclerosis, like many chronic human diseases, including cancer and diabetes, develops slowly over many years. Unlike most other diseases, however, atherosclerosis is often diagnosed only after an acute, fatal event. Of the approximately 700,000 cardiac deaths per year in America, about 60% are "sudden deaths," occurring without any advanced warning of pathology (20). Atherosclerosis starts as "fatty streak" lesions in utero (21) and by the early teens can produce plaques prone to rupture (22). Rupture of unstable atherosclerotic plaques can lead to thrombosis, vascular occlusion, and subsequent myocardial infarction or stroke (23–25).

Atherosclerotic plaques grow in discrete stages consisting of repeated episodes of rupture, thrombosis, and healing (26), leading inevitably to a final event causing complete vascular obstruction (27). A vulnerable plaque is defined as a lesion exhibiting physical and biochemical properties that predispose it to rupture and thrombosis but may not yet be ruptured (26). Typically, these plaques consist of a large lipid core covered by a thin fibrous cap harboring relatively few smooth muscle cells, a population of activated macrophages, and abundant angiogenesis (28). The large lipid core is known to destabilize lesions by directing mechanical stress to the fragile shoulder regions of the plaque (29). Exposure of the lipid core, even through a small localized rupture, can induce the clotting cascade through the interaction of serum clotting factors with locally expressed tissue factor (30).

The lack of smooth muscle cells also weakens the cap (31), facilitating plaque rupture. The accumulation of macrophages as well as other inflammatory cells, which usually secrete high levels of metalloproteinases (MMPs), can undermine the fibrous cap, potentially exposing the thrombotic lipid core (32,33). Upregulation of angiogenesis can lead to erosion of the extracellular matrix and replacement with physically fragile neovascular beds, weakening the fibrous cap and promoting plaque rupture (34–36).

In current clinical practice, the diagnosis and characterization of most atherosclerotic plaques is achieved with invasive X-ray catheterization. Highly stenotic lesions, typically with 50% or greater narrowing of the lumenal diameter, are identified for immediate therapeutic intervention; less-stenotic lesions are generally deemed clinically insignificant. Ironically, these plaques are often the very lesions prone to rupture, leading to heart attack and stroke (37,38).

Stress tests employing nuclear or ultrasound imaging are also extensively used for detection of flow-limiting vascular obstructions during a range of metabolic challenges. Similar to invasive X-ray angiography, however, these techniques are insensitive to plaques with low-grade stenosis, which are those most prone to rupture. Because rupturing atherosclerotic plaques are frequently manifest at various stages in arteries with only modest (40–60%) stenosis (39,40), they remain diagnostically elusive with routine clinical imaging techniques. If recognized and localized, a window of opportunity extending from days to months exists to intervene or stabilize plaques medically before more serious clinical sequelae ensue *(27)*.

The principal difficulty revolves around the fact that atherosclerosis produces numerous plaques throughout the vascular system, and it is not feasible to individually treat each lesion. Of all the less than 50% stenotic lesions, only a small fraction might rupture and lead to clinical events. A significant new opportunity exists for delineating which lesions are prone to rupture and applying therapeutic treatments to only the areas of pathology that pose an immediate danger.

CELLULAR AND MOLECULAR IMAGING

To achieve clinically effective cellular and molecular imaging with MRI, targeted contrast agents must be designed to accomplish long circulating half-life, sensitive and selective binding to the epitope of interest, prominent contrast-to-noise enhancement, acceptable toxicity, ease of clinical use, and applicability with standard commercially available imaging systems. A variety of different types of ligands can be utilized for targeting, including antibodies, peptides, polysaccharides, aptamers, and more.

MRI may enjoy several advantages over the other modalities, such as high resolution, high anatomical contrast, high signal-to-noise ratio (SNR), widespread clinical availability, and lack of ionizing radiation. However, because of comparatively modest contrast enhancement in present usage vs nuclear imaging of localized radioactive tracers, for example, MRI detection can take advantage of novel nanotechnologies to provide sufficient contrast-to-noise features for noninvasive depiction of the molecular signatures of disease.

Because molecular epitopes of interest may reside on or inside of cells in sparse quantities, existing even at low nanomolar or picomolar concentrations, one may require a considerable amplification of the local contrast effect to achieve sufficient diagnostic signal. For example, in the case of paramagnetic agents for T_1-weighted imaging, simple attachment of a gadolinium atom to an antibody as a targeting ligand may not provide enough signal if micromolar concentrations of the lanthanide are required to elicit contrast enhancement based on conventional T_1 relaxation mechanisms (*see* below) *(41,42)*.

Accordingly, accumulation of a high payload of metal-chelate at the site of sparse cellular epitopes more often than not will require binding of a gadolinium-loaded particulate carrier or a nanoparticle. In the case of T_1-weighted (or "hot spot") imaging, it is the surface area of the particle decorated with gadolinium chelate that is critical to deposition of sufficient gadolinium to achieve the micromolar concentrations required. In the case of "cold spot" imaging with superparamagnetic agents, sufficient material can be packed into the core of the nanoparticle to exert a prominent T_2^* effect, producing a localized signal reduction that can be detected with potentially greater sensitivity than is possible with paramagnetic agents.

The rapid growth of nanotechnology and nanoscience is expected to greatly expand the clinical opportunities for magnetic resonance (MR) molecular imaging *(6,7,43)*. Nanotechnology seeks to develop and combine new materials by precisely engineering atoms and molecules to yield new molecular assemblies on the scale of individual cells, organelles, or even smaller components, generally in the range of 1–300 nm. The specific organization of such nanoscale materials is anticipated to confer unique chemical and biological properties based on interactions at their surfaces. These materials might mimic or substitute for many existing features of cell behavior that already operate at the nanoscale level.

Indeed, the National Heart Lung and Blood Institute initiated a Program of Excellence in Nanotechnology, funding Centers of Excellence to develop new approaches to diagnostics and therapeutics based on nanoscience. The National Cancer Institute for some time has sponsored similar research, leading to the inception of their Centers for Cancer Nanotechnology Excellence program. Other government organizations both here and abroad have developed active nanotechnology research and translational agendas *(6)*.

The intent of this research is to develop an array of systems that can serve as biosensors, diagnostic and therapeutic devices, molecular imaging agents, and biomaterials for cell or tissue replacement. Synthesis of such materials may occur from a top-down approach by miniaturizing existing microscopic materials or more likely from a bottom-up approach involving self-assembly of molecules into reproducible and well-defined nanoscale constructs. Some of the nanoscale molecular imaging agents that have been proposed and tested for cardiovascular diagnosis and therapy are described.

SUPERPARAMAGNETIC NANOPARTICLES

Ultrasmall superparamagnetic iron oxide (USPIO) nanoparticles are potent MRI contrast agents. The iron produces strong local disruptions in the magnetic field of MRI scanners, which lead to increased T_2* relaxation. This increased relaxation causes decreased image intensity in areas with iron oxide accumulation, termed *susceptibility artifacts*. When formulated with a dextran coating and a diameter within the range of 15–25 nm, these particles have a long circulating half-life and appear to be sequestered by macrophages in the body. These properties have allowed dextran-coated USPIO nanoparticles to be employed for passive targeted imaging of pathological inflammatory processes, such as unstable atherosclerotic plaques, by MRI *(44)*. For example, USPIO-labeled macrophages have been imaged and localized to unstable and ruptured plaques (75% demonstrating uptake) but not in stable lesions (only 7% showing USPIO uptake) *(45)*.

The imaging protocols are critically important for USPIO detection by MRI. The susceptibility artifacts created by accumulation of USPIOs are most sensitively imaged with T_2*-weighted imaging sequences. T_1-weighted and proton density imaging sequences are far less sensitive to the susceptibility artifacts induced by USPIO uptake in tissues *(45)*. The T_2*-weighted sequences typically utilize gradient echo techniques with long echo times. The long echo time accentuates signal loss caused by the presence of USPIOs, but these sequences also tend to suffer from a low SNR. Often, highly specialized coils, such as phased array coils or application-specific surface coils, are employed to maximize the available SNR *(44,45)*.

Blood vessels are typically surrounded by fatty tissue, which can interfere with imaging structures within the arterial wall. On MRI, fat appears as a bright signal, which often displays a spatial misregistration artifact relative to other tissues in the body, called a *chemical shift artifact*. This artifact can often overlap signals from the vessel wall and obscure the atherosclerotic plaques under investigation. To avoid this problem, imaging sequences employing fat-suppression or selective excitation techniques are used for imaging USPIO uptake *(44–46)*. With these sequences, fat appears dark because its signal is either suppressed or not excited. In a similar manner, bright blood imaging sequences, such as two-dimensional fast, low-angle shot (FLASH) sequences, are often used for detection of USPIOs (45,46). The bright blood signal allows clearer definition of the vessel lumen, and signal voids in the arterial wall caused by USPIO uptake are much easier to distinguish.

In addition to the imaging protocol itself, the choice of imaging time after USPIO injection is critically important. The long circulating half-life of dextran-coated USPIO nanoparticles is necessary to achieve adequate loading into inflammatory cells, but it can also interfere with obtaining high-quality images. Up to approximately 24 hours after USPIO administration, the blood concentration is high enough to create image artifacts (44,45), which can obscure visualization of the vessel wall. On the other hand, too long of a delay (~72 hours) after USPIO injection can result in no detectable susceptibility artifacts.

Besides the sequence dependence for signal detection and the time required for contrast agent clearance from the circulatory system (perhaps 24 hours or more before imaging can be performed), other artifacts exist. The cold spot imaging technique might be confused with other susceptibility artifacts in the image, all of which might be amplified at higher (e.g., 3 T) field strengths. Indeed, cold spots may abound in background tissues, rendering specific diagnosis based on signal loss difficult. A comparative before-and-after image may be required, which would be separated by 24 hours or more, creating difficulties for image registration. Also, for imaging disrupted lesions, intraplaque hemorrhage (a concomitant of microfissures) leads to deposition of heme moieties that may create susceptibility artifacts of their own.

Advances in imaging techniques have enabled hot spot detection of iron oxide-based particles. Exploiting the same inherent dipole of magnetic particles that causes signal dropout on typical MR imaging, Cunningham et al. (47) and Stuber et al. (48) illustrated techniques for off-resonance imaging that can instead produce bright signals in regions surrounding the accumulation of particles. Stemming from similar methods employed for tracking catheters (49), these techniques require specialized excitation pulses that image the water molecules in close proximity to an accumulation of particles. Once optimized, these techniques offer potential for localizing sources of extraneous magnetic dipoles (i.e., superparamagnetic particles) and, via their signal intensity, tracking their size and distribution and providing a method for relative quantification.

PARAMAGNETIC NANOPARTICLES

As an alternative approach, ligand-targeted, lipid-encapsulated, nongaseous perfluorocarbon nanoparticle emulsions have been applied for molecular imaging (11,12,14,50). The nanoparticles can be formulated to carry paramagnetic gadolinium ions and targeted to a number of important biochemical epitopes, such as fibrin, tissue factor, and $\alpha_v\beta_3$-integrin, which allow binding to cell or tissue surfaces (Fig. 1).

Unlike the USPIO agents, the image enhancement characteristics of commercially available paramagnetic contrast agents are too small to visualize the sparse concentrations (e.g., picomolar to nanomolar) of epitopes relevant to molecular imaging. By incorporating vast numbers of paramagnetic complexes (>50,000) onto each particle, the signal enhancement possible for each binding site is magnified dramatically, by a factor of more than 10^6. The increased paramagnetic influence arises from two mechanisms: the relaxivity per particle increases linearly with respect to the number of gadolinium complexes, and the relaxivity of each gadolinium increases because of the slower tumbling of the molecule when

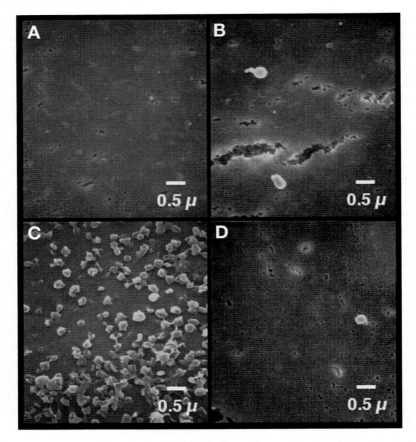

Fig. 1. Scanning electron micrographs (12,000×) of porcine aortic smooth muscle cells known to overexpress cell surface tissue factor in culture. (**A**) Cells exposed to phosphate buffer as a control. (**B**) Cells exposed to unconjugated control emulsion (no targeting ligand). (**C**) Cells exposed to tissue factor-targeted emulsion. (**D**) Cells pretreated with anti-tissue factor antibody and subsequently exposed to tissue factor-targeted emulsion.

attached to the much larger particle. By studying dilutions of nanoparticles in water, we have observed increased T_1 relaxivity with increasing gadolinium payloads (11). We also verified that the increased relaxivity seen in solution corresponded to increased signal intensity on T_1-weighted images of particles bound to fibrin clots (Fig. 2) (11). Thus, improvements in the formulation chemistry can be assessed in simple phantoms of nanoparticle dilutions and verified in models of physiological systems.

The T_1 relaxivity (r_1) of nanoparticles formulated with gadolinium diethylenetriamine-pentaacetic acid *bis*-oleate (51) (Gd-DTPA-BOA) or gadolinium diethylenetriaminepen-taacetic acid-phosphatidylethanolamine (Gd-DTPA-PE) (52) has been measured at selected magnetic field strengths: 0.47, 1.5, and 4.7 T. At all magnetic field strengths, r_1 of the Gd-DTPA-PE formulation was approximately two times greater than for the Gd-DTPA-BOA agent (13), indicating that small adjustments to the molecular configuration of a paramagnetic chelate can substantially improve the fundamental relaxation properties.

Variable-temperature relaxometry measurements have shown that r_1 of the Gd-DTPA-BOA emulsion was largely independent of temperature (13). In contrast, r_1 increased at higher temperatures for the Gd-DTPA-PE emulsion. These temperature-dependent

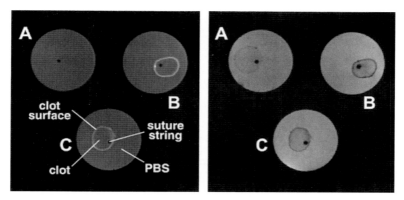

Fig. 2. Cross-sectional T_1-(left) and T_2-(right) weighted spin echo images of cylindrical clots formed on suture strings. Clots were suspended in PBS solution and imaged with a 5-cm birdcage coil. Untreated clot (**A**) showed minimal contrast with PBS solution in both T_1- and T_2-weighted images. With the binding of fibrin-targeted contrast agent on the surfaces of the clots, both treated (**B**) and partially blocked (**C**) clots showed excellent contrast with surrounding PBS solution because of the decrease in both T_1 and T_2 relaxation times.

data suggest that the water exchange rate with the paramagnetic ion is higher for the Gd-DTPA-PE chelate as compared with Gd-DTPA-BOA. At the higher temperature, the r_1 of Gd-DTPA-PE nanoparticles increased because of the faster water exchange and increased kinetic activity. The Gd-DTPA-BOA nanoparticles, however, may experience somewhat restricted water access and did not benefit from the increased kinetic activity of water at the higher temperature. This increased water exchange may result from the elevated position of the chelate relative to the phosphate head group level (i.e., more distant from the particles' surface) for Gd-DTPA-PE nanoparticles *(52)* and likely contributed to the marked increase of the relaxivity of the Gd-DTPA-PE nanoparticles.

Although we have demonstrated that increased relaxivity augments visualization of targeted epitopes, these techniques can only improve molecular imaging to a finite extent. With the use of MRI signal modeling programs, we can theoretically evaluate a range of contrast agent relaxivities at different magnetic field strengths *(42)*. At higher magnetic fields, the SNR increases, leading to increased contrast-to-noise ratio and a lower detectable limit of contrast agent binding. Therefore, we expect that the application of higher clinical field strengths (i.e., 3 T) could considerably improve the performance of current molecular imaging agents and help facilitate adoption of these techniques in clinical practice. In contrast, attempts to increase the intrinsic paramagnetic relaxivity (r_1) of a molecular imaging agent beyond a certain point do not improve the lower detection limit in a linear fashion because potential reductions in T_1 times ultimately encounter asymptotic limits at high relaxivity values, as shown by us *(42)* and others *(53)* (Fig. 3). Accordingly, efforts to enhance the performance of molecular imaging contrast agents through increasing the ionic relaxivity may offer only limited additional benefit. For example, methods that feature contrast agents with two exchangeable water sites might double the relaxivity under certain conditions but not yield the orders of magnitude (10^6) type of improvement that can be gained through the use of high-payload nanoparticles.

The chemistry employed to bind the targeted ligand to the particle surface can also dramatically affect the efficacy of the final contrast agent. In some cases, the active binding site of the ligand may become occupied or obscured after attachment to

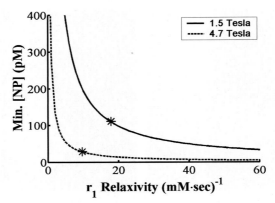

Fig. 3. Minimum predicted nanoparticle concentration necessary for generating visually apparent contrast as a function of relaxivity per gadolinium molecule on the particle. Stars indicate the current formulation values. Note that, as the relaxivity increases, there is a diminishing return on decreasing the minimum concentration needed.

the nanoparticle. Obviously, such agents would yield poor molecular imaging results. In addition, the incorporation of flexible polymer spacers (i.e., polyethylene glycol) between the targeting ligand and the nanoparticle surface may improve targeting efficiency. These flexible "tethers" permit a wider range of motion for the targeting ligand, potentially increasing the likelihood of encountering and binding to the target of interest.

In addition to the number of gadolinium ions per particle, the number of targeting ligands per particle must also be optimized. A nanoparticle with numerous binding ligands (i.e., high ligand valency) tends to provide a more efficacious contrast agent. The combination of ligand valency and binding affinity (i.e., avidity) allows the contrast agent to rapidly and tenaciously bind to the intended biomarker. Incorporating too many targeting ligands on each nanoparticle, however, can in certain cases produce steric hindrance, inhibiting binding to the desired epitope. An excessively dense cover of ligands on the particle surface may also interfere with the relaxivity by impeding free water interaction with the gadolinium complexes.

FLUORINE IMAGING WITH NANOPARTICLES

Alternatively, the signal generated by the fluorine atoms in the perfluorocarbon core of the nanoparticles can be used for either imaging or spectroscopy in certain situations as an alternative or compliment to traditional proton imaging *(14,54)*. Biological tissues contain little endogenous fluorine, so measurement of the fluorine component of targeted particles has the potential for definitive confirmation of particle deposition at the site because the fluorine signal is unique. This avoids many of the issues associated with contrast agents that rely solely on paramagnetic signal amplification on proton images such as partial volume dilution of the signal, confusion with local signal inhomogeneities caused by tissue variation, and the particular scan sequence selected. Furthermore, when looking for paramagnetic agents that have accumulated at low concentrations (e.g., the signal change is small), it may be prudent to acquire images both before and after contrast agent administration to deemphasize the background signal. With fluorine imaging, there is essentially no background, allowing for the possibility of requiring only a single image after contrast agent administration.

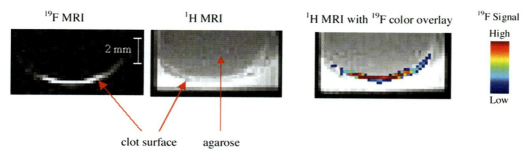

Fig. 4. MR images of a fibrin clot targeted with perfluorocarbon nanoparticles acquired at 4.7 T. The fluorine signal is clearly localized to the clot surface (right), and the fluorine signal (left) is less ambiguous than the proton (middle) for determining where the particles have bound.

The biggest challenge to date for fluorine imaging has been in generating sufficient signal. This problem can be mitigated by using high field strengths (e.g., 3 T or greater) or vastly increasing the concentration of targeted fluorine in the body with various agents *(55,56)*. In the case of molecular imaging with perfluorocarbon particles, the fluorine atoms become localized to the site of interest, allowing them to accumulate at a high concentration and provide enough signal for MRI and spectroscopy. This technique has been demonstrated for imaging of fibrin at 4.7 T (Fig. 4) *(54)*. In addition, the fluorine nuclear magnetic resonance (NMR) spectra that can be acquired from the samples are quantitative for the presence of fluorine atoms. Therefore, by combining imaging and spectroscopy, it may be feasible to generate a quantitative map of bound nanoparticles, which should be representative of the number of epitope-binding sites *(54)*.

Another use for fluorine imaging and spectroscopy of perfluorocarbon particles is in recognizing different targeted moieties on the same sample. Because of differences in their local nuclear environments (e.g., electron shielding, J-coupling, etc.), different fluorine atoms resonate at slightly different frequencies so that they are often readily separable on an NMR spectrum *(57)*. This means that, by using perfluorocarbon nanoparticles formulated with different perfluorocarbon species, it is possible to target them to the same sample and quantify their presence separately with one spectroscopic scan *(54)*. Although spectroscopy will ultimately be most useful for quantification, other techniques allow imaging of the different perfluorocarbon particles as well. These may include frequency-selective excitation so that only the perfluorocarbon species of interest produces a signal or other forms of chemical shift imaging that have been developed for differentiating fat from water in clinical imaging *(58,59)*.

Finally, perfluorocarbons have an interesting interaction with oxygen that may provide another avenue for research into cardiovascular disease with MRI. The R_1 relaxation rate constant (inverse of T_1 relaxation time) of many perfluorocarbon species varies linearly with oxygen content, indicating that they can be used as a sensitive indicator of oxygenation levels *(56,59)*. This feature has been explored extensively for mapping pO_2 concentrations in the lungs *(55,60)* and in tumors *(56,61,62)* but may also extend to other areas of research in the cardiovascular field, particularly in delineating arteries from veins or for highlighting areas downstream of stenosis where pO_2 content would be low *(63)*. Fluorine MRI of perfluorocarbon agents may thus provide a means of producing angiographic images with additional information that may lead to improved diagnosis and treatment *(64)*.

OPTIMIZATION OF MAGNETIC RESONANCE
IMAGING TECHNIQUES

In contradistinction to USPIO agents, which are designed to increase the T_2^* relaxation of targeted tissue, paramagnetic compounds are typically used to increase T_1 relaxation. The T_2^* effect employed with USPIOs is usually visualized as decreased image intensity with T_2^*-weighted MRI. Paramagnetic agents, however, will produce increased tissue signal when interrogated with T_1-weighted MRI. Therefore, the contrast effects of USPIO and paramagnetic agents are very different, and the MRI pulse sequences and parameters are also distinct for the two methods.

The signal level and contrast obtainable with a given sequence depend heavily on the scan parameters employed. For instance, with T_1-weighted imaging, those tissues or samples with a lower T_1 relaxation time produce more signal than those with a higher T_1, providing a means for generating contrast in the image. However, the actual amount of contrast is highly dependent on the repetition time (TR) used in the scanning sequence *(41)*. Given two tissues with known T_1 times, it is possible to optimize the TR to maximize the difference in signal produced between them *(42)*. Scanning with a TR that is 300–400 ms removed from this optimum value can reduce the contrast-to-noise ratio by up to 25%, which is problematic when imaging low concentrations of paramagnetic agents.

From an MRI sequence design perspective, it might be useful to have some knowledge *a priori* of the expected concentration of paramagnetic agent that will accumulate at the site so that the proper scan parameters can be chosen for optimum detection ability. If such information is not known, then one might use fast T_1 mapping sequences, such as Look-Locker EPI, to provide quantitative data *(65)*.

As with the USPIO particles, adequate circulation must be allowed for ligand-targeted nanoparticles to reach and bind to the molecular marker of interest. The pharmacokinetics and pharmacodynamics can be influenced by surface chemistry, in vivo stability, size, and the biological milieu. Approximately 2–3 hours are required to saturate a vascular-accessible biochemical target, reflecting the time required for all blood to complete one passage through a remote vascular bed. The time to maximum signal can be decreased by increasing the amount of contrast agent injected, but the dose is typically limited to the minimum effective dose.

We generally inject 0.5–1.0 mL/kg of perfluorocarbon nanoparticles for animal experiments, which fortunately is much lower than the amount required to generate an appreciable blood pool signal *(13,19)*. This approach avoids the issue of whether the contrast is specifically targeted to the site or just circulating through a region of interest. Such problems can be particularly vexatious for agents with high signal intensity and prolonged half-lives. The dramatic effects of particle composition and chemistry on contrast agent elimination kinetics and the resulting imaging protocol can be appreciated by comparing the optimum imaging time-points of three vastly different contrast agents. For example, $\alpha_v\beta_3$-targeted nanoparticles yield significant MRI contrast signal enhancement within 30 minutes *(66)* to 2 hours after injection *(13,19)* compared with 24 hours for a liposome agent *(67)* and 36 hours for an avidin-DTPA complex *(10)*.

Although bright blood imaging sequences are preferred for distinguishing the negative contrast effects of USPIO accumulation, black blood techniques are better suited for visualization of MRI signal enhancement caused by targeted paramagnetic nanoparticles *(19)*. For instance, one black blood MRI method involves collecting cross-sectional images of a vessel and placing saturation bands on either side of the current imaging plane. These saturation bands null all MRI signals on either side of the imaged slice, including signal from the blood. A short delay is inserted between application of the saturation bands and image data acquisition, allowing the saturated blood to flow into the imaged slice, which provides no signal. By placing saturation bands on both sides of the current slice, both arterial and venous blood appears black on the final image. As with USPIO imaging, the chemical shift artifact from fat can obscure visualization of the vessel wall. Therefore, fat-suppression techniques are often employed to null the fat signal and provide clear delineation of vessel wall anatomy (19).

QUANTIFICATION OF THE MAGNETIC RESONANCE SIGNAL

Although tracking qualitative changes in signal intensity before and after contrast agent administration can provide diagnostic information, the ability to quantify the absolute amount of agent could prove invaluable for following therapy. In the case of targeted imaging, it may be important to characterize the change in molecular binding over the course of drug treatment as a surrogate marker for treatment efficacy. If the drug delivery vehicle is directly linked to the imaging agent, quantification of the concentration of the therapeutic agent delivered to the intended site also is important.

However, unlike traditional nuclear techniques in which the image generated is a direct map of the number of emitting radioisotopes, the signal from MR images is complicated by the presence of magnetic relaxation phenomena. With proton (^{1}H nuclei) imaging, contrast agents serve to increase (paramagnetic) or decrease (superparamagnetic) the signal intensity in the MR image by affecting the relaxation processes of the nearby water molecules. The equations that describe how these agents change the T_1 and T_2 relaxation of tissues as a function of their concentration can be used as inputs to signal-modeling paradigms to predict contrast behavior for the scan sequence parameters used. This approach has been described by Morawski et al. for predicting the minimum concentration of targeted paramagnetic nanoparticles that must bind to a site to produce adequate contrast for diagnosis (42).

However, signal-modeling approaches can be confounded by partial volume dilution effects, the need for a priori estimates of contrast agent concentration, and local inhomogeneities in tissue signal levels. A more accurate method for quantification is the use of MR sequences specifically designed for measuring relaxation times in a given sample. The traditional sequences used, such as inversion recovery and partial saturation recovery, are highly accurate but time consuming.

Much faster variations have been developed including Look-Locker EPI and multiple-angle gradient echo (65,68). These sequences provide quantitative information regarding the degree to which the contrast agent has affected the relaxation parameters, and from these data, one can calculate the concentration of agent that must be present if the intrinsic relaxivity of the agent is known (and does not change after binding). Morawski et al. used this technique to determine the amount of "tissue factor"-targeted nanoparticles bound to a sample of porcine aortic smooth muscle cells that constitutively expressed tissue factor in culture (42). Although this method is more precise than ones employing signal intensity values alone, it still may suffer from inaccuracies related to characterizing the relaxivity of an agent (water exchange rates); crowding of the gadolinium molecules when bound to a surface, reducing access to free water exchange; excessive particle "off rates" in cases of low-avidity/low-valency agents; nonspecific binding; and such, all of which can affect the assumptions under which the quantification is carried out.

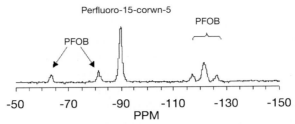

Fig. 5. ^{19}F NMR spectrum of two different nanoparticle formulations, one made with perfluoro-15-crown-5 ether and one made with perfluorooctylbromide (PFOB) as its core component. The peaks of these two perfluorocarbons are readily separable and quantifiable, thus providing a mechanism for quantitative molecular targeting of more than one epitope within the same sample.

Another option for quantification is to use a separate MR signal that is unique, such as fluorine. With ^{1}H imaging, quantification requires characterizing the signal *change* after contrast agent administration. However, if a separate signal that is not present in the sample prior to delivery of the agent used, quantification becomes much more straightforward as the agent is the only signal-producing molecule in the sample. NMR spectroscopy can be utilized to measure the total amount of contrast agent present in a sample, as demonstrated with fibrin-targeted perfluorocarbon nanoparticles bound to clots *(54)*. MRI using fluorine is still subject to variations in relaxation parameters, but in this case all the signal-generating nuclei have the same relaxation times (if pH, temperature, and oxygen content are the same at all locations), so that the images can be quantified. Finally, as discussed, multiple perfluorocarbons with distinct chemical shifts can be quantified and imaged separately, providing a technique for multiple-epitope quantification *(54)* (Fig. 5).

ESTABLISHING TARGET SPECIFICITY

The targeting ability of nanoparticle contrast agents should be validated under controlled experimental conditions. Confirmation of active particle targeting is best achieved with in vivo competition procedures *(13,19)*. Targeted, high-avidity nanoparticles lacking the paramagnetic gadolinium chelate are injected to occupy all available binding sites, but they do not provide MRI signal enhancement. Subsequent injection of targeted paramagnetic nanoparticles will produce image enhancement only through nonspecific and passive particle accumulation if all specific binding sites are occupied. In this manner, we have demonstrated specific molecular imaging of angiogenesis in vasa vasorum of atherosclerotic plaques in cholesterol-fed rabbits and in nascent Vx-2 tumors implanted in the hind limb of rabbits *(69)*. Alternative methods entail use of particles containing nonspecific binding ligands that are known not to bind to the intended target.

SPECIFIC EXAMPLES OF CARDIOVASCULAR IMAGING

Imaging Molecular Epitopes Associated With Unstable or Disrupted Plaque

A *disrupted plaque* is one that already has ruptured, or manifested fissures or erosions, as compared to the more quiescent vulnerable plaque. The *sine qua non* of the disrupted plaque is fibrin deposition: fibrin deposition is one of the earliest signs of plaque rupture or erosion, and it also forms a large part of the core of growing lesions *(70)*.

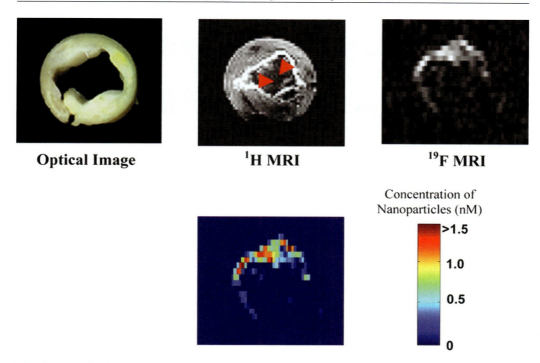

Optical Image   **¹H MRI**   **¹⁹F MRI**

Concentration of
Nanoparticles (nM)

>1.5

1.0

0.5

0

Fig. 6. An excised human carotid endarterectomy sample was treated with fibrin-targeted perfluoro-carbon nanoparticles. The optical image (top, left) shows asymmetrical plaque distribution with areas of fat deposition. The proton MR image shows signal enhancement caused by paramagnetic nanoparticle binding (middle, red arrowheads), and the fluorine projection image shows heterogeneous binding through the sample. Using NMR spectroscopy, the fluorine image can be converted into a map of the nanoparticle binding, corresponding to the number of epitopes (bottom).

The diagnosis of disrupted plaque by detecting small deposits of fibrin in erosions or microfractures could allow characterization of the potential "culprit" lesion before a high-grade stenosis has been formed that is detectable by cardiac catheterization.

The possibility of targeted fibrin imaging with paramagnetic MR contrast agents was first demonstrated by Lanza et al. in 1996 *(71)*. By loading 250-nm perfluorocarbon particles with 50,000–90,000 gadolinium atoms per particle, a substantial amplification of signal was achieved after binding that ultimately allowed detection of fibrin clots both in vitro and in vivo *(7,12)*. Furthermore, the detection of disrupted plaque was illustrated in actual human carotid endarterectomy specimens obtained from patients symptomatic with transient ischemic attacks, stroke, or bruits *(11)* (Fig. 6). In this case, the ligand comprised an antibody fragment highly specific for the E domain of cross-linked fibrin, which can be complexed to the particle either through avidin-biotin linkages or directly linked to the functionalized nanoparticle as we have shown for tissue factor antibodies *(16,17)*.

Epix Pharmaceuticals (Cambridge, MA) utilized phage display methods to produce a peptide ligand specific for fibrin (EP-2104R), which may be useful for imaging thrombi in various body locations *(72–74)*. It contains four Gd-DTPA chelates per peptide moiety and thus provides signal enhancement on an MR image. Despite the low gadolinium load per binding site, the excess of fibrin epitopes in fresh or chronic clots allows accumulation of contrast agent concentrations sufficient to achieve micromolar levels of the lanthanide and thus ready detection of the clot.

Targeted   Non-targeted   Untreated

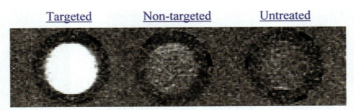

Fig. 7. MR image of smooth muscle cell monolayers treated with tissue factor-targeted paramagnetic nanoparticles. Note the distinct signal enhancement of the treated cell layers as compared to the non-targeted (given particles without the targeting ligand) and the untreated group.

Spuentrup et al. demonstrated the potential of this agent for imaging human clots produced ex vivo and implanted into the left atrium or trapped in the pulmonary arteries of swine *(73,74)*. In both cases, intravenous delivery of EP-2104R produced appreciable contrast in the location of the clots after the signal in the blood pool was sufficiently decreased (1–2 hours). Furthermore, Botnar et al. applied this technique to clots produced in vivo with the use of thrombogenic stents placed in the left coronary artery of swine *(72)*.

Neeman's group reported development of a low molecular weight transglutaminase substrate for imaging fibrin clots *(75)*. Plasma and tissue transglutaminase are instrumental for stabilizing matrix materials such as fibrin in clots through crosslinking selected peptidyl glutamine residues. A peptide seven amino acids long served as the substrate and was linked to Gd-DTPA as the imaging agent. Transglutaminase activity could be detected in both fibrin clots and tumor spheroids at 9.4 T with T_1-weighted sequences.

Tissue factor is a prothrombotic transmembrane glycoprotein expressed within plaques that is upregulated following vascular injury or stent placement and contributes as a mitogen to restenosis *(76)*. Tissue factor in the core of plaques is exposed during plaque rupture and is the proximate cause of local thrombosis that leads to vessel occlusion or distal embolization. Tissue factor imaging has been demonstrated in vivo for molecular imaging with ultrasound and in vitro with MRI *(17,42)*. In fact, the ability to image tissue factor-targeted paramagnetic nanoparticles bound to smooth muscle cell monolayers in cell culture at 1.5 T attests to the potency of nanoparticle agents that carry 50,000 or more gadolinium chelates (Fig. 7).

Angiogenesis

Although fibrin and tissue factor can be utilized to delineate unstable cardiovascular diseases, the $\alpha_v\beta_3$-integrin is a general marker of angiogenesis and plays an important role in a wide variety of disease states *(77)*. The $\alpha_v\beta_3$-integrin is a well-characterized heterodimeric adhesion molecule that is widely expressed by endothelial cells, monocytes, fibroblasts, and vascular smooth muscle cells. In particular, $\alpha_v\beta_3$-integrin plays a critical part in smooth muscle cell migration and cellular adhesion *(78,79)*, both of which are required for the formation of new blood vessels. The $\alpha_v\beta_3$-integrin is expressed on the luminal surface of activated endothelial cells but not on mature quiescent cells *(80)*. We have demonstrated the utility of $\alpha_v\beta_3$-integrin-targeted nanoparticles for the detection and characterization of angiogenesis associated with growth factor expression *(81)*, tumor growth *(69)* (Fig. 8), and atherosclerosis *(19)*.

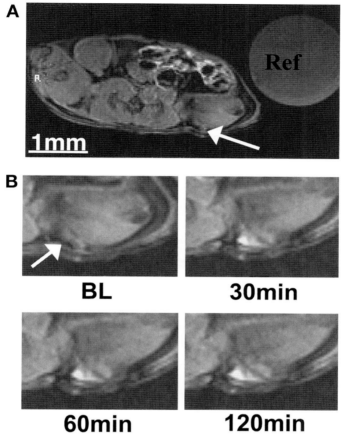

Fig. 8. (A) T_1-weighted MR image (axial view) of athymic nude mouse before injection. Arrow indicates difficult-to-detect implanted C32 tumor (Ref. = Gd-DTPA-doped water in 10-cc syringe). (B) Enlarged section of MR image showing T_1-weighted signal enhancement of angiogenic vasculature of early tumors over 2 hours as detected by $\alpha_v\beta_3$-targeted paramagnetic nanoparticles. BL, baseline image.

Angiogenesis plays a critical role in plaque growth and rupture *(82,83)*. Normal large-caliber arteries in humans receive oxygen and nutrients from blood that is delivered by the adventitial vasa vasorum, not necessarily from the vessel lumen itself. The vasa vasorum carries blood in the same direction as arterial flow and extends perpendicular branches around the vessel wall to supply deep tissues. In regions of atherosclerotic lesions, angiogenic vessels proliferate from the vasa vasorum to meet the high metabolic demands of plaque growth *(84,85)*. Atherosclerosis promotes both inflammation and angiogenesis in the arterial wall, likely via a positive-feedback type of system. Inflammatory cells within the lesion stimulate angiogenesis through local molecular signaling, which in turn promotes neovascular growth, thereby providing an avenue for more inflammatory cells to enter the plaque. This process yields a strong correlation between the extent of plaque angiogenesis and local accumulation of inflammatory cells *(82)*.

Fundamentally, validation of a molecular imaging contrast agent relies on corroboration between MRI signal enhancement and histological staining of the targeted epitope.

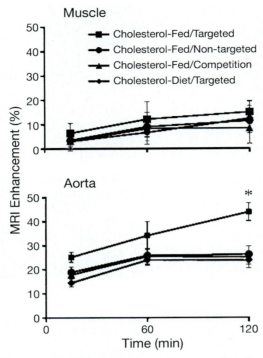

Fig. 9. Quantitative analysis of MRI signal enhancement (percentage change from baseline) from aortic wall (bottom) and skeletal muscle (top) after treatment with $\alpha_v\beta_3$-targeted or control nanoparticles (nontargeted) in cholesterol-fed or normal diet rabbits. * $p < 0.05$ for cholesterol-fed/targeted vs all other groups.

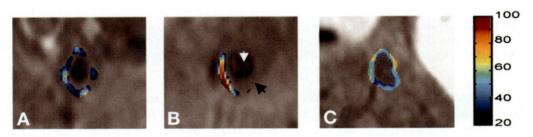

Fig. 10. Percentage enhancement maps (false colored from blue to red) from individual aortic segments at renal artery (**A**), midaorta (**B**), and diaphragm (**C**) 2 hours after injection of $\alpha_v\beta_3$-targeted nanoparticles given to rabbits fed a high-cholesterol diet for 80 days. White arrowhead in (**B**) designates aortic lumen; the black arrowhead points to the aortic wall.

Angiogenic expression of $\alpha_v\beta_3$-integrin was confirmed by co-localized histological staining of $\alpha_v\beta_3$-integrin and platelet endothelial cell adhesion molecule (PECAM), a general endothelial marker. Staining for $\alpha_v\beta_3$-integrin was manifest extensively in the adventitia as a result of marked expansion of vasa vasorum in cholesterol-fed rabbits but much was more sparsely distributed in animals on a control diet *(19)*. Likewise, MRI signal enhancement was widely observed with $\alpha_v\beta_3$-integrin-targeted nanoparticles in the aortic wall of cholesterol-fed rabbits but not control diet animals (Figs. 9 and 10) *(19)*.

Other Plaque Components

Macrophage imaging has been reported with the use of nontargeted USPIOs, first by Schmitz et al. in Watanabe rabbits, and by Reuhm et al. in cholesterol-fed atherosclerotic rabbits *(44,86)*. Because macrophages are abundant in plaques throughout the vascular tree and they are well known to ingest particulate matter, the use of superparamagnetic agents to delineate macrophages and foam cells has been pursued in both animal models and in clinical trials *(87)*. The demonstration of macrophage targeting in vivo in rabbits required a waiting period of 1–3 days to allow for both passive uptake of sufficient numbers of particles and for bloodstream clearance of the long-circulating particles. In general, the susceptibility artifacts produced extended beyond the confines of the plaque macrophages and appeared as heterogeneously distributed signal voids up and down the aorta. In similar clinical trials of patients undergoing carotid endarterectomy by Kooi et al. and Trivedi et al., USPIO particles accumulated in the macrophages in plaques and were optimally imaged as signal reductions at 24 hours after injection *(45,88)*. Kooi also noted that more contrast change was observed for ruptured than for stable plaques.

Fayad's group has reported the development of recombinant paramagnetic high-density lipoprotein (HDL)-like particles that have been shown to enhance atherosclerotic regions in mice deficient in apolipoprotein E *(89)*. These particles are formed through the delipidation of normal isolated human HDL particles, followed by reconstitution with phospholipids and addition of a phospholipid-based conjugate of Gd-DTPA for signal enhancement. With approximately 15–20 molecules of gadolinium included in each 9-nm particle, the signal amplification on a proton MR image is improved. Although the similarity of these particles to native HDL provides a mechanism for nonselective uptake into atherosclerotic regions in vessels, the possibility for inclusion of a targeting ligand into the particle extends the possible uses of this technology for molecular imaging.

This group also has demonstrated the use of conventional nontargeted agents such as gadofluorine, which appears to preferentially label the fatty cores of plaques *(90)*. Gadofluorine is a lipophilic chelate of gadolinium (Gd-DO3A derivative) with a fluorinated side chain that forms 5-nm micelles in aqueous solution and has a higher r_1 relaxivity and longer circulating half-life than traditional Gd-DTPA. The small size and lipophilic nature of this contrast agent allowed it to localize to the lipid-rich areas of plaque in the aorta of rabbits in which lesions were induced with cholesterol feeding and balloon injury. Histological analysis of aortic sections agreed with the MR images, indicating that gadofluorine may be useful in the identification of more plaques with high lipid content by MR.

Myeloperoxidase (MPO) imaging with a paramagnetic substrate has been suggested by the Weissleder group *(91)*. Peroxides are secreted by various cells in plaques as a component of both plaque growth and destabilization, and serum levels have been associated with clinical events *(92)*. By catalyzing the conversion of hydrogen peroxide to hyperchlorite and other reactive molecular species, MPO induces a variety of pathological effects that lead to increased atherosclerosis and possible plaque rupture. Chen et al. were able to generate a gadolinium-containing compound that can also act as a substrate for MPO, leading to free-radical formation and polymerization *(91)*. Polymerization of the gadolinium-containing compound results in marked enhancement of the signal on MR images, indicating that this molecule may be useful for characterizing atherosclerotic lesions.

Stem Cell Imaging

Stem cell imaging with MRI is another emerging area that might fit under the rubric of molecular imaging with targeted nanoparticle contrast agents. In this case, however, the cells are treated with superparamagnetic nanoparticles in vitro and then engrafted into the selected location by local injection. The stem cells exhibit a propensity to endocytosis that can be facilitated with various strategies, including coating the particles with dendrimers, transfection agents, or antibodies/peptides *(93–95)*, which results in the intracellular accumulation of significant amounts of intact nanoparticles that then can exert a local susceptibility effect for detection in vivo. These particles appear to be well tolerated by cells over the long term, although the signal ultimately dissipates as the cells divide and distribute the material or as the particles are catabolized naturally.

Along these lines, Frank, Bulte, and others have demonstrated the clinical utility of stem cell tracking following in vitro preparation with superparamagnetic nanoparticles *(94,96)*. Kraitchman et al. demonstrated the ability to detect and track mesenchymal stem cells injected into necrotic regions of a pig heart at 1.5 T *(97)*. The role of paramagnetic agents is less certain for this purpose because the gadolinium chelates would need to be internalized, and the interaction with free water in the intracellular milieu could blunt fast water exchange and T_1 relaxation, although Crich et al. have shown proof of concept *(98)*.

Nevertheless, the fluorine component of perfluorocarbon emulsions might be utilized to advantage for cell imaging after nanoparticle ingestion. Our group originally demonstrated the capability of detecting small amounts of fluorine either by spectroscopy or by imaging (at 1.5 and 4.7 T) after fibrin-targeted binding of nanoparticles comprising perfluorooctylbromide or crown ether core materials. Subsequently, Ahrens et al. used the crown ether nanoparticles to load dendritic immune cells with no loss of viability and illustrated the use of fluorine imaging at high field strengths (9 T) for tracking cells after local injection *(99)*. The advantage to this approach is that no background signal exists because there is no appreciable amount of fluorine in the body to confound the signal from the targeted cells. If this approach can be transitioned to clinical imaging scenarios, then the ability to image the fluorine component could offer a powerful alternative to T_1- or $T_2/T_2{*}$-weighted proton imaging strategies that avoids nonspecific background signals.

DELIVERING AND MONITORING THERAPY

The potential dual use of nanoparticles for both imaging and site-targeted delivery of therapeutic agents offers great promise for individualizing therapeutics. Although nanoparticulate liposomes already have been approved for use as clinical drug delivery systems (e.g., Abraxane™, Los Angeles, CA; carrying albumin-bound paclitaxel), these agents are passively distributed to their targets, as contrasted with active binding, and they cannot be imaged. Image-based therapeutics with site-selective agents should enable conclusive assurance that the drug is reaching the intended target. Periodic follow-up imaging with the same agents might then provide proof of drug efficacy in individuals against the very molecules selected for targeted imaging. In this manner, patient populations can be "segmented" for hypothetical drug efficacy based not on population statistics or even pharmacogenomic tendencies but on their actual measured responses to therapy.

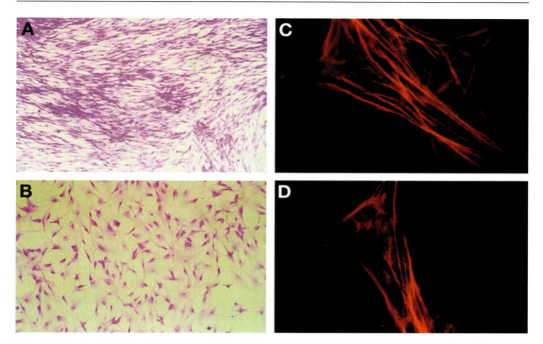

Fig. 11. Routine H&E and immunostaining of α-smooth muscle actin cytoskeleton of porcine vascular smooth muscle cells exposed to control (0.0 mol%) (**A**) and (**C**) and TF-targeted (2.0 mol%) (**B**) and (**D**) doxorubicin-containing nanoparticles. The doxorubicin on the particles greatly decreased the muscle cell proliferation and disrupted the cytoskeleton of many of the remaining cells.

Traditional pharmacokinetic and pharmacodynamic analysis used to predict drug efficacy and toxicity is rooted in monitoring serum concentrations. For simple compartmental analysis, several linked differential equations are used to describe the transport of drug from one compartment (i.e., the serum) to another (i.e., the extracellular space where the drug binds to its target). When bound, the actions of the drug can then be modeled in a variety of ways, including the often-used sigmoid-E_{max} model. In the case of particulate agents, the mechanisms of drug delivery become more complicated such that serum concentrations are not necessarily indicative of the amount of drug accessible to the desired site *(100)*. Furthermore, by targeting the carrier to the tissue of interest, the drug release is also localized to that area, resulting in a much higher effective drug concentration at the site than indicated by serum levels alone. The unique ability to image these particles (e.g., T_1-weighted imaging of paramagnetic nanoparticles) would be of great benefit for calculating local drug concentrations and developing new pharmacokinetic and dynamic paradigms to describe this new class of agents.

As an example of this new paradigm for drug delivery, Lanza et al. treated smooth muscle cells in culture with tissue factor-targeted nanoparticles that were loaded with paclitaxel *(17)*. The smooth muscle cells were harvested from pig aorta and constitutively expressed tissue factor epitopes in vitro. Binding of the drug-free nanoparticles to the cells yielded no alterations in growth characteristics of the cultured cells (Fig. 11). However, when paclitaxel-loaded nanoparticles were applied to the cells, specific binding elicited a substantial reduction in smooth muscle cell proliferation. However, if nontargeted paclitaxel-loaded particles were applied (i.e., no binding of nanoparticles to cells occurred), cell proliferation proceeded as usual. These data indicate that specifically targeted drug-loaded nanoparticles can inhibit cell proliferation, whereas nontargeted particles are innocuous and do not deliver the drug to the cells and exert no effect on cell proliferation or viability. Reports indicate that intravenous delivery of fumagillan-loaded nanoparticles (an antiangiogenic agent) targeted to $\alpha_v\beta_3$-integrin epitopes on vasa vasorum in growing plaques results in marked inhibition of plaque angiogenesis in cholesterol-fed rabbits (101).

Accordingly, the mechanism of drug delivery for highly lipophilic agents such as paclitaxel depends on close apposition between the nanoparticle carrier and the targeted cell membrane and has been described as contact-facilitated drug delivery. In contrast to liposomal drug delivery, the mechanism of drug transport in this case involves lipid exchange or lipid mixing with the targeted cell membrane (102,103). Generally, lipid exchange is a somewhat slow process that depends on the extent and frequency of contact between two lipidic surfaces. When nanoparticles with their lipid monolayer coatings are bound to targeted cell membranes, an opportunity for more rapid lipid exchange occurs because contacts are more frequent, permitting more lipid exchange or even particle-cell fusion (17). We have shown also that the rate of lipid exchange and drug delivery can be greatly increased by the application of safe levels of ultrasound energy that increase the propensity to fusion or enhanced contact between the nanoparticles and the targeted cell membrane by stimulating these interactions between nanoparticles and cell membranes (102,103).

CONCLUSION

The combination of targeted drug delivery and molecular imaging with MRI has the potential to revolutionize the field of cardiology as well as many other fields. The ability to noninvasively characterize disease at the molecular level may provide the necessary added information to direct and monitor treatment in otherwise ambiguous cases (i.e., >50% stenotic lesions). Furthermore, the combination of drug-delivering agents that are also imageable may ultimately permit serial characterization of the targeted epitope expression and determination of treatment efficacy, thereby permitting personalized treatment regimens. Rapid developments in genomics, molecular biology, and nanotechnology have energized the multidisciplinary field of molecular imaging, and we anticipate that clinical applications are just around the corner for these novel agents.

REFERENCES

1. Britz-Cunningham SH, Adelstein SJ. Molecular targeting with radionuclides: state of the science. J Nucl Med 2003;44:1945–1961.
2. Herschman HR. Molecular imaging: looking at problems, seeing solutions. Science 2003;302:605–608.
3. Tsien RY. Imagining imaging's future. Nat Rev Mol Cell Biol 2003;suppl:SS16–SS21.
4. Lanza GM, Wickline SA. Targeted ultrasonic contrast agents for molecular imaging and therapy. Progr Cardiovasc Dis 2001;44:13–31.
5. Lanza GM, Wickline SA. Targeted ultrasonic contrast agents for molecular imaging and therapy. Curr Probl Cardiol 2003;28:625–653.
6. Wickline SA, Sahn DJ, Kerber R, Reichek N, Pennell DJ. Report from the First International Conjoint Conference on Cardiovascular Magnetic Resonance and Echocardiography. J Cardiovasc Magn Reson 2002;4:515–520.
7. Wickline SA, Lanza GM. Nanotechnology for molecular imaging and targeted therapy. Circulation 2003;107:1092–1095.
8. Weissleder R. Molecular imaging: exploring the next frontier. Radiology 1999;212:609–614.

9. Gupta H, Weissleder R. Targeted contrast agents in MR imaging. Magn Reson Imaging Clin N Am 1996;4:171–184.

10. Artemov D. Molecular magnetic resonance imaging with targeted contrast agents. J Cell Biochem 2003;90:518–524.

11. Flacke S, Fischer S, Scott MJ, et al. Novel MRI contrast agent for molecular imaging of fibrin: implications for detecting vulnerable plaques. Circulation 2001;104:1280–1285.

12. Lanza GM, Lorenz CH, Fischer SE, et al. Enhanced detection of thrombi with a novel fibrin-targeted magnetic resonance imaging agent. Acad Radiol 1998;5:S173–S176.

13. Winter PM, Caruthers SD, Yu X, et al. Improved molecular imaging contrast agent for detection of human thrombus. Magn Reson Med 2003;50:411–416.

14. Yu X, Song SK, Chen J, et al. High-resolution MRI characterization of human thrombus using a novel fibrin-targeted paramagnetic nanoparticle contrast agent. Magn Reson Med 2000;44:867–872.

15. Kang HW, Josephson L, Petrovsky A, Weissleder R, Bogdanov A Jr. Magnetic resonance imaging of inducible E-selectin expression in human endothelial cell culture. Bioconjug Chem 2002;13:122–127.

16. Lanza GM, Abendschein DR, Hall CS, et al. In vivo molecular imaging of stretch-induced tissue factor in carotid arteries with ligand-targeted nanoparticles. J Am Soc Echocardiogr 2000;13:608–614.

17. Lanza GM, Yu X, Winter PM, et al. Targeted antiproliferative drug delivery to vascular smooth muscle cells with a magnetic resonance imaging nanoparticle contrast agent: implications for rational therapy of restenosis. Circulation 2002;106:2842–2847.

18. Tiukinhoy SD, Mahowald ME, Shively VP, et al. Development of echogenic, plasmid-incorporated, tissue-targeted cationic liposomes that can be used for directed gene delivery. Invest Radiol 2000;35:732–738.

19. Winter PM, Morawski AM, Caruthers S, et al. Specific molecular imaging of vasa vasorum in early atherosclerosis with alpha(nu)beta(3)–integrin targeted nanoparticles. Circulation 2003;108:168–168.

20. Zheng ZJ, Croft JB, Giles WH, Mensah GA. Sudden cardiac death in the United States, 1989 to 1998. Circulation 2001;104:2158–2163.

21. Napoli C, Glass CK, Witztum JL, Deutsch R, D'Armiento FP, Palinski W. Influence of maternal hypercholesterolaemia during pregnancy on progression of early atherosclerotic lesions in childhood: Fate of Early Lesions in Children (FELIC) study. Lancet 1999;354:1234–1241.

22. Zieske AW, Malcom GT, Strong JP. Natural history and risk factors of atherosclerosis in children and youth: the PDAY study. Pediatr Pathol Molecular Med 2002;21:213–237.

23. Davies MJ, Krikler DM, Katz D. Atherosclerosis: inhibition of regression as therapeutic possibilities. Br Heart J 1991;65:302–310.

24. Davies MJ, Thomas AC. Plaque fissuring—the cause of acute myocardial infarction, sudden ischaemic death, and crescendo angina. Br Heart J 1985;53:363–373.

25. Richardson PD, Davies MJ, Born GV. Influence of plaque configuration and stress distribution on fissuring of coronary atherosclerotic plaques. Lancet 1989;2:941–944.

26. Naghavi M, Libby P, Falk E, et al. From vulnerable plaque to vulnerable patient: a call for new definitions and risk assessment strategies: Part I. Circulation 2003;108:1664–1672.

27. Ojio S, Takatsu H, Tanaka T, et al. Considerable time from the onset of plaque rupture and/or thrombi until the onset of acute myocardial infarction in humans: coronary angiographic findings within 1 week before the onset of infarction. Circulation 2000;102:2063–2069.

28. Mitra AK, Dhume AS, Agrawal DK. "Vulnerable plaques"—ticking of the time bomb. Can J Physiol Pharmacol 2004;82:860–871.

29. Arroyo LH, Lee RT. Mechanisms of plaque rupture: mechanical and biologic interactions. Cardiovasc Res 1999;41:369–375.

30. Petit L, Lesnik P, Dachet C, Moreau M, Chapman MJ. Tissue factor pathway inhibitor is expressed by human monocyte-derived macrophages: relationship to tissue factor induction by cholesterol and oxidized LDL. Arterioscler Thromb Vasc Biol 1999;19:309–315.

31. Kockx MM, De Meyer GR, Buyssens N, Knaapen MW, Bult H, Herman AG. Cell composition, replication, and apoptosis in atherosclerotic plaques after 6 months of cholesterol withdrawal. Circ Res 1998;83:378–387.

32. Newby AC, Zaltsman AB. Fibrous cap formation or destruction—the critical importance of vascular smooth muscle cell proliferation, migration and matrix formation. Cardiovasc Res 1999;41:345–360.

33. Shah PK. Role of inflammation and metalloproteinases in plaque disruption and thrombosis. Vasc Med 1998;3:199–206.

34. de Boer OJ, van der Wal AC, Teeling P, Becker AE. Leucocyte recruitment in rupture prone regions of lipid-rich plaques: a prominent role for neovascularization? Cardiovasc Res 1999;41:443–449.

35. Libby P. Molecular bases of the acute coronary syndromes. Circulation 1995;91:2844–2850.
36. McCarthy MJ, Loftus IM, Thompson MM, et al. Angiogenesis and the atherosclerotic carotid plaque: an association between symptomatology and plaque morphology. J Vasc Surg 1999;30:261–268.
37. Ballantyne CM. Clinical trial endpoints: angiograms, events, and plaque instability. Am J Cardiol 1998;82:5M–11M.
38. Yokoya K, Takatsu H, Suzuki T, et al. Process of progression of coronary artery lesions from mild or moderate stenosis to moderate or severe stenosis: a study based on four serial coronary arteriograms per year. Circulation 1999;100:903–909.
39. Ambrose JA, Tannenbaum MA, Alexopoulos D, et al. Angiographic progression of coronary artery disease and the development of myocardial infarction. J Am Coll Cardiol 1988;12:56–62.
40. Goldstein JA. Multifocal coronary plaque instability. Prog Cardiovasc Dis 2002;44:449–454.
41. Ahrens ET, Rothbacher U, Jacobs RE, Fraser SE. A model for MRI contrast enhancement using T_1 agents. Proc Natl Acad Sci U S A 1998;5:8443–8448.
42. Morawski AM, Winter PM, Crowder KC, et al. Targeted nanoparticles for quantitative imaging of sparse molecular epitopes with MRI. Magn Reson Med 2004;51:480–486.
43. Buxton DB, Lee SC, Wickline SA, Ferrari M, for the Working Group Members. Recommendations of the National Heart, Lung, and Blood Institute Nanotechnology Working Group. Circulation 2003;108:2737–2742.
44. Schmitz SA, Coupland SE, Gust R, et al. Superparamagnetic iron oxide-enhanced MRI of atherosclerotic plaques in Watanabe hereditable hyperlipidemic rabbits. Invest Radiol 2000;35:460–471.
45. Kooi ME, Cappendijk VC, Cleutjens KB, et al. Accumulation of ultrasmall superparamagnetic particles of iron oxide in human atherosclerotic plaques can be detected by in vivo magnetic resonance imaging. Circulation 2003;107:2453–2458.
46. Schmitz SA, Taupitz M, Wagner S, Wolf KJ, Beyersdorff D, Hamm B. Magnetic resonance imaging of atherosclerotic plaques using superparamagnetic iron oxide particles. J Magn Reson Imaging 2001;14:355–361.
47. Cunningham CH, Arai T, Yang PC, McConnell MV, Pauly JM, Conolly SM. Positive contrast magnetic resonance imaging of cells labeled with magnetic nanoparticles. Magn Reson Med 2005; 53:999–1005.
48. Stuber M, Gilson WD, Schaer M, Bulte JW, Kraitchman DL. Shedding light on the dark spot with IRON: a method that generates positive contrast in the presence of superparamagnetic nanoparticles. Proc Intl Soc Magn Reson Med 2005;13:2608.
49. Seppenwoolde JH, Viergever MA, Bakker CJ. Passive tracking exploiting local signal conservation: the white marker phenomenon. Magn Reson Med 2003;50:784–790.
50. Lanza GM, Wallace KD, Scott MJ, et al. A novel site-targeted ultrasonic contrast agent with broad biomedical application. Circulation 1996;94:3334–3340.
51. Cacheris W, Richard T, Grabiak R, Lee A; HemaGen/PFC, assignee. Paramagnetic complexes of N-alkyl-N-hydroxylamides of organic acids and emulsions containing same for magnetic resonance imaging. U.S. patent 5,614,170. March 25, 1997.
52. Grant CW, Karlik S, Florio E. A liposomal MRI contrast agent: phosphatidylethanolamine-DTPA. Magn Reson Med 1989;11:236–243.
53. Button TM, Fiel RJ. Isointense model for the evaluation of tumor-specific MRI contrast agents. Magn Reson Imaging 1988;6:275–280.
54. Morawski AM, Winter PM, Yu X, et al. Quantitative "magnetic resonance immunohistochemistry" with ligand-targeted ^{19}F nanoparticles. Magn Reson Med 2004;52:1255–1262.
55. Huang MQ, Ye Q, Williams DS, Ho C. MRI of lungs using partial liquid ventilation with water-in-perfluorocarbon emulsions. Magn Reson Med 2002;48:487–492.
56. Le D, Mason RP, Hunjan S, Constantinescu A, Barker BR, Antich PP. Regional tumor oxygen dynamics: ^{19}F PBSR EPI of hexafluorobenzene. Magn Reson Imaging 1997;15:971–981.
57. Bovey F, Jelinski L, Mirau P. Nuclear magnetic resonance spectroscopy. San Diego, CA: Academic Press; 1988.
58. Doyle M, Mansfield P. Chemical-shift imaging: a hybrid approach. Magn Reson Med 1987;5:255–261.
59. Noth U, Jager LJ, Lutz J, Haase A. Fast ^{19}F-NMR imaging in vivo using FLASH-MRI. Magn Reson Imaging 1994;12:149–153.
60. Laukemper-Ostendorf S, Scholz A, Burger K, et al. ^{19}F-MRI of perflubron for measurement of oxygen partial pressure in porcine lungs during partial liquid ventilation. Magn Reson Med 2002; 47:82–89.

61. Fan X, River JN, Zamora M, Al-Hallaq HA, Karczmar GS. Effect of carbogen on tumor oxygenation: combined fluorine-19 and proton MRI measurements. Int J Radiat Oncol Biol Phys 2002;54: 1202–1209.

62. Hunjan S, Zhao D, Canstandtinescu A, Hahan EW, Antich PP, Mason RP. Tumor oximetry: demonstration of an enhanced dynamic mapping procedure using fluorine-19 echo planar magnetic resonance imaging the Dunning prostate R3327-At1 rat tumor. Int J Radiat Oncol Biol Phys 2001;49:1097–1108.

63. Shukla HP, Mason RP, Bansal N, Antich PP. Regional myocardial oxygen tension: ^{19}F MRI of sequestered perfluorocarbon. Magn Reson Med 1996;35:827–833.

64. Neubauer AM, Caruthers S, Cyrus T, et al. ^{19}F MRI using perfluorocarbon nanoparticles. Proc Intl Soc Magn Reson Med 2005;13:2705.

65. Gowland P, Mansfield P. Accurate measurement of T_1 in vivo in less than 3 seconds using echo-planar imaging. Magn Reson Med 1993;30:351–354.

66. Schmieder AH, Winter P, Caruthers S, et al. Molecular MR imaging of melanoma angiogenesis with avb3-targeted paramagnetic nanoparticles. Magn Reson Med 2005;53:621–627.

67. Sipkins DA, Cheresh DA, Kazemi MR, Nevin LM, Bednarski MD, Li KC. Detection of tumor angiogenesis in vivo by alphaVbeta3-targeted magnetic resonance imaging. Nat Med 1998;4:623–626.

68. Fram EK, Herfkens RJ, Johnson GA, et al. Rapid calculation of T_1 using variable flip angle gradient refocused imaging. Magn Reson Imaging 1987;5:201–208.

69. Winter PM, Caruthers SD, Kassner A, et al. Molecular imaging of angiogenesis in nascent Vx-2 rabbit tumors using a novel avb3-targeted nanoparticle and 1.5 T MRI. Cancer Res 2003;63:5838–5843.

70. Constantinides P. Plaque fissuring in human coronary thrombosis. J Atheroscler Res 1966;6:1–17.

71. Lanza GM, Lorenz CH, Fischer SE, et al. A novel site targeted emulsion-based MRI contrast agent for detection of thrombus [abstract]. Circulation 1996.

72. Botnar RM, Buecker A, Wiethoff AJ, et al. In vivo magnetic resonance imaging of coronary thrombosis using a fibrin-binding molecular magnetic resonance contrast agent. Circulation 2004;110:1463–1466.

73. Spuentrup E, Fausten B, Kinzel S, et al. Molecular magnetic resonance imaging of atrial clots in a swine model. Circulation 2005.

74. Spuentrup E, Katoh M, Wiethoff AJ, et al. Molecular magnetic resonance imaging of pulmonary emboli with a fibrin-specific contrast agent. Am J Respir Crit Care Med 2005.

75. Mazooz G, Mehlman T, Lai T-S, Greenberg CS, Dewhirst MW, Neeman M. Development of magnetic resonance imaging contrast material for in vivo mapping of tissue transglutaminase activity. Cancer Res 2005;65:1369–1375.

76. Oltrona L, Speidel CM, Recchia D, Wickline SA, Eisenberg PR, Abendschein DR. Inhibition of tissue factor-mediated coagulation markedly attenuates stenosis after balloon-induced arterial injury in minipigs. Circulation 1997;96:646–652.

77. Kerr JS, Mousa SA, Slee AM. Alpha(v)beta(3) integrin in angiogenesis and restenosis. Drug News Perspect 2001;14:143–150.

78. Bishop GG, McPherson JA, Sanders JM, et al. Selective alpha(v)beta-receptor blockade reduces macrophage infiltration and restenosis after balloon angioplasty in the atherosclerotic rabbit. Circulation 2001;103:1906–1911.

79. Corjay MH, Diamond SM, Schlingmann KL, Gibbs SK, Stoltenborg JK, Racanelli AL. alphavbeta3, alphavbeta5, and osteopontin are coordinately upregulated at early time points in a rabbit model of neointima formation. J Cell Biochem 1999;75:492–504.

80. Brooks PC, Stromblad S, Klemke R, Visscher D, Sarkar FH, Cheresh DA. Antiintegrin alpha v beta 3 blocks human breast cancer growth and angiogenesis in human skin. J Clin Invest 1995;96:1815–1822.

81. Anderson SA, Rader RK, Westlin WF, et al. Magnetic resonance contrast enhancement of neovasculature with alpha(v)beta(3)-targeted nanoparticles. Magn Reson Med 2000;44:433–439.

82. Moulton KS, Heller E, Konerding MA, et al. Angiogenesis inhibitors endostatin or TNP-470 reduce intimal neovascularization and plaque growth in apolipoprotien E-deficient mice. Circulation 1999;99:1653–1655.

83. Tenaglia AN, Peters KG, Sketch MH Jr, Annex BH. Neovascularization in atherectomy specimens from patients with unstable angina: implications for pathogenesis of unstable angina. Am Heart J 1998;135:10–14.

84. Wilson SH, Herrmann J, Lerman LO, et al. Simvastatin preserves the structure of coronary adventitial vasa vasorum in experimental hypercholesterolemia independent of lipid lowering. Circulation 2002;105:415–418.

85. Zhang Y, Cliff WJ, Schoefl GI, Higgins G. Immunohistochemical study of intimal microvessels in coronary atherosclerosis. Am J Pathol 1993;143:164–172.

86. Reuhm SG, Corot C, P. V, et al. Magnetic resonance imaging of atherosclerotic plaque with ultrasmall superparamagnetic particles of iron oxide in hyperlipidemic rabbits. Circulation 2001;103:415–422.

87. Corot C, Petry KG, Trivedi R, et al. Macrophage imaging in central nervous system and in carotid atherosclerotic plaque using ultrasmall superparamagnetic iron oxide in magnetic resonance imaging. Invest Radiol 2004;39:619–625.

88. Trivedi RA, U-King-Im JM, Graves MJ, et al. In vivo detection of macrophages in human carotid atheroma: temporal dependence of ultrasmall superparamagnetic particles of iron oxide-enhanced MRI. Stroke 2004;35:1631–1635.

89. Frias JC, Williams KJ, Fisher EA, Fayad ZA. Recombinant HDL-like nanoparticles: a specific contrast agent for MRI of atherosclerotic plaques. J Am Chem Soc 2004;126:16,316–16,317.

90. Sirol M, Itskovich VV, Mani V, et al. Lipid-rich atherosclerotic plaques detected by gadofluorine-enhanced in vivo magnetic resonance imaging. Circulation 2004;109:2890–2896.

91. Chen JW, Pham W, Weissleder R, Bogdanov A Jr. Human myeloperoxidase: a potential target for molecular MR imaging in atherosclerosis. Magn Reson Med 2004;52:1021–1028.

92. Brennan ML, Penn MS, Van Lente F, et al. Prognostic value of myeloperoxidase in patients with chest pain. N Engl J Med 2003;349:1595–1604.

93. Arbab AS, Bashaw LA, Miller BR, Jordan EK, Bulte JW, Frank JA. Intracytoplasmic tagging of cells with ferumoxides and transfection agent for cellular magnetic resonance imaging after cell transplantation: methods and techniques. Transplantation 2003;76:1123–1130.

94. Frank JA, Miller BR, Arbab AS, et al. Clinically applicable labeling of mammalian and stem cells by combining superparamagnetic iron oxides and transfection agents. Radiology 2003;228:480–487.

95. Funovics MA, Kapeller B, Hoeller C, et al. MR imaging of the her2/neu and 9.2.27 tumor antigens using immunospecific contrast agents. Magn Reson Imaging 2004;22:843–850.

96. Bulte JW, Kraitchman DL. Monitoring cell therapy using iron oxide MR contrast agents. Current Pharmaceutical Biotechnology 2004;5:567–584.

97. Kraitchman DL, Heldman AW, Atalar E, et al. In vivo magnetic resonance imaging of mesenchymal stem cells in myocardial infarction. Circulation 2003;107:2290–2293.

98. Crich SG, Biancone L, Cantaluppi V, et al. Improved route for the visualization of stem cells labeled with a Gd-/Eu-chelate as dual (MRI and fluorescence) agent. Magn Reson Med 2004;51:938–944.

99. Ahrens ET, Flores R, Xu HY, Morel PA. In vivo imaging platform for tracking immunotherapeutic cells. Nature Biotechnology 2005 Aug;23(8):983–987.

100. Harashima H, Iida S, Urakami Y, Tsuchihashi M, Kiwada H. Optimization of antitumor effect of liposomally encapsulated doxorubicin based on simulations by pharmacokinetic/pharmacodynamic modeling. J Controlled Release 1999;61:93–106.

101. Winter PM, Morawski AM, Caruthers SD, et al. Antiangiogenic therapy of early atherosclerosis with paramagnetic alpha(v)beta-integrin-targeted fumagillin nanoparticles. J Am Coll Cardiol 2004; 43:322A–323A.

102. Crowder KC, Hughes MS, Marsh JN, et al. Sonic activation of molecularly-targeted nanoparticles accelerates transmembrane lipid delivery to cancer cells through contact-mediated mechanisms: implications for enhanced local drug delivery. Ultrasound Med Biol 2005 Dec;31(12):1693–1700.

103. Crowder KC, Hughes MS, Marsh JN, et al. Augmented and selective delivery of liquid perfluoro-carbon nanoparticles to melanoma cells with noncavitational ultrasound. Honolulu, Hawaii; 2003, pp. 532–535.

30   Cardiac Magnetic Resonance Spectroscopy

Robert G. Weiss, Glenn A. Hirsch, and Paul A. Bottomley

CONTENTS

Magnetic resonance spectroscopy (MRS) is a multinuclear noninvasive tool that offers a window into myocardial metabolism. This chapter reviews the nuclei typically studied with cardiac MRS and the magnetic resonance (MR) techniques used to acquire spatially localized cardiac spectra. We then review the clinical MRS studies of human myocardial metabolism with emphasis on common clinical conditions such as myocardial ischemia, viability, hypertrophy, and heart failure.

METHODS

Magnetic Resonance Spectroscopy

Nuclear magnetic resonance (NMR) can be performed on any nucleus that has an odd number of nucleons. Nuclei that undergo MR in the atoms of a molecule resonate at slightly different frequencies because of variations in the local magnetic field caused by "shielding" from electrons in different chemical bonds on the molecule. The chemical shifts in the resonant frequencies are so small that they are measured in parts per million (ppm) of the main resonant frequency, and careful "shimming" of the magnetic field homogeneity is routinely performed to maximize the ability to detect them. The chemical shifts of different chemical moieties on each molecule result in an NMR signal comprised of one or more discrete resonant frequencies, with the signal intensity at each frequency proportional to the relative abundance of nuclei attached to each moiety. The discrete frequencies and peak ratios are a characteristic of each molecule and are routinely used to identify molecules in modern chemistry. With a suitable calibrating reference signal, the integrated peak areas can be used to determine the absolute concentrations of specific compounds.

From: *Contemporary Cardiology: Cardiovascular Magnetic Resonance Imaging*
Edited by: Raymond Y. Kwong © Humana Press Inc., Totowa, NJ

The plot of the NMR signal intensity as a function of the NMR frequency measured in parts per million relative to the resonant frequency of a reference compound is termed the *NMR spectrum*. The spectrum is typically generated by Fourier transformation (FT) of the transient, time-dependent NMR signal excited by a radio-frequency (RF) magnetic field pulse tuned to the NMR frequency and recorded in the absence of any spatial localization or magnetic resonance imaging (MRI) magnetic field gradients.

Naturally abundant nuclei suitable for performing MRS in biological tissue and the body include hydrogen or protons (^{1}H) *(1,2)*, phosphorus (^{31}P) *(3)*, and, less commonly, carbon (^{13}C) *(4)*. For noninvasive in vivo MRS studies, a number of naturally occurring chemical compounds that appear in the spectrum can be used as chemical shift references. For ^{31}P MRS, the chemical shift reference compound is phosphocreatine (PCr) taken as 0.0 ppm. For in vivo ^{1}H MRS, water at 4.7 ppm, total creatine (CR) at 3.0 ppm, or for brain studies, *n*-acetyl aspartate at 2.0 ppm are routinely used as chemical shift references based on a chemical shift scale with tetramethyl silane at 0.0 ppm.

Spatial Localization

The NMR spectrum from a body placed in a magnet is the sum of all the contributing resonant signals and compounds, undistinguished by location. To obtain a spectrum from a specific tissue, or a discrete portion thereof, the MRS signal must be spatially localized. Just as chemical shift information is encoded as frequency information in the NMR signal, MRI gradients also frequency encode the spatial information. Therefore, to ensure that the frequency-encoded chemical MRS information can be distinguished from the frequency-encoded spatial information, MRI gradients cannot in general be applied during spectral acquisition for the purpose of spatial localization. Instead, spatial encoding with MRI gradients must generally be applied prior to the acquisition.

SURFACE COILS

The simplest approach to achieving localization without any MRI gradients is to place a small NMR receiver coil, a "surface coil," on the body closest to the tissue of interest (e.g., on the human chest over the heart) as a detector *(5)*. Indeed, because of the unavailability of body coils for ^{31}P and ^{13}C, in vivo MRS studies of human hearts have invariably been conducted using surface coils for both excitation and detection.

Surface coils provide an important advantage in signal-to-noise ratio (SNR) over large-volume coils that is critical for the detection of millimolar level metabolites by MRS. The advantage results from the fact that the coils are close to the signal sources of interest. Moreover, they do not pick up the electronic noise from the greater portion of the sample that lies beyond its local region of sensitivity. For example, the SNR advantage realized by a flat 6.5-cm ^{31}P surface coil over a 27-cm diameter head coil has been measured at over sixfold *(6)*.

To achieve the best sensitivity for a surface coil, it should be optimized such that its losses are small compared with the sample loading and designed with a coil diameter roughly equal to the depth of the tissue of interest *(7)*. For cardiac detectors, this results in surface coil diameters of 6–15 cm for the anterior left ventricular (LV) wall. The sensitivities of 15 cm and 6.5 cm for the heart are illustrated in Fig. 1.

With surface coil detection, MRS is preferably excited by a separate, larger RF excitation coil to avoid the spatially dependent spectral distortions that would result from the nonuniform NMR flip angle provided by the surface coil. For ^{1}H MRS, the standard MRI

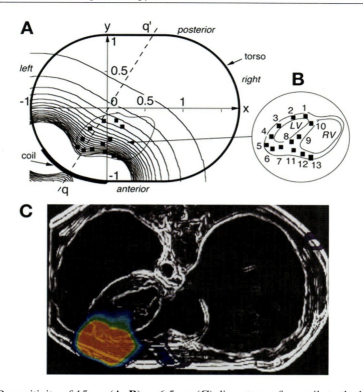

Fig. 1. The MR sensitivity of 15 cm (**A, B**) an 6.5 cm (**C**) diameter surface coils to the heart illustrating the nonuniform reception of surface coils, and the advantage of proximity. (**A**) Model torso with anterior-posterior dimension 0.3 m shows the heart at a location determined by averaging MRI measurements from axial images of adult volunteers lying prone in the magnet, against a flexible 15 cm diameter coil on the lower left side (from Ref. a). The 20 computed contours correspond to 5% to 95% of the sensitivity at the center of a flat 15 cm coil. Inset (**B**) depicts points 1–13 around the LV and anterior RV with sensitivities 16%,19%, 34%, 59%, 86%, 81%, 71%, 53%, 38%, 18%, 82%, 92%, and 97%, respectively. (**C**) Color-coded PCr signal obtained by chemical shift imaging (CSI) acquired with a 6.5 cm surface coil at 1.5Tesla in a comparable location to (**A**), overlaid on an edge detected convention axial MRI (from Ref. b). Sensitivity is limited to the anterior myocardium.
a. Bottomley PA, Luogo-Olivieri CH, Giaquinto R. What is the optimum phased-array coil design for cardiac magnetic resonance? Magn Reson Med 1997;37:591–599.
b. Hardy CJ, Bottomley PA, Rohling KW, Roemer PB. "An NMR phased array for human cardiac ^{31}P spectroscopy". Magn Reson Med 1992;28:54–64.

body coil will provide uniform excitation over the sensitive region of a small surface detector. However, for ^{31}P and ^{13}C MRS, for which there is no body coil and limited broadband power available from the scanner, a second surface coil that is several times larger than the detector coil will serve just as well. The idea is that the larger excite coil will still have a fairly uniform excitation field over the sensitive MRS volume. We have successfully used a 25-cm excite, 6.5-cm receive surface coil set for human cardiac ^{31}P MRS *(8)*.

Nevertheless, the uniformity of the excitation field with such a setup would, unless compensated for, still be inadequate for quantitative work involving the measurement of metabolite ratios, concentrations, or fluxes. To eliminate both the time required to set up or calibrate the excitation pulse and the need to provide spatially dependent corrections for nonuniform excitation, low-angle adiabatic NMR pulses such as BIR4 or BIRP pulses are preferably used for excitation *(9,10)*. Once implemented, these

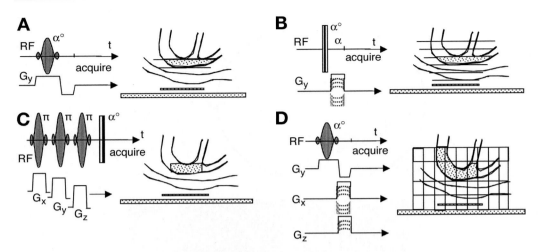

Fig. 2. The DRESS (**A**), ID CSI (**B**), ISIS (**C**), and slice-selective 3D CSI pulse sequences (left) for localizing MRS signals to various voxels in the heart (right; adapted from Ref. *3*). G_x, G_y, and G_z are imaging gradients, and NMR pulses with flip-angles of α or π are applied on the RF channel. With DRESS (**A**), a plane is selectively excited with a single sequence application. The ID CSI method (**B**) requires repeat application on an imaging phase-encoding gradient, G_y, applied in the vertical direction, and the resulting signals are Fourier transformed with respect to G_y amplitude to obtain a set of spectra from all of the slices encoded. The ISIS sequence (**C**) selectively excites a single volume if the signals from all 8 combinations of the *x*, *y*, and *z* selective excitation pulses being applied and not applied, are properly added. In (**D**), an axial slice through the chest is selectively excited, and the remaining two dimensions encoded by the other 2 gradients. The sequence is repeated N = N_xN_y times where N_xN_y is the array size, and a 2D FT with respect to gradient amplitude yields the spatial information.

pulses can simply be turned on and set without requiring any further prescan setup or calibration, and they provide an absolutely constant flip angle over a manyfold variation in excitation field strength.

POSITIONING

With surface coils, accurate positioning is essential because optimum sensitivity is delivered only over a very restricted volume. Placement of surface coils relative to the tissue of interest is therefore invariably done under MRI guidance by performing scout MRI acquisitions prior to MRS. For heart studies, incorrect positioning not only will deleteriously affect sensitivity to the detection of myocardial metabolites, as is evident in Fig. 1, but also will affect the degree of contamination of spectra with MR signal from nearby tissues, especially chest muscle. In this case, sensitivity is also affected by patient orientation because the heart is closer to a coil on the surface of the chest when the subject is lying in a prone position compared to a supine patient position. A prone orientation also minimizes motion artifacts caused by respiratory motion.

The deleterious effect of cardiac motion on the acquisitions is remedied by synchronizing the MRS acquisitions to the cardiac cycle. Even so, it should be noted that, with the exception of spin echo techniques (e.g., PRESS, STEAM), spectral artifacts caused by breathing and cardiac motion are generally much less obvious than in MRI because of

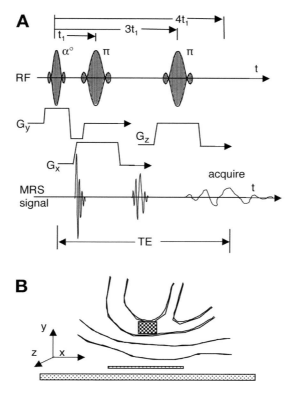

Fig. 3. Spatial localization to a single voxel in the heart using the PRESS method (*12*). A sequence comprised of an $\alpha°$ RF pulse followed by two π RF pulses at times t_1 and $3t_1$ later generate a spin-echo signal centered at time $4t_1$. If each RF pulse is rendered slice selective in each of the orthogonal Cartesian directions by applying *y*-, *x*-, and *z*-gradients, and if the signals between the pulses are crushed by leaving the gradients on, the echo signal will derive from the voxel at the intersection of the 3 slices (**B**).

the much coarser spatial resolution and lower SNR of metabolite MRS *(11)*. By analogy, clinical radionuclide exams have long been performed ungated with little heed paid to physiological motion.

GRADIENT LOCALIZATION

With only surface coils for localization, however carefully they are placed on the chest adjacent to the heart, one cannot seriously claim that the resultant spectra are myocardial spectra. Additional localization is essential. Fortunately, two MRI gradient localization methods that do not use gradients during signal acquisition are directly applicable to MRS. These are selective excitation and phase encoding. Several examples are depicted in Figs. 2 and 3. Selective excitation involves application of an MRI gradient synchronously with a frequency-tailored RF excitation pulse. This results in the excitation of nuclei that lie only in a plane section of the sample oriented orthogonal to the direction of the gradient. The FT of the signal acquired immediately after refocusing the gradient (Fig. 2) is the spectrum from the preselected slice. Spatial localization in the other two dimensions coplanar with the selected slice is afforded by the limited sensitivity of the surface detection coil. This method is known as DRESS for depth-resolved surface coil spectroscopy *(3,5)* (Fig. 2A). The location of the plane is controlled by offsetting the frequency of the selection pulse.

PRESS, STEAM, ISIS

The principal of selective excitation can certainly be extended to three dimensions. If the initial excitation pulse, say, excites a section parallel to the y-axis, it may be followed by two frequency-tailored 180° pulses applied at times t_1 and $3t_1$ after the initial pulse, in the presence of x- and z- gradients. Each 180° pulse generates spin echoes: the echo at $2t_1$ is localized in two dimensions, and the one at $4t_1$ derives from the volume element (voxel) lying at the intersection of the three selected planes. This method is called PRESS for point-resolved surface coil spectroscopy *(12)* (Fig. 3). This method works well when the transverse relaxation time or signal decay time is long compared to the echo time (TE) ($T_2 > 4t_1$), which tends to be true of ^1H MRS but not ^{31}P or ^{13}C, for which, for example, the ^{31}P ATP (adenosine triphosphate) signals are gone by 10–20 ms.

From the standpoint of T_2 decay, the effective time between initial excitation and detection can be reduced to $2t_1$ by making all of the pulses 90° pulses in a method called STEAM for stimulated-echo acquisition mode *(13)*. The time reduction arises because the MRS signal is tipped into the longitudinal plane between the last two pulses, a time window for which T_2 relaxation is not operable. The cost of the shorter STEAM decay time is a factor of two signal loss compared to PRESS owing to the nature of the echo. This is typically still too long to provide full three-dimensional (3D) localization for ^{31}P or ^{13}C and even for ^1H MRS. Thus, signal loss during the 2t or 4t echo delays must be accounted for in any quantification. Note that both PRESS and STEAM are spin echo methods that are also sensitive to motion, which causes the signals to dephase, resulting in a loss in SNR. Cardiac STEAM and PRESS MRS can thus benefit substantially from cardiac and respiratory gating techniques *(14)* or from postacquisition signal processing in which the signals are first phased prior to averaging *(15)*.

If TEs are fatal for localizing short T_2 ^{31}P and ^{13}C signals, then slice-selective pulses can be applied as inversion (180°) pulses in the presence of the x-, y-, and z-gradients prior to the initial excitation in a technique called ISIS, for image-selected in vivo spectroscopy *(16)* (Fig. 2C). However, if they are all applied at once, then the signal following excitation is just the signal sum from the entire sample minus the inverted signals from the inverted slices. This does not equal the signal from the voxel at the intersection of the slices. To obtain the signal from the single voxel at the intersection of the slices, the experiment must be repeated eight times with all combinations of the three inversion pulses turned on and off, with the resultant signals appropriately added and subtracted *(3,16)*. This method is particularly prone to substantial contamination from outside the selected volume, caused by the combined effects of motion during the eight-cycle period, the addition and subtraction of large net signals from the whole of the excited region, and the partial saturation of superficial tissues by the inversion pulses *(17)*.

1D-3D CSI

A deficiency of all these selective excitation methods is that they only permit MRS of a single voxel at a time. To study metabolism in more voxels, PRESS, STEAM, or ISIS must be applied serially, and the SNR that results from studying, say, eight voxels is equal to that of only a single voxel, even though the total exam took eight times as long. This is not the case with the second MRI gradient-based method: phase-encoding gradients.

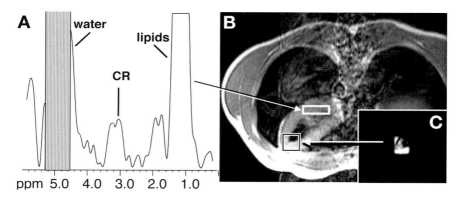

Fig. 4. ^{1}H MRS and MRI data from a normal volunteer (*1*). (**A**) Water suppressed spectrum from a 3 × 1 × 2 cm STEAM voxel from the posterior LV wall (echo time, TE = 15 ms, NEX 128) acquired in 4 minutes. Shading (s = 5 ppm) denotes water suppression. (**B**) Spin echo MRI showing the location of the STEAM voxel. (**C**) Image of STEAM voxel intersecting LV chamber shows that moving blood in the LV chamber and in a blood vessel (black line near top of voxel) does not contribute significantly to the voxel signal.

The phase-encoding gradient is a small gradient pulse applied by one or more of the three Cartesian MRI gradient coils applied immediately after excitation *(3)* (Fig. 2B). The gradient pulse length is typically short, on the order of 0.5–1 ms, to minimize the signal loss caused by T_2 decay. Phase-encoding gradients for each of the *x*-, *y*-, and *z*-gradients can be applied simultaneously. Acquisitions are repeated $N_X × N_Y × N_Z$ times with the amplitude of the *x*-, *y*-, and *z*-gradients each incremented N_X, N_Y, and N_Z times. The 3D FT of the resulting data set with respect to the *x*-, *y*-, and *z*-gradient amplitudes yields a spatially resolved 3D image and spectra from each voxel in the image, obtained from the FT of the time domain signals as in conventional MRS.

This essentially 4D FT technique is called 3D chemical shift imaging (CSI). Because all of the sample contributes to all of the signal all of the time during acquisition, this method yields the maximum SNR per unit time for multiple voxels. For example, because the SNR increases as the square root of the number of acquisitions or scan time, the SNR that results from 3D CSI in the eight-voxel STEAM/PRESS/ISIS study noted above would be √8 times higher for the same resolution, and the T_2 problems of STEAM and PRESS for ^{31}P and ^{13}C are eliminated.

This said, however, $N_X × N_Y × N_Z$ can be a very large number even for a modestly resolved array. A 16 × 16 × 16 array, for instance, would require a minimum of 4096 acquisitions, which, if cardiac gated at a heart rate of 60 beats per minute, would require an untenable 68-minutes scan time regardless of the excellent SNR achieved. Decimating this scan time to something that is practical for patients is most expediently accomplished by modifying the 3D method to two-dimensional (2D) or one-dimensional (1D) versions *(3)*. The 2D version shortens the scan time by limiting the phase encoding to two dimensions, say *X* and *Y* (Fig. 2D). The third, *Z*-dimension is addressed by making the excitation pulse slice selective in the presence of a *z*-gradient. The sequence is repeated $N_X × N_Y$ times, and a 3D FT performed with respect to *x*- and *y*-gradient amplitude and time yields a cross-sectional image with a spectrum in every voxel *(3,18)*.

A drawback of 2D CSI is that the slice-selective excitation pulse can no longer be adiabatic, which may negatively impact quantification when surface coil excitation is used. The 1D CSI version with surface coil detection utilizes only a single phase-encoding gradient to encode slices that are typically oriented parallel to the plane of the surface coil (Fig. 2B). Without selective excitation, adiabatic excitation (9,10) can be reinstated; localization in the other two dimensions, albeit fuzzy, is again afforded by the surface coil sensitivity profile. This sequence with 1-cm resolution and an 8.5-cm receiver can routinely yield useful cardiac ^{31}P spectra from patients in about 5 minutes in a 1.5-T MRI scanner (8,11), enabling various dynamic or flux studies to be performed (19,20).

Cardiac ^1H MRS

As is typical of the rest of the body, the ^1H spectrum from the human heart is dominated by the intense water resonance on which MRI is based, along with variable lipid methylene resonances from $(-CH_2-)_n$ and CH_3 moieties at 1.3 and 0.9 ppm (21), which are a factor of 10 or so less intense. The latter derive from adipose in pericardial fat as well as other mobile fats and lipids. With cardiac water content at 77%, corresponding to a ^1H concentration of 86 M, the water peak is so intense that it typically obliterates millimolar-level signals from metabolites of interest. Accordingly "solvent suppression" NMR methods are applied to attenuate the water and sometimes the lipid signals as well, so that metabolites that nestle between the water and lipid resonances can be quantified (22) (Fig. 4). Typically, water (or fat) suppression involves the addition of chemical-selective NMR saturation pulses applied precisely at the resonant frequency of the water (or fat) signal. These pulses are applied in addition to those required for spatial localization and would normally precede a PRESS or STEAM pulse train.

QUANTIFICATION

With water suppression, the total myocardial creatine pool (CR = PCr plus unphosphorylated creatine, Cr) can be observed and quantified in ^1H spectra via its $\{-N-CH_3\}$ moiety at 3.0 ppm, adjacent to a choline $\{N-(CH_3)_3\}$ moiety (Cho) at 3.2 ppm (1,2,14,23) (Fig. 4). Metabolite quantification first requires obtaining a measure of the area of the corresponding peak, for example, by curve fitting or integration. The concentration of CR is about 25 µmol/g wet tissue weight in normal heart, corresponding to a proton concentration of 75 µmol/g for the $(-N-CH_3)$ moiety. This is approximately 1/1000th of the concentration of tissue water protons (1), so that one might consider introducing a unit for the ratio of the metabolite to (unsuppressed) water signal of a "milli-hoh" (mHOH), with HOH representing water.

Indeed, quantification of CR or Cho from ^1H cardiac spectra is problematic because other resonances that might be used as intensity references (as distinct from chemical shift references) exhibit highly variable intensities—in the case of lipids—or are actually suppressed during the acquisition, as is invariably the case with water. This problem is endemic to ^1H MRS performed outside the brain: the brain is endowed with some other useful endogenous metabolite intensity markers. The approach that we have adopted for heart uses an unsuppressed water signal acquired separately from the same voxel as an intensity reference (1,23). This unfortunately increases the total scan time, although the duration of the water acquisition can be short because its 1000-fold higher SNR is such that little or no signal averaging is necessary.

Adoption of tissue water as an intensity reference requires that water content remain relatively constant for different patients. This is less of a problem than one might imagine. The water content of normal and infarcted cardiac tissue does not change by much more than 1% from 77% by weight (1,23), and even if cardiac tissue were confused

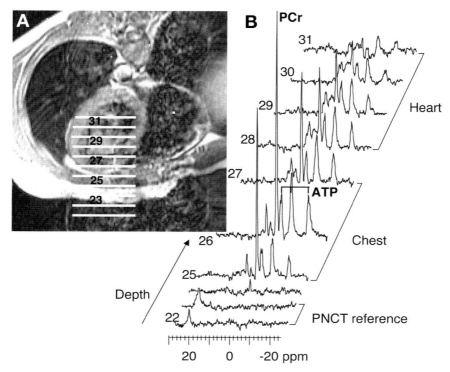

Fig. 5. Typical cardiac-gated data set acquired during a patient exam comprised of an axial MIU to locate the coil and spectra relative to the heart (**A**), and ^{31}P spectra (**B**) acquired as a function of depth with 1 cm resolution(acquisition time, 12.4 minutes). The subject was oriented prone, rotated on the left side. Spectra derive from the same numbered sections annotated in the image. (Adapted from Ref. *34*).

with blood, the comparable blood water content of 80% by weight *(24)* ensures that the error typically would be smaller than the SNR or variability in the CR measurement. The essential constancy of tissue water content in a range 77–80% renders the water ^{1}H peak not only suitable for providing a relative measure of cardiac metabolites via, say, the CR-to-water ratio, but also for determining the absolute concentration of the metabolite *(1,23)*.

For example, the CR concentration is simply equal to two-thirds of the ratio of CR ($-N-CH_3$) signal to the water (H_2O) signal in the same voxel times the water concentration. The only wrinkle in this calculation is that any differences in the NMR relaxation times (T_1, T_2) for the two moieties must be taken into account. Of these, the T_1 correction can be avoided by using a long repetition time, TR (e.g., TR ~ 2 s >> T_1). This leaves a T_2 correction that, unfortunately, cannot be avoided if echo sequences such as STEAM and PRESS localization are used. The T_2 correction involves measuring the loss in signal between the initial excitation pulse and the acquired echo for each of the water and metabolite moieties by varying the TE in repeat acquisitions, fitting the decay, and compensating each of the measured signals for the loss *(1,2,23)*.

Human myocardial triglyceride levels have also been quantified relative to water via the methylene ($-CH_2-$)$_n$ resonances localized by PRESS to the septum to avoid pericardial fat *(25)*. Also, in rats and dogs, resonances associated with deoxy- and oxymyoglobin at 75 ppm and −2.8 ppm that correlate with intracellular pO_2 have been reported *(26,27)*, although this work has not yet been extended to the human heart. The resonance at 75 ppm is so far away from water that no water suppression is needed, and the resonance can be directly excited with chemical-selective NMR pulses.

Cardiac ^{31}P MRS

In addition to a sharp PCr singlet peak taken as a chemical shift reference at 0 ppm, the normal human ^{31}P cardiac spectrum is typically graced by the three phosphate multiplet peaks from ATP at about −2.7 ppm (γ–ATP), −7.8 ppm (α-ATP), and −16.3 ppm (β-ATP). There are variable amounts of phosphodiester at 2–3 ppm; an intracellular pH-dependent inorganic phosphate (Pi) peak at a chemical shift of 3.9–5.1 ppm; two blood 2,3-diphosphoglycerate (DPG) peaks at 5.4 and 6.3 ppm (a typical contaminant from the blood in the ventricular chamber); and possible phosphomonoester (PM) resonances at 6.3–6.8 ppm *(3,5)*. Tissue pH can be measured from the chemical shift of Pi with the aid of a suitable calibration curve *(28)*. Figure 5 shows examples of ^{31}P NMR spectra from a normal human heart.

PCr/ATP Ratios

Metabolite quantification again involves measuring the metabolite peak area and comparing it to a reference. Because PCr and ATP are both energy metabolites and may change with patient condition and because phosphodiester, PM, DPG, and Pi are also variable, there is no reliable endogenous concentration reference in the spectrum unless one assumes a particular value for [ATP]. Both ATP and PCr appear to be 100% NMR visible in 1.5-T MRI scanners, and the ratio of PCr/ATP based on the areas of the PCr and γ–ATP or β-ATP moieties is widely taken as an index of myocardial creatine kinase (CK) metabolic reserve *(3,5)*. The raw PCr/ATP numbers can vary by a factor of two or more within a given study group owing to differences in the T_1's of PCr and ATP. The T_1 differences cause differential saturation when the TR is changed, for example, because of heart rate, when acquisitions are gated synchronous to the heart rate *(3)*. The T_1's of PCr and ATP are quite long at 4.4 seconds for PCr and 2.3 seconds for β-ATP at 1.5 T *(29)*, but there is little evidence that they vary much with disease *(30)*.

To obtain useful cardiac PCr/ATP measurements, the ratios need to be corrected for the differential saturation effect either using standard T_1 values for the metabolites *(29)* or directly measuring the saturation distortion factors by acquiring some fully relaxed data *(30)*. The latter may result in studies in which nothing else gets done because the TR values may need to be increased to more than $3T_1$ or 15 seconds or more for the fully relaxed data. The alternative requires knowledge of the flip angle, which is solved using adiabatic excitation and the known TR or the average heart rate when gating *(29,30)*.

Contamination from skeletal muscle in the chest wall and from blood when voxels intersect the ventricular cavities is another source of intergroup variability in PCr/ATP ratios *(3)*. Because blood contains ATP but no PCr, it reduces the observed PCr/ATP ratio. The amount of blood ATP contaminant can be dealt with by measuring the blood DPG peak and subtracting a proportionate amount from the spectral ATP estimate *(31)*. Because [ATP]/[DPG] is approximately 0.3 in humans, the cardiac PCr/ATP is corrected for blood ATP by subtracting an ATP signal amount corresponding to 0.15 times the integrated DPG signal (remembering it has two phosphates) *(3,31)*. On the other hand, skeletal muscle contamination of heart spectra increases the observed PCr/ATP

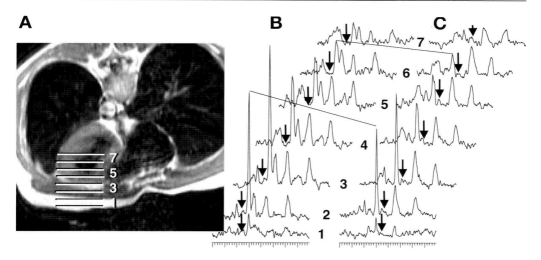

Fig. 6. Cardiac axial spin-echo scout MRI of a normal subject acquired at rest (**A**) with horizontal lines showing the source of two of the four ^{31}P ID CSI data sets of a FAST experiment (*19, 20*), plotted as a function of depth through the chest (spectra 1–7). Arrows on the spectra identify the frequency of the saturating irradiation, which is tuned to the γ-ATP resonance in (**C**), and to a symmetric control location relative to PCr in (**B**). With γ-ATP saturated, the PCr resonances decrease (oblique line) in direct proportion to the forward CK flux (*19*). Each of these ^{31}P data sets was acquired in 6 minutes using 60° adiabatic excitation: the other two data sets for the FAST method (not shown) are each acquired in 12 minutes with a 15° excitation.

ratio because [PCr] in skeletal muscle is about 25 μmol/g compared with about 10 μmol/g in normal heart; [ATP] values in heart and skeletal muscle are essentially the same, at about 5.6 μmol/g. The amount of skeletal tissue contamination can be estimated if PCr/ATP is known (*30*) but generally must be dealt with via careful spatial localization protocols. After corrections for T_1 distortion and blood contamination, a consensus exists for a normal human myocardial PCr/ATP ratio of about 1.83 ± 0.12 (*3*).

CONCENTRATIONS

As with ^{1}H MRS, metabolite ratios measured with ^{31}P MRS can be converted to concentrations with the aid of concentration references. There are basically two approaches: use of a ^{31}P reference (*18,32,33*) or a ^{1}H water reference (*34*). With the former, the absence of an endogenous ^{31}P reference demands that either a reference signal is acquired from a source located outside the body during the MRS exam, or a signal is acquired from the reference in an additional study performed during a separate calibration procedure. With the external reference residing at a different location than the tissue voxel under examination and with surface coil detection, the ratio of metabolite to reference signals requires an additional correction to account for the difference in sensitivity of the surface detection coil at the two locations (*18*) (Fig. 1). With the water reference method, the ^{1}H water signal is acquired with the ^{31}P detector coil from the identical voxel, and no such correction is required. However, an additional calibration is required to determine the ratio of the ^{31}P signal per nucleus to the ^{1}H signal per proton, for example, by measuring the signals in a large volume of phosphate solution (*33*). These methods yield concentrations of 9–10 μmol/g for [PCr] and 5–6 μmol/g in normal human myocardium.

CREATINE KINASE FLUX

The pseudo-first-order forward CK reaction rate for the human heart can also be measured by ^{31}P MRS with a method known as saturation transfer *(35)*. In the forward CK reaction, the phosphate moiety on PCr exchanges with the γ-ATP moiety. The saturation transfer method involves selectively saturating the γ-ATP resonance with a chemical-selective NMR pulse tuned precisely to the γ-ATP resonance frequency, as depicted in Fig. 6. The γ-ATP signal then disappears from the spectrum. Saturated γ-ATP moieties transfer to the PCr resonance via the reverse CK reaction, but, because they are saturated, they cannot contribute any signal to the PCr resonance. At the same time, PCr phosphates transfer to γ-ATP via the forward CK reaction. This outflow of the phosphate signal without a commensurate inflow of unsaturated phosphate reduces PCr, by an amount proportional to the forward rate constant k_f in units of the T_1 of PCr measured in the presence of the saturation, T_1'. Thus, $k_f T_1' = 1 - M_0'/M_0$, where M_0'/M_0 is the ratio of fully relaxed signals acquired with and without the selective irradiation. In practice, M_0 is acquired with saturation directed at +2.7 ppm, symmetrically opposite to γ-ATP on the other side of PCr, as a control.

In practice, performing spatially localized saturation transfer measurements under full-relaxed (long-TR) conditions is not tenable in patients because of time constraints. The measurement, however, can be done with short TR provided appropriate correction is made to M_0' and M_0 for saturation using a technique called FAST (four-angle saturation transfer) *(19)* (Fig. 6). This technique utilizes two acquisitions with adiabatic 15° and 60° excitations with control saturation and another two during γ-ATP saturation. All these can be acquired in about 40 minutes at 1.5 T. The forward product of k_f (s^{-1}) with the PCr concentration {k_f[PCr]} (in units of μmol/g wet weight s^{-1}. Thus, to measure CK flux, the FAST protocol must be followed by one of the concentration measurement protocols discussed. A complete study yielding all the metabolite concentrations, the rate constant, and the flux takes about an hour at 1.5T with 1D CSI. For normal human heart, the forward CK rate constant is about 0.3 s^{-1}, and the flux is about 3 μmol/g wet weight s^{-1} *(20)*.

Cardiac ^{13}C MRS

The only naturally abundant, stable, nonradioactive carbon isotope that meets the NMR condition of having an odd number of nucleons is ^{13}C. Unfortunately, its natural abundance is only about 1% of carbon atoms, which proportionately affects sensitivity. In addition, the natural abundance ^{13}C spectrum from the human heart has a large range of chemical shifts that covers nearly 200 ppm. The latter introduces the practical problem of ensuring that the bandwidth of the NMR excitation pulse is sufficiently large to excite all of the spectral range, a problem that already affects in vivo human ^{31}P MRS, which only has about 20 ppm to cover.

The standard solution is to reduce the NMR pulse width and increase the pulse power. An associated bandwidth problem that arises when slice selection is used for localization is that different resonances in the spectrum will derive from physically different parts of the sample unless high-power short pulses are applied *(4)*. For this reason, use of phase-encoding gradients offers the best approach to spatial localization. In vivo ^{13}C MRS can, however, benefit from simultaneous irradiation at the ^{1}H NMR frequency. The ^{13}C nuclei are coupled to protons so that the irradiation results in the transfer of nuclear magnetization to the ^{13}C nuclei, increasing the signal and SNR by up to a factor equal to the ratio of their NMR frequencies, approximately fourfold. This is known as the nuclear Overhauser effect and can also provide some (albeit lesser) benefit to ^{31}P MRS *(35)*. If the irradiation is continued during the ^{13}C acquisition, then the multiplet structures collapse providing further gains in SNR.

The cardiac ^{13}C MRS spectrum is dominated by fat resonances: $(-CH_2-)_n$ at about 30 ppm and glycerol and carboxyl (–CO) resonances at 170 ppm, although sometimes a glycogen resonance at about 101 ppm is detectable *(4)*. Because of its low natural abundance, use of ^{13}C-enriched substrates, or even substrates labeled with hyperpolarized ^{13}C, may provide access for tracer studies of glycolytic and tricarboxylic acid cycle metabolism. Although many labeled ^{13}C MRS studies have been performed in animals (e.g., *36,37*), human cardiac applications with ^{13}C-labeled substrates have yet to be reported.

CLINICAL STUDIES WITH CARDIAC MAGNETIC RESONANCE SPECTROSCOPY

Myocardial Infarction

Bottomley et al. were the first to study cardiac high-energy phosphate metabolism in patients with anterior myocardial infarction (MI) *(38)*. Approximately 1 week after the onset of symptoms, cardiac-gated, ^{31}P MR DRESS was performed, and significant reductions in the PCr-to-Pi ratio and elevations in the Pi-to-ATP ratio were observed. However, contamination of the Pi resonances by other phosphate compounds, including blood DPG, precluded precise spectral quantification of Pi and pH determination. These findings demonstrated that localized ^{31}P MRS can directly detect changes in myocardial energy metabolism in the clinical setting following MI.

The effect of infarct transmurality on energetics was later studied by Mitsunami et al. *(39)*. They also used DRESS ^{31}P MR techniques and compared the findings in patients with Q-wave myocardial infarction (QMI), those patients with non-Q-wave myocardial infarction (NQMI), and those in healthy subjects *(39)*. The infarct extent score was determined by ^{201}Tl scintigraphy. Although no significant differences were found among the three groups in the relative PCr/ATP ratio, significant reductions were observed in the absolute amount of PCr (normalized by a standard HMPT for QMI patients, $p \ll 0.05$, and in ATP for QMI and NQMI patients, $p \ll 0.01$) compared with controls. These results suggested that reductions in high-energy phosphate levels in infarcted nonviable myocardium, detected by ^{31}P MRS, may be useful in evaluating myocardial viability following infarction. This was also the first clear demonstration that metabolite pool sizes, rather than relative ratios such as that afforded by the PCr/ATP ratio, may better reflect the extent of metabolic abnormalities.

Another important study of myocardial viability was reported by Yabe et al., who also measured PCr and ATP contents rather than just ratios *(32)*. Forty-one subjects with left anterior descending critical disease were characterized on the basis of exercise ^{201}Tl scintigraphy: a reversible ^{201}Tl defect group (RD[+]) who demonstrated redistribution and a fixed ^{201}Tl defect group (RD[–]). PCr content was significantly decreased in patients with both reversible and fixed ^{201}Tl defects compared with healthy controls, and ATP content was decreased significantly only in subjects with fixed thallium defects. These observations showed that the measurement of ATP content in the human heart by ^{31}P NMR may be a clinically important method for distinguishing viable and nonviable myocardium.

The use of newer 3D acquisition techniques may now enable measures of high-energy phosphates with ^{31}P MRS from the inferior LV wall in people. Beer et al. used an acquisition weighted, [31]P 3D CSI sequence to study patients with a history of inferior MI *(40)*. By orienting the array along the LV short axis, spectra with adequate SNR could be obtained from 25-mL voxels located over the inferior wall, and reduced high-energy phosphates were observed there in patients with inferior MI *(40)*. Unfortunately, metabolic information from the posterior LV wall has not been routinely available from ^{31}P MRS at 1.5 T.

A different metabolic approach for detecting viability after MI involves the detection of total creatine with ^{1}H MRS *(1)*. This approach offers higher sensitivity than ^{31}P MRS detection of PCr or ATP, and this higher sensitivity can in turn be used to acquire data from smaller voxels, including those remote from the anterior wall. The ^{1}H nucleus generates intrinsically about sixfold more MR SNR per nucleus than the ^{31}P nucleus at a constant field strength (assuming sample noise is dominant); the ^{1}H nuclei are more abundant. As noted in "Cardiac ^{1}H MRS" above, the concentration of proton concentration on the –CH_3 moiety of creatine (CR) resonating at 3.0 ppm is roughly 75 µmol/g in normal tissue compared to approximately 10 µmol/g for the PCr phosphate moiety. Thus, ^{1}H MRS detection of myocardial CR can potentially offer SNR advantages in the realm of 40-fold over the detection of PCr by ^{31}P MRS, although these gains have not yet been fully realized. Quantification of skeletal *(41)* and cardiac *(23)* muscle CR content by ^{1}H MRS has been validated and shown to be independent of fiber orientation *(42)*.

In the human heart, ^{1}H MRS spectra can be obtained in 6 minutes from voxels as small as 8 mL *(1)*, and the normal concentration of myocardial total CR is approximately 28 µmol/g *(1)*. In a cohort of patients with a history of MI and nonviable myocardium, total creatine was reduced by approximately 65% from that in noninfarcted regions and that observed in healthy individuals *(1)*. In contrast to ^{31}P MRS studies to date, ^{1}H MR spectra have been obtained from the posterior wall of the human heart *(1,2)*. Thus, ^{1}H MRS detection of total creatine offers a new avenue for metabolically characterizing myocardial viability throughout the entire LV in patients with MI.

Stunned Myocardium

Cardiac high-energy phosphates are reduced during experimental and clinical ischemia *(8,43,44)*. If the recovery of myocardial high-energy phosphates following ischemia is incomplete or delayed, then this could theoretically contribute to the dysfunction that is observed in postischemic "stunned" myocardium. Although rapid recovery of high-energy phosphates and a normal PCr/ATP has been reported in most animal models of stunning *(45–47)*, the phenomenon had not been studied in humans.

Kalil-Filho et al. used ^{31}P MRS to measure cardiac high-energy phosphates in postischemic stunned human myocardium by studying 29 patients with a first anterior MI who underwent successful reperfusion within 6 hours of the onset of chest pain *(48)*. In regions that demonstrated spontaneous improvement in function between early (day 4) and late (days 30–40) studies (stunned myocardium), the myocardial PCr/ATP at the early time was similar to that of healthy control subjects and similar to that of the same patients measured at the late time *(48)*. The study had a 90% power to detect a 9% difference. Thus, in stunned human myocardium, as previously observed in experimental models of stunning, the recovery of high-energy phosphates is rapid and complete, suggesting that reduced relative high-energy phosphates cannot account for the depressed mechanical function observed at that time.

Myocardial Ischemia

The feasibility of combining ^{31}P MRS with a stress test to detect ischemia metabolically was explored, and indeed transient stress-induced reductions in myocardial high-energy phosphates can be detected in patients with critical coronary disease. Weiss et al. studied cardiac high-energy phosphates with ^{31}P MRS before, during, and after continuous isometric handgrip exercise *(8)*. Isometric handgrip exercise did not induce changes in the cardiac PCr/ATP in age-matched healthy subjects or in patients with nonischemic heart disease. However, patients with critical lesions in arteries supplying the anterior wall had a significant 35% reduction in the PCr/ATP during stress, which later improved after the exercise stopped. Following successful revascularization (balloon angioplasty or bypass surgery), the cardiac PCr/ATP no longer declined during stress *(48)*. The decrease in cardiac PCr/ATP ratio during handgrip exercise in patients with coronary disease reflects a transient imbalance between oxygen supply and demand in myocardium with compromised blood flow and metabolic evidence of inducible ischemia. Exercise testing with ^{31}P MRS appears to be a specific method for assessing the effect of ischemia on myocardial high-energy phosphate metabolism and for monitoring the response to ischemic therapies *(49)*.

Those findings were confirmed and expanded by Yabe et al., who related cardiac ^{31}P MRS stress observations with viability measures by ^{201}Tl scintigraphy *(50)*. They also observed no significant reduction in the cardiac PCr/ATP in healthy subjects during handgrip stress and reported a 40% exercise-induced decline in PCr/ATP in patients with critical disease and a reversible ^{201}Tl defect. In contrast, in patients with nonviable myocardium (fixed anterior ^{201}Tl defect), the ratio was lower at rest and did not change with exercise stress. The most likely explanation is that patients with fixed defects had reductions in total PCr and ATP *(32)*, and that the PCr/ATP ratio from the residual myocardium is unchanged during stress. These results are consistent with the view that ^{31}P MRS with handgrip exercise testing is a specific method for detecting reversible myocardial ischemia.

Because ^{31}P MRS stress testing appeared to provide a specific means to detect myocardial ischemia, Buchthal et al. *(51)* used this approach to study patients with chest pain but no significant epicardial coronary disease. Some have speculated that microvascular disease may cause exercise-induced ischemia even in the absence of epicardial coronary disease in this population. Buchthal et al. reported that a small subset (~20%) of the Women's Ischemia Syndrome Evaluation (WISE) study had a significant decline in cardiac PCr/ATP during isometric exercise, akin to that observed in patients with coronary disease. Women with chest pain, no coronary disease, and an abnormal ^{31}P MRS stress test have similar major cardiovascular outcomes (e.g., higher rates of anginal hospitalization, repeat catheterization, and greater treatment costs) to those of women with coronary disease and significantly higher rates than those with a normal ^{31}P MRS stress test *(52)*. Thus, an abnormal ^{31}P MRS stress test consistent with ischemia is uncommon in women without coronary disease but, when present, may predict future cardiovascular outcomes.

Chronic Heart Failure

Because high-energy phosphate metabolism is absolutely required to maintain normal myocardial contractile function, it has been hypothesized that abnormal energy metabolism could contribute to contractile dysfunction in heart failure or that the failing heart is energy "starved" *(53,54)*. In fact, abnormalities in myocardial high-energy phosphates have been reported in nearly all animal models of heart failure *(55–58)*. What is the evidence that abnormal high-energy phosphate metabolism underlies human heart failure?

Most studies have found a reduced cardiac PCr/ATP at rest in patients with dilated cardiomyopathy (DCM) and heart failure. In 1990, Schaefer et al. reported a modestly lower cardiac PCr/ATP ratio in heart failure patients that was not statistically significantly different from that in healthy subjects *(59)*. The next year, Hardy and collaborators were the first to report significant reductions in the myocardial PCr/ATP ratio in adults with DCM and heart failure *(31)*. These mean reductions of approximately 18% were observed at rest in both ischemic and nonischemic heart failure.

In 1992, Neubauer et al. reported lower PCr/ATP in dilated DCM and found a significant inverse correlation between the PCr/ATP ratio and the New York Heart Association (NYHA) class *(60)*. There was no clear correlation between PCr/ATP and LV ejection fraction (EF) or fractional shortening. Patients with heart failure were followed for several years following the initial ^{31}P MRS study, and the cardiac PCr/ATP ratio was a better predictor of overall and cardiovascular survival than LVEF or NYHA class *(61)*. Other investigators have also reported reduced cardiac PCr/ATP in heart failure *(62,63)* and, in uncommon instances for which the Pi resonance could be identified, lower PCr/Pi *(64)*. Thus, abnormalities in cardiac PCr/ATP have been observed at rest in patients with moderate-to-severe heart failure, and such metabolic abnormalities may predict outcomes and survival.

Although a 20% or so reduction in cardiac PCr/ATP is commonly observed in patients with heart failure, it is not clear that such a modest reduction would be sufficient to cause contractile dysfunction. Several energetic factors are commonly listed as potential metabolic causes of contractile dysfunction in heart failure, and they include ATP depletion, increased [ADP] ([adenosine 5′-diphosphate]) and reduced $\Delta G_{\sim ATP}$ (the free energy of ATP hydrolysis), and reduced CK flux *(54,65)*. Modest ATP loss (20–30%) occurs in severe human heart failure *(66,67)*, but this degree of ATP depletion is not caused by the K_m of most ATP-requiring reactions and thus not a likely explanation for contractile dysfunction in heart failure.

Beer et al. were the first to use ^{31}P MRS to measure myocardial PCr and ATP absolute concentrations in human heart failure *(33)*. They reported a 35% reduction in cardiac [ATP], a 50% loss of [PCr], and a 25% reduction in PCr/ATP of borderline significance in 10 patients with DCM, nearly all in NYHA class III. [PCr], and to a lesser extent [ATP], correlated with EF and volumes. The authors concluded that PCr/ATP underestimates changes in high-energy phosphate levels. In addition, Nakae et al. measured total creatine concentrations [CR] in patients with DCM and heart failure *(2)*. They observed a 40% reduction in [CR] in DCM and found that [CR] correlated positively with EF and negatively with B-type natriuretic peptide *(2)*.

A new method to quantify ATP flux in the human heart was developed and used to address the other potential metabolic causes of contractile dysfunction in heart failure listed in this section. As described in the Methods section, the method FAST relies on magnetization transfer techniques and employs them for the first time in a time-efficient manner that can be tolerated by normal volunteers and patients. This technique underwent theoretical (68,69) and experimental (19) validation, producing identical results to classic saturation transfer techniques. In the normal human heart, the rate of ATP production through CK, the main energy reservoir of the heart is approximately 3 μmol/g/second, which is 7–10 times that of the rate of ATP generation through oxidative phosphorylation (20).

In patients with mild-moderate heart failure, although [ATP] was not significantly depleted and [PCr] was reduced by only 20%, the rate of ATP flux through CK was reduced by 50% in heart failure (20). Because the ratio of CK flux to that of oxidative phosphorylation should exceed unity if CK acts as a temporal or spatial ATP buffer ("shuttle"), the new observation from this study that the ratio of CK flux to oxidative phosphorylation approaches unity in patients with severe heart failure, or those with moderate heart failure during stress, offers a potential metabolic explanation for contractile dysfunction in heart failure.

In addition, the CK pseudo-first-order rate constant K_{for} in some settings parallels changes in [ADP] such that an observed 35% reduction in K_{for} in heart failure predicts lower rather than higher [ADP] in human heart failure because of DCM (20). If [ADP] is calculated by the classic CK equilibrium reaction using recent ^1H MRS measures of Cr from human heart failure (2), lower [ADP] is also predicted (20). A lower [ADP] would result in an increased, not reduced, $\Delta G_{\sim ATP}$, whereas ATP depletion, higher [ADP], and lower $\Delta G_{\sim ATP}$ have been postulated as potential energetic contributors to mechanical failure in heart failure. Thus, we do not have evidence indicating that higher [ADP] and lower ΔG play a significant role in human heart failure and DCM.

Instead, reduced CK flux is the most prominent energetic abnormality in patients with heart failure, and the magnitude of the CK reduction is theoretically sufficient to impair contractile function (20). Thus, new magnetization transfer techniques that allow measurement of ATP turnover can be used in clinical settings, provide more insight than relative or absolute pool measures, and generate novel mechanistic insights into heart failure.

Left Ventricular Hypertrophy

LV hypertrophy (LVH) can arise from genetic mutations or result as a consequence of pressure overload, such as from hypertension or valvular aortic stenosis. Familial LVH is inherited in about half of cases, whereas other cases spontaneously arise from new genetic mutations.

Jung et al. described myocardial metabolic abnormalities in patients with LVH (70) and subsequently compared cases of asymptomatic familial vs spontaneous cases of hypertrophic cardiomyopathy (HCM) LVH. They found that PCr/ATP ratios were significantly lower (14%) and P_i/PCr ratios significantly greater (46%) in those with familial HCM LVH despite similar LV masses between the two groups (71). More extensive research will be necessary to identify those genetic mutations that lead to metabolic abnormalities prior to the onset of clinical symptoms in some LVH cases but not others. These findings in human familial LVH parallel previous results from a mouse model of familial LVH that indicate that energetic abnormalities were a consequence of a myosin mutation rather than myocardial hypertrophy alone (72).

Several other studies have similarly reported low PCr/ATP at rest in LVH (64,73–75). When pH was detectable, pH was lower in LVH in some (64) but not all reports (70). LVH from chronic pressure overload is adaptive and clinically prevalent but is associated with a 10-fold increased risk for future congestive heart failure (CHF) (76,77). Chronic pressure overload leads to increased myocardial energetic demand, and a mismatch between energy supply and demand may eventually progress from an asymptomatic individual to one with heart failure. In patients with clinical symptoms from aortic stenosis, the resting PCr/ATP ratio is lower at rest compared to those with aortic stenosis and no symptoms *(78)*.

In animal models of LVH *(57,79)* and clinical LVH *(78,80,81)*, reduced PCr/ATP ratios have also been reported. The CK reaction is the prime myocardial energy reservoir, and alterations in CK flux as measured by ^{31}P MRS magnetization transfer techniques are greater than those seen with the PCr/ATP ratio in animal models of chronic pressure overload LVH *(57,82)*.

Given the presence of normal and abnormal myocardial energetics in asymptomatic individuals with LVH but myocardial energetic abnormalities in CHF, it is conceivable that metabolic abnormalities may precede the onset of symptoms from CHF. However, the cross-sectional nature of these studies precludes definitive evidence of this progression from metabolic abnormality to clinically apparent CHF with LVH. Prospective studies with serial measurements of cardiac energetics, potentially including those with interventions to improve symptoms or regression of LVH, would further clarify this hypothesis.

Transplanted Hearts

Animal studies have shown a relationship between reductions in the myocardial PCr/ATP ratio and the histological evidence of transplant rejection *(83–85)* as well as the ability to predict the development of histological evidence of rejection over the next few days *(83)*. However, the mechanism for altered metabolism in experimental transplant rejection remains unknown. Although those experimental studies raised hopes that ^{31}P MRS may be a noninvasive means to follow transplant rejection, unfortunately human studies have failed to show a close relationship between the myocardial PCr/ATP ratio and the severity of transplant rejection *(86–88)*.

The first publication to describe cardiac high-energy phosphates following human cardiac transplantation and relate them to histological evidence of rejection was reported by Bottomley et al. from 1 to 6 years after transplantation *(86)*. Patients with mild rejection had reduced cardiac PCr/ATP compared with those of normal subjects, but ^{31}P MRS could not distinguish mild from moderate histological rejection and could therefore not distinguish patients who required augmented therapy for rejection. Van Dobbenburgh et al. also found that PCr/ATP did not correlate with transplant rejection severity but instead convincingly showed that time after transplantation affected PCr/ATP *(87)*. Buchthal et al. studied acute rejection in the first month after transplantation *(88)* and found low PCr/ATP; however, the reduction did not correlate with histological rejection severity in the current or future biopsies. Thus, abnormalities in resting cardiac high-energy phosphate levels do not appear to predict acute or chronic transplant rejection in patients.

Van Dobbenburg et al. also studied the energy metabolism in excised human donor hearts with ^{31}P MRS before implantation *(89)*. The PCr/ATP, PM/ATP, and PCr/Pi ratios at the time of reperfusion correlated with the cardiac index 1 week after transplantation. Caus et al. also studied explanted donor hearts with ^{31}P MRS prior to transplantation and reported that a score based on the PCr/Pi ratio and pH predicted outcomes and the need for inotropic support *(90)*. Taken together, these observations suggest that functional recovery after the human heart transplantation is related to the metabolic condition of the hypothermic donor heart, and that ^{31}P MRS may help guide the use of grafts from marginal donors.

SUMMARY

In conclusion, MRS provides a noninvasive means to study myocardial metabolism. In fact, ^{31}P MRS is the only method for noninvasively quantifying human myocardial high-energy phosphate metabolism. Future technological advances in MRS must focus on efforts to improve the sensitivity of the technique to augment spatial resolution and metabolite detection. With these in hand, one could envisage a clinical role for metabolic imaging of high-energy phosphates (91–93) or Cr (41), performed in conjunction with routine cardiac MRI techniques, as described in other chapters. Meanwhile, the opportunity to now noninvasively study metabolite flux or turnover will likely provide critical new mechanistic insights that are not accessible to MRS studies of the metabolite pool sizes alone.

REFERENCES

1. Bottomley PA, Weiss RG. Creatine depletion in non-viable, infarcted myocardium measured by noninvasive MRS. Lancet 1998;351:714–718.
2. Nakae I, Mitsunami K, Omura T, et al. Proton magnetic resonance spectroscopy can detect creatine depletion associated with the progression of heart failure in cardiomyopathy. J Am Coll Cardio 2003;42:1587–1593.
3. Bottomley PA. MR spectroscopy of the human heart: the status and the challenges. Radiology 1994;191:593–612.
4. Bottomley PA, Hardy CJ, Roemer PB, Mueller OM. Proton-decoupled, Overhauser-enhanced, spatially localized carbon-13 spectroscopy in humans. Magn Reson Med 1989;12:348–363.
5. Bottomley PA. Noninvasive study of high-energy phosphate metabolism in human heart by depth-resolved ^{31}P NMR spectroscopy. Science 1985;229:769–772.
6. Bottomley PA. A practical guide to getting NMR spectra in vivo. In: Budinger TF, Margulis AF, eds. Medical magnetic resonance imaging and spectroscopy, a primer. Berkeley, CA: Society for Magnetic Resonance in Medicine; 1986 p. 81–95
7. Vesselle H, Collin E. The signal-to-noise ratio of nuclear magnetic resonance surface coils and application to a lossy dielectric cylinder model. IEEE Trans Biomed Eng 1995;42:497–520.
8. Weiss RG, Bottomley PA, Hardy CJ, Gerstenblith G. Regional myocardial metabolism of high-energy phosphates during isometric exercise in patients with coronary artery disease. N Engl J Med 1990;323:1593–1600.
9. Garwood M, Ke Y. Symmetric pulses to induce arbitrary flip-angles with compensation for RF inhomogeneity and resonance offsets. J Magn Reson 1991;94:511–525.
10. Bottomley PA, Ouwerkerk R. BIRP, an improved implementation of low-angle adiabatic (BIR-4) excitation pulses. J Magn Reson 1993;103A:242–244.
11. Bottomley PA, Hardy CJ. Strategies and protocols for clinical ^{31}P research in the heart and brain. Phil Trans R Soc Lond A 1990;333:531–544.
12. Bottomley PA. Spatial localization in NMR spectroscopy in vivo. Ann N Y Acad Sci 1987;508:333–348.
13. Bruhn H, Frahm J, Gyngell ML, Merboldt KD, Hanicke W, Sauter R. Localized proton NMR spectroscopy using stimulated echoes: application to human skeletal muscle in vivo. Magn Reson Med 1991;17:82–94.
14. Felblinger J, Jung B, Slotboom J, Boesch C, Kreis R. Methods and reproducibility of cardiac/respiratory double-triggered (1)H-MR spectroscopy of the human heart. Magn Reson Med 1999;42:903–910.
15. Gabr R, Sathyanarayana S, Schar M, Weiss RG, Bottomley PA. On restoring motion-induced signal loss in single-voxel magnetic resonance spectra. Magn Reson Med 2006;56:754–760.
16. Ordidge RJ, Connelly A, Lohman JAB. Image-selected in vivo spectroscopy (ISIS)—a new technique for spatially selective NMR-spectroscopy. J Magn Reson 1986;66:283–294.
17. Lawry TJ, Karczmar GS, Weiner MW, Matson GB. Computer simulation of MRS localization techniques: an analysis of ISIS. Magn Reson Med 1989;9:299–314.
18. Bottomley PA, Hardy CJ, Roemer PB. Phosphate metabolite imaging and concentration measurements in human heart by nuclear magnetic resonance. Magn Reson Med 1990;14:425–434.

19. Bottomley PA, Ouwerkerk R, Lee RF, Weiss RG. The four-angle saturation transfer (FAST) method for measuring creatine kinase reaction rates in vivo. Magn Reson Med 2002;47:850–863.

20. Weiss RG, Gerstenblith G, Bottomley PA. ATP flux through creatine kinase in the normal, stressed, and failing human heart. Proc Natl Acad Sci U S A 2005;102:808–813.

21. Den Hollander JA, Evanochko WT, Pohost GM. Observation of cardiac lipids in humans by localized ^{1}H magnetic resonance spectroscopic imaging. Magn Reson Med 1994;32:175–180.

22. Bottomley PA, Edelstein WA, Foster TH, Adams WA. In vivo solvent suppressed localized hydrogen nuclear magnetic resonance spectroscopy: a window to metabolism? Proc Natl Acad Sci USA 1985;82:2148–2152.

23. Bottomley PA, Weiss RG. Noninvasive localized MR quantification of creatine kinase metabolites in normal and infarcted canine myocardium. Radiology 2001;219:411–418.

24. Snyder WS, Cook MJ, Nasset ES, Karhausen LR, Howells GP, Tipton IH. Repot of the task group on reference man. In: International Commission on Radiological Protection No. 23. Oxford, UK: Pergamon Press, 1984 pp. 280–285.

25. Jason S, Reingold JS, McGavock JM, et al. Determination of triglyceride in the human myocardium by magnetic resonance spectroscopy: reproducibility and sensitivity of the method. Am J Physiol 2005;289:E935–E939.

26. Kreutzer U, Wang DS, Jue T. Observing the ^{1}H NMR signal of the myoglobin Val-Ell in myocardium: an index of cellular oxygenation. Proc Natl Acad Sci USA 1992;89:4731–4733.

27. Chen W, Zhang J, Eljgelshoven MH, et al. Determination of deoxymyoglobin changes during graded myocardial ischemia: an in vivo ^{1}H NMR spectroscopy study. Magn Reson Med 1997;38:193–197.

28. Gadian DG. In: Nuclear magnetic resonance and its applications to living systems. Oxford, UK: Oxford University Press; 1982 p. 32.

29. Bottomley PA, Ouwerkerk R. Optimum flip-angles for exciting NMR with uncertain T_1 values. Magn Reson Med 1994;32:137–141.

30. Bottomley PA, Hardy CJ, Weiss RG. Correcting human heart ^{31}P NMR spectra for partial saturation. Evidence that saturation factors for PCr/ATP are homogeneous in normal and diseased states. J Magn Reson 1991;95:341–355.

31. Hardy CJ, Weiss RG, Bottomley PA, Gerstenblith G. Altered myocardial high-energy phosphate metabolites in patients with dilated cardiomyopathy. Am Heart J 1991;122:795–801.

32. Yabe T, Mitsunami K, Inubushi T, Kinoshita M. Quantitative measurements of cardiac phosphorus metabolites in coronary artery disease by ^{31}P magnetic resonance spectroscopy. Circulation 1995; 92:15–23.

33. Beer M, Seyfarth T, Sandstede J, et al. Absolute concentrations of high-energy phosphate metabolites in normal, hypertrophied, and failing human myocardium measured noninvasively with ^{31}P SLOOP magnetic resonance spectroscopy. J Am Coll Cardiol 2002;40:1267–1274.

34. Bottomley PA, Atalar E, Weiss RG. Human cardiac high-energy phosphate metabolite concentrations by 1D-resolved NMR spectroscopy. Magn Reson Med 1996;35:664–670.

35. Bottomley PA, Hardy CJ. Proton Overhauser enhancements in human cardiac phosphorus NMR spectroscopy at 1.5 T. Magn Reson Med 1992;24:384–390.

36. Degani H, Laughlin MR, Campbell S, Shulman RG. Kinetics of creatine kinase in heart: a ^{31}P NMR saturation- and inversion-transfer study. Biochemistry 1985;24:5510–5516.

37. Weiss RG, Chacko VP, Glickson JD, Gerstenblith G. Comparative ^{13}C and ^{31}P NMR assessment of altered metabolism during graded reductions in coronary flow in intact rat hearts. Proc Natl Acad Sci USA 1989;86:6426–6430.

38. Bottomley PA, Herfkens RJ, Smith LS, Bashore TM, Altered phosphate metabolism in myocardial infarction detected by p–31 MR spectroscopy. Radiology 1986;165:703–707.

39. Mitsunami K, Okada M, Inoue T, Hachisuka M, Kinoshita M, Inubushi T. In vivo ^{31}P nuclear magnetic resonance spectroscopy in patients with old myocardial infarction. Jpn Circ J 1992;56:614–619.

40. Beer M, Spindler M, Sandstede J, et al. Detection of myocardial infarctions by acquisition-weighted ^{31}P-MR spectroscopy in humans. J Magn Reson Imaging 2004;20:798–802.

41. Bottomley PA, Lee Y, Weiss RG. Total creatine in muscle: imaging and quantification with proton MR spectroscopy. Radiology 1997;204:403–410.

42. Gao F, Bottomley PA, Arnold C, Weiss RG. The effect of muscle orientation on quantification of muscle creatine by ^{1}H MR spectroscopy. MRI 2003;21:561–566.

43. Gadian DG, Hoult DI, Radda GK, Seeley PJ, Chance B, Barlow C. Phosphorus nuclear magnetic resonance studies on normoxic and ischemic cardiac tissue. Proc Natl Acad Sci USA 1976;73:4446–4448.

44. Jacobus WE, Taylor GJ, Hollis DP, Nunnally RL. Phosphorus nuclear magnetic resonance of perfused working rat hearts. Nature 1977;265:756–758.

45. Zimmer SD, Ugurbil K, Michurski SP, et al. Alterations in oxidative function and respiratory regulation in the post-ischemic myocardium. J Biol Chem 1989;264,21:12,402–12,411.

46. Neubauer S, Hamman BL, Perry SB, Bittl JA, Ingwall JS. Velocity of the creatine kinase reaction decreases in postischemic myocardium: a ^{31}P-NMR magnetization transfer study of the isolated ferret heart. Circ Res 1988;63,1:1–15.

47. Weiss RG, Gerstenblith G, Lakatta EG. Calcium oscillations index the extent of calcium loading and predict functional recovery during reperfusion in rat myocardium. J Clin Invest 1990;85:757–765.

48. Kalil-Filho R, de Albuquerque CP, Weiss RG, et al. Normal high energy phosphate ratios in "stunned" human myocardium. J AM Coll Cardiologe 1997;30:1228–1232.

49. Najjar SS, Bottomley PA, Schulman SP, et al. Effects of a pharmacologically-induced shift of hemoglobin-oxygen dissociation on myocardial energetics during ischemia in patients with coronary artery disease. J Cardiovasc Magn Reson 2005;7:657–666.

50. Yabe T, Mitsunami K, Okada M, Morikawa S, Inubushi T, Kinoshita M. Detection of myocardial ischemia by ^{31}P magnetic resonance spectroscopy during handgrip exercise. Circulation 1994; 89:1709–1716.

51. Buchthal SD, Den Hollander JA, Merz C, et al. Abnormal myocardial phosphorus-31 nuclear magnetic resonance spectroscopy in women with chest pain but normal coronary angiograms. N Engl J Med 2000;342:829–835.

52. Johnson BD, Shaw LJ, Buchthal SD, et al. Prognosis in women with myocardial ischemia in the absence of obstructive coronary disease: results from the National Institutes of Health-National Heart, Lung, and Blood Institute-Sponsored Women's Ischemia Syndrome Evaluation (WISE). Circulation 2004;109:2993–2999.

53. Ingwall JS. Is cardiac failure a consequence of decreased energy reserve? Circulation 1993;87:VII-58–VII–62.

54. Ingwall JS, Weiss RG. Is the failing heart energy starved? On using chemical energy to support cardiac function. Circ Res 2004;95:135–145.

55. Tian R, Nascimben L, Kaddurah-Daouk R, Ingwall JS. Depletion of energy reserve via the creatine kinase reaction during the evolution of heart failure in cardiomyopathic hamsters. J Mol Cell Cardiol 1996;28:755–765.

56. Ye Y, Wang C, Zhang J, et al. Myocardial creatine kinase kinetics and isoform expression in hearts with severe LVH hypertrophy. Am J Physiol 2001;281:H376–H386.

57. Ye Y, Gong G, Ochiai K, Liu J, Zhang J. High-energy phosphate metabolism and creatine kinase in failing hearts: a new porcine model. Circulation 2001;103:1570–1576.

58. Gong G, Liu J, Liang P, et al. Oxidative capacity in failing hearts. Am J Physiol 2003;285:H541–H548.

59. Schaefer S, Gober JR, Schwartz GG, Twieg DB, Weiner MW, Massie B. In vivo phosphorus-31 spectroscopic imaging in patients with global myocardial disease. Am J Cardiol 1990;65:1154–1161.

60. Neubauer S, Krahe T, Schindler R, et al. [31]P magnetic resonance spectroscopy in dilated cardiomyopathy and coronary artery disease: altered cardiac high-energy phosphate metabolism in heart failure. Circulation 1992;86:1810–1818.

61. Neubauer S, Horn M, Cramer M, et al. Myocardial phosphocreatine-to-ATP ratio is a predictor of mortality in patients with dilated cardiomyopathy. Circulation 1997;96:2190–2196.

62. Hansch A, Rzanny R, Heyne J-P, Leder U, Reichenbach JR, Kaiser WA. Noninvasive measurements of cardiac high-energy phosphate metabolites in dilated cardiomyopathy by using ^{31}P spectroscopic chemical shift imaging. Eur Radiol 2005;15:319–323.

63. Conway MA, Allis J, Ou voerkerk R, Niioka T, Rajagopalan B, Radda GK. Detection of low phosphocreatine to ATP ration failing hypertrophied human myocardium by 31 p magnetic resonance spectroscopy Lancet 1991;338;978–976.

64. deRoos A, Doornbos J, Luyten PR, Osterwaal LJMP, van der Wall EE, Den Hollander JA. Cardiac metabolism in patients with dilated and hypertrophic cardiomyopathy: assessment with proton-decoupled P-31 MR spectroscopy. J Magn Reson Imaging 1992;2:711–719.

65. Katz AM. Is the failing heart energy depleted? Cardiol Clin 1998;16:633–644.

66. Starling RC, Hammer DF, Altschuld RA. Human myocardial ATP content and in vivo contractile function. Mol Cell Biochem 1998;180:171–177.

67. Nascimben L, Ingwall JS, Pauletto P, et al. Creatine kinase system in failing and nonfailing human myocardium. Circulation 1996;94:1894–1901.

68. Ouwerkerk R, Bottomley PA. On neglecting chemical exchange effects when correcting in vivo (31)P MRS data for partial saturation. J Magn Reson 2001;148:425–435.

69. Ouwerkerk R, Bottomley PA. On neglecting chemical exchange when correcting in vivo (31)P MRS data for partial saturation: commentary on: "Pitfalls in the measurement of metabolite concentrations using the one-pulse experiment in in vivo NMR." J Magn Reson 2001;149:282–286.

70. Jung W, Sieverding L, Breuer J, et al. ^{31}P NMR Spectroscopy detects metabolic abnormalities in asymptomatic patients with hypertrophic cardiomyopathy. Circulation 1998;97:2536–2542.

71. Jung WI, Hoess T, Bunse M, et al. Differences in cardiac energetics between patients with familial and nonfamilial hypertrophic cardiomyopathy. Circulation 2000;101:E121.

72. Spindler M, Saupe KW, Christe ME, et al. Diastolic dysfunction and altered energetics in the αMHC[403/+] mouse model of familial hypertrophic cardiomyopathy. J Clin Invest 1998;101:1775–1783.

73. Masuda Y, Tateno Y, Ikehira H, et al. High-energy phosphate metabolism of the myocardium in normal subjects and patients with various cardiomyopathies: the study using ECG gated MR spectroscopy with a localization technique. Jpn Circ J 1992;56:620–626.

74. Sakuma H, Takeda K, Tagami T, et al. [31]P MR spectroscopy in hypertrophic cardiomyopathy: comparison with 2011T myocardial perfusion imaging. Am Heart J 1993;125:1323–1328.

75. Rajagopalan B, Blackledge MJ, McKenna WJ, Bolas N, Radda GK. Measurement of phosphocreatine to ATP ratio in normal and diseased human heart by ^{31}P magnetic resonance spectroscopy using the rotating frame-depth selection technique. Ann N Y Acad Sci 1987;508:321–332.

76. Grossman W. Cardiac hypertrophy: useful adaptation or pathologic process? Am J Med 1980; 69:576–584.

77. Levy D, Garrison RJ, Savage DD, Kannel WB, Castelli WP. Prognostic implications of echocardiographically determined left ventricular mass in the Framingham Heart Study. N Engl J Med 1990; 322:1561–1566.

78. Conway MA, Allis J, Ouwerkerk R, Niioka T, Rajagopalan B, Radda GK. Detection of low phosphocreatine to ATP ratio in failing hypertrophied human myocardium by ^{31}P magnetic resonance spectroscopy. Lancet 1991;338:973–976.

79. Massie B, Schaefer S, Garrcia J, et al. Myocardial high-energy phosphate and substrate metabolism in swine with moderate left ventricular hypertrophy. Circulation 1995;91:1814–1823.

80. Okada M, Mitsunami K, Yabe T, Morikawa S, Inubushi T. Influence of aging and hypertrophy on the human heart: concentrations of phosphorus metabolites measured by ^{31}P NMR spectroscopy. Circulation 1992;86:I–694.

81. Lamb HJ, Beyerbacht HP, van der Laarse A, et al. Diastolic dysfunction in hypertensive heart disease is associated with altered myocardial metabolism. Circulation 1999;99:2261–2267.

82. Bittl JA, Balschi JA, Ingwall JS. Contractile failure and high-energy phosphate turnover during hypoxia: ^{31}P-NMR surface coil studies in living rat. Circ Res 1987;60:871–878.

83. Fraser CD, Chacko VP, Jacobus WE, Baumgartner WA. Early phosphorus 31 nuclear magnetic bioenergetic changes potentially predict rejection in heterotopic cardiac allografts. J Heart Transplant 1990;9:197–204.

84. Canby RC, Evanochko WT, Barrett LV, et al. Monitoring the bioenergetics of cardiac allograft rejection using in vivo P-31 nuclear magnetic resonance spectroscopy. J Am Coll Cardiol 1997;9:1067–1074.

85. Lukes DJ, Madhu B, Kjellstrom C, et al. Decreasing ratios of phosphocreatine to β-ATP correlates to progressive acute rejection in a concordant mouse heart to rat xenotransplantation model. Scand J Immunol 2001;53:171–175.

86. Bottomley PA, Weiss RG, Hardy CJ, Baumgartner WA. Myocardial high-energy phosphate metabolism and allograft rejection in patients with heart transplants. Radiology 1991;181:67–75.

87. Van Dobbenburgh JO, DeGroot MA, DeJonge J, et al. Myocardial high-energy phosphate metabolism in heart transplant patients is temporarily altered irrespective of rejection. NMR Biomed 1999;12:515–524.

88. Buchthal SD, Noureuil TO, Den Hollander JA, et al. ^{31}P-magnetic resonance spectroscopy studies of cardiac transplant patients at rest. J Cardiovasc Magn Reson 2000;2:51–56.

89. Van Dobbenburgh JO, Lahpor JR, Woolley SR, de Jonge N, Klopping C, Van Echteld CJ. Functional recovery after human heart transplantation is related to the metabolic condition of the hypothermic donor heart. Circulation 1996;94:2831–2836.

90. Caus T, Kober F, Mouly-Bandini A, et al. ^{31}P MRS of heart grafts provides metabolic markers of early dysfunction. Eur J Cardiothorac Surg 2005;28:576–580.

91. Hetherington HP, Luney DJ, Vaughan JT, et al. 3D ^{31}P spectroscopic imaging of the human heart at 4.1 T. Magn Reson Med 1995;33:427–431.

92. Twieg B, Meyerhoff DJ, Hubesch B, et al. Phosphorus-31 magnetic resonance spectroscopy in humans by spectroscopic imaging: localized spectroscopy and metabolite imaging. Magn Reson Med 1989;12:291–305.

93. Hardy CJ, Bottomley PA, Rohling KW, Roemer PB. An NMR phased array for human cardiac ^{31}P spectroscopy.1992;28:54–64.

31 Assessment of Arterial Elasticity by Cardiovascular MRI

Christopher J. Hardy

INTRODUCTION

Although some of the energy of left ventricular contraction produces forward blood flow during systole, the majority is briefly stored as potential energy in the distended arteries. During diastole, this energy is then reconverted into forward flow as the arteries contract *(1,2)*. This serves to ease the load on the left ventricle, promote coronary artery perfusion, and maintain forward flow to the peripheral vessels. In Otto Frank's original "Windkessel" model *(3)*, the arterial system acts as an elastic chamber in which diastolic pressure decays exponentially with a time constant determined by total arterial resistance and capacitance or compliance. Later refinements to this model include the addition of an inductance, or blood inertia, term and the division of the arterial tree into smaller Windkessel elements in analogy to a transmission line *(4,5)*. Systemic arterial compliance is dominated by the aorta, which contributes over 60% of the total value *(6)*.

Reduced compliance of the large central arteries has been found to correlate with age *(7–9)* and with pathological states, such as coronary artery disease *(8–11)*, hypertension *(12–16)*, heart failure *(17,18)*, and connective tissue disorders, including Marfan syndrome *(19–24)*. Decreased compliance has a number of adverse consequences. It results in a loss of buffering in cardiac pressure pulsation, leading to elevated systolic pressure and reduced diastolic pressure. It also increases the pulse wave velocity, which leads to early arrival of reflected pressure waves in end-systole, adding to the peak pressure and reducing forward blood flow. Higher pulse pressure can in turn lead to increased ventricular loading *(25,26)* and hypertrophy and is a major risk factor in

From: *Contemporary Cardiology: Cardiovascular Magnetic Resonance Imaging*
Edited by: Raymond Y. Kwong © Humana Press Inc., Totowa, NJ

coronary artery disease (27). Meanwhile, the decreased diastolic pressure leads to a reduction in coronary perfusion.

Arterial compliance is typically determined either directly by measuring the change in vessel cross-sectional area and blood pressure over the cardiac cycle or indirectly by measurement of the pulse wave velocity along the vessel. The former method has been implemented with use of ultrasound (28) or cine X-ray angiography (29) and the latter with Doppler ultrasound (30), arterial applanation tonometry (31,32), or micromanometers on catheters (33). However, ultrasound methods as applied to the aorta suffer from limited acoustic windows and difficulty in achieving accurate spatial registration between different measurements. Applanation tonometry is not applicable to the central vasculature, projective X-ray techniques do not give accurate vessel cross sections, and catheterization is invasive.

MAGNETIC RESONANCE DETERMINATION OF ARTERIAL ELASTICITY

During each pulse wave in an artery, a hysteresis curve of vessel diameter vs pressure is traced. The arterial compliance can be represented as the slope at each point along this curve and tends to become smaller at higher pressures (34). This nonlinear behavior results from the fact that different components of the vessel wall have different elastic properties, with elastin primarily determining compliance at low pressures and with fully stretched collagen fibers causing higher stiffness at high pressures (35). Reduction in the elasticity of the arterial wall caused by aging or pathology results in a diameter–pressure curve that is shifted downward and has lower slope at any given pressure. In practice, when measuring arterial compliance it is common to simplify matters by considering differences only between end-systolic and end-diastolic pressures and dimensions.

There are a number of related metrics for arterial elasticity. The stiffness index or β-index (28,34) is given as

$$\beta = \frac{\ln(P_s/P_d)}{(d_s - d_d)/d_d},$$ (1)

where P_s and P_d are systolic and diastolic pressures, respectively, and d_s and d_d are the corresponding systolic and diastolic vessel diameters. Regional compliance (8) RC can be expressed as the change in local vessel volume per unit change in pressure:

$$RC = L(A_s - A_d)/(P_s - P_d),$$ (2)

where A_s and A_d are the local systolic and diastolic arterial cross-sectional areas, respectively, and L is the chosen length of vessel (e.g., 1 cm). Perhaps the most direct measure of elasticity is the distensibility (36) D, which is given as the relative change in vessel cross-sectional area over pulse pressure:

$$D = \frac{(A_s - A_d)}{A_d \, (P_s - P_d)}.$$ (3)

Because not only the size but also the shape of the lumen can change over the cardiac cycle, direct area measurements are preferable to calculations from the diameter (37).

These metrics consider the overall local stiffness of the artery as a tube. To relate this to the elastic material properties of the arterial wall, the ratio of wall thickness h to vessel diameter d_d can be incorporated *(36)* to yield the incremental Young's modulus E:

$$E = \frac{1}{D(h/d_d)} = \frac{(P_s - P_d)\, d_d^2}{(d_s - d_d)\, 2h}.$$ (4)

Here, we have assumed that the wall behaves like a thin, homogeneous membrane. The accuracy of any in vivo determination of Young's modulus is typically limited by the precision with which h can be measured.

One drawback to these direct determinations of arterial distensibility is that they require knowledge of the local pulse pressure in the vessel. For the central vasculature, this can only be determined invasively using an intravascular pressure transducer or estimated from remote sphygmomanometer measurements, which tend to significantly overestimate central pressures in adult humans *(38)*.

An alternative, indirect method for calculating arterial distensibility that avoids this problem uses measurement of the pulse wave velocity V_{pw}. For an incompressible fluid in a completely rigid vessel, pressure and flow changes would be instantly transmitted down the vessel, but for an artery with compliant walls, the pressure wave distends the vessel and travels along it at a finite velocity. V_{pw} can be related to distensibility by a variant of the Moens-Korteweg equation *(4)*:

$$D = 1/\left(\rho V_{pw}^2\right),$$ (5)

where the blood density ρ can be taken as constant at 1.057 ± 0.007 g cm^{-3} in normal subjects *(39)* and is expected to show only small variations even among patients.

The pulse wave velocity is typically determined by measuring the time delay Δt of the flow wave between upstream and downstream locations with relative separation Δs that is known. However, the apparent wave velocity is increased by motion of the blood and so must be corrected by subtracting the instantaneous blood velocity V_b at the point on the velocity waveform where the time measurement is made *(4)*:

$$V_{pw} = \frac{\Delta s}{\Delta t} - V_b.$$ (6)

If the foot of the velocity wave is used as the reference point, then the blood velocity correction term can be dropped:

$$V_{pw} = \frac{\Delta s}{\Delta t}.$$ (7)

Use of the foot also has the advantage of avoiding contributions from any reflected waves, which arrive later in the waveform.

A variety of magnetic resonance (MR) methods have been published for determining arterial distensibility, but they all fall into two categories: direct determination via measurement of cross-sectional area changes and indirect determination through measurement of the pulse wave velocity.

MAGNETIC RESONANCE CROSS-SECTIONAL AREA MEASUREMENT

MR measurements of aortic compliance were first performed by Mohiaddin et al. *(8,10)*, who used a spin echo pulse sequence to acquire end-systolic and end-diastolic images perpendicular to the midpoints of the ascending aorta, the aortic arch, and the descending thoracic aorta. They then manually outlined the lumen of the aorta and calculated the change in area between diastole and systole. They found a mean change of 30% for normal subjects under the age of 50 years and determined the reproducibility of the area measurements to be 6%. This method was also used to measure distensibility of the pulmonary arteries in nine normal volunteers *(40)*. Average values, expressed as percentage change in cross-sectional area, were 25.6 ± 10.7 for the main pulmonary artery, 21.4 ± 10.7 for the right pulmonary artery, and 24.5 ± 7.8 for the left pulmonary artery.

Two subsequent studies used cine gradient echo magnetic resonance imaging to perform measurements of aortic area over the cardiac cycle *(37,41)*. One of these *(41)* concluded spin echo imaging provided superior results to gradient echo, especially if optimized spatial saturation pulses and flow compensation were used to improve contrast between lumen and wall. The other *(37)* concluded gradient echo imaging was best, particularly when low tip angles (20–30°) and higher spatial resolution (0.5–1.2 mm) were used and when signal thresholding was employed before outlining cross-sectional areas. This study also noted that cine gradient echo has the advantage of providing high-time-resolution time sequences over the cardiac cycle, allowing one to choose the cardiac phases at which vessel distension is minimized and maximized in each subject.

Two additional studies of aortic compliance have since been carried out, each performing a more systematic analysis of spin echo *(42)* or gradient echo *(43)* techniques. The first of these *(42)* measured short- and long-term reproducibility for the spin echo method in 47 healthy volunteers. Long-term reproducibility in 24 subjects was determined to be $3 \pm 7\%$ (SE). Short-term reproducibility in 15 subjects was $7 \pm 6\%$ and improved to $2 \pm 5\%$ when the scan protocol was modified to incorporate two averages and to improve spatial resolution. Comparison with the gradient echo method revealed a 35% lower value of compliance than the spin echo method, and the authors attributed this to problems distinguishing the blood–wall boundary in their gradient echo technique.

The second study *(43)* performed aortic compliance measurements using a cine gradient echo sequence and an automated snake-based edge detection algorithm to determine cross-sectional areas. Standard gradient echo imaging was compared with a balanced steady-state free precession (SSFP) variant, with a pulse wave velocity technique included as an additional standard for comparison. The study found a relative error in the measurement of compliance of 7% for both standard gradient echo and balanced SSFP methods. The pulse wave velocity results were more consistent with balanced SSFP (Pearson correlation coefficient of 0.94) than with the standard gradient echo (coefficient 0.88). This was attributed to the improved blood–wall contrast of balanced SSFP relative to standard gradient-echo.

Another study used a three-dimensional double-inversion fast spin echo pulse sequence with selective volume excitation to acquire black blood images of the carotid arteries at end-systole and mid- to end-diastole in 10 normal volunteers *(44)*. From these, distensibility was determined as a function of position along the carotid artery. Relative changes in cross-sectional area ranged from 9 to 23% among the 10 subjects,

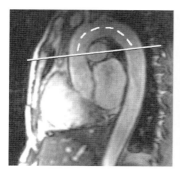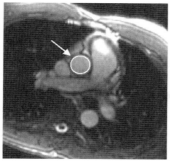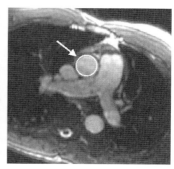

Fig. 1. (A) Oblique sagittal view of aorta of normal volunteer, used to prescribe transverse slice (straight line) for balanced SSFP cine data sets of aorta. Vessel areas are then determined from contours (arrows) traced on end-diastolic **(B)** and end-systolic **(C)** time frames and used, along with pulse-pressure measurements, to determine vessel distensibility.

and increased distensibility was found in the carotid bulb relative to the common carotid. This method has the advantage of showing not only expansion of the lumen area along the vessel, but also changes in the geometry of the vessel wall or deviation of the lumen shape from circular that may occur in diseased vessels.

Figure 1 illustrates the use of one variant of the area method to measure aortic distensibility in a normal volunteer. An oblique sagittal image was first acquired and a plane prescribed (line, Fig. 1A) orthogonal to the aorta, in this case at the level of the bifurcation of the pulmonary artery. Cine imaging was then performed using a balanced SSFP gradient echo pulse sequence, and aortic area was measured at end-diastole (Fig. 1B) and end-systole (Fig. 1C). Local pulse pressure was estimated from peripheral sphygmomanometric measurements, and the distensibility was determined from Eq. 3.

MAGNETIC RESONANCE PULSE WAVE VELOCITY MEASUREMENT

Phase Contrast Methods

Mohiaddin et al. first measured aortic pulse wave velocity in 20 healthy volunteers using a cine gradient echo pulse sequence with and without bipolar gradients to encode through-plane blood velocity *(9)*. Images, including cross sections of the mid-ascending and mid-descending thoracic aorta, were acquired as a function of time after the cardiac *R* wave in a plane orthogonal to the aorta at the level of the bifurcation of the pulmonary artery. The instantaneous flow in liters per second was calculated from the aortic cross-sectional area and the mean blood velocity within that area. V_{pw} was determined from Eq. 7, where the transit time Δt was measured from the foot of the flow wave in the mid-ascending and mid-descending aorta, and the distance between the two points Δs was determined by manually drawing a line along the center of the aorta in an oblique sagittal image.

A variation on this technique used retrospective gating to avoid phase distortions and omitted the non-velocity-encoded reference to reduce imaging time *(45)*. Residual phase variations were removed by subtracting the phase of data acquired at the beginning of the cardiac cycle, where only small blood flow occurs. This method allowed for the acquisition of two or three slices with a time resolution of 3 ms, in a total measurement time of 11 minutes or less. The uncertainty in the determination of pulse wave velocity

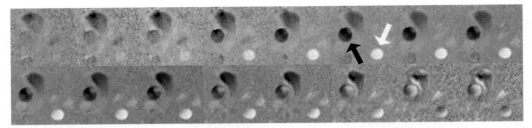

Fig. 2. Selected time frames from cine phase contrast data set showing blood flow in ascending (e.g., black arrow) and descending (e.g., white arrow) aorta. Signal is integrated over vessel lumen for each time frame to determine net flow. Slices are from the same level prescribed in Fig. 1A.

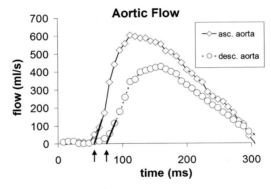

Fig. 3. Plots of blood flow vs time in the ascending (solid line, diamonds) and descending (dashed line, circles) aorta, taken from data set of Fig. 2. Time delay (arrows) is measured from the foot of the flow wave in the two curves and divided by the distance between the vessel sections (curved line in Fig. 1A).

from a two-slice measurement was determined to be around 15% in a flow phantom and somewhat higher in humans.

In a more recent variation, multislice oblique imaging was performed with the aorta in plane and with two-directional velocity encoding applied in plane to yield flow curves over 10 different segments of the aorta *(46)*.

Figure 2 shows a series of time frames from a cine phase contrast data set acquired from a normal volunteer, from the same plane prescribed in Fig. 1A, and with flow encoding applied in the through-plane direction. The ascending aorta can be seen as the region of cranial flow indicated by dark pixels (black arrow) and the descending aorta as the region of caudal flow indicated by bright pixels (white arrow). Integrating signals over the area of the lumen in each time frame yields the flow curves shown in Fig. 3 for ascending and descending aorta. The time delay between the two flow waves, taken at the foot, can be measured and divided by the distance between positions along the mid-line of the aorta (Fig. 1a) to determine pulse wave velocity.

To reduce scan times and increase spatial resolution, an ECG-gated phase contrast pulse sequence was developed *(47)* in which selection of one or more slices was replaced by the excitation of a pencil-shaped region *(48,49)* (Fig. 4) running along the artery. A bipolar velocity-encoding pulse was then played out, followed by a readout gradient, both in the direction of the pencil axis. The sequence was reiterated on the

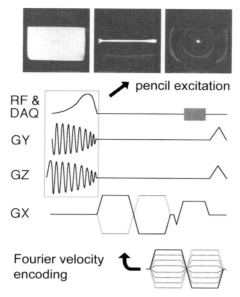

Fig. 4. Phase contrast MR M-mode pulse sequence used to measure aortic pulse wave velocity. Initial 2D-selective pulse excites pencil-shaped region shown at top (left: image of uniform phantom; center: side view of pencil; right: end view of pencil). In Fourier velocity-encoded variant (bottom), the bipolar gradient pulse is stepped through multiple levels instead of only two, and resulting data undergo Fourier transformation in the velocity-encoding dimension.

next electrocardiographic (ECG) trigger, with the polarity of the bipolar pulse inverted, and the signals from the two acquisitions were subtracted.

This sequence was repeated over multiple cardiac phases, with a time resolution of 20–30 ms, to produce a scrolling display of position along the vessel vs time, in which image intensity is proportional to blood velocity. The effective time resolution was improved to 2 ms by staggering the gating delay by 2-ms intervals and interleaving the results, yielding a total scan time of around 32 heartbeats. The pulse wave velocity was then the slope of the leading edge of the velocity trace.

Figure 5 shows the results of this technique in a normal volunteer (top) and in a patient with an aortic aneurysm secondary to Marfan syndrome (bottom). Validation of this method in a flow phantom revealed a reproducibility of less than 0.2% and good agreement with pressure catheter measurements performed in the same phantom *(50)*.

Fourier Velocity-Encoding Methods

Unlike phase contrast methods, Fourier velocity encoding enables measurement of the distribution of velocities within a voxel *(51,52)*, which can improve visualization of the flow wave as it propagates along an artery. A number of pulse sequences have been developed that use this feature, including one that combines Fourier velocity encoding with comb excitation of multiple slices *(53)*. In one example, five slices were simultaneously excited orthogonal to the femoral artery at 4-cm intervals. Fourier velocity encoding was applied in the slice direction. The comb excitation pulse was designed to increment the phase of each slice by a different amount for each bipolar velocity-encoding pulse, resulting in a plot of velocity vs position in which the velocity spectra from the various slices are stacked vertically in the velocity dimension. This sequence was

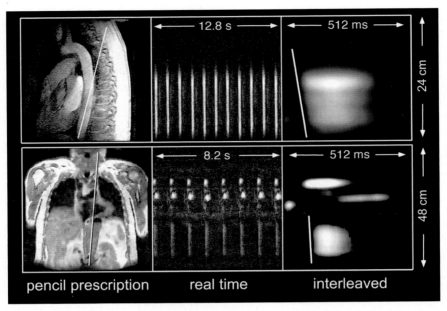

Fig. 5. Phase contrast M-mode data sets from descending aortas of (top) normal volunteer and (bottom) patient with aortic aneurysm secondary to Marfan syndrome. Slope of leading edge of flow gives pulse wave velocity, which is 340 cm/second in normal volunteer (top right) and 1600 cm/second in Marfan patient (bottom right).

repeatedly played out at multiple phases of the cardiac cycle, resulting in a movie of blood velocities in which the velocity wave can be seen to propagate from slice to slice. From this, a distensibility of 1.7×10^{-6} cm s^2/g was calculated for the femoral artery of a 35-years-old normal volunteer.

Another ECG-gated method combined Fourier velocity encoding with pencil excitation to produce movies of blood velocity distributions similar to Doppler M-mode results (54). The pulse sequence was similar to an earlier one (47), except that the bipolar velocity-encoding gradient was stepped to a new value on each ECG trigger, typically through a total of 16 steps (Fig. 4, bottom), and the resulting signals were Fourier transformed to produce a velocity spectrum on the horizontal axis as a function of position along the pencil on the vertical axis (Fig. 6). To improve the time resolution to around 6 ms, the trigger delay was incremented four times, by 6 ms each time, and the frames were interleaved.

The results can be played as a movie loop in which the velocity wave can be seen to propagate across the frame. The location of the foot of the wave in each frame is determined by measuring the intersection point with the horizontal (zero-velocity) axis. A best fit is then calculated of foot position vs time, and the pulse wave velocity is taken from the slope of this line. The total scan time is typically around 64 heartbeats. This method has the added benefit of illuminating details of blood flow, including helical flow patterns distal to the aortic arch, and retrograde flow through damaged cardiac valves.

Single-Heartbeat Methods

In patients who have irregular heartbeats, many of the above ECG-gated techniques can become degraded, with either ghosting or irregular motion in the velocity waveforms.

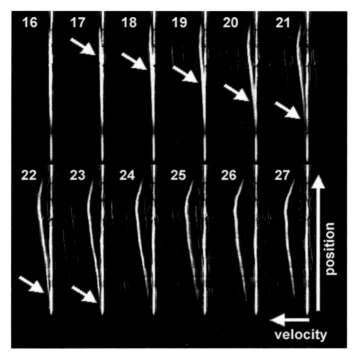

Fig. 6. Frames 16–27 from Fourier velocity-encoded M-mode data set from descending aorta of normal volunteer, showing propagation of foot of flow wave (arrows) down the aorta. Field of view (vertical axis) was 240 cm zoomed to 190 cm; time per frame was 3.6 ms; wave velocity was 550 cm/second.

A number of techniques have been developed that address this problem by generating wave velocity information essentially within a single heartbeat, although they are often used over a period of several heartbeats and the results averaged.

In one study, phase encoding was omitted to produce a real-time projective pulse sequence *(55)*. The slice-selection gradient, which was orthogonal to the vessel of interest, was timed to encode the flow velocity in the slice direction into a phase change. This pulse sequence was rapidly interleaved between an upstream and a downstream slice to produce two images of position vs time in which systolic blood flow appears as bright phase changes in the projection of the vessel. Because the vessel signal is contaminated by contributions from static spins within the same projection, a correction technique was employed to subtract the stationary signal. Pulse wave velocity was calculated from the timing difference in the foot of the velocity wave between the two slices and the distance between them. In 15 volunteers, the value in the abdominal aorta averaged around 3–4 m/second with an uncertainty of 0.6 m/second.

In another projective technique *(56,57)*, contamination from static tissue was substantially reduced in part by the use of an ECG-gated presaturation sequence consisting of repeated sinc-cos RF pulses in the presence of a rotating gradient field. This produced an annular saturation region with an unaffected central region encompassing the aorta. The measurement portion of the pulse sequence was then repeatedly played out. This consisted of simultaneous excitation of an upstream and a downstream slice, both orthogonal to the vessel, followed by readout along the slice-select direction. The resulting signal is a projection in which four discrete peaks can be seen corresponding to the static and moving spins from each of the two slices. The peak separation between each static/moving pair was then used to calculate blood velocity in the corresponding slice at that time point. Because the measurement sequence is repeatedly played out, a curve of blood velocity vs time can be generated for each slice. The wave velocity was then calculated by taking the separation between the midpoints of the rising waveforms and applying Eq. 6. In 10 normal volunteers, the mean wave velocity in the thoracic aorta was 591 cm/second, and the reproducibility was 7.6%. A high degree of correlation was found ($R = 0.95$) between this method and a more conventional phase velocity two-dimensional (2D) mapping technique.

Another single-heartbeat projective technique (58) used dual-band saturation of the regions on either side of the aorta followed by 2D selective excitation of a column centered in the aorta to reduce contamination of the blood signal by surrounding static tissue. Between saturation and excitation, a SPAMM (spatial modulation of magnetization) tagging sequence was applied to sinusoidally modulate the signal along the aorta. After excitation, a train of 128 first-moment-nulled gradient echoes was collected. The result was an image of position along the aorta vs time, in which the propagating flow wave can be seen as periodic bright bands that start horizontal but then in succession tail down as the foot of the velocity wave reaches each band. The wave velocity is then the slope of the line connecting the inflection points of each of the bands. In four normal volunteers under the age of 30 years, the average wave velocity was 4.2 m/second, and the uncertainty was 0.5–0.9 m/second.

A related ECG-gated single-heartbeat method improved the spatial resolution by use of a comb-excitation pulse to tag nine locations along the artery of interest (59,60). A train of 64 gradient echoes, which sample the signal with 2-ms time resolution, followed this. To reduce contamination from static signals in this projective technique, spatial presaturation was applied to the region posterior to the aorta prior to excitation and readout. This resulted in an image of position along the vessel vs time, similar to that of the SPAMM method, only with narrower bright bands. In five normal volunteers aged 22–72 years, the pulse wave velocity ranged from 4.1 to 9.8 m/second and the measurement uncertainty from 0.5 to 1.1 m/second.

Indirect Methods

A number of groups have developed indirect MR methods for determining pulse wave velocity. These typically correlate properties of extended portions of the flow waveform rather than just timing the motion of its foot. For example, one group performed phase contrast velocity imaging of multiple sections of the aorta and then estimated aortic compliance by correlating the second-order spatial and temporal derivatives of blood velocity over most of the cardiac cycle (61,62) according to the equation

$$V_{pw} = \sqrt{\frac{\partial^2 V_b}{\partial t^2} \bigg/ \frac{\partial^2 V_b}{\partial z^2}} \qquad (8)$$

The accuracy of this method was 16% for vessels with compliance exceeding 0.37% per mmHg, with errors reaching as high as 46% in less-flexible arteries (61). Wave velocities between 360 and 473 cm/second were measured in three pigs (62), compared with values of 400–485 cm/second determined by timing the foot of the wave. Micromanometer measurements produced an average value that was 42 ± 35 cm/second

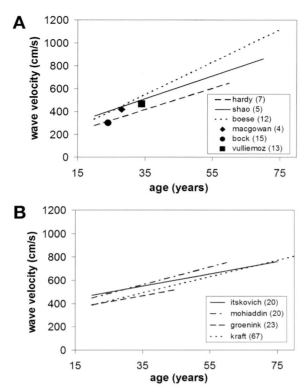

Fig. 7. Plots of pulse wave velocity vs age in normal descending aorta, from MR studies with **(A)** fewer than 20 subjects and **(B)** 20 subjects or more. Study first authors and number of subjects are listed in keys.

higher than the values determined from Eq. 8. Pressure waveforms were also derived from the wave velocity measurements and changes in cross-sectional area and agreed well with the micromanometer waveforms.

Another study used ECG-gated phase contrast imaging of a slice orthogonal to the ascending and descending aorta at a location 5 cm above the aortic valve *(63)*. Aortic cross-sectional areas were determined from the magnitude images, and flow was extracted from the phase images by summing the volume flow of each pixel within the aorta. Pulse wave velocity was then calculated by plotting flow vs area over the cardiac cycle and taking the average slope of the line in early systole. Thus,

$$V_{pw} = \Delta Q / \Delta A, \tag{9}$$

where ΔQ is the change in flow, and ΔA is the change in area. In 13 young healthy volunteers, the average wave velocity in the ascending aorta was determined to be 4.9 ± 1.1 (SD) m/second compared to 4.4 ± 0.9 m/second using a foot-to-foot measurement and 6.7 ± 1.4 m/second using brachial pulse pressure measurement and Eqs. 3 and 5. A paired *t*-test showed no significant difference with the foot-to-foot method and a highly significant difference with the brachial pressure method, with the latter discrepancy assigned to the use of brachial measurements to approximate aortic pressures.

Figure 7 shows aortic pulse wave velocity as a function of age as measured in 10 different MR studies on normal volunteers. The key shows study by first author along with the number of subjects scanned in each case. The average values range from around 3–4 m/second in 20-years-olds to 7–8 m/second in 70-years-olds. The standard deviation in values within each age tertile (young, middle, aged) has been found to average around 20% in apparently healthy subjects (60). Equation 5 can be used to compare the pulse wave velocities in Fig. 7 to aortic distensibility values. Thus, a pulse wave velocity of 4 m/second corresponds to a distensibility of 7.9×10^{-3} mmHg^{-1}, and a value of 8 m/second corresponds to a distensibility of 2.0×10^{-3} mmHg^{-1}.

CLINICAL STUDIES

MR has been used to measure aortic distensibility in a number of different cardiovascular diseases, including hypertension (12–15), coronary artery disease (8,11,64), heart failure (17,18), and Marfan syndrome (20–23,65,66) and related diseases (24). Most of these studies used cine gradient echo imaging (11–15,17–19,21–24,65) to calculate systolic and diastolic cross-sectional areas. In addition, one group used phase contrast magnetic resonance imaging to measure aortic pulse wave velocities (21,23,65) in Marfan patients.

In most MR studies of hypertension, aortic distensibility was significantly decreased (13–15), with, for example, values of 2.5 ± 0.4, 2.2 ± 0.4, $2.3 \pm 0.4 \times 10^{-3}$ mmHg^{-1} vs 7.0 ± 1.6, 5.1 ± 0.3, $7.3 \pm 0.8 \times 10^{-3}$ mmHg^{-1} in control subjects ($p < 0.05$) in ascending, thoracic descending, and abdominal aorta, respectively (14). This same study also found that systolic blood pressure ($R = -0.662$, $p = 0.000007$), left ventricular mass ($R = -0.484$, $p = 0.0067$), and abdominal visceral fat ($R = -0.416$, $p = 0.023$) were inversely related to aortic distensibility, with intracellular free magnesium showing a positive correlation ($R = 0.712$, $p = 0.006$ in brain). In a study of pulmonary hypertension, the fractional change in cross-sectional area of the pulmonary arteries was significantly reduced (16) from 23 to 8% ($p > 0.005$). Although pulse pressure was not measured, it is likely to be higher, if anything, in patients, which would reduce distensibility further relative to normal controls.

In two MR studies of patients with coronary artery disease (8,11), significantly reduced aortic distensibility was found (e.g., 2.9 ± 1.6 and $2.7 \pm 1.1 \times 10^{-3}$ mmHg^{-1} in ascending and descending aortas, respectively, of patients vs 6.5 ± 3.1 and $4.5 \pm 2.5 \times 10^{-3}$ mmHg^{-1}, $p < 0.05$, in controls; 11), although in one of the studies this effect appeared to be most pronounced in patients under the age of 50 years (8). Preliminary findings from a third study of patients with risk factors for coronary atherosclerosis revealed a significant correlation of pulse wave velocity with pulse pressure but not with plaque burden in the aorta (64). Normalized aortic diameter increased with plaque burden, suggesting positive aortic remodeling in this population.

In two other MR studies, aortic distensibility was significantly decreased in patients with diastolic (18) and systolic (17) heart failure and correlated with peak exercise oxygen consumption. For instance, in older subjects (age ≥ 60 years) with systolic heart failure, distensibility of the proximal aorta was $0.5 \pm 0.4 \times 10^{-3}$ mmHg^{-1} vs $2.2 \pm 1.2 \times 10^{-3}$ mmHg^{-1} ($p < 0.002$) in healthy subjects in the same age range (17). Aortic distensibility was also significantly correlated with peak VO$_2$ ($R = 0.80$, $p < 0.0001$), suggesting that increased aortic stiffness may contribute to exercise intolerance in patients with heart failure caused by left ventricular systolic dysfunction and may thus serve as a therapeutic target for this disease.

MR studies of Marfan syndrome generally found significantly decreased aortic distensibility in patients *(19,20,22,65,66)*, even at an early age *(19)*. For example, Groenink et al. found distensibilities of 3.0 ± 2.6, 3.4 ± 1.9, 5.1 ± 2.0, and $3.8 \pm 2.2 \times 10^{-3}$ mmHg^{-1} at four different levels extending from ascending to abdominal aorta vs 4.4 ± 2.2, 4.6 ± 1.5, 5.4 ± 2.3, and $5.2 \pm 3.4 \times 10^{-3}$ mmHg^{-1} at the same levels in normal controls (with p values of 0.03, 0.01, >0.5, and 0.02, respectively) *(65)*. Likewise, pulse wave velocity measurements between neighboring levels in the same study showed significantly increased values of 4.4 ± 1.1, 6.7 ± 2.2, and 5.5 ± 1.5 m/second vs 3.8 ± 0.7, 4.6 ± 0.9, and 4.5 ± 0.9 m/second in controls ($p = 0.01$, < 0.001, 0.003, respectively) in all regions of the aorta. A long-term study of 78 Marfan patients showed that the combined measurement of distensibility and diameter had value in predicting progressive dilatation of the aorta *(23)*. Another study showed that β-blocker therapy increased aortic distensibility in Marfan patients but not in normal controls *(21)*.

CONCLUSIONS

Distensibility of the large central arteries, primarily the aorta, serves to buffer cardiac pressure pulsation and maintain forward blood flow to the peripheral vessels while easing the load on the left ventricle and promoting coronary perfusion. Loss of aortic compliance because of disease results in increased pulse pressure, which can lead to long-term medial damage as well as cardiac pressure overload and hypertrophy. MR provides an accurate noninvasive means of measuring arterial compliance and thus may help assess cardiovascular risk and monitor treatment.

Of the two main MR methods for determining arterial compliance, the cross-sectional area method and the pulse-wave velocity method, the latter has the advantage of not requiring the estimation of local blood pressure. Although a variety of MR methods have been developed for determining pulse wave velocity, the most widely available is the gradient echo-based cine phase contrast pulse sequence, which can be used to measure arterial flow at multiple times and locations. Most clinical MR studies to date have used either this method (sometimes in its balanced SSFP or phase contrast variants) or direct distensibility measurement via the cine gradient echo method to determine cross-sectional area changes over the cardiac cycle. MR provides a robust noninvasive means of determining arterial stiffness, with high potential for further improvements in technology.

REFERENCES

1. Firmin DN, Mohiaddin RH, Underwood SR, Longmore DB. Magnetic resonance imaging: a method for the assessment of changes in vascular structure and function. J Hum Hypertens 1991;5(suppl 1);31–40.
2. Metafratzi ZM, Efremidis SC, Skopelitou AS, De Roos A. The clinical significance of aortic compliance and its assessment with magnetic resonance imaging. J Cardiovasc Magn Reson 2002;4:481–491.
3. Frank, O. Die theorie der pulswellen. Z Biol 1926;85:91–130.
4. Milnor WR. Hemodynamics. 2nd ed. Baltimore, MD: Williams and Wilkins; 1989.
5. Greenwald, SE. Pulse pressure and arterial elasticity. QJM 2002;95:107–112.
6. Stergiopulos N, Segers P, Westerhof N. Use of pulse pressure method for estimating total arterial compliance in vivo. Am J Physiol 1999;276:H424–H428.
7. Learoyd BM, Taylor MG. Alterations with age in the viscoelastic properties of human arterial walls. Circ Res 1966;18:278–292.
8. Mohiaddin RH, Underwood SR, Bogren HG, et al. Regional aortic compliance studied by magnetic resonance imaging: the effects of age, training, and coronary artery disease. Br Heart J 1989;62:90–96.
9. Mohiaddin RH, Firmin DN, Longmore DB. Age-related changes of human aortic flow wave velocity measured noninvasively by magnetic resonance imaging. J Appl Physiol 1993;74:492–497.

10. Bogren HG, Mohiaddin RH, Klipstein RK, et al. The function of the aorta in ischemic heart disease: a magnetic resonance and angiographic study of aortic compliance and blood flow patterns. Am Heart J 1989;118:234–247.

11. Matsumoto Y, Honda T, Hamada M, Matsuoka H, Hiwada K. Evaluation of aortic distensibility in patients with coronary artery disease by use of cine magnetic resonance. Angiology 1996;47:149–155.

12. Di Renzi P, De Santis M, Fedele F, Passariello R. [Evaluation of aortic distensibility using cine-MR before and after antihypertensive treatment with calcium antagonists and ACE-inhibitors]. Cardiologia 1993;38:779–784.

13. Honda T, Yano K, Matsuoka H, Hamada M, Hiwada K. Evaluation of aortic distensibility in patients with essential hypertension by using cine magnetic resonance imaging. Angiology 1994;45:207–212.

14. Resnick LM, Militianu D, Cunnings AJ, et al. Direct magnetic resonance determination of aortic distensibility in essential hypertension: relation to age, abdominal visceral fat, and *in situ* intracellular free magnesium. Hypertension 1997;30:654–659.

15. Toikka JO, Niemi P, Ahotupa M, et al. Decreased large artery distensibility in borderline hypertension is related to increased in vivo low-density lipoprotein oxidation. Scand J Clin Lab Invest 2002;62: 301–306.

16. Bogren HG, Klipstein RH, Mohiaddin RH, et al. Pulmonary artery distensibility and blood flow patterns: a magnetic resonance study of normal subjects and of patients with pulmonary arterial hypertension. Am Heart J 1989;118:990–999.

17. Rerkpattanapipat P, Hundley WG, Link KM, et al. Relation of aortic distensibility determined by magnetic resonance imaging in patients > or = 60 years of age to systolic heart failure and exercise capacity. Am J Cardiol 2002;90:1221–1225.

18. Hundley WG, Kitzman DW, Morgan TM, et al. Cardiac cycle-dependent changes in aortic area and distensibility are reduced in older patients with isolated diastolic heart failure and correlate with exercise intolerance. J Am Coll Cardiol 2001;38:796–802.

19. Savolainen A, Keto P, Hekali P, et al. Aortic distensibility in children with the Marfan syndrome. Am J Cardiol 1992;70:691–693.

20. Adams JN, Brooks M, Redpath TW, et al. Aortic distensibility and stiffness index measured by magnetic resonance imaging in patients with Marfan's syndrome. Br Heart J 1995;73:265–269.

21. Groenink M, de Roos A, Mulder BJ, Spaan JA, van der Wall EE. Changes in aortic distensibility and pulse wave velocity assessed with magnetic resonance imaging following β-blocker therapy in the Marfan syndrome. Am J Cardiol 1998;82:203–208.

22. Fattori R, Bacchi Reggiani L, Pepe G, et al. Magnetic resonance imaging evaluation of aortic elastic properties as early expression of Marfan syndrome. J Cardiovasc Magn Reson 2000;2:251–256.

23. Nollen GJ, Groenink M, Tijssen JG, Van Der Wall EE, Mulder BJ. Aortic stiffness and diameter predict progressive aortic dilatation in patients with Marfan syndrome. Eur Heart J 2004;25:1146–1152.

24. Van Kien PK, Mathieu F, Zhu L, et al. Mapping of familial thoracic aortic aneurysm/dissection with patent ductus arteriosus to 16p12.2-p13.13. Circulation 2005;112:200–206.

25. Wilcken DE, Charlier AA, Hoffman JI, Guz A. Effects of alterations in aortic impedance on the performance of the ventricles. Circ Res 1964;14:283–293.

26. Urschel CW, Covell JW, Sonnenblick EH, Ross J Jr, Braunwald E. Effects of decreased aortic compliance on performance of the left ventricle. Am J Physiol 1968;214:298–304.

27. Franklin SS, Khan SA, Wong ND, Larson MG, Levy D. Is pulse pressure useful in predicting risk for coronary heart Disease? The Framingham Heart Study. Circulation 1999;100:354–360.

28. Dart AM, Lacombe F, Yeoh JK, et al. Aortic distensibility in patients with isolated hypercholesterolaemia, coronary artery disease, or cardiac transplant. Lancet 1991;338:270–273.

29. Merillon JP, Motte G, Fruchaud J, Masquet C, Gourgon R. Evaluation of the elasticity and characteristic impedance of the ascending aorta in man. Cardiovasc Res 1978;12:401–406.

30. Dahan M, Paillole C, Ferreira B, Gourgon R. Doppler echocardiographic study of the consequences of aging and hypertension on the left ventricle and aorta. Eur Heart J 1990;11(suppl G):39–45.

31. Kelly R, Hayward C, Avolio A, O'Rourke M. Noninvasive determination of age-related changes in the human arterial pulse. Circulation 1989;80:1652–1659.

32. Vaitkevicius PV, Fleg JL, Engel JH, et al. Effects of age and aerobic capacity on arterial stiffness in healthy adults. Circulation 1993;88:1456–1462.

33. Ting CT, Chang MS, Wang SP, Chiang BN, Yin FC. Regional pulse wave velocities in hypertensive and normotensive humans. Cardiovasc Res 1990;24:865–872.

34. Kuecherer HF, Just A, Kirchheim H. Evaluation of aortic compliance in humans. Am J Physiol Heart Circ Physiol 2000;278:H1411–H1413.

35. Roach MR, Burton AC. The reason for the shape of the distensibility curves of arteries. Can J Biochem Physiol 1957;35:681–690.
36. Caro CG, Pedley TJ, Schroter RC, Seed WA. The mechanics of the circulation. Oxford, UK: Oxford University Press; 1978.
37. Chien D, Saloner D, Laub G, Anderson CM. High resolution cine MRI of vessel distension. J Comput Assist Tomogr 1994;18:576–580.
38. Karamanoglu M, O'Rourke MF, Avolio AP, Kelly RP. An analysis of the relationship between central aortic and peripheral upper limb pressure waves in man. Eur Heart J 1993;14:160–167.
39. Snyder WS, Cook MJ, Nasset ES, Karhausen LR, Howells GP, Tipton IH. Report of the Task Group on Reference Man. Oxford, UK: Pergamon Press; 1975.
40. Paz R, Mohiaddin RH, Longmore DB. Magnetic resonance assessment of the pulmonary arterial trunk anatomy, flow, pulsatility and distensibility. Eur Heart J 1993;14:1524–1530.
41. Buonocore MH, Bogren H. Optimized pulse sequences for magnetic resonance measurement of aortic cross sectional areas. Magn Reson Imaging 1991;9:435–447.
42. Forbat SM, Mohiaddin RH, Yang GZ, Firmin DN, Underwood SR. Measurement of regional aortic compliance by MR imaging: a study of reproducibility. J Magn Reson Imaging 1995;5:635–639.
43. Krug R, Boese JM, Schad LR. Determination of aortic compliance from magnetic resonance images using an automatic active contour model. Phys Med Biol 2003;48:2391–2404.
44. Crowe LA, Gatehouse P, Yang GZ, et al. Volume-selective 3D turbo spin echo imaging for vascular wall imaging and distensibility measurement. J Magn Reson Imaging 2003;17:572–580.
45. Boese JM, Bock M, Schoenberg SO, Schad LR. Estimation of aortic compliance using magnetic resonance pulse wave velocity measurement. Phys Med Biol 2000;45:1703–1713.
46. Grotenhuis HB, Westenberg JJM, Doornbos J, et al. In-plane pulse wave velocity with MRI in ischemic heart disease: validation of a new technique. Society for Cardiovascular Magnetic Resonance 8th Annual Meeting, San Francisco, January 21–23, 2005. J Cardiovasc Magn Reson 2005;7:120–121.
47. Hardy CJ, Bolster BD, McVeigh ER, Adams WJ, Zerhouni EA. A one-dimensional velocity technique for NMR measurement of aortic distensibility. Magn Reson Med 1994;31:513–520.
48. Pauly J, Nishimura D, Macovski A. A k-space analysis of small tip-angle excitation. J Magn Reson 1989;81:43–56.
49. Hardy C, Cline H. Broadband nuclear magnetic resonance pulses with two-dimensional spatial selectivity. J Appl Phys 1989;66:1513–1516.
50. Bolster BD Jr, Atalar E, Hardy CJ, McVeigh ER. Accuracy of arterial pulse-wave velocity measurement using MR. J Magn Reson Imaging 1998;8:878–888.
51. Redpath TW, Norris DG, Jones RA, Hutchison JM. A new method of NMR flow imaging. Phys Med Biol 1984;29:891–895.
52. Feinberg DA, Crooks LE, Sheldon P, Hoenninger J 3rd, Watts J, Arakawa M. Magnetic resonance imaging the velocity vector components of fluid flow. Magn Reson Med 1985;2:555–566.
53. Dumoulin CL, Doorly DJ, Caro CG. Quantitative measurement of velocity at multiple positions using comb excitation and Fourier velocity encoding. Magn Reson Med 1993;29:44–52.
54. Hardy CJ, Bolster BD Jr, McVeigh ER, Iben IE, Zerhouni, EA. Pencil excitation with interleaved Fourier velocity encoding: NMR measurement of aortic distensibility. Magn Reson Med 1996;35:814–819.
55. Bock M, Schad LR, Muller E, Lorenz WJ. Pulsewave velocity measurement using a new real-time MR-method. Magn Reson Imaging 1995;13:21–29.
56. Itskovich VV, Kraft KA, Fei DY. Rapid aortic wave velocity measurement with MR imaging. Radiology 2001;219:551–557.
57. Kraft KA, Itskovich VV, Fei DY. Rapid measurement of aortic wave velocity: in vivo evaluation. Magn Reson Med 2001;46:95–102.
58. Macgowan CK, Henkelman RM, Wood ML. Pulse-wave velocity measured in one heartbeat using MR tagging. Magn Reson Med 2002;48: 115–121.
59. Shao X, Fei DY, Kraft KA. Rapid measurement of pulse wave velocity via multisite flow displacement. Magn Reson Med 2004;52:1351–1357.
60. Kraft KA, Shao X, Arena R, Fei DY. Proceedings of 13th Meeting of International Society for Magnetic Resonance in Medicine; Miami Beach, FL; 2005; p. 601.
61. Urchuk SN, Plewes DB. A velocity correlation method for measuring vascular compliance using MR imaging. J Magn Reson Imaging 1995;5:628–634.
62. Urchuk SN, Fremes SE, Plewes DB. In vivo validation of MR pulse pressure measurement in an aortic flow model: preliminary results. Magn Reson Med 1997;38:215–223.

63. Vulliemoz S, Stergiopulos N, Meuli R. Estimation of local aortic elastic properties with MRI. Magn Reson Med 2002;47:649–654.

64. Auseon AJ, Tran T, Garcia AM, Hardy CJ, Valavalkar P, Moeschberger M, Raman SV. Aortic pathophysiology by cardiovascular magnetic resonance in patients with clinical suspicion of coronary artery disease. J Cardiovase Magn Reson 2007;9:43–48.

65. Groenink M, de Roos A, Mulder BJ, et al. Biophysical properties of the normal-sized aorta in patients with Marfan syndrome: evaluation with MR flow mapping. Radiology 2001;219:535–540.

66. Oosterhof T, Nollen GJ, van der Wall EE, et al. Comparison of aortic stiffness in patients with juvenile forms of ascending aortic dilatation with vs without Marfan's syndrome. Am J Cardiol 2005; 95:996–998.

32 Interventional Cardiovascular MRI

Robert J. Lederman

INTRODUCTION

Interventional cardiovascular magnetic resonance imaging (iCMR) is potentially revolutionary because of the exquisite tissue and blood imaging afforded to guide therapeutic procedures. By making small compromises in spatial or temporal resolution, and with little or no modifications to commercial high-performance magnetic resonance imaging (MRI) systems, images can be acquired and displayed almost instantaneously to operators. This may be useful simply to avoid ionizing radiation during conventional catheter-based procedures, especially in children. Perhaps more important, iCMR promises to enable more advanced procedures not otherwise possible without open surgical exposure.

APPEAL OF INTERVENTIONAL MAGNETIC RESONANCE IMAGING FOR CARDIOVASCULAR PROCEDURES

X-ray fluoroscopy is widely available and is used to drive a wealth of catheter-based and minimally invasive cardiovascular and noncardiovascular interventions. Other procedures are guided by external or invasive ultrasound (i.e., transesophageal or intravascular), external or invasive electrical (i.e., basket catheters) or electromagnetic position mapping (i.e., NOGA), alone or in tandem with X-ray.

From: *Contemporary Cardiology: Cardiovascular Magnetic Resonance Imaging*
Edited by: Raymond Y. Kwong © Humana Press Inc., Totowa, NJ

To change the primary image guidance modality away from X-ray would require a more favorable risk-benefit profile or would require applications not otherwise possible with X-ray. For certain applications, iCMR is likely to meet these requirements.

iCMR does not expose patients or operators to ionizing radiation. Children with congenital cardiovascular disease suffer excess risk of late malignancy after exposure to ionizing radiation. They also are prone to multiple catheter-based treatments, subjecting them to higher cumulative radiation exposure. Similarly, iCMR does not require radiation protection for operators and staff. Lead aprons worn during X-ray procedures are associated with career-threatening musculoskeletal injuries.

iCMR, by virtue of imaging soft tissue, blood spaces, and catheter devices simultaneously, may enable procedures not readily accomplished under X-ray guidance. In preclinical experiments, iCMR has been shown to guide and track targeted cell delivery into or around myocardial infarctions, to guide atrial septal puncture, and to guide connection of portal and systemic venous circulations. iCMR is under development in preclinical systems to guide cardiac valve replacement, repair, and extra-anatomic bypass, procedures that in the past would have required surgical exposure. In some settings, iCMR may provide safety advantages over conventional image guidance, such as revealing vascular perforation or rupture more rapidly.

TECHNICAL ISSUES

Pulse Sequences

iCMR is possible because of the same technical advances that enable MRI of moving cardiac structures. Newer hardware with homogeneous magnetic fields and with rapidly switching magnetic gradients permit repetition times (TRs) shorter than 3 ms, generating over 300 distinct echoes per second. The most widely used pulse sequences are steady-state free precession (SSFP, also known as balanced fast field echo, true FISP [fast imaging with steady-state precession], and FIESTA) because of the relatively high signal-to-noise ratio (SNR) generated with short TRs. T_1 and T_2 contrast and blood signal can be altered using intermittent magnetization preparation pulses. Gradient echo techniques, used especially to enhance magnetic susceptibility artifacts, can be equally fast but usually have inferior SNR. Although fast spin echo techniques are available, they are limited by higher heat absorption during prolonged imaging sequences.

"Interventional" pulse sequences alter the compromise between temporal and spatial resolution in favor of speed *(1)*. Compared with X-ray imaging, which typically uses 1024×1024 pixel images at 15 frames/second, a typical iCMR image will be 192×128 pixels at 8 frames/second. Because of enhanced tissue imaging, the relative information content in these small-matrix iCMR images is comparable to larger-matrix X-ray images.

Undersampling refers to image creation with less-than-complete data sets. iCMR images can be undersampled further to increase temporal resolution. Multiple methods can be combined, including incomplete phase sampling of frequency space (*k*-space), and sampling of incomplete echoes. Because opposite quadrants of frequency space are symmetric, missing portions can be synthesized using algorithms such as homodyne correction.

Alternative frequency space sampling trajectories also can employ undersampling. For example, frequency space can be sampled radially so that each echo intersects the center frequency *(2)*. Radial trajectories intrinsically oversample the center of frequency space and undersample the outer frequencies. As a result, an image created using radial sampling may have comparable information to an image reconstructed with more echoes using classic rectilinear (or Cartesian) sampling of frequency space. Other groups advocate "spiral" sampling of frequency space to provide the advantages both of rectilinear and radial sampling.

Postprocessing

MRI uses high-sensitivity receivers to detect minute radio-frequency (RF) emissions. As a result, traditional diagnostic MRI uses prolonged acquisitions to generate high-resolution images with adequate SNR. Images are reconstructed by complex computations of frequency data, which for diagnostic studies traditionally have been reconstructed and reviewed off-line. However, iCMR requires on-line reconstruction of images even while additional images are acquired. This requires faster computational hardware and efficient image-processing algorithms. The rapid creation of serial images with short latency is called real-time MRI (rtMRI). Investigational iCMR systems are capable of rtMRI at 8 frames/second with an acquisition-to-display latency of 250 ms or less, compared with less than 100 ms for X-ray fluoroscopy. Fortunately, in practice we find this latency to be nearly imperceptible during catheter manipulation in vivo.

Other image-processing techniques can improve real or perceived temporal resolution of rtMRI. In echo sharing, echoes are recycled over multiple images. For example, using 2:1 echo sharing and rtMRI, a given image updates only half of the frequency space data (using all of the odd lines from the last rectilinear image and using only new data for even lines). Imaging speed is effectively doubled (but not temporal resolution).

Parallel imaging techniques exploit the fact that differently located receiver coils each have different "perspectives." This is analogous to the enhanced imaging afforded by binoculars compared with monocular telescopes. Such techniques, bearing monikers such as simultaneous acquisition of spatial harmonics (SMASH) and sensitivity encoding (SENSE), require multiple hardware receiver channel systems, special receiver coils with reduced crosstalk, and dramatically increased computational horsepower. In practice, they readily increase frame rate two- to threefold or more.

Creative interleaving of radial or rectilinear echoes can permit variable or "sliding" window image reconstructions consisting of few (high temporal resolution) or many (high spatial resolution) echoes using the same data during continuous MRI. The two reconstructions can even be displayed simultaneously.

MRI Features Especially Useful for iCMR

Most commercial MRI systems provide rtMRI functionality using SSFP with interactive graphics slice prescription during continuous scanning. For many labs, investigational implementations copy raw MRI data, after each echo, from the scanner to an external computer system. Bidirectional computer communications can be implemented to permit scan control from the external computer as well as nearly instantaneous image reconstruction.

Our labs have found several additional features to be especially valuable in conducting preclinical and clinical iCMR. Perhaps most important is the ability independently to process signals from individual receiver channels, especially those attached to intravascular devices (*see* next section). Specifically, this permits signals from device channels, such as intravascular guidewires or endocardial injection needles, to be displayed in color (Fig. 1). This simple modification provides high user confidence in rtMRI procedural guidance. It has proven helpful also to be able to alter gain settings for each

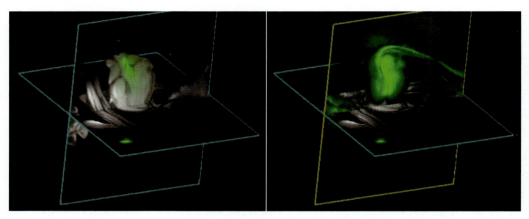

Fig. 1. Demonstration of multislice imaging. Two slices are acquired together and displayed in their true 3D relationship. This also demonstrates the problem of out-of-plane catheters. On the left, the heart is visualized in multiple concurrent imaging planes while a transaortic myocardial injection needle is manipulated. The guiding catheter is colored green. The distal end of the catheter is outside the selected imaging plane and is therefore not visible. On the right, "projection mode" is activated in the coronal view so that the entire length of the guiding catheter can be visualized. This functionality is possible with catheters incorporating active receiver coils. (From ref. *77*.)

channel interactively, much as operators adjust gain on intravascular or transthoracic ultrasound devices.

Other features we have found useful include the ability to toggle the following on and off: electrocardiographic gating to suspend cardiac motion, saturation prepulse to enhance the appearance of gadolinium during intra-arterial injections, inside devices, or hyperenhanced myocardium. Image acceleration, such as with echo sharing, is toggled interactively. Similarly, it has proven useful to apply subtraction masks for interactive digital subtraction MRI. The interaction also can be automated. For example, the group at Case Western Reserve University automatically reduces the field of view or increases temporal resolution during rapid device motion; the pictures may be fast but blurry during coarse device movements but slow and sharp during fine device positioning *(3)*. Similarly, the field of view may be large during rapid movement or small during fine positioning.

Our investigational interventional procedures are guided by multiple slices acquired and displayed in rapid succession. We have found it useful to display a three-dimensional (3D) volume rendering of the slices to convey their relative position. Updates of individual slices can be paused or reactivated to speed the frame rate of other slices. This type of display also can be enhanced by interactive user point marking to identify important anatomical features or targets, the ability to make measurements on-line and the ability to combine with prior road map images to make rapid before-after comparisons (Fig. 1).

iCMR operators have two general imaging approaches. For some applications, rtMRI is directed at target pathology while devices are manipulated in or out of the desired target slice. Alternatively, the rtMRI slice can automatically track catheter movements and alter the slice prescription to always keep the desired catheter device in view while changing the view of the neighboring anatomy. Ideally, both imaging techniques should be available to the operator. We have found a projection mode feature useful during

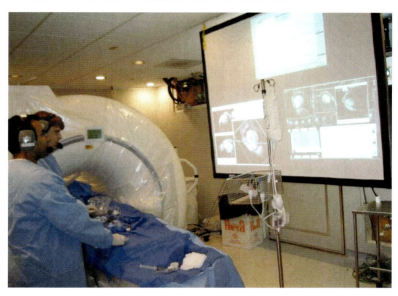

Fig. 2. A view of the iCMR suite during a procedure. The operators wear noise-suppression headsets with fiber-optic microphones and watch images projected from shielded projectors.

catheter manipulations within target slices. When parts of catheter devices move outside these selected slices, they appear "lost." By toggling projection mode (which switches to thick-slice or sliceless imaging), the catheter can be "found" and manipulated back into the target slice. Combining an adaptive projection mode with multislice 3D rendering has been especially useful (Fig. 1).

LOGISTICS AND SAFETY: ASSEMBLING A CLINICAL INTERVENTIONAL MAGNETIC RESONANCE IMAGING SUITE

Constructing a clinical laboratory suitable for iCMR procedures is fairly straightforward but requires a degree of customization *(4)*. Once configured, the laboratory resembles conventional X-ray fluoroscopy suites (Fig. 2).

Transportation, Evacuation, Bailout, and Resuscitation

All major systems manufacturers provide turnkey installation of combined X-ray/MRI (XMR) systems consisting of single- or biplane X-ray fluoroscopy system, clinical 1- to 3-T MRI system, the capacity to transport patients rapidly and safely between the modalities, and X-ray and RF shielded doors that permit the two imaging systems to be used independently when they are not used together. We believe combined XMR installations are both useful and cost-effective in providing adjunctive and bailout treatment environment during the early years of translation of iCMR from animals to human subjects. Moreover, the incremental cost over two separate labs is fairly low, consisting only of the barrier doors and the intermodality patient transport system.

For oe noteworthy logistical point, at present transfemoral access may best be obtained using X-ray guidance for backup. In a combined XMR system, arterial access is obtained under X-ray, and the patient is then transferred rapidly into the MRI system for further procedure conduct.

Communications

rtMRI is loud. Even in newer "acoustically shielded" systems, the acoustic noise is sufficiently loud that unassisted verbal communication is impossible, and protective headsets are necessary to avoid occupational injury. Several imperfect commercial solutions are available using nonmagnetic staff headsets and pneumatic or fiber-optic transmission lines. We use a custom solution combining highly directional fiber-optic microphones and sound-suppressing headsets. The directional microphones permit verbal communications on an open channel.

Unless patients always will be under general anesthesia, there must be a second communications channel, as well as the ability for staff to switch between channels to address each other or the patient. We believe this functionality is essential for safe management of patients undergoing conscious sedation.

Video Display

Excellent video display is readily accomplished. We use three different video displays: one for instantaneous hemodynamics, one mirroring the host computer for scanner control, and one for rtMRI display. Popular display options include in-lab shielded liquid crystal digital (LCD) displays, either floor or ceiling mounted. Some LCD projectors, especially with terminators applied to unused inputs, emit little or no RF noise in the lab. Unmodified or shielded in-lab LCD projectors can be positioned inside the lab or can project from outside the lab through suitably designed waveguides (large conductive cylinders installed across the RF shield that allow nonconductive materials to pass freely) and can project onto inexpensive aluminum-framed projector screens.

Sterility

Sterile procedure during iCMR procedures is similar to other procedures. In our laboratories, before transfer from X-ray to MRI systems, we cover the sterile patient access site (usually groin area) with a large sterile drape, especially to protect that site while surface MRI coils are placed. We enclose surface coils in sterile plastic bags and interventional coil connectors in sterile plastic sheaths marketed to enclose intravascular ultrasound connectors. Finally, we line the MRI bore and controls with adhesive clear plastic drapes.

Safety

iCMR procedures require standard operating procedures that are an extension of those applied for standard noninvasive MRI procedures.

Suites need to be designed to minimize trips by "circulating" staff members across the RF barrier to gather devices. Opening the door, interrupting the RF barrier, usually interferes with the iCMR procedure by introducing excessive noise into images. This requires both circulating staff and disposable devices to be positioned inside the iCMR room.

Contingency plans must exist to avoid introducing ferrous "missiles" into the iCMR suite. As during conventional MRI, the risk seems highest during emergencies. Of particular note are the dangers of cardiac defibrillation inside the high magnetic field. Not only can the defibrillator console become a missile if not adequately secured, but also discharging the defibrillator current can generate sufficient force to knock staff off their feet. As during standard MRI, contingency plans should be in place rapidly to evacuate the patient outside the field during emergencies.

A great deal of biomechanical patient care equipment is commercially available for operation in the MRI suite, including patient monitoring equipment, intravenous solution pumps, and mechanical ventilators. Such equipment still should be tested and marked as safe for operation inside the high magnetic field. All other ferrous materials that are deemed essential must be tethered outside the high field line if they must remain inside the scanning room.

As for conventional MRI, interventional staff must be specifically trained, and new MRI interventions must be rehearsed. Some iCMR teams require staff to wear special pocketless clothing to prevent them from introducing ferrous missiles into the scanner (5).

A surprisingly large number of lines are connected to the patient, and their management should be planned in advance. They are enumerated here for effect: (1) oxygen and other gases; (2) mechanical ventilation; (3) oximetric detector; (4) microphone; (5) headset; (6) multiple intravenous lines; (7) intra-arterial pressure transducer connectors; (8) interventional fluid manifold, including contrast, flush, and waste lines; (9) urinary catheters; (10) electrocardiography leads for MRI and for bailout X-ray; (11) surface MRI coil connectors; (12) intravascular MRI coil connectors. These should be arranged so that no inadvertent loops are formed of conductive materials, and so that conductive materials are kept away from the wall of the MRI bore, both of which can contribute to heating. The lines also should be organized so that the patient can be evacuated rapidly without disrupting and disconnecting them.

Do We Need a Shorter-Bore MRI System to Conduct iCMR Procedures?

In short, no, a shorter-bore MRI system for iCMR procedures is not needed. For transfemoral arterial access, the length of conventional 1.5-T MRI bores (150 cm) does not significantly interfere with catheter manipulations in adults. Femoral artery puncture and transjugular access are indeed inconvenient inside the MRI bore and may best be conducted under conventional X-ray guidance. Shorter-bore (120-cm) 1.5-T MRI systems are now commercially available and may reduce these obstacles. Shorter-bore MRI systems also may reduce patient anxiety and claustrophobia and may facilitate intraprocedural nursing care and observation. However, shorter bore MRI systems may require some MRI performance compromises; these questions have not yet been answered.

CATHETER DEVICES

X-ray fluoroscopic interventional devices are conspicuous because they attenuate X-ray photons. Most off-the-shelf devices are intrinsically conspicuous under X-ray; others incorporate heavy metals like barium or platinum. Catheter devices usually incorporate ferrous materials (such as wire braiding) to make them rigid and torque resistant. By contrast, under standard (hydrogen proton) MRI, structures are conspicuous because they contain excited proton spins. Off-the-shelf catheter devices, designed for X-ray, usually distort the MR image because the ferrous materials destroy the local magnetic field.

Devices rendered "MR compatible" by having ferrous materials removed are also rendered invisible because they still do not contain water protons. Attempts to coat or fill catheter devices with gadolinium-type contrast agents have for the most part been unsuccessful because not enough excited proton spins are able to interact with the gadolinium-type "relaxation" agent. Moreover, MR-compatible guidewire materials such as nitinol are electrically conductive; when long enough to be clinically useful, they are vulnerable to rapid heating from the MRI radio energy excitation, much as they would be inside a microwave oven. Table 1 and Fig. 3 provide an overview of general approaches to making catheter devices visible under MRI.

"Passive" catheter devices are the simplest and are visualized based on their intrinsic material properties. Most passive devices are visible because they do not contain water protons and therefore appear black using most MRI pulse sequences. Tracking dark devices can be challenging using MRI because the darkness can be difficult to spot when it is diluted (or volume averaged) in a larger imaging slice. The dark spots can be enhanced by adding small amounts of metal to create "blooming" or magnetic susceptibility artifacts (Fig. 3a). These artifacts can make the passive device appear larger than the actual size and can even obscure surrounding tissue detail. Guidewires and catheters (6–8) have been made out of nonmetallic polymers (Fig. 3b), and even clinical procedures have been conducted using passive CO_2-filled balloon catheters (5,9,10).

We prefer to use MRI catheter devices that are modified to incorporate MRI receiver coils or antennae. These so-called active catheter devices become highly visible when they are attached to the MRI scanner hardware because they accentuate nearby excited water protons. Early designs were intended for high-resolution tissue imaging or spectroscopy (11–17) of nearby tissue. In their simplest designs, the entire length or "profile" of active catheters is made conspicuous (18–23). In addition, these profile design active catheters can help visualize the devices even if they move outside the selected scanning plane (Fig. 1). Profile design active catheters generally are imaged along with target tissue and require no modification of imaging pulse sequences. Active catheter coils can be attached to separate receiver channels in the MRI system, analogous to separate audio channels in stereo audio systems, and images deriving from catheters can be assigned colors that help to distinguish them from surrounding structures in 2D or 3D space (Fig. 3c). When active guidewires are combined with passive catheters or balloons filled with dilute gadolinium MRI contrast, the pair become readily visible.

Another type of active catheter design, embedding tracking microcoils, is used to track individual points on the catheter during MRI (16,24–26). Tracking microcoil catheters require a slight modification of the MRI pulse sequences, a small number of intermittent nonselective excitations to localize the microcoils in space and calculate their position on the image. The microcoil location usually is depicted as a crosshair overlaid on the image (Figs. 3d,e and 4). These tracking microcoil systems are simple and effective but unfortunately cannot depict the full length of catheter devices unless the catheter contains dozens of them.

Active catheter designs require conductive connections to the MRI scanner. These tend to heat if longer than 50–80 cm. Several teams have developed circuitry for detuning or decoupling these transmission lines (27–31) or have developed alternative transmission lines such as fiber optics (32–35). One profile design, loopless active decoupled and detuned guidewire, the Surgi-Vision 0.030 in. × 100 cm guidewire, has U.S. Food and Drug Administration marketing approval for invasive intravascular MRI in humans (4,36,37). The limitation of this device is that the receiver sensitivity falls to zero at the distal tip, so the distal tip becomes difficult to visualize. The Surgi-Vision device is therefore imperfect for navigating tortuous or stenotic vasculature under rtMRI. Improved designs have not yet been commercialized (23).

Table 1
General Approaches to Make Catheter Devices Conspicuous Under MRI

Approach	Advantages	Disadvantages	Solutions	Examples
Passive devices: Catheter materials directly influence MR image	Simple and inexpensive View device by imaging device in tissue context Reduced technical and regulatory requirements	Visibility is reduced Susceptibility markers (steel, dysprosium) destroy nearby signal	Conductive lines, if present, can heat	Can work in combination with active devices (e.g., passive balloon over active guidewire) Gd-filled balloon (*42–46*) CO_2-filled balloon (*5,9,10*) Gd-filled catheter (*47,48*) Nitinol stent (*46,49–53*)
Active "profile" devices: Catheter incorporates an MRI receiver coil ("antenna") along much of its length and is imaged along with target tissue	View device by imaging device in tissue context Can use special MRI features: color highlighting, projection mode, plane tracking	Potential heating Less visible at tip than at shaft ("loopless" designs) "Profile" of devices is blurry compared with sharp profile of devices under X-ray or sharp "points" using active tracking devices	Detuning and decoupling can prevent heating Coils can enhance tip visibility	Surgi-Vision Intercept 0.030-in. guidewire coil (*4,36,37*)
Active tracking coil devices: Catheter incorporates small MRI receiver coils that can be tracked with simple pulse sequences alternating with MRI pulse sequences	Points on device can be visualized rapidly and accurately Points can be tracked without imaging to increase speed or reduce absorbed RF	Useful in automatic scan control (plane tracking, etc.)	"Synthesized" points might deviate from "true" location on image Number of points is usually limited Requires "special" MRI pulse sequences, a minor modification Can be combined with other approaches	Massachusetts General Hospital/General Electric electrophysiology mapping system (*54*)

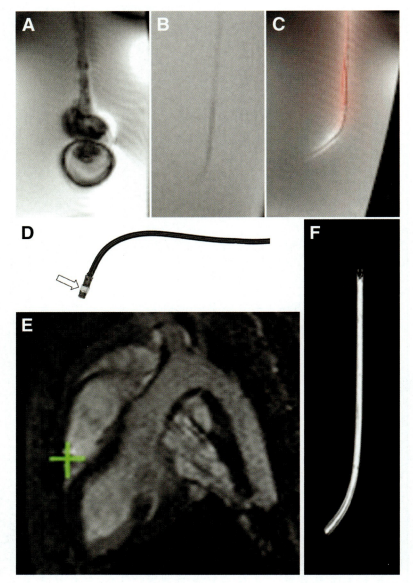

Fig. 3. A comparison of representative catheter designs for iCMR. **(A)** A traditional X-ray catheter, which incorporates stainless steel braid for strength. The steel distorts the MR image and has the potential to heat, as it would in a microwave oven. **(B)** The same passive catheter without steel braids, rendering it nearly invisible even in vitro. **(C)** The same catheter shape in an active profile design, incorporating an MRI receiver coil to make it visible. **(D)** A tracking microcoil design catheter incorporating a microcoil near the tip. The 3D position of the microcoil can be tracked rapidly and indicated using computer-synthesized crosshairs (green) as it is moved into the right ventricle of the animal shown in **(E)** (Courtesy of Michael Bock, DKFZ, Heidelberg.) The rest of the catheter is not visible under MRI. **(F)** A catheter incorporating a "wireless" inductively coupled receiver coil (courtesy of Harald H. Quick, University Essen, Germany) that can be visualized as a bright signal using MRI. (From ref. *91*.)

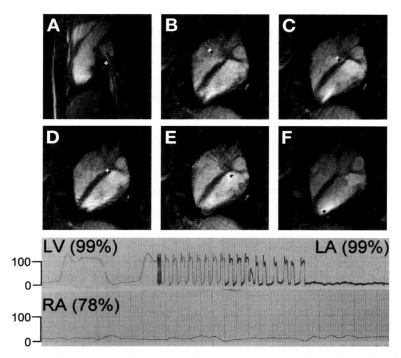

Fig. 4. Diagnostic cardiovascular catheterization in swine using a tracking microcoil active catheter. The + marker overlaid on the image indicates the tip of the catheter as it advances from the inferior vena cava (**A**) into the right atrium (**B**), (**C**) and across septal defect (**D**) into the left atrium (**E**) and left ventricle (**F**). Hemodynamic tracings and oxyhemoglobin saturation are displayed on the lower panels during pullback. (From ref. *69* with permission.)

Two teams have reported "wireless" active catheters or stents *(38–41)*, which are inductively coupled with the MRI system (Fig. 3f) Theoretically, these can be exploited to enhance later noninvasive imaging, for example, of restenosis or of captured thromboemboli.

Of note, several of these approaches to enhance device visibility can be combined. For example, an interventional MRI system could include an active-profiling guidewire that incorporates tracking microcoils near the tip to enhance distal visibility and a passive balloon incorporating passive platinum marker bands when deflated and filled with dilute gadolinium when inflated used together to deliver an inductively coupled stent-graft device. Such devices are available today.

The main barrier to further clinical translation of iCMR is the limited availability of clinical-grade active devices. Nevertheless, a wide range of prototype applications have been demonstrated in animals.

APPLICATIONS

Applications Suited to iCMR

Certain applications lend themselves to iCMR development. Target anatomical structures that are relatively immobile or slowly moving (such as peripheral arteries) are attractive because MR images can be updated slowly and therefore can have higher SNR or spatial resolution. Large or thick-walled structures (such as aorta) are attractive because they contain many proton spins and can be imaged with high SNR, and contrast mechanisms might be available readily to distinguish them from neighboring structures. Structures that can be contained within a single imaging plane (such as straight segments of iliac arteries) can be imaged rapidly, compared with tortuous structures such as coronary arteries, which are difficult to image in real time.

The ventricular myocardium is an attractive target despite its high degree of cardiac and respiratory motion because it is a large, thick-walled structure that is readily depicted (using SSFP MRI) in high contrast compared with the blood space. Conversely, thin-walled structures, such as myocardial atria, are difficult to visualize even using segmented (non-real-time) MRI.

Applications Unsuited to iCMR: Coronary Artery Disease

The SNR of proton MRI is too low to provide temporal resolution (33–66 ms) at anywhere near the spatial resolution (200 μm) currently enjoyed by X-ray fluoroscopy operators conducting complex coronary interventions in heavily diseased, even occluded, coronary arteries using 0.014-in. (0.35-mm) guidewires. Barring unforeseen technical breakthroughs, meaningful coronary artery interventions are not likely to be conducted using MRI.

That said, Spuentrup et al. *(55)* demonstrated navigation and delivery of passively visualized stainless steel stents in the coronary arteries of healthy swine. The devices and target proximal coronary arteries were readily visible using SSFP at 1.5 T despite cardiac motion and the small size of these structures.

Peripheral Vascular Disease

The most straightforward iCMR applications, transluminal angioplasty *(43,44,56–58)* and stent deployment *(46,49,50,53,59,60)*, have been conducted in numerous animal models. Similarly, investigators have reported placement of vena cava filters *(61–63)* and even transcatheter visceral embolization of, for example, renal parenchyma *(64,65)*. These are important proofs of concept toward clinical development. Indeed, a few human examples of peripheral artery angioplasty and stenting have been reported. For the most part, these represent straightforward axial displacement of devices requiring little interactive image guidance.

iCMR also offers the convenience of using a single imaging modality to determine reference vessel size. X-ray guided angioplasty requires adjunctive intravascular ultrasound to determine arterial wall characteristics (including media-to-media diameter). However, even in simple angioplasty and stenting, iCMR offers a potential safety advantage over conventional X-ray. Raval et al. *(46)* conducted iCMR-guided stenting of aortic coarctation in a pig model. Continuous imaging of both target pathology and devices immediately revealed catastrophic aortic rupture when deliberately oversize devices were employed. Early recognition offers the only opportunity to treat this life-threatening complication effectively.

Perhaps more compelling are applications that exploit the ability of MRI to visualize vascular spaces not conspicuous using MRI. In a pig model of chronic total occlusion of peripheral arteries, Raval et al. *(66)*, used iCMR to navigate a recanalizing guidewire. These trajectories cannot be determined using X-ray because the occluded lumen cannot fill with contrast. iCMR permitted the operators to traverse complex occlusions while remaining within the walls of the target operator. This can be especially important in recanalization of tortuous peripheral artery occlusions, such as those found in the pelvis.

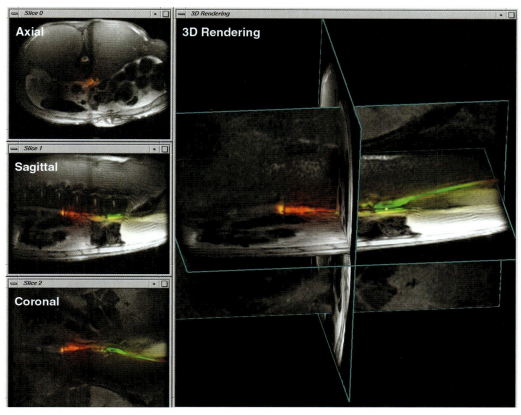

Fig. 5. Multislice 3D display of active aortic endograft positioned using iCMR in a pig model of abdominal aortic aneurysm. (Courtesy of Venkatesh K. Raman.)

Aortic aneurysm disease often entails complex tortuous 3D structures that are difficult to visualize using projection X-ray. iCMR might provide a single-modality solution to procedure planning, device deployment, and anatomical and hemodynamic assessment of catheter-based (endograft) treatment of aortic aneurysm. In a simple pig model, Raman et al. *(67)* demonstrated all of these steps using custom active stent graft devices. Endograft treatment under MRI restored a normal lumen contour and restored laminar flow. Moreover, MRI demonstrated device apposition to the target aortic wall and allowed interrogation for endoleak (Fig. 5 and 6). The team at University Hospital Essen in Germany has elegantly applied iCMR to guide the placement of stent grafts in an animal model of thoracic aortic dissection *(68)*. They used unmodified, passive stent graft devices. MRI clearly revealed the true and false lumena of the dissected aorta, guided stent-graft deployment, and demonstrated stent-graft obliteration of the false lumen. This was another excellent example of the intrinsic value of simultaneous tissue and device imaging using real-time MRI (Fig. 7).

Cardiac Procedures

The University of California, San Francisco (UCSF) group *(69)* has reported a comprehensive diagnostic cardiac catheterization procedure in a porcine model of atrial septal defect using iCMR. They used catheters containing tracking microcoils embedded near

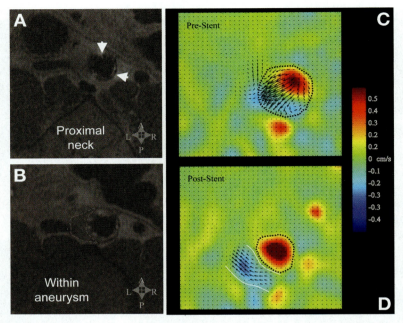

Fig. 6. MRI showing apposition **(A)** of aortic endograft and **(B)** aneurysm exclusion in pig model of abdominal aortic aneurysm. Before endograft deployment, vector flow map **(C)** shows turbulent in-plane flow; endograft deployment restores laminar flow **(D)** through aorta. (From ref. *67*.)

the tip. They were easily able to accomplish left and right heart catheterization, including continuous intracavitary pressure monitoring and blood sampling (Fig. 4). They also incorporated phase contrast MRI into their procedures for the determination of shunt ratios. Other groups have reported rtMRI catheter manipulation using selective arteriography using, for example, tracking microcoil-based catheters for selective carotid artery catheterization *(70)*, passive catheters over active guidewires for selective coronary arteriography *(71)*, or active catheters for selective visceral artery catheterization *(72)* in swine.

Several groups have deployed passively visualized nitinol occluder devices to treat porcine models of atrial septal defect *(73)* and thereafter to assess hemodynamics using phase contrast MRI *(74,75)*.

Kuehne et al. *(76)* reported preliminary experience deploying a passively visualized nitinol-based aortic valve prosthesis from a transfemoral approach in healthy swine. Theirs is a good demonstration of the value of combined tissue and device imaging for the precise placement of critical prosthetic devices (Fig. 8).

Our lab *(77,78)* and others *(79–82)* have used iCMR to deliver cells and other materials into specified targets in normal and infarcted animal hearts. We have found it particularly useful to interleave multiple slices during iCMR and to render them in 3D to represent their true geometric relationship. This technology provides "exposure" of the inside of the beating heart even better than does open-chest surgery (Fig. 9). Targeting can be based on wall motion, delayed hyperenhancement (infarction), perfusion defects, strain maps, or any other contrast mechanism selected. When the injectate includes a contrast agent, real-time MRI can interactively depict the intramyocardial dispersion of the injected materials. This can be valuable for confirming successful delivery, for ensuring confluence of treated volumes, and for avoiding inadvertently overlapping injections.

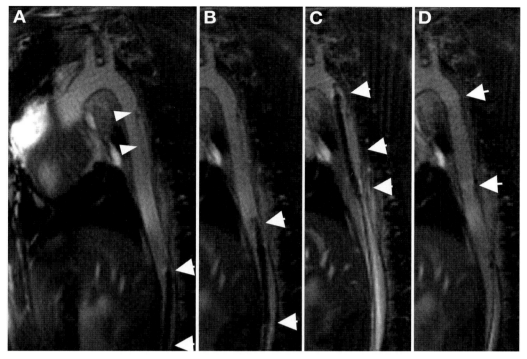

Fig. 7. Endograft treatment of thoracic aortic dissection in a pig model using a commercially available passive device. **(A)** Baseline aortic dissection. The dissection is depicted with arrowheads. **(B)** The endograft is advanced retrograde from the iliac artery. The tip of the endograft (arrows) approaches the inferior aspect of the dissection, inside the true lumen. **(C)** The endograft is in final position before deployment. **(D)** Most of the false lumen is obliterated after endograft delivery. (Courtesy of Holger Eggebrecht, MD, and Harald H. Quick, PhD, University Hospital Essen, Germany.)

Image-Guided Cardiac Electrophysiology

A range of therapeutic cardiac electrophysiology procedures are conducted using catheter techniques without compelling image guidance. Rough endocardial surface maps are generated using electromagnetic mapping techniques, but these provide only road maps that do not account for respiratory and other dynamic changes in cardiac wall location. Most catheter-based ablation procedures are ultimately guided by multi-channel intracardiac electrograms. Alternatively, image-guided myocardial ablation is currently conducted under direct surgical exposure *(83)*. iCMR might provide similar "exposure" for image-guided transcatheter ablation of cardiac arrhythmia. MRI may be particularly useful for visualizing lines of continuity (corresponding to functional electrophysiological block) after delivery of ablative energy.

The group at Johns Hopkins University (Baltimore, MD) has reported preliminary catheter tracking experiments using active catheters that acquire filtered local intracardiac electrograms *(84)*. They also have characterized ablated myocardium over time *(85)* (Fig. 10). The team at Massachusetts General Hospital (Boston, MA), in collaboration with General Electric, presented animal experiments positioning electrophysiology catheters in an MRI system and overlaying these positions onto high-resolution cardiac images *(54)* (Fig. 11).

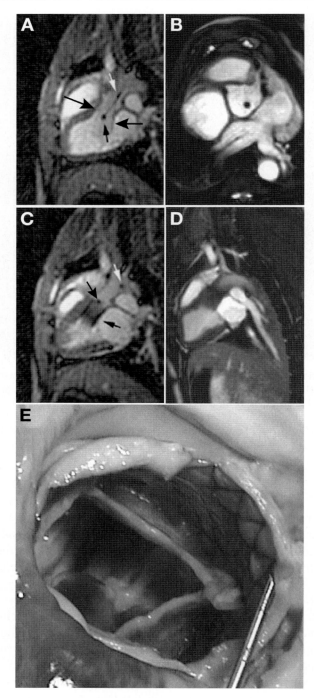

Fig. 8. iCMR deployment of a passive self-expanding valve-stent in the aortic valve position of a healthy pig. **(A)** Long-axis view of the stent-valve during deployment. Proximal (small white arrow) and distal (small black arrow) indicate the passive markers of the stent delivery system before deployment. **(B)** A short-axis view at the level of the coronary ostia. The proximal marker of the delivery system appears in the center of the aortic root. **(C)** The system immediately after deployment. The valve abuts the anterior mitral valve leaflet, and the delivery system is withdrawn into the

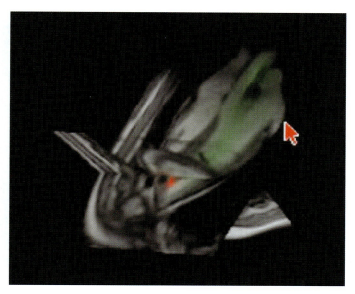

Fig. 9. Multislice view of targeted myocardial injection of iron-labeled mesenchymal stromal cells into a small myocardial infarction. This is a rotated view showing both long and short axis of the myocardium. The injection-guiding catheter is colored green, and the needle tip is colored red. The injected cells appear as a black spot beyond the tip of the needle.

Transseptal and Extra-anatomic Communications

iCMR may even enable interventions outside normal lumen spaces. Arepally et al. *(86)* conducted image-guided puncture of the cardiac interatrial septum, a procedure currently conducted primarily using tactile feedback under X-ray. Our lab conducted similar septal puncture followed by balloon septostomy and MRI assessment of the resulting small intracardiac shunts *(87)*. Although similar guidance is afforded by intracardiac or transesophageal ultrasound, these are important preclinical steps toward more elaborate procedures guided by MRI.

Using a unique double-doughnut MRI configuration containing an integrated flat-panel X-ray fluoroscopy system, Kee et al. have conducted preclinical *(51)* and clinical *(88)* transjugular intrahepatic portosystemic shunt procedures. Even in this proof-of-concept experiment, MRI reduced the number of transhepatic needle punctures compared with historical controls. Arepally et al. conducted even more adventurous preclinical experiments in creating a catheter-based mesocaval shunt outside the liver capsule *(89)*.

This sort of extra-anatomic bypass, once made available to nonsurgeons, has the potential to revolutionize mechanical revascularization.

Early Human iCMR procedures

Several groups have begun investigational human iCMR procedures. Razavi et al. *(5)* at Kings College in London have conducted diagnostic cardiac catheterization in children

Fig. 8. *(Continued)* aortic root, as indicated by the passive markers. **(D)** The final position of a stent-valve in the aortic position and **(E)** the valve *in situ* during necropsy, viewed from the incised aortic root. (Courtesy of Titus Kuehne, German Heart Institute, Berlin.)

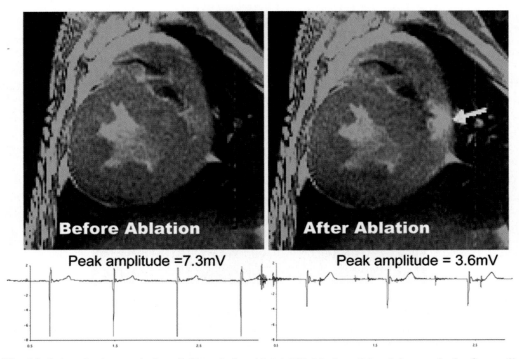

Fig. 10. Spin echo images before (left) and after (right) RF ablation of the right ventricular free wall (arrow). Lower panels are corresponding intracardiac electrograms showing reduced voltage after ablation. (Courtesy of Henry R. Halperin, MD, Johns Hopkins University.)

using a combined XMR environment. The same group is conducting X-ray fused with MRI (XFM) procedures, in which prior MRI data sets are combined with real-time X-ray fluoroscopy (XRF) to conduct therapeutic procedures. Kuehne et al. also have conducted diagnostic cardiac catheterization procedures using passive catheter devices under rtMRI *(10).*

Three groups have reported invasive imaging of peripheral artery atheromata using profile design active guidewire receiver coils *(4,36,37).* In the report by Dick et al. *(4),* we concluded this guidewire design adds little to surface coils for diagnostic MRI of atherosclerosis but might have value in delivering interventional devices using iCMR. A team in Regensburg, Germany, has conducted high-quality selective intra-arterial MR angiography *(90)* and has reported preliminary revascularization procedures using passive devices in the iliac *(52)* and femoral *(45)* arteries. The team at Stanford has conducted iCMR-assisted transjugular intrahepatic portosystemic shunt procedures in patients *(88)* in a novel hybrid double-doughnut X-ray/MRI system. Numerous additional investigational human iCMR procedures are now under way at several medical centers around the world.

CONCLUSION: WILL iCMR EVER BE WIDELY ADOPTED?

Advocates promote the development of iCMR for the sake of reduction of radiation exposure to patients, especially young patients who are anticipated to require a large cumulative radiation exposure during diagnostic and therapeutic procedures; reduction

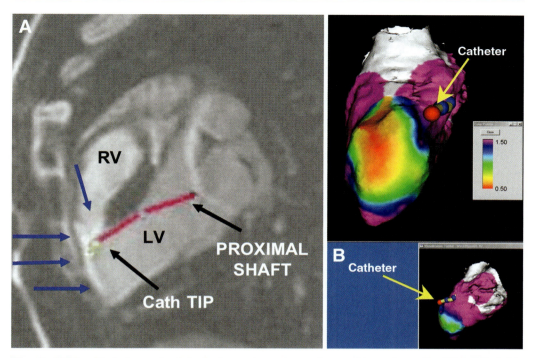

Fig. 11. MRI-guided electrophysiological mapping using active-tracking microcoils. **(A)** MRI of this porcine model of healed myocardial infarction reveals the hyperenhanced anterior wall scar (blue arrows), to which an MRI-compatible mapping catheter was manipulated in a real-time fashion. **(B)** A left ventricular substrate map is generated by displaying sinus rhythm electrogram amplitude values onto a 3D rendering of the chamber. (Courtesy of Vivek Y. Reddy, MD, Massachusetts General Hospital.)

of radiation exposure to operators and staff, who endure a large cumulative radiation exposure during their careers; reduction of patient exposure to toxic radiocontrast, which is important in a minority of patients with moderate-severe renal disease; and to eliminate the requirement that staff wear heavy protective lead garments, which are associated with a high incidence of chronic musculoskeletal injury. Detractors argue that iCMR represents a costly and cumbersome alternative to procedures that otherwise are conducted rapidly and efficiently under X-ray guidance and occasionally enhanced with adjunctive ultrasound. Detractors also argue that, despite any potential benefit, the large capital outlays and expected higher marginal cost of disposable (catheter) equipment are simply unjustifiable. These arguments are less tenable. Existing XMR facilities are constructed that permit each imaging system to be used independently of the other. The only incremental expense over separate angiography and MRI systems is the cost of the intermodality transfer table and the barrier doors connecting the systems.

As described, the chief obstacle to further development of iCMR is the limited availability of clinical-grade catheter devices suitable for MRI. This in turn discourages wider deployment of XMR or iCMR systems. That said, clinical iCMR appears feasible using available technology, and further investigational procedures are under way worldwide. Competing technology is under development to guide minimally invasive procedures using real-time or road map (retrospective) images from multiple imaging modalities, including X-ray, computed tomography, 3D ultrasound, electromagnetic position mapping, and MRI.

However, iCMR may prove superior because use of a single modality, 3D anatomy, composition, function, and hemodynamics can be combined. iCMR can provide surgical-grade exposure to guide nonsurgical minimally invasive procedures. This has the potential to revolutionize the conduct of minimally invasive image-guided treatments.

ACKNOWLEDGMENTS

This work was supported by NIH Z01-HL005062-03 CVB. Thanks to Venkatesh K. Raman for his thoughtful comments.

REFERENCES

1. Duerk JL, Butts K, Hwang KP, Lewin JS. Pulse sequences for interventional magnetic resonance imaging. Top Magn Reson Imaging 2000;11:147–162.
2. Peters DC, Korosec FR, Grist TM, Block WF, Holden JE, Vigen KK, Mistretta CA. Undersampled projection reconstruction applied to MR angiography. Magnetic Resonance in Medicine 2000;43:91–101.
3. Elgort DR, Wong EY, Hillenbrand CM, Wacker FK, Lewin JS, Duerk JL. Real-time catheter tracking and adaptive imaging. J Magn Reson Imaging 2003;18:621–626.
4. Dick AJ, Raman VK, Raval AN, et al. Invasive human magnetic resonance imaging during angioplasty: feasibility in a combined XMR suite. Catheter Cardiovasc Interv 2005;64:265–274.
5. Razavi R, Hill DL, Keevil SF, Miquel ME, et al. Cardiac catheterisation guided by MRI in children and adults with congenital heart disease. Lancet 2003;362:1877–1882.
6. Bakker CJ, Hoogeveen RM, Weber J, van Vaals JJ, Viergever MA, Mali WP. Visualization of dedicated catheters using fast scanning techniques with potential for MR-guided vascular interventions. Magn Reson Med 1996;36:816–820.
7. Bakker CJ, Bos C, Weinmann HJ. Passive tracking of catheters and guidewires by contrast-enhanced MR fluoroscopy. Magn Reson Med 2001;45:17–23.
8. Buecker A, Spuentrup E, Schmitz-Rode T, et al. Use of a nonmetallic guide wire for magnetic resonance-guided coronary artery catheterization. Invest Radiol 2004;39:656–660.
9. Miquel ME, Hegde S, Muthurangu V, Corcoran BJ, Keevil SF, Hill DL, Razavi RS. Visualization and tracking of an inflatable balloon catheter using SSFP in a flow phantom and in the heart and great vessels of patients. Magn Reson Med 2004;51:988–995.
10. Kuehne T, Yilmaz S, Schulze-Neick I, et al. Magnetic resonance imaging guided catheterisation for assessment of pulmonary vascular resistance: in vivo validation and clinical application in patients with pulmonary hypertension. Heart 2005;91:1064–1069.
11. Kantor HL, Briggs RW, Balaban RS. In vivo ^{31}P nuclear magnetic resonance measurements in canine heart using a catheter-coil. Circ Res 1984;55:261–266.
12. Martin AJ, Plewes DB, Henkelman RM. MR imaging of blood vessels with an intravascular coil. J Magn Reson Imaging 1992;2:421–429.
13. Hurst GC, Hua J, Duerk JL, Cohen AM. Intravascular (catheter) NMR receiver probe: preliminary design analysis and application to canine iliofemoral imaging. Magn Reson Med 1992;24:343–357.
14. Kandarpa K, Jakab P, Patz S, Schoen FJ, Jolesz FA. Prototype miniature endoluminal MR imaging catheter. J Vasc Interv Radiol 1993;4:419–427.
15. Atalar E, Bottomley PA, Ocali O, et al. High resolution intravascular MRI and MRS by using acatheter receiver coil. Magn Reson Med 1996;36:596–605.
16. Hillenbrand CM, Elgort DR, Wong EY, et al. Active device tracking and high-resolution intravascular MRI using a novel catheter-based, opposed-solenoid phased array coil. Magn Reson Med 2004;51:668–675.
17. Worthley SG, Helft G, Fuster V, et al. A novel nonobstructive intravascular MRI coil: in vivo imaging of experimental atherosclerosis. Arterioscler Thromb Vasc Biol 2003;23:346–350.
18. Ladd ME, Erhart P, Debatin JF, et al. Guidewire antennas for MR fluoroscopy. Magn Reson Med 1997;37:891–897.
19. Ocali O, Atalar E. Intravascular magnetic resonance imaging using a loopless catheter antenna. Magn Reson Med 1997;37:112–118.
20. Atalar E, Kraitchman DL, Carkhuff B, et al. Catheter-tracking FOV MR fluoroscopy. Magn Reson Med 1998;40:865–872.

21. Burl M, Coutts GA, Herlihy DJ, et al. Twisted-pair RF coil suitable for locating the track of a catheter. Magn Reson Med 1999;41:636–638.

22. Rivas PA, Nayak KS, Scott GC, et al. In vivo real-time intravascular MRI. J Cardiovasc Magn Reson 2002;4:223–232.

23. Susil RC, Yeung CJ, Atalar E. Intravascular extended sensitivity (IVES) MRI antennas. Magn Reson Med 2003;50:383–390.

24. Dumoulin CL, Souza SP, Darrow RD. Real-time position monitoring of invasive devices using magnetic resonance. Magn Reson Med 1993;29:411–415.

25. Leung DA, Debatin JF, Wildermuth S, et al. Intravascular MR tracking catheter: preliminary experimental evaluation. AJR Am J Roentgenol 1995;164:1265–1270.

26. Ladd ME, Zimmermann GG, McKinnon GC, et al. Visualization of vascular guidewires using MR tracking. J Magn Reson Imaging 1998;8:251–253.

27. Ladd ME, Quick HH. Reduction of resonant RF heating in intravascular catheters using coaxial chokes. Magn Reson Med 2000;43:615–619.

28. Lee C, McNamara C, Viohl I, inventors; Surgi-Vision, assignee. Connector and guidewire connectable thereto. U.S. patent 6,714,809, 2004.

29. Yeung CJ, Susil RC, Atalar E. RF safety of wires in interventional MRI: using a safety index. Magn Reson Med 2002;47:187–193.

30. Serfaty JM, Yang X, Foo TK, Kumar A, Derbyshire A, Atalar E. MRI-guided coronary catheterization and PTCA: a feasibility study on a dog model. Magn Reson Med 2003;49:258–263.

31. Weiss S, Vernickel P, Schaeffter T, Schultz V, Gleich B. A safe transmission line for interventional devices. Paper presented at: Fifth International MRI Symposium; Boston, MA; 2004.

32. Wong EY, Zhang Q, Duerk JL, Lewin JS, Wendt M. An optical system for wireless detuning of parallel resonant circuits. J Magn Reson Imaging 2000;12:632–638.

33. Konings MK, Bartels LW, van Swol CF, Bakker CJ. Development of an MR-safe tracking catheter with a laser-driven tip coil. J Magn Reson Imaging 2001;13:131–135.

34. Eggers H, Weiss S, Boernert P, Boesiger P. Image-based tracking of optically detunable parallel resonant circuits. Magn Reson Med 2003;49:1163–1174.

35. Weiss S, Schaeffter T, Brinkert F, Kuhne T, Bücker A. [An approach for safe visualization and localization of catheter during MR-guided intravascular procedures]. Z Med Phys 2003;13: 172–176.

36. Hofmann LV, Liddell RP, Eng J, et al. Human peripheral arteries: feasibility of transvenous intravascular MR imaging of the arterial wall. Radiology 2005;235:617–622.

37. Larose E, Yeghiazarians Y, Libby P, et al. Characterization of human atherosclerotic plaques by intravascular magnetic resonance imaging. Circulation 2005;112:2324–2331.

38. Quick HH, Kuehl H, Kaiser G, Bosk S, Debatin JF, Ladd ME. Inductively coupled stent antennas in MRI. Magn Reson Med 2002;48:781–790.

39. Kivelitz D, Wagner S, Schnorr J, et al. A vascular stent as an active component for locally enhanced magnetic resonance imaging: initial in vivo imaging results after catheter-guided placement in rabbits. Invest Radiol 2003;38:147–152.

40. Kuehne T, Fahrig R, Butts K. Pair of resonant fiducial markers for localization of endovascular catheters at all catheter orientations. J Magn Reson Imaging 2003;17:620–624.

41. Quick HH, Zenge MO, Kuehl H, et al. Interventional magnetic resonance angiography with no strings attached: wireless active catheter visualization. Magn Reson Med 2005;53:446–455.

42. Paetzel C, Zorger N, Bachthaler M, et al. Feasibility of MR-guided angioplasty of femoral artery stenoses using real-time imaging and intraarterial contrast-enhanced MR angiography. Rofo 2004;176:1232–1236.

43. Godart F, Beregi JP, Nicol L, et al. MR-guided balloon angioplasty of stenosed aorta: in vivo evaluation using near-standard instruments and a passive tracking technique. J Magn Reson Imaging 2000;12:639–644.

44. Omary RA, Frayne R, Unal O, et al. MR-guided angioplasty of renal artery stenosis in a pig model: a feasibility study. J Vasc Interv Radiol 2000;11:373–381.

45. Paetzel C, Zorger N, Bachthaler M, et al. Magnetic resonance-guided percutaneous angioplasty of femoral and popliteal artery stenoses using real-time imaging and intra-arterial contrast-enhanced magnetic resonance angiography. Invest Radiol 2005;40:257–262.

46. Raval AN, Telep JD, Guttman MA, et al. Real-time magnetic resonance imaging-guided stenting of aortic coarctation with commercially available catheter devices in Swine. Circulation 2005;112: 699–706.

47. Unal O, Korosec FR, Frayne R, Strother CM, Mistretta CA. A rapid 2D time-resolved variable-rate *k*-space sampling MR technique for passive catheter tracking during endovascular procedures. Magn Reson Med 1998;40:356–362.

48. Omary RA, Unal O, Koscielski DS, et al. Real-time MR imaging-guided passive catheter tracking with use of gadolinium-filled catheters. J Vasc Interv Radiol 2000;11:1079–1085.

49. Kuehne T, Saeed M, Higgins CB, et al. Endovascular stents in pulmonary valve and artery in swine: feasibility study of MR imaging-guided deployment and postinterventional assessment. Radiology 2003;226:475–481.

50. Buecker A, Neuerburg JM, Adam GB, et al. Real-time MR fluoroscopy for MR-guided iliac artery stent placement. J Magn Reson Imaging 2000;12:616–622.

51. Kee ST, Rhee JS, Butts K, et al. 1999 Gary J. Becker Young Investigator Award. MR-guided transjugular portosystemic shunt placement in a swine model. J Vasc Interv Radiol 1999;10:529–535.

52. Manke C, Nitz WR, Djavidani B, et al. MR imaging-guided stent placement in iliac arterial stenoses: a feasibility study. Radiology 2001;219:527–534.

53. Feng L, Dumoulin CL, Dashnaw S, et al. Feasibility of stent placement in carotid arteries with real-time MR imaging guidance in pigs. Radiology 2005;234:558–562.

54. Reddy V, Malchano Z, Dukkipati S, et al. Interventional MRI: electroanatomical mapping using real-time MR tracking of a deflectable catheter [abstract]. Heart Rhythm 2005;2:S279–S280.

55. Spuentrup E, Ruebben A, Schaeffter T, Manning WJ, Gunther RW, Buecker A. Magnetic resonance–guided coronary artery stent placement in a swine model. Circulation 2002;105:874–879.

56. Wildermuth S, Dumoulin CL, Pfammatter T, Maier SE, Hofmann E, Debatin JF. MR-guided percutaneous angioplasty: assessment of tracking safety, catheter handling and functionality. Cardiovasc Intervent Radiol 1998;21:404–410.

57. Yang X, Bolster BD Jr, Kraitchman DL, Atalar E. Intravascular MR-monitored balloon angioplasty: an in vivo feasibility study. J Vasc Interv Radiol 1998;9:953–959.

58. Buecker A, Adam GB, Neuerburg JM, et al. Simultaneous real-time visualization of the catheter tip and vascular anatomy for MR-guided PTA of iliac arteries in an animal model. J Magn Reson Imaging 2002;16:201–208.

59. Dion YM, Ben El Kadi H, Boudoux C, et al. Endovascular procedures under near-real-time magnetic resonance imaging guidance: an experimental feasibility study. J Vasc Surg 2000;32:1006–1014.

60. Wacker FK, Hillenbrand C, Elgort DR, Zhang S, Duerk JL, Lewin JS. MR imaging-guided percutaneous angioplasty and stent placement in a swine model: Comparison of open- and closed-bore scanners. Acad Radiol 2005;12:1085.

61. Bartels LW, Bos C, van Der Weide R, Smits HF, Bakker CJ, Viergever MA. Placement of an inferior vena cava filter in a pig guided by high-resolution MR fluoroscopy at 1.5 T. J Magn Reson Imaging 2000;12:599–605.

62. Bücker A, Neuerburg JM, Adam GB, et al. Real-time MR guidance for inferior vena cava filter placement in an animal model. J Vasc Interv Radiol 2001;12:753–756.

63. Frahm C, Gehl HB, Lorch H, et al. MR-guided placement of a temporary vena cava filter: technique and feasibility. J Magn Reson Imaging 1998;8:105–109.

64. Bücker A, Neuerburg JM, Adam G, Glowinski A, van Vaals JJ, Gunther RW. [MR-guided coil embolisation of renal arteries in an animal model]. Rofo 2003;175:271–274.

65. Fink C, Bock M, Umathum R, et al. Renal embolization: feasibility of magnetic resonance-guidance using active catheter tracking and intraarterial magnetic resonance angiography. Invest Radiol 2004;39:111–119.

66. Raval AN, Karmarkar PV, Guttman MA, et al. Real-time MRI-guided endovascular recanalization of chronic total arterial occlusion in a swine model. Circulation 2006 Feb 28; 113(8):1101–1107.

67. Raman VK, Karmarkar PV, Guttman MA, et al. Real-time magnetic resonance-guided endovascular repair of experimental abdominal aortic aneurysm in swine. J Am Coll Cardiol 2005;45:2069–2077.

68. Eggebrecht H, Quick HH. Personal communication; 2005.

69. Schalla S, Saeed M, Higgins CB, Martin A, Weber O, Moore P. Magnetic resonance-guided cardiac catheterization in a swine model of atrial septal defect. Circulation 2003;108:1865–1870.

70. Feng L, Dumoulin CL, Dashnaw S, et al. Transfemoral catheterization of carotid arteries with real-time MR imaging guidance in pigs. Radiology 2005;234:551–557.

71. Omary RA, Green JD, Schirf BE, Li Y, Finn JP, Li D. Real-time magnetic resonance imaging-guided coronary catheterization in swine. Circulation 2003;107:2656–2659.

72. Quick HH, Kuehl H, Kaiser G, et al. Interventional MRA using actively visualized catheters, TrueFISP, and real-time image fusion. Magn Reson Med 2003;49:129–137.

73. Buecker A, Spuentrup E, Grabitz R, et al. Magnetic resonance-guided placement of atrial septal closure device in animal model of patent foramen ovale. Circulation 2002;106:511–515.

74. Rickers C, Jerosch-Herold M, Hu X, et al. Magnetic resonance image-guided transcatheter closure of atrial septal defects. Circulation 2003;107:132–138.

75. Schalla S, Saeed M, Higgins CB, Weber O, Martin A, Moore P. Balloon sizing and transcatheter closure of acute atrial septal defects guided by magnetic resonance fluoroscopy: assessment and validation in a large animal model. J Magn Reson Imaging 2005;21:204–211.

76. Kuehne T, Yilmaz S, Meinus C, et al. Magnetic resonance imaging-guided transcatheter implantation of a prosthetic valve in aortic valve position: feasibility study in swine. J Am Coll Cardiol 2004;44: 2247–2249.

77. Dick AJ, Guttman MA, Raman VK, et al. Magnetic resonance fluoroscopy allows targeted delivery of mesenchymal stem cells to infarct borders in swine. Circulation 2003;108:2899–2904.

78. Lederman RJ, Guttman MA, Peters DC, et al. Catheter-based endomyocardial injection with real-time magnetic resonance imaging. Circulation 2002;105:1282–1284.

79. Corti R, Badimon J, Mizsei G, et al. Real time magnetic resonance guided endomyocardial local delivery. Heart 2005;91:348–353.

80. Karmarkar PV, Kraitchman DL, Izbudak I, et al. MR-trackable intramyocardial injection catheter. Magn Reson Med 2004;51:1163–1172.

81. Krombach GA, Pfeffer JG, Kinzel S, Katoh M, Gunther RW, Buecker A. MR-guided percutaneous intramyocardial injection with an MR-compatible catheter: feasibility and changes in T_1 values after injection of extracellular contrast medium in pigs. Radiology 2005;235:487–494.

82. Saeed M, Lee R, Martin A, et al. Transendocardial delivery of extracellular myocardial markers by using combination X-ray/MR fluoroscopic guidance: feasibility study in dogs. Radiology 2004;231: 689–696.

83. Hazel SJ, Paterson HS, Edwards JR, Maddern GJ. Surgical treatment of atrial fibrillation via energy ablation. Circulation 2005;111:e103–e106.

84. Susil RC, Yeung CJ, Halperin HR, Lardo AC, Atalar E. Multifunctional interventional devices for MRI: a combined electrophysiology/MRI catheter. Magn Reson Med 2002;47:594–600.

85. Lardo AC, McVeigh ER, Jumrussirikul P, et al. Visualization and temporal/spatial characterization of cardiac radiofrequency ablation lesions using magnetic resonance imaging. Circulation 2000;102:698–705.

86. Arepally A, Karmarkar PV, Weiss C, Rodriguez ER, Lederman RJ, Atalar E. Magnetic resonance image-guided trans-septal puncture in a swine heart. J Magn Reson Imaging 2005;21:463–467.

87. Raval AN, Karmarkar PV, Guttman MA, et al. Real-time MRI guided atrial septal puncture and balloon septostomy in swine. Cath Cardiovasc Intervent 2006 Apr; 67(4):637–643.

88. Kee ST, Ganguly A, Daniel BL, et al. MR-guided transjugular intrahepatic portosystemic shunt creation with use of a hybrid radiography/MR system. J Vasc Interv Radiol 2005;16(2 pt 1):227–234.

89. Arepally A, Kamarkar P, Weiss C, Atalar E. Percutaneous MR-guided transvascular access of the mesenteric venous system-study in a swine model. Radiology 2006 Jan; 238(1):113–118.

90. Paetzel C, Zorger N, Seitz J, et al. Intraarterial contrast material-enhanced magnetic resonance angiography of the aortoiliac system. J Vasc Interv Radiol 2004;15:981–984.

91. Lederman RJ. Cardiovascular interventional magnetic resonance imaging. Circulation 2005;112: 3009–3017.

INDEX